Exercise Physiology

Integrating Theory and Application

William J. Kraemer, PhD

Professor
Department of Kinesiology
Neag School of Education
Department of Physiology and Neurobiology
University of Connecticut
Storrs, Connecticut

Steven J. Fleck, PhD

Professor and Chair
Department of Sport Science
Colorado College
Colorado Springs, Colorado

Michael R. Deschenes, PhD

Professor and Chair
Department of Kinesiology and Health Sciences
The College of William & Mary
Williamsburg, Virginia

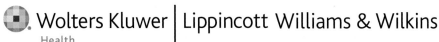

Wolters Kluwer | Lippincott Williams & Wilkins
Health

Philadelphia · Baltimore · New York · London
Buenos Aires · Hong Kong · Sydney · Tokyo

Acquisitions Editor: Emily Lupash
Product Manager: Andrea M. Klingler
Development Editor: David Payne
Marketing Manager: Allison Powell
Designer: Teresa Mallon
Compositor: Aptara Corp.

First Edition

Copyright © 2012 Lippincott Williams & Wilkins, a Wolters Kluwer business

351 West Camden Street
Baltimore, MD 21201

Two Commerce Square
2001 Market Street
Philadelphia, PA 19103

Printed in China

Library of Congress Cataloging-in-Publication Data

Kraemer, William J., 1953–
 Exercise physiology : integrating theory and application / William J. Kraemer, Steven
J. Fleck, Michael R. Deschenes.—1st ed.
  p. cm.
 Includes bibliographical references and index.
 ISBN 978-0-7817-8351-4 (alk. paper)
 1. Exercise—Physiological aspects—Textbooks. 2. Clinical exercise physiology—Textbooks. I. Fleck, Steven J.,
1951– II. Deschenes, Michael R. III. Title.
 QP301.K654 2012
 612'.044—dc22

                                    2010043274

To purchase additional copies of this book, call our customer service department at **(800) 638-3030** or fax orders to **(301) 824-7390**. For other book services, including chapter reprints and large quantity sales, ask for the Special Sales department.

For all other calls originating outside of the United States, please call **(301) 714-2324.**

Visit Lippincott Williams & Wilkins on the Internet: **http://www.lww.com.** Lippincott Williams & Wilkins customer service representatives are available from 8:30 am to 6:00 pm, EST, Monday through Friday, for telephone access.

9 8 7 6 5 4 3 2 1

DISCLAIMER

Care has been taken to confirm the accuracy of the information present and to describe generally accepted practices. However, the authors, editors, and publisher are not responsible for errors or omissions or for any consequences from application of the information in this book and make no warranty, expressed or implied, with respect to the currency, completeness, or accuracy of the contents of the publication. Application of this information in a particular situation remains the professional responsibility of the practitioner; the clinical treatments described and recommended may not be considered absolute and universal recommendations.

 The authors, editors, and publisher have exerted every effort to ensure that drug selection and dosage set forth in this text are in accordance with the current recommendations and practice at the time of publication. However, in view of ongoing research, changes in government regulations, and the constant flow of information relating to drug therapy and drug reactions, the reader is urged to check the package insert for each drug for any change in indications and dosage and for added warnings and precautions. This is particularly important when the recommended agent is a new or infrequently employed drug.

 Some drugs and medical devices presented in this publication have Food and Drug Administration (FDA) clearance for limited use in restricted research settings. It is the responsibility of the health care providers to ascertain the FDA status of each drug or device planned for use in their clinical practice.

 To purchase additional copies of this book, call our customer service department at (800) 638-3030 or fax orders to (301) 223-2320. International customers should call (301) 223-2300.

 Visit Lippincott Williams & Wilkins on the Internet: http://www.lww.com. Lippincott Williams & Wilkins customer service representatives are available from 8:30 am to 6:00 pm, EST.

To my mother, Jewell; my late father, Ray; and my sister, Judy:
I thank you for the love and nurturing in my life.
To my children, Daniel, Anna, and Maria: your love
and support, and your very lives, have given meaning to
my own. To my wife Joan for her love and support when taking
on all of life's challenges.
—WILLIAM J. KRAEMER

To my mother, Elda; father, Marv; brothers, Marv and Glenn;
sisters, Sue and Lisa; and their families for their support in all
aspects of my career and life. To my wife, Maelu, for her
support and understanding throughout our life together,
but especially during the time necessary
to complete a textbook.
—STEVEN J. FLECK

To my mother for showing me unconditional love. To my father
for always having faith in me. To Jennifer and Gabrielle, my
two beautiful girls whom that I love so very much and who make
me so anxious to come home at the end of each day.
—MICHAEL R. DESCHENES

Preface

The vision for this textbook is a bit different from others in the field today. It is directed toward undergraduate students, many of whom will not go immediately on to graduate school but will be taking positions as personal trainers, strength and conditioning specialists, fitness instructors, exercise technicians, physical therapy assistants, athletic trainers, wellness educators, recreational fitness specialists, or health and physical education teachers. Our goal is to capture the interest and excitement of students. We want students to become fascinated with how the body works and its responses to exercise. We want students to understand how one can train to improve performance and we want them to be interested in the basic physiological mechanisms that allow these training adaptations to occur in different structures and their specific functions. With the popularity of sports we want students to understand the physiological basis of sport performance and conditioning. Furthermore, we want them to understand the vital health benefits of exercise and physical activity during the life span and for special populations.

It is our experience that textbooks in the field today are too overwhelming for many undergraduate students to deal with or for the professor to cover in one semester. Almost every topic in exercise physiology has had a host of scientific papers and books written about them, and the real temptation we wanted to avoid was growing this text into a graduate-level book with deep dimensions of detail. In many scenarios, students cannot connect these concepts to the practical applications when called upon to do so in their jobs. For example, a high school high jumper may ask, How should I stretch before an attempt in a meet? Or, a client may ask his or her personal trainer, Can I really get a six pack set of abs in 6 weeks like I saw on this infomercial last night? Explanations and choices made in these scenarios and many others reflect the level of educational experiences and training. In *Exercise Physiology: Integrating Theory and Application* we emphasize a fundamental understanding of the exercise physiology that surrounds such practical questions. Our aim is to integrate basic exercise physiology as key elements to help the students understand what the answers may be to various questions and understand how to find these answers using a research-based perspective to help the students find the facts and evaluate information in today's society. We want our students to understand the body's acute responses to exercise stress, building on this with an understanding of how the body adapts to exercise and environmental stresses. We integrate how these concepts relate to the array of practical job outcomes in which students will quickly find themselves; they need to be able to understand exercise physiology from a practical perspective so that they can apply it to their various working environments. With this professional preparation, it is our hope that students will be better able to take on the challenges and solve the problems they will face as young professionals.

The approach of this text will allow for a linked understanding of central concepts that exercise professionals need to know. Although chapters have domains of content, we cross-reference information and do not corral content in only one area. Adaptations to exercise weave throughout the book as standard feature, rather than limiting adaptations to a single chapter. We take advantage of the interest students have in nutrition, improved training, or losing weight, and use a number of examples in each area to integrate topics across the different chapters. Utilizing the student's long-term memory by connecting the physiology to an example or an overall context is vital in this process. We used our experiences as a diverse group of authors to give examples of practical applications to help the students in their study of exercise physiology.

This textbook is for undergraduate courses in exercise science, including exercise physiology, but it may well be adapted for other courses in which this type of information is important for student's professional preparation. Having all taught exercise physiology at the college level for many years, we wanted to make it as easy as possible for the professors to use this text as a pivot point from which to expand upon with their own style and expertise. We hope that it will facilitate inquiry and interest in the field and enhance professional preparation and knowledge-based practice for students.

FEATURES

Exercise Physiology: Integrating Theory and Application contains many pedagogical features that will help students remember and apply the material presented to them. At the beginning of each chapter, **Chapter**

Objectives highlight the main points of the chapter and what important information the students should focus on as they read through the content presented. The **Introduction** gives a brief overview of the topic discussed in and the point of the chapter.

Within each chapter there are various boxes meant to help students bridge the gap between learning, understanding, and application. **Quick Review boxes** use brief, bulleted topic points to highlight important material. **Did You Know? boxes** provide more detailed information about a topic that may be above and beyond the scope of the chapter to help students expand their knowledge base. **Applying Research boxes** describe in-depth how research findings can be applied in real-life situations that students may encounter in practice. **Practical Questions from Students boxes** provide answers to popular questions, giving detailed explanations about topics or issues that students may find difficult. **An Expert View boxes** give firsthand opinions and perspectives of experts in the field related to content presented in the chapter. Finally, **Case Studies** provide scenarios and questions, along with options of how you might respond to those scenarios, along with rationale. These are meant to provoke discussion and expand students' critical thinking.

At the end of each chapter, an extensive list of **Review Questions** provides the students with a chance to apply what they have learned and assess their knowledge through fill-in-the-blank, multiple choice, true/false, short answer, and critical thinking questions. A **Key Terms list** at the end of each chapter provides definitions of important terminology with which students should become familiar.

ADDITIONAL RESOURCES

Exercise Physiology: Integrating Theory and Application includes additional resources for both instructors and students that are available on the book's companion Web site at http://thepoint.lww.com/KraemerExPhys.

Instructors

Approved adopting instructors will be given access to the following additional resources:

- Brownstone test generator
- Answers to the in-text Review Questions
- PowerPoint lecture outlines
- Image bank
- WebCT and Blackboard cartridge

Students

Students who have purchased *Exercise Physiology: Integrating Theory and Application* have access to the following additional resources:

- Interactive Quiz Bank
- Animations

In addition, purchasers of the text can access the searchable Full Text by going to the book's Web site at http://thePoint.lww.com. See the inside front cover of this text for more details, including the passcode you will need to gain access to the Web site.

WILLIAM J. KRAEMER, PhD
STEVEN J. FLECK, PhD
MICHAEL R. DESCHENES, PhD

User's Guide

Exercise Physiology: Integrating Theory and Application was created and developed to explain how one can train to improve performance, the knowledge of which builds off of an understanding of the basic physiological mechanisms that allow these training adaptations to occur in different structures and their specific functions. The book also aims to help students comprehend the vital health benefits of exercise and physical activity during the life span and for special populations. Please take a few moments to look through this User's Guide, which will introduce you to the tools and features that will enhance your learning experience.

Chapter Objectives highlight the main points of the chapter and what important information the students should focus on as they read through the content presented.

The **Introduction** gives a brief overview of the topic discussed in and the point of the chapter.

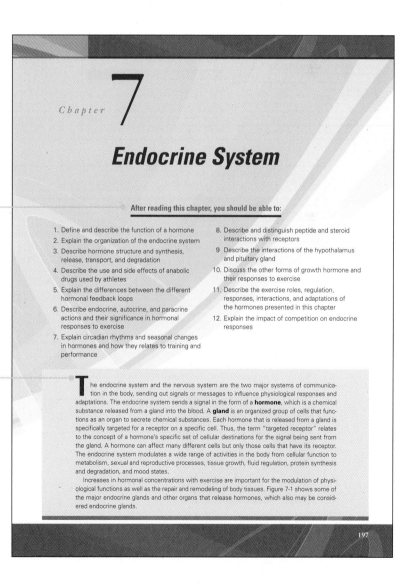

Chapter 7

Endocrine System

After reading this chapter, you should be able to:

1. Define and describe the function of a hormone
2. Explain the organization of the endocrine system
3. Describe hormone structure and synthesis, release, transport, and degradation
4. Describe the use and side effects of anabolic drugs used by athletes
5. Explain the differences between the different hormonal feedback loops
6. Describe endocrine, autocrine, and paracrine actions and their significance in hormonal responses to exercise
7. Explain circadian rhythms and seasonal changes in hormones and how they relates to training and performance
8. Describe and distinguish peptide and steroid interactions with receptors
9. Describe the interactions of the hypothalamus and pituitary gland
10. Discuss the other forms of growth hormone and their responses to exercise
11. Describe the exercise roles, regulation, responses, interactions, and adaptations of the hormones presented in this chapter
12. Explain the impact of competition on endocrine responses

The endocrine system and the nervous system are the two major systems of communication in the body, sending out signals or messages to influence physiological responses and adaptations. The endocrine system sends a signal in the form of a **hormone**, which is a chemical substance released from a gland into the blood. A **gland** is an organized group of cells that functions as an organ to secrete chemical substances. Each hormone that is released from a gland is specifically targeted for a receptor on a specific cell. Thus, the term "targeted receptor" relates to the concept of a hormone's specific set of cellular destinations for the signal being sent from the gland. A hormone can affect many different cells but only those cells that have its receptor. The endocrine system modulates a wide range of activities in the body from cellular function to metabolism, sexual and reproductive processes, tissue growth, fluid regulation, protein synthesis and degradation, and mood states.

Increases in hormonal concentrations with exercise are important for the modulation of physiological functions as well as the repair and remodeling of body tissues. Figure 7-1 shows some of the major endocrine glands and other organs that release hormones, which also may be considered endocrine glands.

197

Quick Review

- The reversible binding of oxygen to hemoglobin accounts for 98% of the oxygen transported by blood.
- The sigmoidal shape of the oxyhemoglobin disassociation curve ensures near-maximal formation of oxyhemoglobin at the lungs even when the atmospheric partial pressure of oxygen decreases. It also ensures that small changes in partial pressure result in release of oxygen at active tissue.
- Changes in temperature and acidity shift the oxyhemoglobin disassociation curve, causing greater delivery of oxygen to muscle tissue during exercise.
- Three methods are responsible for carbon dioxide transport, but 70% of carbon dioxide is transported in the form of bicarbonate.
- The transport of oxygen and that of carbon dioxide is linked by the formation of carbaminohemoglobin and the buffering of hydrogen ions by hemoglobin, which decrease hemoglobin's affinity for oxygen.

bicarbonate ion for a chloride ion is termed the **chloride shift**.

The hydrogen ion produced is bound to the globin part of hemoglobin. So, hemoglobin acts as a buffer and helps maintain normal acidity (pH) within the red blood cell. Hemoglobin's buffering of hydrogen ions reduces its affinity for oxygen. So, the buffering of hydrogen ions triggers the Bohr effect or moves the oxyhemoglobin disassociation curve to the right. At the tissue level, this results in the release of oxygen from hemoglobin so that it is available for metabolism.

The bicarbonate reaction can proceed in either direction. At the lungs, where Pco_2 is low within the alveoli, carbon dioxide diffuses out of solution, disturbing the balance of the bicarbonate reaction and causing this reaction to proceed in the direction of the production of carbon dioxide and water. Additionally, oxygenation of hemoglobin causes it to lose its affinity for hydrogen ions. Thus, they are available for the production of carbonic acid, which because of the low Pco_2, disassociates into carbon dioxide and water. So, the release of oxygen by hemoglobin at tissue is linked to the transport of carbon dioxide by hemoglobin, and the release of carbon dioxide by hemoglobin at the lungs is linked to oxygenation of hemoglobin.

GAS EXCHANGE AT THE MUSCLE

Gas exchange at the muscle or any tissue occurs due to differences in Po_2 and Pco_2 between the tissue and capillary blood (Fig. 6-7). All of the factors previously described concerning partial pressure differences and blood transport of oxygen and carbon dioxide apply to capillary gas exchange at the tissue level. The amount of oxygen delivered to tissue can be calculated using the Fick principle and the arterial-venous oxygen difference (see "Oxygen Delivery to Tissue" section in Chapter 5). Once oxygen has diffused into tissue, an oxygen carrier molecule (myoglobin) within muscle assists in its transport to the mitochondria.

Myoglobin is an oxygen transport molecule similar to hemoglobin except that it is found within skeletal and cardiac muscle. Myoglobin reversibly binds with oxygen, and its role is to assist in the passive diffusion of oxygen from the cell membrane to the mitochondria. Because the rate of diffusion slows exponentially as distance is increased, myoglobin located between the membrane and the mitochondria actually results in two smaller diffusion distances rather than a single long one. As a result, the transit time of oxygen across the muscle fiber to the mitochondria is significantly reduced.

Different from hemoglobin, myoglobin contains only one iron molecule, whereas hemoglobin contains four iron molecules. Muscle that appears reddish contains large amounts of myoglobin, whereas muscles that appear white contain small amounts of myoglobin. The concentration of myoglobin within a muscle fiber varies with the muscle fiber type (see Chapter 3). Myoglobin concentration is high in type I muscle fibers with a high aerobic capacity (slowtwitch), whereas type IIa (fast-twitch) and type IIx (fast-twitch) muscle fibers contain an intermediate and a limited amount of myoglobin, respectively.

In addition to speeding up the diffusion of oxygen across the muscle fiber, myoglobin functions as an oxygen "reserve" at the start of exercise. Even with the anticipatory rise (see "Effects of Exercise on Pulmonary Ventilation," below) in breathing rate prior to the beginning of exercise, there is a lag in oxygen delivery to muscle. During this period, the oxygen bound to myoglobin helps to maintain the oxygen requirements of muscle that is becoming active. Upon the cessation of exercise, myoglobin oxygen must be replenished and is a small component of the oxygen deficit (see Chapter 2).

Although myoglobin and hemoglobin are similar in chemical structure, one difference between these two molecules is that myoglobin has a much steeper oxygen disassociation curve and approaches 100% oxygen saturation at a much lower Po_2 (30 mm Hg). Because of these factors, myoglobin releases its oxygen at very low levels of Po_2, which is important because within the mitochondria of active muscle, the Po_2 can be as low as 2 mm Hg. Thus, myoglobin's oxygen disassociation curve allows it to transport oxygen at the lower levels of Po_2 (40 mm Hg) found within skeletal muscle.

Quick Review

- Gas exchange at tissue occurs due to partial pressure differences in oxygen and carbon dioxide between the tissue and the blood.
- Myoglobin, a molecule similar to hemoglobin, transports oxygen from the cell membrane to the mitochondria for use in aerobic metabolism.

Quick Review boxes use brief, bulleted topic points to highlight important material.

Did You Know? boxes provide more detailed information about a topic that may be above and beyond the scope of the chapter to help students expand their knowledge base.

Box 6-3 DID YOU KNOW?

Common Types of Anemia

Anemia is a deficiency in the number of red blood cells or of their hemoglobin content, or a combination of these two factors. Anemia results in a decrease in the ability to transport oxygen and so can affect endurance or aerobic capabilities. Symptoms of anemia include pallor, easy fatigue, breathlessness with exertion, heart palpitations, and loss of appetite. Iron deficiency can result in anemia and is the most common type of anemia. It most commonly occurs due to an insufficient intake of iron in the diet or impaired iron absorption. However, iron-deficient anemia can also occur because of hemorrhage or increased iron needs, such as during pregnancy.

Sports anemia refers to reduced hemoglobin concentrations that approach clinical anemia (12 and 14 g·dL⁻¹ of blood in women and men, respectively) caused by the performance of physical training. Although physical training does result in a small loss of iron in sweat, loss of hemoglobin caused by increased destruction of red blood cells, and possibly gastrointestinal bleeding with distance running sports, anemia is typically not caused by these factors. Physical training, including both aerobic training and weight training, results in a plasma volume increase of up to 20% during the first several days of training. This plasma volume increase parallels the decrease in hemoglobin concentration.[1,2] The total amount of hemoglobin within the blood does not significantly change, but due to the increase in plasma volume, hemoglobin concentration decreases. After several weeks of training, hemoglobin concentrations and hematocrit return toward normal. Thus, sports anemia is normally a transient event and less prevalent than once believed.[3]

References

1. Deruisseau KC, Roberts LM, Kushnick MR, et al. Iron status of young males and females performing weight training exercise. Med Sci Sports Exerc. 2004;36:241–248.
2. Schumacher YO, Schmid A, Grathwohl D, et al. Hematological indices of iron status of athletes in various sports and performances. Med Sci Sports Exerc. 2002;34:869–875.
3. Wright LM, Klein M, Noakes TD, et al. Sports anemia: a real or apparent phenomenon in endurance trained athletes. Int J Sports Med. 1992;13:344–347.

(Fig. 6-8). At the lungs, where there is a high Po_2, hemoglobin binds oxygen, forming oxyhemoglobin, and becomes 100% saturated with oxygen. When hemoglobin is 100% saturated with oxygen, it is carrying the maximal amount of oxygen possible. At tissues where oxygen is used for aerobic metabolism, there is a low Po_2 and hemoglobin releases oxygen or becomes less than 100% saturated, with hemoglobin being converted to deoxyhemoglobin.

The oxyhemoglobin disassociation curve is sigmoidal, or has an "S" shape. This shape offers advantages to hemoglobin becoming both oxyhemoglobin at the lungs and deoxyhemoglobin at the tissue level. First, at a Po_2 ranging from 90 to 100 mm Hg, oxygen saturation is above 97% and the curve is quite flat, meaning there is only a small change in oxygen saturation when a change in Po_2 occurs. Po_2 at the lungs is approximately 105 mm Hg, ensuring that 100% oxygen saturation occurs, but even if Po_2 decreases to as low as 90 mm Hg, little change in oxygen saturation would occur. This is physiologically important because it ensures that close to 100% saturation takes place at the lungs even if Po_2 at the lungs decreases due to factors such as assent to moderate altitude.

The oxyhemoglobin disassociation curve has a very steep slope from 0 to 40 mm Hg Po_2. At active tissue, where Po_2 is low, this portion of the curve ensures that for a small change in Po_2 a very large change in oxygen saturation will take place, meaning oxygen will be more readily released and available to the tissue. This portion of the curve is critical for the supply of oxygen to tissue during exercise, when Po_2 at the tissue level decreases. At rest, tissue needs little oxygen and approximately 75% of the oxygen remains bound to hemoglobin, meaning 25% of the oxygen is released to tissues. During exercise, only approximately 10% of the oxygen remains bound to hemoglobin, so 90% of the oxygen carried by hemoglobin is released to tissues. Other factors, in addition to the sigmoid shape of the oxyhemoglobin disassociation curve, help to ensure adequate oxygen delivery to tissue during exercise.

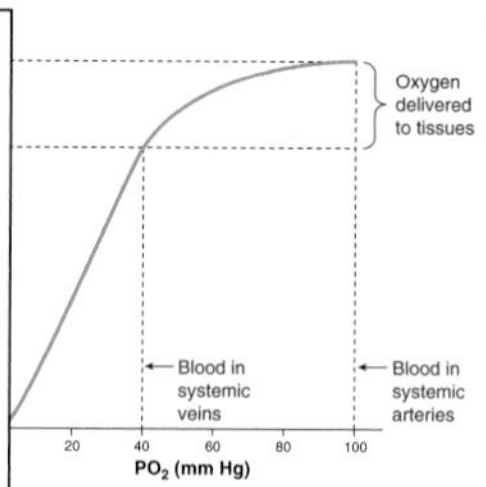

. The oxyhemoglobin disassociation curve depicts ...nship between hemoglobin saturation with oxygen ...rtial pressure of oxygen. The difference in oxygen ...etween the lungs and tissue is the amount of oxygen ... the tissue.

The **hypothalamus** is one of the most important regulatory parts of the brain, influencing a host of different physiological functions involved in exercise, including thirst, body temperature, blood pressure, water balance, and endocrine function. It has been called the homeostatic center of the brain. The hypothalamus is vital as a relay center for incoming neural signaling. Because the brain controls bodily function, injury to the brain, such as concussion due to sports participation, has very serious ramifications (Box 4-1). Likewise developmental disabilities such as Down syndrome also affect mental and movement abilities (Box 4-2).

Spinal Cord

The spinal cord is a tubular bundle of nerves that is part of the central nervous system, arising from the brain. It is enclosed and protected by vertebra making up the vertebral column, and each level has nerves that come out of it to different target organs. Nerves related to muscle functions are shown in Figure 4-5. Information is passed from the higher brain centers to the peripheral target tissues, such as muscle. In addition, local circuits from a particular spinal cord level out to the periphery and back can also be operational for sensory (e.g., reflex to heat) and motor activities featuring local repetitive movements, such as running at a set speed.

The spinal cord is also the site of reflex actions. A reflex action is an involuntary response to a stimulus. Typically, a reflex involves a stimulation of a sensory neuron, which brings information to the spinal cord. In the spinal cord, it connects with an efferent neuron, which, in turn, causes a response in the periphery. Reflexes can be both simple and complex. The simplest reflex is the monosynaptic reflex, an example of which is the tendon jerk reflex or tendon tap reflex. Figure 4-6 shows the classical "knee-jerk" reflex when the patellar tendon is struck with a direct mechanical tap. We depend upon reflexes, not only during daily activities, but also during sports events, and even when sleeping, to respond to our environment without thinking about it. For example, the consequences of placing a hand on a hot stove could be severe if one had to take the time to consider the stimulus and consciously devise a response before pulling it off.

The patellar reflex is a bit different from other reflexes because it is mediated by what is called a monosynaptic reflex, and no interneuron connection is involved. Most

Box 4-2 APPLYING RESEARCH

Neurological and Motor Function: Movement Behaviors in Down Syndrome

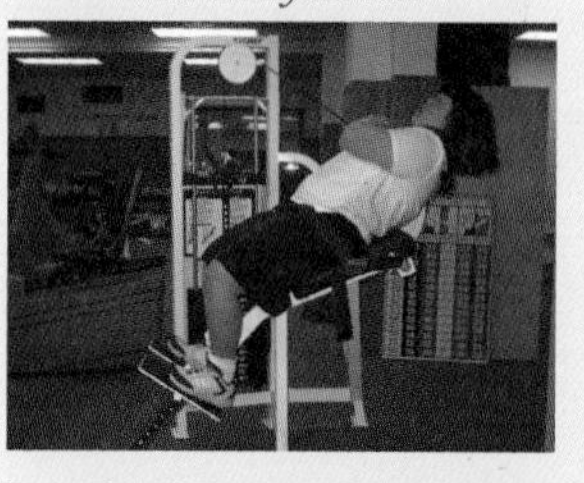

Down syndrome, or trisomy 21, is a genetic alteration caused by presence of an extra chromosome on the 21st human chromosome. It was named after the British physician who described it in 1866. The condition has been characterized by a combination of differences in body size and structure depending upon the penetration of the third chromosome on the phenotypic characteristic examined. Thus, a wide range of differences can occur even within people with Down syndrome.

Interestingly, for years it was thought that the careful movement and rigidity of locomotion was a result of this phenotypic penetration, or interference with normal motor neuron function. In 1994, Latash's research group concluded:

"This study supports the idea that subjects with Down syndrome can use patterns of muscle activation that are qualitatively indistinguishable from those used by individuals who are neurologically normal. With appropriate training, individuals with Down syndrome achieved similar levels of motor performance to that described in the literature for individuals who are neurologically normal."

Much of the movement inhibition was due to protective behaviors (e.g., limiting arm swing because such a movement had resulted in pain from hitting something in everyday movements) carefully reinforced to avoid injury. The importance of practicing new exercise and sport skills to reinforce the the idea that one could safely move in a new range of motion without the fear of pain or injury cannot be underestimated when working with people with Down syndrome, as seen with many athletes in "Special Olympics." This also might be very important in everyday movement tasks in the home and at work. Thus, what appeared as a neurological disorder was in fact a learned protective behavior to prevent injury and ensure survival.

Further Readings

Almeida GL, Corcos DM, Latash ML. Practice and transfer effects during fast single-joint elbow movements in individuals with Down syndrome. Phys Ther. 1994;74(11):1000–1012.

Latash ML, Anson JG. Synergies in health and disease: Relations to adaptive changes in motor coordination. Phys Ther. 2006;86(8):1151–1160.

Applying Research boxes describe in-depth how research findings can be applied in real-life situations that students may encounter in practice.

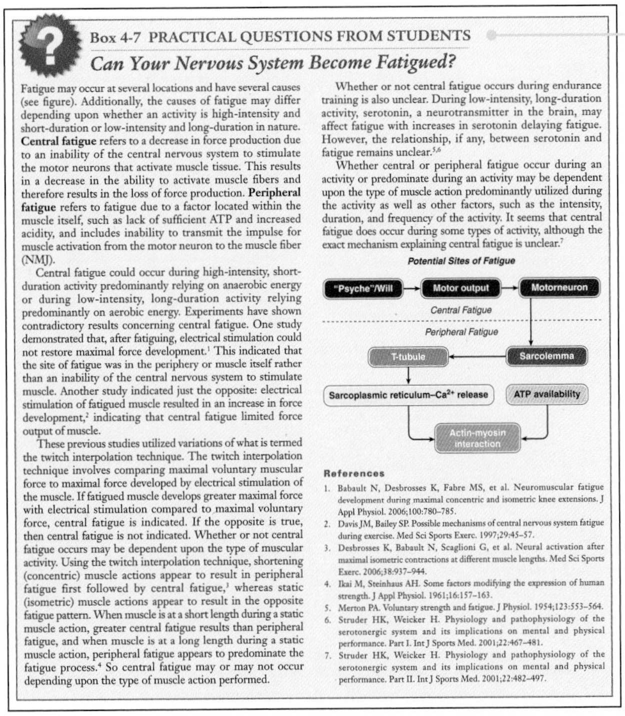

Box 4-7 PRACTICAL QUESTIONS FROM STUDENTS
Can Your Nervous System Become Fatigued?

Fatigue may occur at several locations and have several causes (see figure). Additionally, the causes of fatigue may differ depending upon whether an activity is high-intensity and short-duration or low-intensity and long-duration in nature. **Central fatigue** refers to a decrease in force production due to an inability of the central nervous system to stimulate the motor neurons that activate muscle tissue. This results in a decrease in the ability to activate muscle fibers and therefore results in the loss of force production. **Peripheral fatigue** refers to fatigue due to a factor located within the muscle itself, such as lack of sufficient ATP and increased acidity, and includes inability to transmit the impulse for muscle activation from the motor neuron to the muscle fiber (NMJ).

Central fatigue could occur during high-intensity, short-duration activity predominantly relying on anaerobic energy or during low-intensity, long-duration activity relying predominantly on aerobic energy. Experiments have shown contradictory results concerning central fatigue. One study demonstrated that, after fatiguing, electrical stimulation could not restore maximal force development.[1] This indicated that the site of fatigue was in the periphery or muscle itself rather than an inability of the central nervous system to stimulate muscle. Another study indicated just the opposite: electrical stimulation of fatigued muscle resulted in an increase in force development,[2] indicating that central fatigue limited force output of muscle.

These previous studies utilized variations of what is termed the twitch interpolation technique. The twitch interpolation technique involves comparing maximal voluntary muscular force to maximal force developed by electrical stimulation of the muscle. If fatigued muscle develops greater maximal force with electrical stimulation compared to maximal voluntary force, central fatigue is indicated. If the opposite is true, then central fatigue is not indicated. Whether or not central fatigue occurs may be dependent upon the type of muscular activity. Using the twitch interpolation technique, shortening (concentric) muscle actions appear to result in peripheral fatigue first followed by central fatigue,[3] whereas static (isometric) muscle actions appear to result in the opposite fatigue pattern. When muscle is at a short length during a static muscle action, greater central fatigue results than peripheral fatigue, and when muscle is at a long length during a static muscle action, peripheral fatigue appears to predominate the fatigue process.[4] So central fatigue may or may not occur depending upon the type of muscle action performed.

Whether or not central fatigue occurs during endurance training is also unclear. During low-intensity, long-duration activity, serotonin, a neurotransmitter in the brain, may affect fatigue with increases in serotonin delaying fatigue. However, the relationship, if any, between serotonin and fatigue remains unclear.[5,6]

Whether central or peripheral fatigue occur during an activity or predominate during an activity may be dependent upon the type of muscle action predominantly utilized during the activity as well as other factors, such as the intensity, duration, and frequency of the activity. It seems that central fatigue does occur during some types of activity, although the exact mechanism explaining central fatigue is unclear.[7]

Potential Sites of Fatigue

References
1. Babault N, Desbrosses K, Fabre MS, et al. Neuromuscular fatigue development during maximal concentric and isometric knee extensions. J Appl Physiol. 2006;100:780–785.
2. Davis JM, Bailey SP. Possible mechanisms of central nervous system fatigue during exercise. Med Sci Sports Exerc. 1997;29:45–57.
3. Desbrosses K, Babault N, Scaglioni G, et al. Neural activation after maximal isometric contractions at different muscle lengths. Med Sci Sports Exerc. 2006;38:937–944.
4. Ikai M, Steinhaus AH. Some factors modifying the expression of human strength. J Appl Physiol. 1961;16:157–163.
5. Merton PA. Voluntary strength and fatigue. J Physiol. 1954;123:553–564.
6. Struder HK, Weicker H. Physiology and pathophysiology of the serotonergic system and its implications on mental and physical performance. Part I. Int J Sports Med. 2001;22:467–481.
7. Struder HK, Weicker H. Physiology and pathophysiology of the serotonergic system and its implications on mental and physical performance. Part II. Int J Sports Med. 2001;22:482–497.

Practical Questions from Students boxes provide answers to popular questions, giving detailed explanations about topics or issues that students may find difficult.

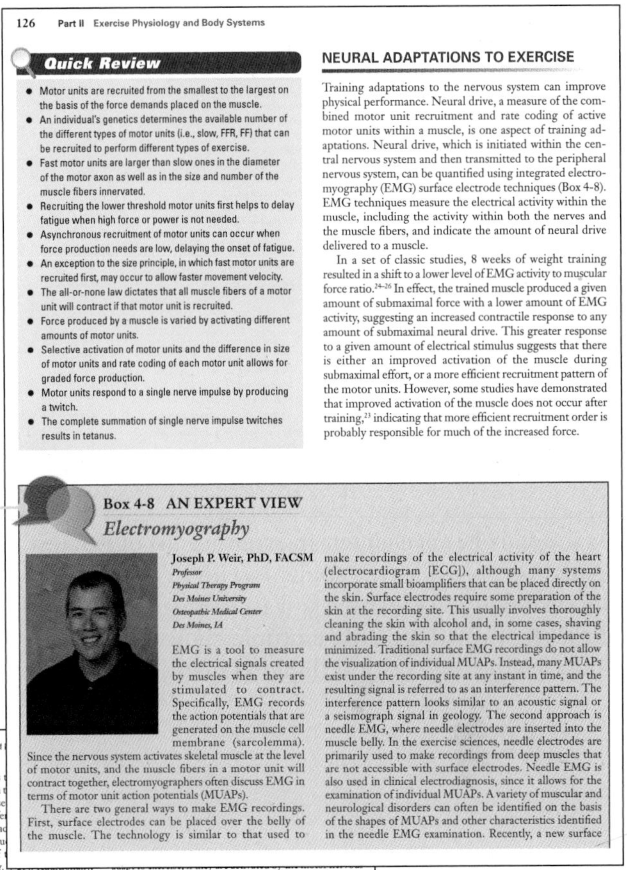

An Expert View boxes give firsthand opinions and perspectives of experts in the field related to content presented in the chapter.

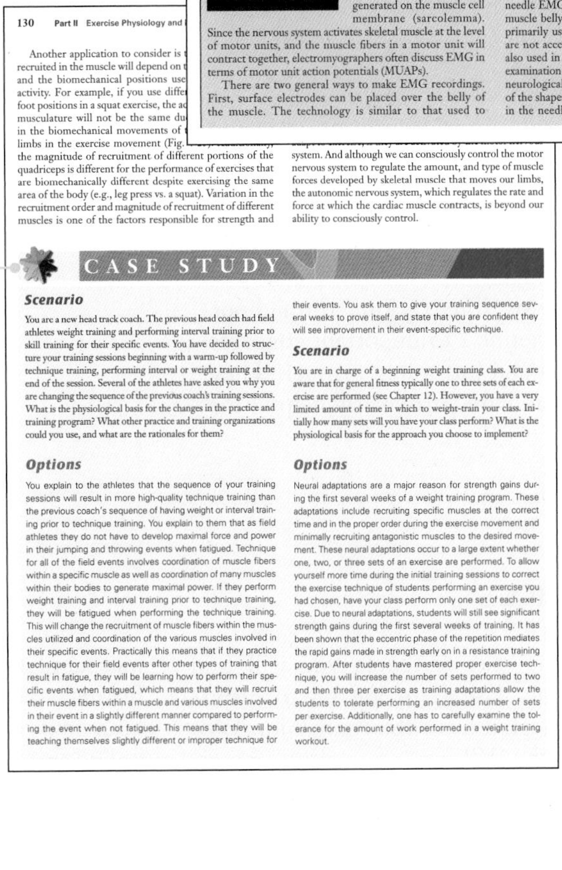

Case Studies provide scenarios and questions, along with options of how you might respond to those scenarios, along with rationale. These are meant to provoke discussion and expand students' critical thinking.

---

126   Part II   Exercise Physiology and Body Systems

Quick Review

- Motor units are recruited from the smallest to the largest on the basis of the force demands placed on the muscle.
- An individual's genetics determines the available number of the different types of motor units (i.e., slow, FFR, FF) that can be recruited to perform different types of exercise.
- Fast motor units are larger than slow ones in the diameter of the motor axon as well as in the size and number of the muscle fibers innervated.
- Recruiting the lower threshold motor units first helps to delay fatigue when high force or power is not needed.
- Asynchronous recruitment of motor units can occur when force production needs are low, delaying the onset of fatigue.
- An exception to the size principle, in which fast motor units are recruited first, may occur to allow faster movement velocity.
- The all-or-none law dictates that all muscle fibers of a motor unit will contract if that motor unit is recruited.
- Force produced by a muscle is varied by activating different amounts of motor units.
- Selective activation of motor units and the difference in size of motor units and rate coding of each motor unit allows for graded force production.
- Motor units respond to a single nerve impulse by producing a twitch.
- The complete summation of single nerve impulse twitches results in tetanus.

NEURAL ADAPTATIONS TO EXERCISE

Training adaptations to the nervous system can improve physical performance. Neural drive, a measure of the combined motor unit recruitment and rate coding of active motor units within a muscle, is one aspect of training adaptations. Neural drive, which is initiated within the central nervous system and then transmitted to the peripheral nervous system, can be quantified using integrated electromyography (EMG) surface electrode techniques (Box 4-8). EMG techniques measure the electrical activity within the muscle, including the activity within both the nerves and the muscle fibers, and indicate the amount of neural drive delivered to a muscle.

In a set of classic studies, 8 weeks of weight training resulted in a shift to a lower level of EMG activity to muscular force ratio.[24–26] In effect, the trained muscle produced a given amount of submaximal force with a lower amount of EMG activity, suggesting an increased contractile response to any amount of submaximal neural drive. This greater response to a given amount of electrical stimulus suggests that there is either an improved activation of the muscle during submaximal effort, or a more efficient recruitment pattern of the motor units. However, some studies have demonstrated that improved activation of the muscle does not occur after training,[23] indicating that more efficient recruitment order is probably responsible for much of the increased force.

Box 4-8 AN EXPERT VIEW
Electromyography

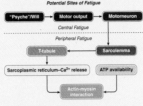

Joseph P. Weir, PhD, FACSM
Professor
Physical Therapy Program
Des Moines University
Osteopathic Medical Center
Des Moines, IA

EMG is a tool to measure the electrical signals created by muscles when they are stimulated to contract. Specifically, EMG records the action potentials that are generated on the muscle cell membrane (sarcolemma). Since the nervous system activates skeletal muscle at the level of motor units, and the muscle fibers in a motor unit will contract together, electromyographers often discuss EMG in terms of motor unit action potentials (MUAPs).

There are two general ways to make EMG recordings. First, surface electrodes can be placed over the belly of the muscle. The technology is similar to that used to make recordings of the electrical activity of the heart (electrocardiogram [ECG]), although many systems incorporate small bioamplifiers that can be placed directly on the skin. Surface electrodes require some preparation of the skin at the recording site. This usually involves thoroughly cleaning the skin with alcohol and, in some cases, shaving and abrading the skin so that the electrical impedance is minimized. Traditional surface EMG recordings do not allow the visualization of individual MUAPs. Instead, many MUAPs exist under the recording site at any instant in time, and the resulting signal is referred to as an interference pattern. The interference pattern looks similar to an acoustic signal or a seismograph signal in geology. The second approach is needle EMG, where needle electrodes are inserted into the muscle belly. In the exercise sciences, needle electrodes are primarily used to make recordings from deep muscles that are not accessible with surface electrodes. Needle EMG is also used in clinical electrodiagnosis, since it allows for the examination of individual MUAPs. A variety of muscular and neurological disorders can often be identified on the basis of the shapes of MUAPs and other characteristics identified in the needle EMG examination. Recently, a new surface

---

130   Part II   Exercise Physiology and

Another application to consider is t... recruited in the muscle will depend on t... and the biomechanical positions use... activity. For example, if you use diff... foot positions in a squat exercise, the a... musculature will not be the same du... in the biomechanical movements of t... limbs in the exercise movement (Fig. ...). ... the magnitude of recruitment of different portions of the quadriceps is different for the performance of exercises that are biomechanically different despite exercising the same area of the body (e.g., leg press vs. a squat). Variation in the recruitment order and magnitude of recruitment of different muscles is one of the factors responsible for strength and

... system. And although we can consciously control the motor nervous system to regulate the amount, and type of muscle forces developed by skeletal muscle that moves our limbs, the autonomic nervous system, which regulates the rate and force at which the cardiac muscle contracts, is beyond our ability to consciously control.

CASE STUDY

Scenario

You are a new head track coach. The previous head coach had field athletes weight training and performing interval training prior to skill training for their specific events. You have decided to structure your training sessions beginning with a warm-up followed by technique training, performing interval or weight training at the end of the session. Several of the athletes have asked you why you are changing the sequence of the previous coach's training sessions. What is the physiological basis for the changes in the practice and training program? What other practice and training organizations could you use, and what are the rationales for them?

Options

You explain to the athletes that the sequence of your training sessions will result in more high-quality technique training than the previous coach's sequence of having weight or interval training prior to technique training. You explain to them that as field athletes they do not have to develop maximal force and power in their jumping and throwing events when fatigued. Technique for all of the field events involves coordination of muscle fibers within a specific muscle as well as coordination of many muscles within their bodies to generate maximal power. If they perform weight training and interval training prior to technique training, they will be fatigued when performing the technique training. This will change the recruitment of muscle fibers within the muscles utilized and coordination of the various muscles involved in their specific events. Practically this means that if they practice technique for their field events when fatigued or after other types of training that result in fatigue, they will be learning how to perform their specific events when fatigued, which means that they will recruit their muscle fibers within a muscle and various muscles involved in their event in a slightly different manner compared to performing the event when not fatigued. This means that they will be teaching themselves slightly different or improper technique for

their events. You ask them to give your training sequence several weeks to prove itself, and state that you are confident they will see improvement in their event-specific technique.

Scenario

You are in charge of a beginning weight training class. You are aware that for general fitness typically one to three sets of each exercise are performed (see Chapter 12). However, you have a very limited amount of time in which to weight-train your class. Initially how many sets will you have your class perform? What is the physiological basis for the approach you choose to implement?

Options

Neural adaptations are a major reason for strength gains during the first several weeks of a weight training program. These adaptations include recruiting specific muscles at the correct time and in the proper order during the exercise movement and minimally recruiting antagonistic muscles to the desired movement. These neural adaptations occur to a large extent whether one, two, or three sets of an exercise are performed. To allow yourself more time during the initial training sessions to correct the exercise technique of students performing an exercise you had chosen, have your class perform only one set of each exercise. Due to neural adaptations, students will still see significant strength gains during the first several weeks of training. It has been shown that the eccentric phase of the repetition mediates the rapid gains made in strength early on in a resistance training program. After students have mastered proper exercise technique, you will increase the number of sets performed to two and then three per exercise as training adaptations allow the students to tolerate performing an increased number of sets per exercise. Additionally, one has to carefully examine the tolerance for the amount of work performed in a weight training workout.

CHAPTER SUMMARY

The nervous system interacts with every physiological system in the body. Neural signals, presented in the form of electrical activity, transmit information about the body's external and internal environments. These signals not only allow for normal resting homeostatic function of the body, they also allow the body to achieve an aroused physiological state or "fight-or-flight" response during intense exercise or physiological stress.

The brain and spinal cord make up the central nervous system, which functions as the primary controller of all of the body's actions. The peripheral nervous system includes nerves not in the brain or spinal cord and connects all parts of the body to the central nervous system. The peripheral (sensory) nervous system receives stimuli, the central nervous system interprets them, and then the peripheral (motor) nervous system initiates responses. The somatic nervous system controls functions that are under conscious voluntary control, such as skeletal muscles. The autonomic nervous system, mostly motor nerves, controls functions of involuntary smooth muscles and cardiac muscles and glands. The autonomic nervous system provides almost every organ with a double set of nerves—the sympathetic and parasympathetic nervous systems. These systems generally, but not always, work in opposition to each other (e.g., the sympathetic system increases the heart rate and the parasympathetic system decreases it). The sympathetic system activates and prepares the body for vigorous muscular activity, stress, and emergencies, whereas the parasympathetic system lowers arousal, and predominates during normal or resting situations. The nervous system controls movement by controlling muscle activity. To control the force produced by a muscle, the number of motor units recruited and rate coding of each motor unit can be varied. The performance of virtually all activities and sport skills requires the proper recruitment of motor units to develop the needed force in the correct order and at the right time. Training-induced adaptations of the nervous system are the basis of skill training for any physical activity, and serve to improve physical performance. In the next chapter, we will also see that the nervous system is important for cardiovascular function.

REVIEW QUESTIONS

Fill-in-the-Blank

1. The _____ nerves stimulate the heart rate to speed up while the _____ nerves stimulate it to slow down.

2. Motor units made up of _____ fibers are typically recruited first due to the _____ recruitment thresholds of their neurons.

3. When a threshold level of activation is reached in a motor unit, _____ of the muscle fibers in the motor unit will be activated; if the threshold level is not achieved, _____ of the muscle fibers in the motor unit will be activated.

4. The complete summation of nerve impulse twitches is called _____, which results in the maximal force a motor unit can develop.

5. The rapidity at which action potentials are fired down the motor axon helps control the force produced by a motor unit. This process is called _____.

Multiple Choice

1. Which of the following is true concerning a neuron?
   a. Dendrites carry impulses toward the cell body
   b. Axons carry impulses away from the cell body
   c. The axon hillock is between the axon and the cell body
   d. One neuron controls all the muscle fibers in a motor unit
   e. All of the above

2. Which of the following is true of a motor unit?
   a. Smaller and larger motor units are able to produce the same amount of maximal force.
   b. On average, for all of the muscles in the body, about 100 neurons control a muscle fiber.
   c. The number of muscle fibers in a motor unit depends on the amount of fine control required for its function.
   d. Motor units that stretch the lens of the eye contain 1000 muscle fibers.
   e. A motor unit consists of a beta motor neuron and its associated skeletal muscle fibers.

3. Which of the following is NOT true of saltatory conduction?
   a. It allows the action potential to "jump" from one Node of Ranvier to the next.
   b. It increases the velocity of nerve transmission.
   c. It conserves energy.
   d. It occurs only in unmyelinated nerves.
   e. It uses the movement of different ions.

4. Which of the following is, or are, exceptions to the size principle of recruitment?
   a. Recruit high-threshold type II motor units first
   b. Not recruiting low-threshold motor units first
   c. Recruiting slow prior to fast motor units
   d. None of the above
   e. a and b

5. Which of the following is NOT true of fast-fatigable motor units?
   a. They have large motor axons
   b. They feature type I muscle fibers
   c. They feature type IIX muscle fibers
   d. Of the three types of motor units, they develop the most force

True/False

1. The fight-or-flight response is brought about by the stimulation of the sympathetic branch of the autonomic nervous system.

2. All muscle fibers of a single motor unit are of the same type (i.e. I, IIA, or IIX).

3. During an action potential, repolarization occurs prior to depolarization.

4. An increase in maximal neural drive to a muscle increases force.

5. Slow motor units are made up of type I muscle fibers.

Short Answer

1. Provide and explain an example of a positive feedback loop during exercise.

2. Explain the different stages of the action potential, that is, depolarization and repolarization, and the movement of ions that occurs in each.

3. What is the advantage of the size principal of motor unit recruitment during an activity like jogging slowly?

4. Are all muscle fibers recruited when a light weight is lifted? Explain why or why not.

5. What contributes to training-induced changes in muscle strength with no significant hypertrophy of the muscle?

Critical Thinking

1. Describe what causes resting membrane potential in an axon or neuron, and then discuss how the movement of ions causes an action potential.

2. Discuss neural adaptations that could increase physical performance.

KEY TERMS

acetylcholine: a neurotransmitter released at motor synapses and neuromuscular junctions, active in the transmission of nerve impulses

action potential (nerve impulse): an impulse in the form of electrical energy that travels down a neuron as its membrane changes from −70 mV to +30 mV back to −70 mV due to the movement of electrically charged ions moving in and out of the cell

all-or-none law: when a threshold level for activation is reached, all of the muscle fibers in a motor unit are activated; if the threshold of activation is not met, none of the muscle fibers are activated

alpha (α) motor neuron: a neuron that controls skeletal muscle activity; it is composed of relatively short dendrites that receive the information, a cell body, and long axons that carry impulses from the cell body to the neuromuscular junction, which interfaces with the muscle fiber

asynchronous recruitment: alternating recruitment of motor units when force production needs are low

autonomic nerves (motor neurons): nerves of the autonomic nervous system, outside of the central nervous system

axon: part of a neuron that carries an impulse from the cell body to another neuron or target tissue receptor (e.g., muscle); it is sometimes referred to as a nerve fiber

axon hillock: the part of a neuron where the summation of incoming information is processed, if threshold is reached an impulse is transmitted down the axon

cell body (soma): the part of a neuron that contains the nucleus, mitochondria, ribosomes, and other cellular constituents

central nervous system: brain and spinal cord

cerebellum: part of the unconscious brain; regulates muscle coordination and coordinates balance and normal posture

cerebrum: a region of the brain consisting of the left and right hemispheres that is important for control of conscious movements

dendrite: part of a neuron that receives information (impulses) and sends it to the cell body

depolarization: a reduction in the polarity from resting membrane potential (−70 mV) to a more positive value (+30 mV) of a neuron's membrane

energy transformation: the conversion of one form of energy to another; in the transmission of an action potential, electrical energy is transformed into chemical energy to cross a synapse or neuromuscular junction

excitability: ability of a neuron or muscle fiber to respond to an electrical impulse

homeostasis: the ability of an organism or cell to maintain internal equilibrium by adjusting its physiological processes to keep function within physiological limits at rest or during exercise

hypothalamus: the homeostatic center of the brain; regulates metabolic rate, body temperature, thirst, blood pressure, water balance, and endocrine function

interneurons: special neurons located only in the central nervous system that connect one neuron to another neuron

ligand: a neurotransmitter, hormone, or other chemical substance that interacts with a receptor protein

local conduction: conduction of nerve impulses in unmyelinated nerves in which the ionic current flows along the entire length of the axon

medulla oblongata: part of the unconscious brain; regulates the heart, breathing, and blood pressure and reflexes such as swallowing, hiccups, sneezing, and vomiting

motor cortex: an area in the frontal lobe of the brain responsible for primary motor control

motor (efferent) neurons: a neuron that carries impulses from the central nervous system to the muscle

motor unit: an alpha motor neuron and its associated muscle fibers

multiple motor unit summation: a method of varying the force produced by a muscle by activating different numbers of motor units within the same muscle

myelin sheath: white covering high in lipid (fat) content that surrounds axons, provides insulation, and maintains electrical signal strength of the action potential as it travels down the axon

myelinated: nerve axons possessing a myelin sheath

Na⁺–K⁺ pump: an energy-dependent pumping system that restores the resting membrane potential by actively removing Na⁺ ions

---

> At the end of each chapter, an extensive list of **Review Questions** provides the students with a chance to apply what they have learned and assess their knowledge through fill-in-the-blank, multiple choice, true/false, short answer, and critical thinking questions.

> A **Key Terms list** at the end of each chapter provides definitions of important terminology with which students should become familiar.

> **High-quality, four-color illustrations** throughout the text help to draw attention to important concepts in a visually stimulating and intriguing manner. They help to clarify the text and are particularly helpful for visual learners.

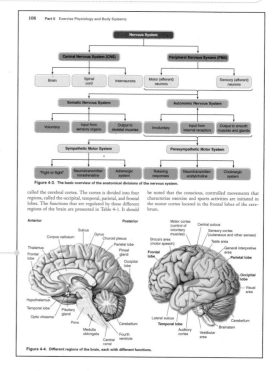

Figure 4-3. The basic overview of the anatomical divisions of the nervous system.

called the cerebral cortex. The cortex is divided into four regions, called the occipital, temporal, parietal, and frontal lobes. The functions that are regulated by these different regions of the brain are presented in Table 4-1. It should be noted that the conscious, controlled movements that characterize exercise and sports activities are initiated in the motor cortex located in the frontal lobes of the cerebrum.

Figure 4-4. Different regions of the brain, each with different functions.

STUDENT RESOURCES

Inside the front cover of your textbook, you will find your personal access code. Use it to log on to http://thePoint.lww.com/KraemerExPhys—the companion Web site for this textbook. On the Web site, you can access various supplemental materials available to help enhance and further your learning. These assets include an interactive quiz bank and animations, as well as the fully searchable online text.

Reviewers

Christopher Bussell, PhD
Head of Sport Science
School of Science and Technology
Nottingham Trent University
England, UK

Sandra Chu, MS, BPHE, CEP
Course Instructor
Personal Fitness Trainer Certificate Program
Faculty of Continuing Education and Extension
Mount Royal University
Calgary, AB

Gregory B. Dwyer, PhD, FACSM
Professor
Exercise Science
East Stroudsburg University of Pennsylvania
East Stroudsburg, PA

Scott A. Eide, MS, CSCS
Health & Fitness Department Coordinator
Minnesota School of Business
Waite Park, MN

William Farquhar, PhD
Associate Professor
Kinesiology and Applied Physiology
University of Delaware
Newark, DE

Jim Fluckey
Health Kinesiology
Texas A&M University
College Station, TX

Jennifer L. Gordon, DPE
Adjunct Professor
Exercise Science/Biology
Manchester Community College
Manchester, CT
Springfield Technical Community College
Springfield, MA
Quinnipiac University
Hamden, CT

Brian Hand, PhD, CSCS
Assistant Professor
Kinesiology
Towson University
Towson, MD

Craig A. Harms, PhD
Professor
Department of Kinesiology
Kansas State University
Manhattan, KS

Glyn Howatson, PhD
Senior Lecturer & Laboratory Director
School of Life Science
Northumbria University
Newcastle-upon-Tyne, UK

Kimberly Huey, PhD
Associate Professor
Pharmacy and Health Sciences
Drake University
Des Moines, IA

Michael G. Hughes, PhD
Senior Lecturer in Sport & Exercise Physiology
Cardiff School of Sport
University of Wales Institute
Cardiff, UK

Colin Iggleden
University of Portsmouth
Portsmouth, UK

Jennifer M. Jakobi, PhD
Professor
Human Kinetics, Faculty of Health and Social Development
University of British Columbia
Kelowna, BC

Greg Kandt, EdD, RCEP, CSCS
Associate Professor
Health and Human Performance
Fort Hays State University
Hays, KS

Michelle L. Komm, BSE, DC
Educator
Health Sciences
Pinnacle Career Institute
Kansas City, MO

Michael R. Kushnick, PhD, HFS
Associate Professor of Exercise Physiology
School of Applied Health Sciences
Ohio University
Athens, OH

Ian Lahart
University College Birmingham
Birmingham, UK

C. Matthew Lee, PhD
ACSM Registered Clinical Exercise
   Physiologist and Clinical Exercise Specialist
Associate Professor
Kinesiology
San Francisco State University
San Francisco, CA

Joseph R. Libonati, PhD
Assistant Professor
School of Nursing
University of Pennsylvania
Philadelphia, PA

Jacalyn J. Roert-McComb, PhD, FACSM
Professor in Exercise Physiology
Certified Clinical ACSM Program
   Director & Clinical Exercise Specialist
Health, Exercise, and Sport Sciences
Texas Tech University
Lubbock, TX

Timothy D. Mickleborough, PhD, FACSM
Associate Professor
Kinesiology
Indiana University
Bloomington, IN

Nicole Mullins, PhD, HFS, CSCS
Associate Professor, Exercise Science
Human Performance & Exercise Science
Youngstown State University
Youngstown, OH

Ian Newhouse, PhD
Professor
School of Kinesiology
Lakehead University
Thunder Bay, ON

Allen C. Parcell, PhD
Associate Professor
Exercise Sciences
Brigham Young University
Provo, UT

Ajay Patel, BSc, MHK
Division Chair—Health Sciences
Human Kinetics
Langara College
Vancouver, BC

David J. Pavlat, EdD, CSCS, CHFS
Associate Professor and Chair
Exercise Science
Central College
 Pella, IA

Brian Pritschet, PhD
Professor
Kinesiology & Sports Studies
Eastern Illinois University
Charleston, IL

Alison Purvis, PhD
Principal Lecturer in Sport and Exercise Physiology
Sport Department
Sheffield Hallam University
Sheffield, UK

Wendy Repovich, PhD, FACSM
Director, Exercise Science
Physical Education, Health & Recreation
Eastern Washington University
Cheney, WA

Steven E. Riechman, PhD, MPH, FACSM
Assistant Professor
Health and Kinesiology, Intercollegiate Faculty of Nutrition
Texas A&M University
College Station, TX

Emma Ross
Brunel University
Uxbridge, UK

Brian Roy, PhD
Professor
Centre for Muscle Metabolism and Biophysics
Brock University
St. Catharines, ON

Daniel G. Syrotuik, PhD
Professor & Vice Dean
University of Alberta
Edmonton, AB

Rene Vandenboom, PhD

Associate Professor
Physical Education and Kinesiology
Brock University
St. Catharines, ON

Pat R. Vehrs, PhD, FACSM

Associate Professor
Exercise Sciences
Brigham Young University
Provo, UT

Benjamin Wax Jr, PhD

Assistant Professor
Kinesiology
Mississippi State University
Mississippi State, MS

Heather E. Webb, PhD, ATC

Assistant Professor
Department of Kinesiology
Mississippi State University
Starkville, MS

Gary Werhonig, MS

ACSM Certified Clinical Exercise Specialist
Associate Lecturer
Kinesiology and Health
University of Wyoming
Laramie, WY

John C. Young, PhD, FACSM

Professor and Chair
Kinesiology and Nutrition Sciences
University of Nevada, Las Vegas
Las Vegas, NV

Acknowledgments

This book was written with the vision of helping young professionals see the value of science in their lives and to enhance their professional practice. As overwhelming as it is, such an undertaking requires a team of highly competent professionals dedicated to its success. For this we thank all of the exceptional professionals at Lippincott Williams & Wilkins for their encouragement and belief each step of the way.

To Ms. Emily Lupash, Acquisitions Editor, who saw the passion in our belief in this book and helped to make it a reality. To Ms. Andrea Klingler, Product Manager, for her day-to-day pragmatic persistence, kindness, and patience with us in this writing and development process; we could not have done it without you. To Mr. David Payne, Development Editor, for his extensive editorial work in the development of each chapter—you shared our dedication to excellence and application. To the other members of the Lippincott team: Allison Powell, Marketing Manager; Teresa Mallon, Design Coordinator; Jen Clements, Art Director—we thank you and your teams for your passion and dedication to this project.

To Dr. Maren Fragala, one of my (WJK) former doctoral fellows, for her help and support in getting this book out of the dock with her daily intellectual exchanges and reading of the material. To all of our departmental colleagues at the University of Connecticut, Colorado College, and The College of William & Mary: we thank you for your support and encouragement during the demanding process of developing this book. To all of our clinical, coaching, and scientific colleagues in our field: we thank you for being the inspiration of our professional lives and supporting such an integrated approach to exercise physiology.

And, to all of our current and previous graduate and undergraduate students who have allowed us to see the joy of discovery, gain new insights into teaching, and how taking knowledge to practice can work: we thank you. This book reflects your accumulated influence.

WILLIAM KRAEMER
STEVEN FLECK
MICHAEL DESCHENES

Contents

PART I

Foundations of Exercise Physiology

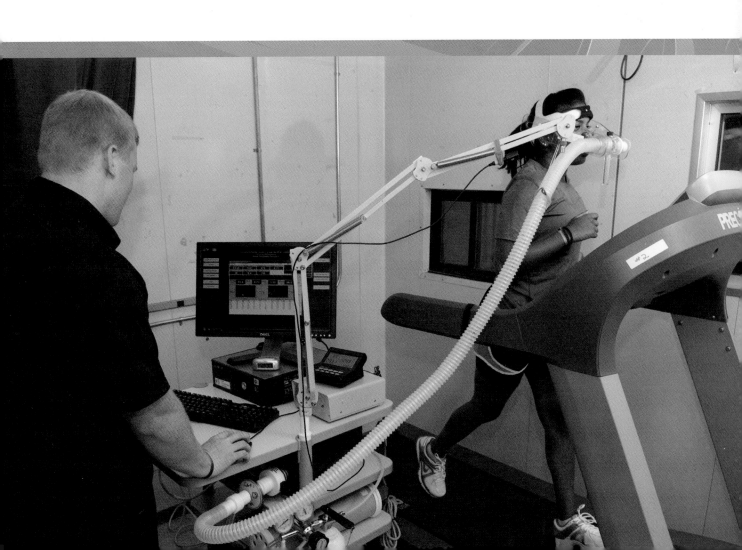

1

Applying Research to Everyday Exercise and Sport

After reading this chapter, you should be able to:

1. Describe the research process
2. Distinguish and classify types of research
3. Explain the difference between facts that are based on scientific versus unscientific practices
4. Read and comprehend a research paper
5. Evaluate sources of information
6. Explain the process of peer review
7. Interpret and extract research findings in context

Did you ever wonder, "What type of cardio program works best to improve aerobic fitness?" or "What might be the best way to train with weights?" or "What are the effects of competing in a cross-country race at altitude?" or "What actually happens to the muscle when you use different types of training programs?" or "What is the best way to lose body fat?" Such curiosity and questioning is what research is all about.

The goal of research is to find answers to questions. If there is no question, then there is no basis for research. The answers to some questions already exist from prior published investigations in scientific journals. Other questions may require further experimentation by scientists to provide new data. New data from research studies provide answers to questions and help to expand our understanding of a topic. Figure 1-1 provides an overview of the research process.

Many questions can be answered by searching for studies on a topic in the scientific literature. Many journals exist in the field of exercise and sport science, with even more in the associated fields of nutrition, physiology, medicine, and epidemiology (Box 1-1). This type of search requires a basic understanding of the research process and how to read a research paper, both of which we will address in this chapter.

Furthermore, this chapter presents unscientific methods that should be avoided, introduces you to the scientific literature, and outlines the components of an original investigative study. Finally, the chapter covers how you can extract practical applications for your day-to-day work from research.

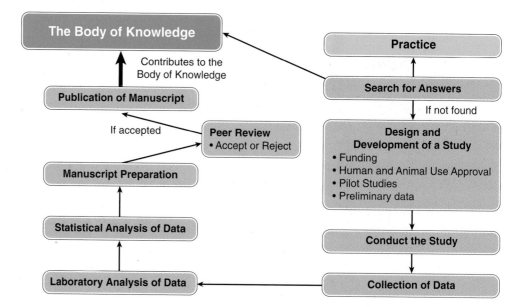

Figure 1-1. **The research process involves several related steps.** A major goal of research is to add to a field of study's body of knowledge.

INTRODUCTION TO RESEARCH

Research begins with experiments conducted following the scientific method, in which data are collected, hypotheses are tested, and answers to specific questions are obtained (Fig. 1-1). Analysis of the accumulated results of many such experiments leads to facts, theories, and principles. Finally, research may be divided into two general categories: basic and applied research (Box 1-5 and Box 1-6).

Before we get into the research process used in experimental studies, it is important to understand the following limitations of research:

1. There is no such thing as the perfect study.
2. No one study can tell you the whole story.
3. Every study has a specific context for why it was done and has potential limits in terms of its generalization to similar situations.
4. Many times research findings are not black and white but rather gray in terms of their practical application. This requires the professional to have an open mind and practice the "art of the profession" by using experience, good judgment, and common sense in the choices that are made from interpolation or extrapolation of research findings.

Box 1-1 APPLYING RESEARCH

Selected Peer-Reviewed Journals in Exercise and Sport Science

1. American Journal of Sports Medicine
2. Applied Physiology, Nutrition, and Metabolism
3. Australian Journal of Science and Medicine in Sport
4. British Journal of Sports Medicine
5. Canadian Journal of Applied Physiology
6. Clinical Journal of Sport Medicine
7. Clinical Exercise Physiology
8. Clinics in Sports Medicine
9. Current Sports Medicine Reports
10. European Journal of Applied Physiology
11. Exercise and Sport Sciences Reviews
12. International Journal of Sport Nutrition and Exercise Metabolism
13. International Journal of Sports Medicine
14. Isokinetics and Exercise Science
15. Journal of Applied Biomechanics
16. Journal of Applied Physiology
17. Journal of Athletic Training
18. The Journal of Orthopaedic and Sports Physical Therapy
19. Journal of Physical Activity & Health
20. The Journal of Sports Medicine
21. The Journal of Sports Medicine and Physical Fitness
22. Journal of Sports Sciences
23. Journal of Strength and Conditioning Research
24. Medicine and Science in Sports and Exercise
25. Medicine and Sport Science
26. Pediatric Exercise Science
27. Research Quarterly for Exercise and Sport
28. Scandinavian Journal of Medicine & Science in Sports
29. Sports Biomechanics
30. Sports Medicine

Box 1-2 APPLYING RESEARCH

Should Stretching Be Part of a Warm-Up?

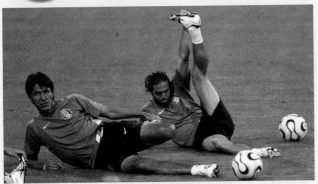

No one study can explain everything about a particular topic of interest. Furthermore, every study has a context as it relates to its dependent variables so that an answer to a question may be different depending upon the conditions of the experiment. Coaches and athletes have been stretching as a part of their warm-up prior to athletic competition and conditioning sessions for years. The theory was that it would reduce the risk of injury and help one prepare for activity. Flexibility training has been documented to improve the range of motion, but whether it should be part of a warm-up has now been questioned.

From the 1970s to the 1990s, occasional research reports questioned the use of flexibility training as part of a warm-up, but it takes time for a body of study to accumulate and impact practice. As the topic became more popular and the research requirements relatively inexpensive, more and more research studies started to accumulate data suggesting that stretching may not prevent injury or help with performance. In fact, research studies started to show that static stretching may be detrimental to performance by decreasing force production possibly due to the reduction in muscle activation and central nervous system inhibitory mechanisms. In addition, both static and proprioceptive neuromuscular facilitation stretchings were shown to produce deficits in muscle force and power production due

also to deformation or stretching of the elastic component in the muscle (i.e., connective tissue), reducing the impact of the stretch-shortening cycle and increasing central nervous system inhibitory mechanisms.

Conversely, dynamic or ballistic stretching, which was considered taboo for years, was shown to be an effective method to enhance dynamic performance when used as a warm-up activity. So, the question of when to stretch and what kind of stretching to perform has become an important decision for coaches and athletes to consider. Research is now being conducted on all aspects of stretching as part of a warm-up to optimize performance. This is one example of how research starts to impact practice. So, you have to make some decisions. What would you do? What is the most prudent approach to take if you had to warm-up your athletes before a workout or competition? What kind of stretching should be used? How long before a competition or workout should stretching be performed, if at all? What would you do with the current state of knowledge on this question? How would you match the studies to your specific circumstances?

Further Readings

Bradley PS, Olsen PD, Portas MD. The effect of static, ballistic, and proprioceptive neuromuscular facilitation stretching on vertical jump performance. J Strength Cond Res. 2007;21(1):223–226.

Cramer JT, Housh TJ, Weir JP, et al. The acute effects of static stretching on peak torque, mean power output, electromyography, and mechanomyography. Eur J Appl Physiol. 2005;93(5-6):530–539.

Marek SM, Cramer JT, Fincher AL, et al. Acute effects of static and proprioceptive neuromuscular facilitation stretching on muscle strength and power output. J Athl Train. 2005;40(2):94–103.

Rubini EC, Costa AL, Gomes PS. The effects of stretching on strength performance. Sports Med. 2007;37(3):213–224.

Shrier I. Stretching before exercise does not reduce the risk of local muscle injury: a critical review of the clinical and basic science literature. Clin J Sport Med. 1999;9(4):221–227.

Young WB, Behm DG. Effects of running, static stretching and practice jumps on explosive force production and jumping performance. J Sports Med Phys Fitness. 2003;43(1):21–27.

5. Most of the time a study will raise more questions than it will answer.
6. Realize that things change and new findings can alter age-old concepts and principles and therefore change the approach to a particular topic (Box 1-2 and Box 1-3).

Steps of the Scientific Method

Essentially, the scientific method consists of a number of basic steps in generating data to provide a factual basis for answers to questions:

1. *What is the question?* First, the scientist must make observations on a phenomenon or group of phenomena

that generate questions regarding why, how, when, who, which, or where.

2. *What do we know from the body of knowledge already accumulated in the form of published studies?* The scientist examines studies in the literature to see whether the question(s) can be answered with existing information.

3. *If the question cannot be specifically answered, then one has to construct a hypothesis.* A hypothesis is an educated guess as to what might happen in an experiment based on the literature or anecdotal observations (e.g., what you or others have observed to be true). The hypothesis should answer the original question and be able to be tested using measurable variables.

Box 1-3 APPLYING RESEARCH

Rethinking a Hypothesis

It is important to understand that a hypothesis is only one concept or guess as to how things work. Any understanding about something in research is based on the conditions (independent variables) that affect the outcome variables (dependent variables) or our ability to measure a phenomenon. Rethinking a hypothesis revolves around the concept that alternatives can exist. In research, we essentially test what is called a "null hypothesis," or a condition in which there will be no differences in any comparisons. When differences do exist, then we have to reject the null and accept what is called an alternative hypothesis based on the conditions that produced it. Rethinking a hypothesis is nothing more than testing the viability of an alternative hypothesis with different conditions. For example, fat intake may be bad if associated with high carbohydrate intakes, but may be its impact is not negative when associated with low carbohydrate intake. Paradigm shifts in hypotheses are many times difficult, as they go against what has been thought to be true for years. Therefore, it is obvious why confusion can exist in the lay community because of what appears to be contradictory research or advice. Understanding the scientific process as a professional in exercise science allows you to provide insights into the interpretation of research findings and their generalization.

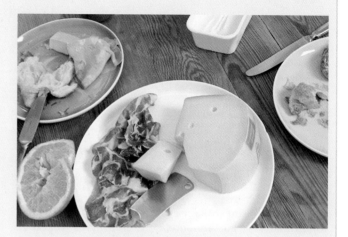

Further Readings

Lofgren I, Zern T, Herron K, et al. Weight loss associated with reduced intake of carbohydrate reduces the atherogenicity of LDL in premenopausal women. Metabolism. 2005;54(9):1133–1141.

Wood RJ, Fernandez ML, Sharman MJ, et al. Effects of a carbohydrate-restricted diet with and without supplemental soluble fiber on plasma low-density lipoprotein cholesterol and other clinical markers of cardiovascular risk. Metabolism. 2007;56(1):58–67.

4. *Test the hypothesis by doing an experiment.* A properly designed experiment should be conducted to collect data to test the validity of the hypothesis. This experimentation, though seemingly simple, is the primary pursuit of graduate students in the sciences and of scientists. Obviously, the more specific the research conditions are to the specific population or conditions in which you are interested, the greater the possibility of application to a specific situation. For example, if you are interested in developing a strength program specifically for older men and are conducting an experiment to determine what exercises will result in the greatest absolute strength gains, older men should serve as subjects in the experiment, not younger men.

5. *Analyze the data and draw a conclusion.* After the data are collected, they must be analyzed statistically to determine whether the hypothesis was supported or not. The experiment will either support or reject the hypothesis, and the question is answered within the context of the experimental conditions (e.g., men or women, age range, training status) and can be applied in both general and specific manners (Box 1-3). In other words, did you guess right and are there now facts to support or reject the hypothesis and answer the original question?

6. *Communicate the results.* The outcome of a study is validated only when it has been published in a **peer-reviewed journal**—one in which studies are evaluated by the scientists' peers and are accepted or rejected on the basis of accuracy, interpretation, general scientific procedures, adequacy of methodology, and strength of data (Box 1-1). As muscle physiologist Philip Gollnick once said, "Work unpublished is work not done and work unpublished is work that does not exist."

Unscientific Methods

Unfortunately, answers to questions are many times derived from unscientific methods. Such methods can sometimes generate correct answers but often lead to a "disconnect" between perception and reality. Although it is not possible to base every decision on a scientific study, professionals should be aware of unscientific methods and the questionable facts they can produce. Below are some unscientific approaches to finding answers *to questions*. You might recognize some of these approaches through your experiences with your friends, teachers, and coaches (Box 1-4).

Intuition

Intuition means the ability to know something without any reasoning. The answer to the question is *sensed* or felt to be right, independent of any previous experience or empirical knowledge. Although intuition is often used in the decision-making process in a profession, even science, it must be recognized for what it is, a guess or a hypothesis.

Box 1-4 DID YOU KNOW?
Batting Rituals

Have you ever noticed the series of preparatory rituals a baseball player will go through before stepping up to bat? These include taking an exact number of practice swings, adjusting a cap, touching each uniform letter, rubbing a medallion, motioning the sign of the cross, and tapping the plate a certain number of times with the bat. For example, before every pitch, former Los Angeles Dodgers first baseman Nomar Garciaparra would step out of the batters' box, adjust his armband on the right arm, tap home plate with the bat, touch his helmet bill, touch the end of the bat, again touch the helmet bill, make the sign of the cross, balance the bat on the right shoulder, adjust the right batting glove with his left hand, dig his cleat into the dirt, cross the right hand over his left as it tugs on the left-hand glove, repeat several times, twist and sink one cleat at a time into the dirt, and circle his bat several times in a counterclockwise direction. In fact, the former Cleveland Indian first baseman Mike Hargrove became known as the "the human rain delay" since he had so many time-consuming elements in his batting ritual. Some may call these prebatting preparatory rituals superstition, whereas players believe that their batting rituals help them concentrate for the upcoming pitch. Since hitting a baseball has been considered the most difficult task in sports, concentration and precision are critical. While these rituals do not have a scientific basis, do you think they are important for sports performance?

One might have a gut feeling about something, but that feeling may in fact be based on many prior experiences and an understanding of the science surrounding the question. Using it as a tool might be part of the "art" for the decision-making process, but one has to make sure that there is some factual basis underlying the intuitive feeling. Without that, intuition can be misleading and wrong. Here are a number of intuitions, all of which are incorrect:

1. I think our weight-training workout should use only single-joint exercises.
2. I think it would be a good idea to eat a steak before a football game.
3. I think it would be a good idea to statically stretch right before my last attempt in the high jump.
4. I think the early morning is the best time to have a competition.
5. I think it is too stressful for women to run a marathon.
6. I think if a woman lifts weights, she will get too big.
7. I think you can never drink too much water during a long distance race.

Tradition

Tradition is the idea that "we have always done it this way and have been successful, so there is no need to change." This type of approach to problem solving is hit or miss, depending on the factual basis of the tradition. In sports, it is common and usually has few or no negative effects. For example, American football helmets may keep the same logo for years as a part of their school's tradition. It is when outdated traditions cross the line and violate the current science and factual understanding on a topic that concerns begin to arise. For example, not having enough water breaks needed for proper hydration during sport practice or practicing in the heat of the day because that is the way it has always been done. Traditions need to be evaluated for their scientific efficacy and current factual basis. Below are some other examples of concepts based on tradition:

1. A player rubs the school's mascot before every home game in the belief that this will result in a win.
2. The same warm-up routine is used for every game.
3. A player will always eat the same pregame meal.
4. Only one type of interval training program is used.

Trial and Error

Trial and error is commonly used to find an answer. This approach is basically to try an action and see whether it elicits the outcome desired. A common approach in many areas of exercise and sport, it can be thought of as "miniexperiments." If scientific facts and an understanding of a topic are used in conjunction with this approach, it can prove efficient. However, caution must always be used with this approach, as random trials are not always optimal and may even be harmful.

This approach is popular because not all individuals respond as the average or mean response. Thus, individual athletes try different methods of diet or training and see how it works for them. People often turn to this method as an alternative when there is a lack of scientific investigation on a certain topic. To address the issue of "responders" and "nonresponders" to a treatment, many investigations now show the responses of each subject in addition to the mean response to allow the reader to see the variability of the individual responses (see Fig. 1-2 for an example). Examples of trial and error methods are given below. Think about the factual basis for each, how one would pick a starting point, and what might be some negative effects of using this approach to finding an answer. Also think about what it means if not all individuals respond in a similar manner.

1. Trying different diets to see which one works
2. Trying a running pace to see whether it elicits the heart rate response desired for an exercise prescription

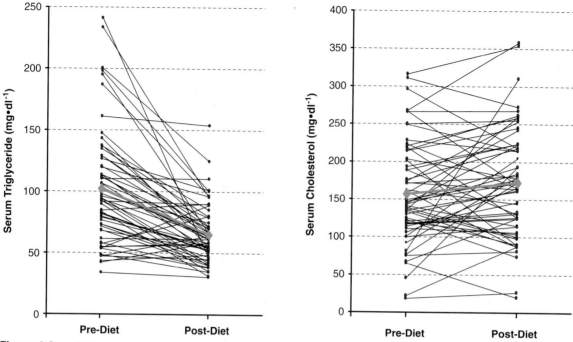

Figure 1-2. Individual responses to an experimental treatment can vary. Individual responses of serum triglyceride and cholesterol to a low-carbohydrate diet vary—some individuals show an increase, others a decrease, and some no change. The *blue line* indicates the group mean.

3. Trying to lift a weight to see whether it allows the desired number of repetitions in the exercise prescription
4. Trying to ingest a certain amount of protein to see whether it helps in building muscle
5. Trying to run at race pace in the heat without previous exposure to heat

Bias

Bias is typically thought of in a negative manner, as it is a preference or an inclination that many times can inhibit impartial answers to a question. If your bias is based on scientific fact, then it can be positive. Conversely, if you come to conclusions based on factors other than factual evidence, then bias may be detrimental to the decision-making process. The following are examples of bias. Consider whether there is any factual basis for each and what negative impacts each might have if it is factually incorrect.

1. It is my bias that only men should participate in ice hockey.
2. It is my bias that our team should be fully hydrated the night before and prior to a competition.
3. It is my bias that only this approach to training is correct.
4. It is my bias that women should not train with weights.
5. It is my bias that athletes need to work harder.
6. It is my bias that the effects of cold weather are all in the mind.
7. It is my bias that competing at 2,200 meters in elevation will not affect our performances in the field events at a track meet.
8. It is my bias that every member of the team should train the same way.

Authority

Answering a question based on some authorities' views can be positive or negative depending on the qualifications, factual basis, and/or historical relevance of the authority. An old article in a medical journal by a physician who cautions against too much exercise in fear of athletes getting enlarged hearts is one example of a poor authority on which to base decisions. The information on the adaptations and functional interpretation of cardiac muscle with exercise training is outdated. One must carefully scrutinize an authority's qualifications, the context for the answer provided, the timeliness of the information, and other known facts. With new research constantly appearing, what was authoritative a few years ago may not be so now. The following are some examples of what might be called "authorities in the field." Consider the positive aspects, as well as reasons for caution, in following such authorities.

1. A professional strength and conditioning coach commenting on diet practices of players
2. A registered dietician commenting on the exercise program that best produces changes in aerobic performance and fat loss
3. A Hall of Fame American football coach commenting on the best method for conditioning a team
4. A Hall of Fame basketball coach commenting on the best method to motivate a team for a big game
5. A professor in exercise science commenting on the best way to hydrate a player prior to a soccer match
6. A World Cup soccer player commenting on how to prepare for a game at altitude

7. A 1991 classic textbook on exercise science
8. A classic peer-reviewed manuscript in a highly reputable journal in exercise science from 1999
9. Your mother telling you not to eat before you go swimming

Rationalistic Method

This approach is based on using reasoning to produce facts. Its efficacy is based on the veracity of the assumptions made and their factual basis. Reasoning is a solid method for making decisions, but creating knowledge based on reasoning alone is not a valid approach to science because absurd outcomes can result. The key factor of this process is the truth of the premises being put forth and their relationship to each other. The following are a few examples of using the rationalistic method to come to a conclusion. Determine the realistic answers that are derived from such an approach and evaluate the efficacy of each.

1. American football players are big (major premise).
    John is big (minor premise).
    John is a football player (conclusion).
2. National Football League linemen typically weigh more than 300 pounds.
    Jim plays as a lineman at a small college and weighs 240 pounds.
    Jim will not be a lineman in the National Football League.
3. Growth hormone is a 22-kD polypeptide.
    Analysis of growth hormone in the blood shows other molecular weight forms of the hormone.
    Other variants of the hormone must exist.
4. Weight loss is a function of the amount of calories taken in and the amount of calories expended.
    A diet equated for total calories but high in protein and fat produces more weight loss than a diet high in carbohydrates and low in fat.
    Not all calories from food have the same impact on metabolism.

Empirical Method

The empirical method is based on one's observations and experience. This method, of course, is a part of the scientific method itself, in that it involves the collecting of data. However, to the degree that our observations and experiences are based on our own personal contexts, what works for us may not be relevant to others and may not be what others need from us as professionals. The use of the empirical method is often seen in coaching, the military, and in the strength and conditioning profession. The adage, "well if it worked for me, then it will work for you," is the thought process that has led to a lot of misinformation. Again, depending upon the background, qualifications, and factual basis of an individual's experiences, use of the empirical method may or may not work. For example, in exercise prescription, it can obviate principles of exercise specificity training and individualization of conditioning programs. Examples of the empirical method are listed below. What are the factual matches or mismatches to such approaches?

1. A soccer coach tells the team that he did not wear insulated clothing in cold rainy weather and therefore the team will not be issued any thermal gear.
2. A physician tells a patient that weight training should not be a part of a cardiac rehabilitation program, as it has never been done in his/her medical practice.
3. A cross-country coach tells the team that she lifted weights in her all-American career as a cross-country runner, so every team member will perform a sport-specific weight-training program as part of their program.
4. A captain in the army tells the company that he ran in boots and had no problems, so all company runs will be done in boots.
5. A golf professional says that she/he sees no need to lift weights for golfing as it might hurt your game, and she/he never lifted.
6. A swim coach says that she/he used to swim 20,000 meters a day, so the team will do the same.

Myth

Myths, or widely held but unfounded beliefs, are another unscientific source of answers. Some myths in exercise are due to the marketing and advertising of equipment and products. From sport drinks to exercise machines, myths related to their origin, use, and efficacy have developed and flourished. Differentiating the myth from the facts is an important factor in optimizing the decision-making process and any problem solving that must occur. Ultimately, decisions must be tempered by the factual evidence that exists in the literature.

Facts, Theory, and Principles

In the next step of the scientific process, results from individual experiments lead to the establishment of facts, theories, and principles. **Facts** are observational data that are confirmed repeatedly by many independent and competent observers. However, facts are not without context.

Quick Review

- The scientific method is a series of steps used to provide a factual basis to answer research questions.
- Many times in exercise and sports science, answers to questions arise from unscientific methods.
- Differentiating facts based on scientific methods versus those from unscientific methods is important for optimal approaches and decision-making processes for programs in exercise and sport.

It might be a fact that under certain conditions something is good for you, but under other circumstances it is bad. For example, water is needed for optimal health and performance to prevent one from becoming dehydrated. On the other hand, drinking too much water before, during, and after an endurance race can be detrimental to health, causing hyponatremia—dilution of electrolytes in the body affecting organ function—or even death.

A **theory** is typically a conceptual framework of ideas or speculations regarding a certain topic, ideally, based on experimental facts. In the scientific context, it has been described as "a comprehensive explanation based upon a given set of data that has been repeatedly confirmed by observation and experimentation and has gained general acceptance within the scientific community but has not yet been decisively proven."[2] One commonly hears that in science theories can never really be proven, only disproven. Again, one needs to keep context in mind. There is always the possibility that a new observation or experiment will conflict with a long-standing theory (such as "water is always good for you") and that we will have to think about things differently, at least in some contexts. As more facts become available, a theory must be modified to reflect this. Thus, theories can change.

From facts and theories are derived many of the guiding **principles** for our approach to a problem or behaviors in a certain situation. Principles are derived from theories that are less likely to change. So what is the definition of a principle? Principles describe how something should be done, the rules that explain a physiological process, or guidelines that should be adhered to for optimal performance of a task, such as exercise prescription. In exercise science, examples of principles include the principle of exercise specificity and the principle of progressive overload. Each of these describes guidelines for various aspects of exercise prescription. Exercise physiology also has many principles that describe function, such as homeostasis. Many professional guidelines related to physiology and exercise prescription are based upon facts generated from research that lead to theories that help to develop guiding principles. Like theories, principles too are modified to address the emerging new facts in a field of study, from care of injuries in athletic training to understanding the role of exercise on pituitary function in exercise physiology.

Basic and Applied Research

Research may be classified as basic and applied, both of which have their place in understanding exercise. The goal of basic research is to gain a greater understanding of the topic under study, without regard to how this information will be specifically applied. It is aimed at expanding knowledge rather than solving a specific, pragmatic problem and is typically driven by a scientist's curiosity or interest in a scientific question (Box 1-5). However, it does have the potential to lead to revolutionary advancements in our lives.

For example, two of the most popular imaging techniques used in the study of exercise's effects on muscle and bone are nuclear magnetic resonance spectroscopy and magnetic resonance imaging. Basic research starting in the late 1940s provided the genesis for these technologies, which we have all come to see as commonplace in both clinical evaluations and scientific study.

Conversely, applied research is designed to solve practical problems of the real world, rather than to acquire knowledge for knowledge's sake.[3] It might be said that the goal of applied science is to improve the human condition. In the case of exercise, the goal is to improve our understanding of its many benefits and how to use it so that we may achieve greater benefits from its use and prescription (Box 1-6). This has been a primary motivation of much of the research in exercise and sport science over the past 50 years. Research has led to a host of exercise guidelines to help people gain the benefits of exercise training.

Ultimately, there is a continuum of knowledge that spans from basic to applied science, with scientists working across the research continuum. Some work on basic genetic, cellular, and molecular mechanisms, and others work in the more applied area of research. This continuum exists, too, in the scientific literature of exercise and sport science. Scientists use basic research techniques in cell and molecular biology to study the mechanisms that mediate the adaptations observed in applied studies. For example, when an endurance training program leads to a higher maximal oxygen consumption value and a faster 10-kilometer race time, what cellular or physiological mechanisms mediate this phenomenon? Basic techniques are then used to study how this occurs. One interesting challenge for basic scientists studying mechanisms is what does applied science indicate is the most effective type of training. If the exercise prescription is not effective, studying the effects at the cellular level will have little meaning. Thus, the exercise program used in basic science studies is vital for establishing the external validity or importance of the study.

For example, if a scientist studies the cellular effects of endurance training but does not understand how to design an effective aerobic endurance training program that decreases 10-kilometer run time, he or she may choose an ineffective program that results in little or no change in 10-kilometer run time and no cellular changes. The conclusion of the study would be that endurance training causes no cellular changes, but really no cellular changes occurred because the training program was not effective. The conclusion of the study would need to be that *this particular* aerobic endurance training program had no influence on 10-kilometer race times and resulted in no cellular changes. This underscores the importance of reading a study with attention to the context. Each study contributes to our understanding but must be put into the paradigm for a scientific approach based on the conditions under which it took place. For instance, no one would prescribe a very low-intensity aerobic training

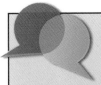

Box 1-5 AN EXPERT VIEW
Role of Basic Research in Exercise Science

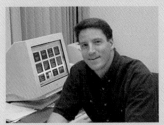

Scott E. Gordon, PhD, FACSM
Associate Professor; Department of
Exercise and Sport Science
East Carolina University
Greenville, NC

What is the importance of basic research to the field of exercise physiology and its advancement? The answer to this question may not be evident to a nonscientist. Generally speaking, pure basic research is driven by humankind's curiosity for exploration and expansion of knowledge without immediate or obvious benefits of the resulting knowledge. This lies at the opposite end of the continuum from pure applied research, the results of which are many times obvious and immediately applicable. Frequently, the potential future application of any single basic research experiment cannot be foreseen. Nevertheless, basic research and applied research are inherently linked, because basic research collectively forms the foundation on which to build and understand applied research.

In a biological science, such as exercise physiology, basic research typically explores phenomena occurring at the cellular, molecular, and genetic levels, especially with respect to how cells respond to a change in their immediate environment. For instance, exactly how and why do muscle fibers sense and respond to varying stimuli, such as hormonal alterations, energy requirements, substrate (fuel) availability, or changes in tension placed upon the cell by exercise contractions? What "signaling molecules" inside the cell allow the muscle fiber to respond to these stimuli and how does the cell alter expression of its genes (DNA), RNA, and protein molecules as a result? Exactly where inside and outside the cell do these mechanisms occur, and what role does microanatomical structure play in the correct function of these mechanisms? Taken independently, the answers to the above questions do not tell a complete story. However, the fact is that every physical movement experienced by a person, as well as every bodily adaptation to exercise training, is a result of thousands of different molecules acting in a coordinated fashion throughout various cells and tissues of the body.

Exercise physiologists using basic research techniques typically do an excellent job of integrating cellular, molecular, and genetic findings and linking them to applied function. Take the example of an elite marathoner. On the applied level, it is easy to observe that he or she has a great capacity for endurance exercise performance, but basic research has now shown us that this ability stems from a combination of specific cellular, molecular, and genetic mechanisms. Optimal endurance exercise performance requires a molecular make-up inside and outside of the muscle fibers that optimizes many factors such as oxygen and substrate delivery to the exercising muscles, ability of the bioenergetic pathways within the muscle fiber to generate energy while avoiding fatiguing conditions, calcium handling by the sarcoplasmic reticulum and calcium-dependent proteins that is appropriate to slow contractions, and the use of energy by the myosin head and other energy-dependent processes that is appropriate to slower but more continuous contractions. All of these factors are controlled at the molecular level and vary with each person's genetics; thus, each individual is different with respect to his or her endurance capacity and ability to respond to endurance training. Alternatively, different molecular and genetic make-ups optimize a person's ability to perform or respond to sprint or resistance exercise training. In some cases, even a difference in one nucleotide of one chromosome (called "a single nucleotide polymorphism," or SNP) can play a large role in somebody's exercise performance or training response.

An impactful role of basic research in exercise physiology is the determination of mechanisms responsible for the beneficial health effects of physical activity. In the United States and elsewhere in the world, a sedentary lifestyle is highly associated with the large incidence of metabolic syndrome, which consists of the interrelated conditions of obesity, type 2 diabetes, and various forms of cardiovascular disease. It is well-known that regular physical activity can prevent or delay the incidence of these and a vast number of other unhealthy conditions, yet many of the molecular mechanisms by which this occurs are still unclear. Because many conditions precipitated by physical inactivity are chronic, the targeted reduction of risk factors earlier in life can be a key to early prevention. Determining molecular-level risk factors affected by exercise interventions can allow us to individually optimize training regimens to target and reduce these risk factors before an overt disease becomes apparent, and thus potentially prevent or delay the disease altogether. In addition, determining the molecular mechanisms underlying the effect of physical activity on health would provide a scientific basis for devising dietary supplements, prescription drugs, gene medicine strategies, cell therapies, or other methods to produce beneficial health effects in those individuals for whom exercise is perhaps impossible, such as extremely frail or obese individuals or patients with spinal cord injuries.

In summary, tremendous basic research progress in the field of exercise physiology has been made with the advent of new molecular tools over the past 30 years. This research has helped us to better understand the mechanisms underlying the body's response to acute exercise as well as exercise training, both with respect to human performance and human health. Moreover, the rapidly evolving research technology being made available to scientists will undoubtedly lead to a much greater understanding of the human body's response to exercise on the cellular, molecular, and genetic levels in the very near future.

Further Reading

Booth FW, Chakravarthy MV, Gordon SE, et al. Waging war on physical inactivity: using modern molecular ammunition against an ancient enemy. J Appl Physiol. 2002;93(1):3–30.

Box 1-6   AN EXPERT VIEW

Role of Applied Research in Exercise Science

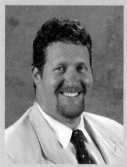

Jay R. Hoffman, PhD, FACSM, FNSCA
Professor, Sports Science
College of Education
The University of Central Florida
Orlando, FL

The basis of our knowledge in strength and conditioning is grounded in scientific principle. It is the product of basic sciences such as biology, physics, and chemistry that are combined to an applied field of study such as exercise science with specific emphasis in physiology, biomechanics, or biochemistry. Our understanding of physiological responses to training is critical in working with athletes and assisting them in the development of realistic training goals and providing critical feedback during evaluation. Without the use of science we would be unable to effectively evaluate the efficacy of various training paradigms, critically examine an assortment of ergogenic aids and nutritional supplements, or understand the physiological, psychological, and biomechanical requirements necessary for success in specific sports.

What makes applied research so special is that it bridges the gap between science and application. It allows the coach to understand how to help athletes maximize performance, or perhaps as important, understand limitations of performance. Such information can assist coaches and athletes in setting realistic training goals and performance expectations. It may also provide assistance in setting more objective criteria used for team selection. Applied research provides tools for the coach to use to minimize risk for injury, to reduce the risk of fatigue and overtraining, and achieve peak performance at the appropriate time. Most scientists are comfortably working in laboratories and using laboratory measures to assess human performance. This type of science and data collection has an important role in increasing our scientific understanding of human performance. However, applied scientists are equally adept at using the playing fields and courts as their laboratory. The examination of athletes within their competitive environment provides a more specific understanding of the needs and stresses of the sport and also provides data that coaches may readily comprehend. In addition, the ability and desire to delineate information collected in both field- and laboratory-based research is a responsibility that the applied scientist must accept. Timely communication to the coach and athlete will allow them to use this information to enhance their understanding of the needs of their sport and when applicable to develop appropriate training paradigms. An example of this is seen in the study published by Hoffman and colleagues in 2002 in the journal *Medicine and Science in Sports and Exercise*.[1] This research examined the biochemical, endocrine, and performance changes during an actual competitive collegiate football game. It was the first time that athletes playing football were examined in real time and provided important information concerning power decrements and biochemical and endocrine markers of muscle damage and exercise stress.

The bridge that spans science and sport though does go in two directions. Coaches and athletes often question the effectiveness of various training methods or specific nutritional supplements. Their curiosity often raises important questions that generate specific research ideas for scientists. This two-way communication is integral in spawning the impetus for new research projects.

Examples of how applied research is used in improving athletic performance can be seen in the studies that have emanated from my laboratory and others I have worked at during my career. Different training paradigms for both in-season and off-season conditioning programs have been examined over the past few years. Examples of such studies include the investigation of linear and nonlinear periodization techniques in both in-season and off-season conditioning programs for football players, comparison of Olympic and traditional power lifting training programs in the off-season conditioning program of football players, and the effect of ballistic exercises (i.e., jump squats and bench press throws) on power development in strength/power athletes. In addition, examination of new training modalities, such as thick bars and resistive running on treadmills, has also been used to provide important information on exercise performance. Results of these studies have been used to format training programs in subsequent seasons. In addition, various nutritional supplements such as protein drinks, creatine and β-alanine combinations, and pre-exercise high-energy drinks have been examined in experienced strength trained athletes to determine the efficacy of these supplements in this population. The critical component attributing to the success of the research performed in my laboratory has been in the ability to rapidly delineate the results of these studies to the coaching staff and athletes. These lines of communication provide positive reinforcement for continued research and generate additional ideas for subsequent study. It also provides support for continued cooperation between coaches and applied scientists.

Reference

1. Hoffman JR, Maresh CM, Newton RU, et al. Performance, biochemical, and endocrine changes during a competitive football game. Med Sci Sports Exerc. 2002;34(11):1845–53.

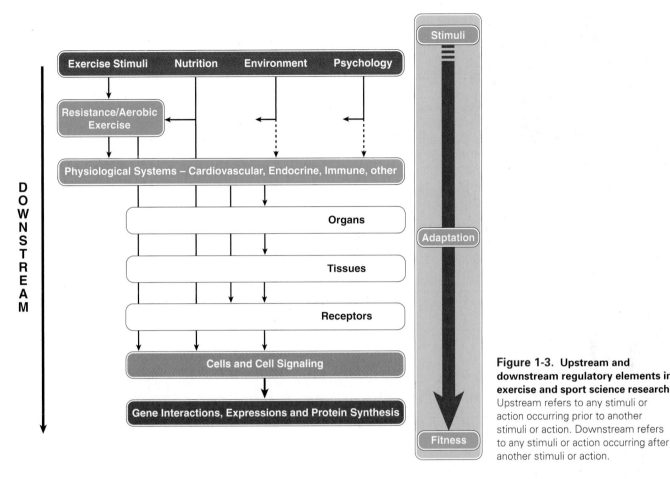

Figure 1-3. Upstream and downstream regulatory elements in exercise and sport science research. Upstream refers to any stimuli or action occurring prior to another stimuli or action. Downstream refers to any stimuli or action occurring after another stimuli or action.

program if the goal was to bring about cellular adaptations that result in improved 10-kilometer race times. Figure 1-3 overviews the basics of upstream and downstream regulatory elements in exercise and sport science research. The decisions made as to the type of exercise prescriptions that will be used in an acute exercise workout or training program will have an impact on the training outcome, such as improved performance and the physiological systems that adapt to result in improved performance. Thus, it is important that basic scientists understand applied research and vice versa.

Types of Research

In addition to the basic and applied designations discussed above, research can be further classified in several ways. First, research can be classified on the basis of the venue in which it is conducted, such as in the field or in the laboratory. Research can also be classified as being qualitative or quantitative in its approach, and various types of study designs can be used. In the quantitative approach to research, numerical data are collected to explain, predict, and/or show control of a phenomenon, and statistical analysis is used with deductive reasoning—reasoning from the general to the specific. It includes descriptive research, correlational research used to predict the relationship of variables,

cause-effect research, and experimental research. The qualitative approach to a study involves the collection of narrative-type data and is typically not used extensively in exercise science research but rather in the social sciences (e.g., to understand attitudes of male coaches toward women in the weight room). This approach requires analysis and coding of data for the production of verbal synthesis, which is an inductive reasoning process, reasoning from the specific to the general. Qualitative research studies are also referred to as ethnographic research, meaning that they are involved in the study of current events rather than past events. It involves the collection of extensive narrative data (nonnumerical data) on many variables over an extended period of time in a natural setting. Case studies that focus on a single subject population or interviews with a small group of individuals can also be used in qualitative research designs.

Some examples of qualitative studies are as follows:

1. A case study of parental involvement in after-school fitness programs
2. A multicase study of children who eat properly and are not obese, despite low income and living in an urban center
3. Examining the attitudes of men who are strength coaches toward women athletes

Another form of qualitative research is historical research, the study of past events. The following are a few examples of historical research:

1. Factors leading to Title IX legislation involving women and sport
2. The historical impact on racial equality in Division I basketball of the win by Texas Western's basketball team, coached by Don Haskins, who won the national title starting five black players for the first time in the national championship game
3. The contributions of Dr. Gary A. Dudley, a renowned researcher to the field of muscle physiology

Next, we will focus on the types of research most relevant to the exercise scientist: field and laboratory research, descriptive research, and experimental research.

Field and Laboratory Research

Research can be conducted in a variety of venues, from a highly controlled laboratory, such as a metabolic ward, to a field event, such as a wrestling match in a gymnasium. Laboratory research takes place in specific, controlled laboratory environments, where a potentially greater control of conditions is possible, whereas field research may take place in classrooms, gymnasiums, athletic fields, a space shuttle, at a marathon course, or under water. Often, people believe that field research is inferior to laboratory research, but in reality it all goes back to the ability to answer a question (Box 1-7). For example, it would be difficult to understand the physiological arousal just prior to walking out to center court in the finals of the U.S. Open tennis competition in a laboratory. Thus, whatever venue

Box 1-7 APPLYING RESEARCH

Quantifying and Qualifying Physical Activity Patterns in the Field Versus the Laboratory: A Challenge for Researchers

We are constantly hearing changing public health recommendations for the amount of moderate and vigorous physical activity required for health and fitness. Basic recommendations from the American College of Sports Medicine and the American Heart Association in 2007 were:

- Do moderately intense cardiovascular exercise 30 minutes a day, 5 days a week.

OR

- Do vigorously intense cardiovascular exercise 20 minutes a day, 3 days a week

AND

- Do 8 to 10 strength-training exercises, 8 to 12 repetitions for each exercise, twice a week.

Did you ever stop to think about how physical activity is quantified or qualified? Physical activity is any bodily movement produced by skeletal muscles that results in an expenditure of energy, which includes household, occupational, transportational, and leisure time activity. As you can imagine, this presents a challenge for researchers. To maximize control, physical activity and energy expenditure might best be measured in a metabolic ward, but considering feasibility, this may not be most appropriate for research, considering that it would be impossible for an individual to carry out the activities of daily living while confined to a metabolic ward. In addition, the expense and labor would further prohibit its feasibility.

Considering this, several other evaluation techniques have been developed and tested to measure physical activity. These techniques include direct observational rating scales, portable metabolic devices, doubly labeled water, self-reported physical activity logs, diaries and surveys, pedometers to measure

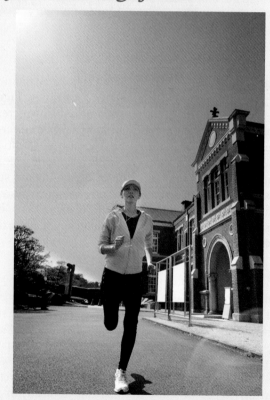

number of steps taken, accelerometers to quantify the intensity of vertical displacements, and heart rate monitoring techniques. Considering feasibility, reality, and control, which techniques would you consider to be most ideal to evaluate physical activity in different populations?

is needed to address the question is the appropriate setting for the experiment, and in any case, the conditions should be carefully noted. Experimental quality is not a function of the venue but rather of the experimental design and controls that are needed to answer a question. Thus, both field and laboratory research can play a very important role in advancing both basic and applied research.

Descriptive Research

Descriptive research is typically used to describe different phenomena without getting at the reasons for how and why something occurs. From the perspective of many scientists, this is not a very exciting type of research, as it does not give any insights into the mechanisms of action that mediate the phenomenon. Yet, it does have a place. For example, a type of descriptive research might be to characterize the performance and body composition profiles of NBA basketball players, Olympic marathon runners, or World Cup soccer players. Although such data may not explain how their bodies adapted to allow them to perform at such a high levels, the profile of characteristics may act to give some insights into the physical capabilities needed to perform at these levels. It might also give the scientist interested in basic mechanisms a clue as to what variables to examine to understand such performances. Descriptive research provides only a profile of a particular set of conditions (e.g., workout A versus workout B) or individuals (e.g., college versus high school basketball players), without any real insights into mechanisms of action that mediate the variables studied or give a cause and effect understanding. Some examples of descriptive research studies are as follows:

1. Body composition and size of the NFL Indianapolis Colts
2. Comparison of the physiological responses of level treadmill running with uphill treadmill running
3. The physiological responses to watching a college basketball game
4. The effects of 6 weeks of detraining on strength and power

Another form of descriptive research is **correlational research.** It is important to understand that correlation does not indicate causality. Thus, something can be correlated but have little to do with causal factors. A great example of this is the role of lactic acid and the changes in pH. Although lactic acid is predictive, it is not a causal factor in the reduction in pH with strenuous exercise.[7] Correlational research attempts to determine whether and to what degree a relationship exists between two or more quantifiable (numerical) variables. When two variables are correlated you can use the relationship to predict the value of one variable for a subject if you know that subject's value for the other variable. Correlation implies prediction but not causation. The investigator frequently uses a correlation coefficient to report the results of correlational research.

Some examples of descriptive correlational research are the following:

1. The relationship between weight training and self-esteem values in young athletes
2. The relationship between the resistance level on an elliptical trainer and heart rate response
3. The relationship between cortisol changes in the blood and anxiety prior to exercise

Experimental Research

The majority of studies in science are experimental in nature. Such research requires manipulation of the experimental variables in the hopes of understanding how something works. There are two major classes of variables in any experimental design. **Independent variables** are held constant and define the context and conditions of the experiment. Typical independent variables concern the population studied (age, sex, percent body fat) and study parameters (environmental temperature, altitude). **Dependent variables** are the measurements, such as oxygen consumption or strength, that will either respond or not respond to the experimental manipulations of the independent variables. Although both descriptive and experimental research designs have independent and dependent variables, experimental research attempts to use different independent variables to intentionally modulate the dependent variables to gain understanding of the cause and effect mechanisms at work. This type of research usually involves group comparisons. The groups in the study make up the values of the independent variable, for example, sex (male vs. female), age (young vs. old), or race (Caucasian vs. African American). Ultimately, the difference between descriptive and experimental research is that experimental research designs are used for the controlled testing of causality processes of a system or phenomenon. So, it is important to understand that it is not the measurements that determine whether the study is experimental or descriptive research but the design of the experiment, which determines the ability to gain an understanding of cause and effect. Below are some examples of cause-effect, experimental research studies:

1. The effect of branch amino acid supplement timing on protein synthesis.
2. The effect of time of day on growth hormone pulsatility.
3. The effect of hydration status on muscle force production.
4. The influence of heat on core temperature in walking versus running
5. The effect of microgravity on type II muscle fibers in rats
6. The effects of a low-carbohydrate diet on blood lipids

Quick Review

- The principles explaining physiological processes and guiding exercise prescriptions are based on facts and theories that must be considered in context, or the conditions under which the information was obtained.
- In exercise and sports science, there is a continuum of knowledge and research that spans from the basic to applied.
- Research can be classified as qualitative (which includes historical) and quantitative (which includes descriptive, correlational, cause-effect, and experimental).
- Descriptive research focuses on characterizing variables.
- Experimental research involves manipulating experimental variables to understand how something works.

THE SCIENTIFIC LITERATURE

The scientific literature is the accumulation of all published research from original investigations using the scientific method and reviews of these studies.[8] The scientific literature provides the factual basis and context for approaches and answers to questions. It does not contain answers to every question but, when skillfully used by professionals, can act as a basic compass to provide direction in addressing a problem, help to give insights into questions, help to explain many of the underlying mechanisms of action in exercise, and set a standard for optimal decision making for the many professions in exercise and sport science, as evidenced in the move toward evidence-based practices.

As our knowledge base expands, this increase in **evidence-based practice** will be seen in many professions, including exercise and sport science, to improve practice. Evidence-based practice is an approach in which the best evidence possible or the most appropriate information available is used to make decisions (Box 1-8).

Search Engines

With the proliferation of scientific information, search engines have become a critical tool in researching the scientific literature. A search engine is a set of computer programs that search for Web documents by key words or phrases. Today, a host of search engines such as Google, Bing, and Yahoo exist, which allow access to information databases. The problem with these programs is that they often list a multitude of Web sites or "hits," many of which are of questionable veracity. It is not uncommon for a personal trainer's fitness client to come to them with information from the Internet about exercise training and fitness programs, asking the personal trainer, "What about this program or that program? What is best?" So, from physicians to personal trainers, professionals are faced with the challenge of evaluating information coming at them each day, whether as a result of their own literature or information searches of others'.

Of more relevance to healthcare professionals, however, are two more specialized search engines. The most common search engine used in medical sciences is **PubMed** (Box 1-9). PubMed is a service of the U.S. National Library of Medicine that includes more than 17 million citations from MEDLINE and other life science and biomedical journals dating back to the 1950s, including exercise journals.

Box 1-8 PRACTICAL QUESTIONS FROM STUDENTS

What is Evidence-Based Practice?

Evidence-based practice is a process using the scientific facts to direct the conduct of professional practices in a field. The goal is for the reliable, precise, and well thought-out use of the field's best evidence in decision making. This process includes a number of steps. For example, an exercise prescription should be based on factual understanding of the exercise process. The process involves the formulation, clarification, and categorization of questions related to the exercise modality of interest (e.g., endurance training or weight training). One must search and gather information for the best available evidence on the topic, evaluate it, and then apply the information in the prescription process. The sources of such information are original research reports, comprehensive reviews, summaries, commentaries, systematic reviews, meta-analyses, and published guidelines.

For many areas in exercise science, this is a growing body of work. The major challenges to using this approach are related to the quality of the evidence available on the practice.

Further Readings

Brownson RC, Gurney JG, Land GH. Evidence-based decision making in public health. J Public Health Manag Pract. 1999;5(5):86–97.

Cavill N, Foster C, Oja P, et al. An evidence-based approach to physical activity promotion and policy development in Europe: contrasting case studies. Promot Educ. 2006;13(2):104–111.

O'Neall MA, Brownson RC. Teaching evidence-based public health to public health practitioners. Ann Epidemiol. 2005;15(7):540–544.

Shrier I. Stretching before exercise: an evidence based approach. British J. Sports Med. 2000;34:324–325.

Box 1-9 PRACTICAL QUESTIONS FROM STUDENTS

How Do You Do a PubMed Search?

Your university's library Web site should have a link to the PubMed database: http://www.ncbi.nlm.nih.gov/pubmed/

If you are unsure how to access it, ask your reference librarian. Many universities even offer workshops on how to use their reference databases. Often your library will have an online subscription to many of the journals in which you are interested, where you can directly access the pdf version of the article from a link in PubMed. The PubMed database provides the most up-to-date access to the literature in the scientific and medicine fields.

In PubMed there are many ways to conduct a search, such as by subject, by author, by date, and by publication type. Also, there are many options to limit a search to find exactly what you need.

Key Word Search

To conduct a basic search by key word, the first step is to identify the key concepts in your research question. For example, to find citations about responses to resistance training in children, you might enter the significant terms (resistance training and children) into the search box. Once you press the "search" button, a list of references related to your key words should appear for you to browse.

Author Search

It is also sometimes useful to search by an author's name. For example, if you were interested in a listing of all of the papers that Dr. William J. Kraemer published, you could enter the author's name in the format of last name followed by initials "Kraemer WJ" into the search box. A listing of papers that Dr. William J. Kraemer authored or coauthored will appear.

Boolean Operators

Boolean operators are used to combine concepts in your search. They are AND, OR, and NOT (Note: **CAPITALIZATION is REQUIRED**).

AND: Combines search terms so that each result contains *all* of the terms. AND is used to narrow searches.

Find: exercise AND children

(Finds records containing **both** terms *exercise* and *children*.)

Find: peptide F AND Kraemer WJ

(Finds records containing the subject *peptide F* and that are written by *W.J. Kraemer*.)

OR: Combines search terms so that each result contains at least one of the terms. OR is used to broaden searches. OR is very useful for grouping synonyms or variant spellings of a single concept.

Find: strength training OR resistance training

(Finds records containing **at least one** of the terms *strength training* or *resistance training*.)

NOT: Excludes terms so that each result will not contain the term that follows the not operator. NOT is used to focus searches.

Find: flexibility NOT passive stretching

(Finds records containing the term *flexibility* but **not** the term *passive stretching*.)

Limits: The limits option provides a way to further specify your search. With this tab, you are able to limit your search by publication type, language, age group, human or animal subjects, gender, and/or date of publication.

PubMed includes links to full text articles and other related resources. This is a free service and is provided at most college and universities' libraries. Another search engine, **SportDiscus**, is the world's leading database in sport, health, fitness, and sports medicine, and provides an even more focused research tool for those in these fields (Box 1-10).

Types of Studies

As has been developed in the above sections, a host of different types of studies can be found in the scientific literature. The most prominent manuscript making up the scientific literature is the **original investigation.** An original investigation uses the scientific method and generates new data based on hypothesis testing. This type of study in its many different forms is the basis of our knowledge, especially in biomedical and life sciences. While new research

data are presented in original investigations, other types of scientific publications contribute to the exercise and sport science literature. Scientific reviews that synthesize the existing literature on a topic can provide important new insights and conclusions based on the available original investigations. Such reviews can be done using statistical analysis of the literature (i.e., meta-analysis), evidence-based ranking of the literature, or opinion reviews. Case studies (e.g., examining the training protocol of an Olympic Gold Medalist) examining a specific situation that would not be possible to replicate in a group of subjects also provide insights. Symposium publications represent a series of papers that were presented at a scientific meeting allowing many more readers to benefit who were not in attendance. The key factor in these types of publications is that they are peer reviewed which most Internet commentaries and blogs are not.

Box 1-10　PRACTICAL QUESTIONS FROM STUDENTS

Is Finding an Article on PUBMED Easy?

Finding an article on PUBMED is actually very easy. See if you can find the article **Kraemer WJ, Patton JF, Gordon SE, et al. Compatibility of high-intensity strength and endurance training on hormonal and skeletal muscle adaptations. J Appl Physiol. 1995;78(3):976–989** on PUBMED.

1. Try your search by key words using key words from the abstract of article
2. Try limiting your search to:
   - humans
   - males
   - English
   - adult
3. Try your search by author name
4. Try using Boolean operators to combine your key words and author name

Abstract: Thirty-five healthy men were matched and randomly assigned to one of four training groups that performed high-intensity strength and endurance training (C; $n = 9$), upper body only high-intensity strength and endurance training (UC; $n = 9$), high-intensity endurance training (E; $n = 8$), or high-intensity strength training (ST; $n = 9$). The C and ST groups significantly increased one-repetition maximum strength for all exercises ($P < 0.05$). Only the C, UC, and E groups demonstrated significant increases in treadmill maximal oxygen consumption. The ST group showed significant increases in power output. Hormonal responses to treadmill exercise demonstrated a differential response to the different training programs, indicating that the underlying physiological milieu differed with the training program. Significant changes in muscle fiber areas were as follows: types I, IIa, and IIc increased in the ST group; types I and IIc decreased in the E group; type IIa increased in the C group; and there were no changes in the UC group. Significant shifts in percentage from type IIb to type IIa were observed in all training groups, with the greatest shift in the groups in which resistance trained the thigh musculature. This investigation indicates that the combination of strength and endurance training results in an attenuation of the performance improvements and physiological adaptations typical of single-mode training.

Peer-Review Process

After a scientist completes a study, it must be published for it to become a part of the body of knowledge (see Fig. 1-4). Each journal has it own set of author guidelines and format that must be adhered to when submitting a paper for publication, but it must involve the peer-review process. When an author submits a paper to a scientific journal, the editor or editor-in-chief sends it out to be rigorously reviewed by other scientists, or "peers," who are experts in that field. The reviewers' task is to read and examine the paper for any missing information, questions on data interpretation, and what are called fatal flaws in the experimental design or methods (e.g., no control group or improper measurement technique). They will make a recommendation to the editor as to whether the paper is worthy of publication. Each reviewer will either suggest accept, accept with revisions, or reject, based on analysis of the paper. The editor typically follows the reviewers' recommendations, and, if there is disagreement, meaning one reviewer suggests rejection whereas the other does not, a third reviewer is requested or the editor makes the final decision concerning whether to publish or not publish the article. Ultimately, it is the editor's responsibility to accept or reject a paper, and the reviewers just make recommendations.

The review process is done in either a **single-blind** or a **double-blind** fashion. In a single-blind review process, the reviewers know who the authors of the paper are but the authors do not know who is reviewing the paper. In the double-blind review process, neither party is known to the other. In more rare cases, some journals use an open review process, in which all parties know the identities of all others (Box 1-11). Arguments can be made in favor of each

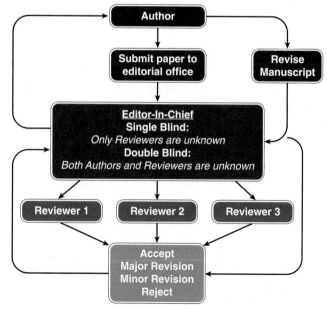

Figure 1-4. The peer-review process involves a series of steps to help insure the quality of published articles. Most articles go through one or two revisions before publication.

Box 1-11 PRACTICAL QUESTIONS FROM STUDENTS

What Do Reviewers Actually Look for When They Review an Article?

A reviewer will typically begin the review process by browsing the abstract of the article to get a general idea of what the paper is about, what type of paper it is, and how it compares to earlier research in the area.

Next, the reviewer will typically read the article with a critical eye focused primarily on understanding the rationale, logic, and science. The overall goal of the reviewer is to judge the *integrity* of the science. This judgment is made by examining the quality of the reasoning and by the applicability of the scientific principles and knowledge. Reviewers will also make an important judgment on the *novelty* of the idea and the contribution of the work to advancing the field. Essentially, an article with scientific integrity that presents new information to the field, without any inherent fatal flaws in the methodology, data, or conclusions, will have a chance of being published, as long as the selected journal is deemed appropriate for the topic of the study.

The reviewer will look for overall flaws in the scientific method, such as:

- Were there any contradictions in the paper?
- Did the author's conclusion fit the data? Or, was the conclusion unwarranted?
- Is it biologically plausible (does it seem possible based on some mechanism)?
- Were any inappropriate extrapolations made?

- Did the authors use circular reasoning?
- Did the research appear to be a pursuit of a trivial question?
- Were the statistical analyses appropriate?
- Was the presentation sound?
- Were there any redundancies, irrelevancies, or unnecessary excursions?
- Were terms adequately defined?
- Was the article written in a clear and focused manner?
- Was the logic behind the investigation explicit?
- Were methodological limitations addressed in the discussion?
- Does the discussion address all discrepancies or agreements between their results and those of other researchers?
- Are there misleading or inaccurate statements from citations?

The reviewer will then typically write up the blinded review, meaning that the authors will not know who wrote the review. The review will generally begin with major comments based on the overall rationale and design of the study. The reviewer will then offer more specific comments, line by line in the paper. If the reviewer determines that the paper is an important contribution to the literature and is scientifically sound, he or she will usually recommend a chance for revision. If it is determined that the paper is not worthy of publication, the reviewer will recommend it be rejected for publication.

---

process, but typically manuscripts are blinded to remove prejudice or conflict in the process.

Typical publication acceptance rates range from 10% to 40%, so all papers are not accepted and many manuscripts have to be resubmitted to other journals until a proper fit for the data is found. If experimental errors or fatal flaws exist, they will be exposed by the peer-review process, and the editor will not allow the paper to be published. The process of publication is a rigorous demand of the academic life for professors at universities or scientists working in industry or government. The process is also not perfect. This is evidenced by the fact that a Nobel Laureate once had a paper rejected by the journal *Science* and ultimately

published it in another journal, and it was that paper that won him the Nobel Prize.

Information Accuracy and Decision Making

Given the massive amount of information now available via the Internet and the variability of its quality, it is more important than ever to evaluate the accuracy and applicability of information when conducting research. From **anecdotal observation** (i.e., facts based on casual observations rather than rigorous scientific study) to controlled laboratory research, the ability to analyze information is critical to your approach and decision making in the exercise and sport science fields.

Information needed to make a decision should have several characteristics. It should be relevant to your question, accurate, timely, complete, and simple enough to be clearly interpreted. Below are a number of steps to follow when evaluating information to make decisions:

1. What are the goals of the program or needs of the individual?
2. From a needs analysis, what decisions have to be made?

Quick Review

- Scientific literature is the accumulation of published original investigations based on the scientific method.
- The peer-review process involves rigorous critique of the submitted manuscript by expert scientists in the field to determine whether the paper is suitable for publication.

Quick Review

- The evolution of the Internet has both increased the volume of information available and created a need for professionals to learn how to better evaluate the information.
- Techniques to evaluate the efficacy of information involve using fundamental principles and laws and evaluating the context of the information or data.

3. What information is needed to make a decision?
4. What is the minimal amount of information needed to make a decision?
5. How accurate is the information being provided and how specific is it to the situation to which it is to be applied?
6. What is its historical context and applicability to the current question or problem?
7. What is the most accurate information? Start with the most accurate information, in the form of principles and laws fundamental to the topic.

ANATOMY OF A STUDY

To read a study with some understanding, it is important to understand each section in a typical scientific manuscript. Each section of a study contains part of the story related to the scientific method, with the authors' interpretation of their data at the end of the paper.

Introduction

The primary purpose of the introduction is to develop the hypothesis that will be tested by the research design. This is done with a concise and logical review of the scientific literature that had led the authors to develop a specific hypothesis. The question and the problem that are being addressed by the investigation need to be clear and evident to the reader. The introduction can be a challenging part of the paper to write, as it sets up the entire project's context and importance. Support for a specific hypothesis should also be obvious to the reader. It is important that in this section the author addresses any potential criticisms and major debates that might surround the problem, hypothesis, methods, and/or question. This section ends with an obvious purpose statement of the study, if the author has been attentive to its development.

Methods

The methods section is important because it helps other scientists understand what was done and gives them the ability to replicate the study. It is also the section that gives the reader the context and conditions of the study. This is where the independent variables of the study that were held constant to set up the study design and the dependent variables measured are explained in detail. The methods section of a paper has very detailed and specific information as to the type of subjects, the specific types of equipment used, the order and explanations of the procedures used, and how the resulting data were analyzed statistically to test the hypothesis of the study. Furthermore, all studies need to include a notice that an Institutional Review Board or Ethics Committee approved the project, whether it is an animal or human study. In the case of human research, it is also important that it be noted that informed consent was obtained after the participants were informed of the potential risks and benefits of the investigation.

The methods section of the paper should explain the authors' approach to the problem, showing how their research design can test the hypothesis and answer the question posed in the introduction. This includes appropriate rationales for the selection of various independent variables and the dependent variables. Procedures must be described in such detail that someone could replicate the study. A methods section should take the reader through the study, giving a sense of the flow and order of the procedures. This section typically ends with the explanation and rationales for the statistical procedures that were used to analyze the data generated. Finally, the authors define the level of statistical significance, which is typically an alpha level of $P \leq 0.05$.

Results

As many scientists will tell you, if the design and methods of the study are strong, the results will carry the day and be the most important section of the article. The results section is where the paper comes alive. Here is where the findings are presented. As previously noted, it is becoming more and more evident that subjects may not all respond in a similar manner and, therefore, although it is important to show means and standard deviations, individual data for the responses of subjects are now being presented to give the reader a feel for the overall patterns of response for all of the subjects.

Discussion

The discussion section of the paper is where the investigators show the paper's importance, interpret the results, and relate it to the existing scientific literature. This gives the paper context and meaning. The discussion will answer the questions brought up in the introduction. It will also

Quick Review

- Publication of research is considered the end point of the scientific method.
- A manuscript contains sections (Introduction, Methods, Results, Discussion) that follow the scientific method.

address what new questions have been raised in the process of undertaking the study and what now needs to be done in future research.

EXTRACTING THE PRACTICAL APPLICATIONS

Ultimately, the practicing professional is interested in extracting the information from studies that might be of help to keep his or her decision-making process, methods, and techniques on the cutting edge of his or her profession. Keeping an open mind is vital in this process because new research can produce changes in one's approach to a problem. Thus, how we do our job is always a "work in progress," if we continue to read and apply the current research.

Understanding the Context of the Study

It is important to understand the context of a study to see how it applies to a particular situation. The context of the study is vital for interpretation of the results and their practical applications. For example, as a junior high school basketball coach, you might be interested in how to train your players to improve their vertical jump. A study that used junior high school basketball players and tested various training methods from plyometric training to weight training to a combination of these methods would be ideal to get a sense of what results one might expect in a group of players of this age. If in reading the literature you find that there are studies only on high school and college-age athletes, you may be faced with the challenge of interpreting the application of the findings to your junior high athletes. So, here is where it is important to understand the context of the study which is related to the independent and dependent variables.

Independent Variables

Recall that independent variables are those factors controlled or selected by the investigator to be held constant. These variables might be manipulated to see whether they alter the dependent variables' response and to gain an understanding of its impact (e.g., temperature, type of training program, gender). Interestingly, a variable that is not controlled in an experiment but has an independent effect is called a "confounding variable," as it muddies up the interpretation because of a lack of control or documentation. For example, you look at the impact of muscle soreness on 5-kilometer run time but find that temperature and humidity were not similar for all testing sessions. The results might be explained by the environmental conditions and not necessarily by the amount of muscle soreness. Thus, control and awareness of the influencing factors are always an important aspect of a scientific investigation. Ideally,

for the results of a study to be applied to a specific situation or group of people, the independent variables of the study should match the situation and population as closely as possible.

Typical independent variables include the following:

- Age
- Sex
- Training status
- Temperature
- Body mass
- Body fat
- Menstrual status
- Nutrient intakes
- Altitude

Dependent Variables

A dependent variable, also called "a response variable," is what is measured in response to the set of independent variables in the research project. Different from the independent variable, the dependent variable can typically not be controlled but acts as the outcome variable for the study. The **validity** and **reliability** of a variable is important. A measure has validity if it measures what it is supposed to measure. For example, palpation of the carotid artery in the neck to count the number of pulses that occur in a 1-minute time span, although not directly measuring heart contractility, is a valid measure to determine the beats per minute of the heart, or heart rate. This is because such a method has been experimentally validated with direct measures of heart rate. Reliability relates to how consistent a measurement is in repeat measurements. If you measure a 40-yard dash (36.7 meters) time on Monday and again on Wednesday, the numbers should be similar. In research terms, the variance should be no greater than about 5% between the two values for the measurement to be accurate. Interestingly, a valid measure must be reliable, but a reliable measure need not be valid.

A few examples of dependent variables are as follows:

- Time to run a 40-yard dash
- Core temperature
- Heart rate
- Oxygen consumption
- 1-repetition maximum strength
- Peak torque
- Power
- Concentration of lactate in the blood
- Cross-sectional area of a muscle fiber

Basic Direction for Choices and Action

Reading the research literature provides a basic direction for action. For example, should stretching be used as a warm-up activity prior to 100-meter sprint? In trying to answer this question, the first place to look is relevant articles in the scientific literature. In addition, books written by authorities in the field should be consulted. This results in a complete background on the topic, so an informed decision can be made. Ultimately, whatever information is used to make a decision should be timely, have the proper context, be valid, and be possible to implement from a practical perspective. This cycle of research and application fosters the professional and intellectual maturity needed for cutting-edge methodologies.

CASE STUDY

Scenario

You are trying to evaluate the efficacy of a dietary supplement you read about in a muscle magazine to help the men and women you train at the local health club, who range in age from 18 to 76 years. The article claims that this herbal supplement can dramatically improve strength. You look up the reference cited and read the research paper. This study examined the effects of the herbal supplement on a resistance training program performed by a Division I collegiate women's soccer team. Twenty women performed a periodized preseason resistance training program for 12 weeks. Each woman took the supplement before and after each workout. After 12 weeks, 1-repetition maximum (1 RM) for the bench and squat improved. The authors concluded that the supplement improved strength. Does the research support the claim of the advertisement for this supplement to improve strength?

Options

It is important to carefully read and critique the paper for the quality and efficacy of the experimental design and to ensure that the conclusions are supported by the results. The subjects are women, and thus the conclusions can be generalized to college-aged women. Can they be generalized to men or women of other ages? You question the experimental design of the study and its interpretation because there was no control group. How would this impact the conclusions in the paper? Specifically, with no control group, would it be possible to distinguish the specific contribution of the supplement from the training program? What about the use of a "placebo" to determine the influence of psychology in the strength improvements observed? These factors make the conclusion that the herbal supplement increases strength highly suspect.

Scenario

As a former college runner and exercise science major, your local running club has asked you to be involved with the club's Race Organization Committee. At the first meeting about the club's annual marathon race, concerns are expressed as to the potential for heat illness because the race is held in late May and it can be hot and humid despite the race being in St. Louis, Missouri. All of the needed measures are discussed consistent with the American College of Sports Medicine Position Stand on "Exertional Heat Illness." In addition, cold water/ice baths are available to use for those suspected of having heat exhaustion or heat stroke. One member of the committee states that to know whether or not a person should be dunked in a cold-water bath, a temperature measurement apart from an intestinal or rectal measure should be used. Several different temperature monitors are proposed. Upon hearing about this, you remember a study that questioned the use of many of these inexpensive devices to measure body temperature. You tell the committee that a real concern might exist and that some runners might have their temperature underestimated and thus treatment may well be missed with this type of triage method in general. What might you propose?

Options

You go back and carefully review the paper on the different methods of measurement used to assess body temperature. You confirm that in the 2009 article by Ganio et al., according to their methods, rectal, gastrointestinal, forehead, oral, aural, temporal, and axillary temperatures were measured with commonly used temperature devices. Temperature was measured before and 20 minutes after entering an environmental chamber, every 30 minutes during a 90-minute treadmill walk in the heat, and every 20 minutes during a 60-minute rest in mild environmental conditions. The authors stated that the validity and reliability of a device were assessed with various statistical measures to compare the measurements using each device compared with rectal temperature. A device was considered invalid if the mean bias (average difference between rectal and device temperatures) was more than ±0.27°C (±0.50°F). The tested devices showed the following results: forehead sticker (0.29°C [0.52°F]), oral temperature using an inexpensive device (−1.13°C [−2.03°F]), temporal temperature measured according to the instruction manual (−0.87°C [−1.56°F]), temporal temperature using a modified technique (−0.63°C [−1.13°F]), oral temperature using an expensive device (−0.86°C [−1.55°F]), aural temperature (−0.67°C [−1.20°F]), axillary temperature using an inexpensive device (−1.25°C [−2.24°F]), and axillary temperature using an expensive device (−0.94°C [−1.70°F]). Measurement of intestinal temperature had a mean bias of −0.02°C (−0.03°F). From these data, what might you suggest to the race committee for use as a temperature monitor? What device might be considered valid for such a use as part of a race safety program?

Quick Review

- Research is progressive because new findings constantly change the way things are done in a particular area of exercise and sport science.
- The ability to interpret and evaluate research in context is critical to understanding and applying the findings.
- Independent variables in research are the variables that are controlled by the investigator.
- Dependent variables in research are the outcome variables of the study.

A Continuum of Possibilities

With the multitude of possible independent variables, all studies are dependent on their context. This is what leads the lay public to be confused when new studies come out that seem to contradict what was thought to be true. In fact, studies that contradict each other may both be true under different circumstances, meaning under different sets of independent variables. Thus, a continuum of possibilities exists in the interpretation of research.

It is also important to keep in mind what qualifies an individual as a scientist. Think about it: Would you consider an individual who studies science and extensively reads scientific publications a true scientist? Or, would you consider a scientist to be an individual with an expert knowledge of science who continually performs research by applying the scientific method to answer new research questions and advance the field beyond what we already know? Many would consider the performance of research an important characteristic of a true scientist. As this chapter has emphasized, experimentation and dissemination of research findings are critical components of the scientific method. Thus, true scientists actually produce science, theories, and hypotheses leading to scientific facts and principles.

CHAPTER SUMMARY

Research plays an important role in advancing any profession. Paradigms of practice are developed with the use of scientific laws, principles, theories, and concepts derived from research. Beyond laws, the interpretation and development of principles, theories, and concepts are all subject to change, as new studies are published constantly. Research increases our understanding of a topic and results in practices that are based on the scientific method. Practitioners in exercise and sport science can use research to stay on the cutting edge of knowledge and advance their practice. Understanding research also allows appreciation of the impressive amount of knowledge that does exist in exercise and sport science, which will be discussed in the many chapters that follow.

REVIEW QUESTIONS

Fill-in-the-Blank

1. When interpreting facts, theories, and principles, it is important to consider the _____, or the conditions under which the observations were made.

2. In exercise and sports science, _____ should be used to make decisions based on the most appropriate information available.

3. _____ are facts based on observations rather than scientific research.

4. _____ variables are variables that are set constant and are defined as the conditions of the study, whereas _____ variables are the measures made.

5. _____ of a measure evaluates how well it measures what it is supposed to measure, whereas _____ evaluates how consistent a measure is from time to time.

Multiple Choice

1. What process seeks to reevaluate hypotheses, concepts, and principles?
   a. Scientific process
   b. Iterative process
   c. Peer-review process
   d. Correlational process
   e. Quantitative process

2. Which of the following is the best example of a qualitative research design?
   a. Body composition and size of NFL players
   b. The effects of training on endurance running performance
   c. Examining women athletes' attitudes toward male coaches
   d. The effects of 6 weeks of training on muscle strength
   e. The relationship between muscle size and strength

3. For research to become part of the scientific literature, it must ____.
   a. pass the peer-review process
   b. be accepted by the editor of the journal
   c. be free of fatal flaws
   d. be considered a proper fit for the specific journal
   e. all of the above

4. Which of the following statements is true regarding dependent variables?
   a. Dependent variables are controlled by the investigators.
   b. Dependent variables are altered to see how they affect independent variables.
   c. Dependent variables are also called confounding variables.
   d. Dependent variables are held constant in the study.
   e. Dependent variables are the outcome variables of the study.

5. Which of the following is the best example of a dependent variable in a study evaluating the responses to a training program?
   a. Sex
   b. Age
   c. Environmental temperature
   d. 1-repetition maximum strength
   e. Altitude

True/False

1. It is possible to conduct a perfect study.
2. Bias always leads to wrong answers to a question.
3. In a double-blind review the authors know who the reviewers are.
4. In the peer-review process, it is the responsibility of the reviewers to accept or reject the paper, whereas the editor offers recommendations for acceptance or rejection.
5. In a scientific manuscript, the introduction section should contain a clear statement of the purpose of the investigation.

Short Answer or Matching

1. Explain whether basic or applied research is more important in exercise and sports science.
2. Explain how the empirical method has efficacy in the scientific method but can also be used as an unscientific method.
3. Explain the purpose of the discussion section of a scientific manuscript, and specify what information it should contain.
4. Match the following terms with their correct definitions (currently mismatched).

| Theory | Observational data that are confirmed repeatedly by many independent and competent observers |

Hypothesis	A conceptual framework of ideas or speculations regarding a certain topic which may or may not be based on experimental facts
Fact	An explanation of a physiological process, or guidelines that should be adhered to for optimal performance of a task
Principle	An educated guess as to what might be expected to happen

5. Match the following terms with their correct definitions (currently mismatched).

Authority	The ability to know something without any reasoning
Trial and error	Answering a question based on what has always been done
Tradition	Trying an action to see whether it elicits the desired outcome
Intuition	A preference that can inhibit impartial answers to questions
Bias	Person answering a question based on qualifications, and/or historical relevance

KEY TERMS

anecdotal observation: facts based on casual observations rather than rigorous scientific study
body of knowledge: the sum of published studies on a topic
dependent variables: measures made during a research project
descriptive research: research examining a topic but not the reasons for how and why something occurs
double-blind review: a peer-review process in which the authors do not know who the reviewers are and the reviewers do not know who the authors are
evidence-based practice: an approach in which the best evidence possible, or the most appropriate information available, is used to make decisions
facts: observational data that are confirmed repeatedly and by many independent and competent observers
hypotheses: best guesses as to the answer to a question based on existing knowledge
independent variables: variables that are constant and defined as the conditions of the study
original investigation: a new research project using the scientific method that generates new data based on hypothesis testing
peer-reviewed study: published research project that goes through the peer-review process
principles: facts derived from theories that are not likely to change
PubMed: a search engine used in medical sciences that is a service of the U.S. National Library of Medicine and includes more than 17 million citations from life science and biomedical journals, including exercise science journals
reliability: the ability of test results to produce consistency of a measurement at different times

scientific method: an organized set of steps to test hypotheses and answer research questions used to develop the body of knowledge in the scientific literature

single-blind review: a peer-review process in which the authors of the paper do not know who the reviewers are but the reviewers do know who the authors are

SportDiscus: a database search engine of sport, health, fitness, and sports medicine journals

validity: ability of a test to measure what it purports to measure

theory: a conceptual framework of ideas or speculations regarding a certain topic, ideally, based on experimental facts

REFERENCES

1. Baumgartner TA, Strong CH. Conducting and Reading Research in Health and Human Performance. Dubuque, IA: Wm, C. Brown & Benchmark, 1994.
2. Berg KE, Latin RW. Essentials of Research Methods in Health, Physical Education, Exercise Science and Recreation. 2nd ed. Baltimore, MD: Lippincott Williams & Wilkins, 2004.
3. Ganio MS, Brown CM, Casa DJ, et al. Validity and reliability of devices that assess body temperature during indoor exercise in the heat. J Athl Train. 2009;44(2):124–135.
4. McNeil DA, Flynn MA. Methods of defining best practice for population health approaches with obesity prevention as an example. Proc Nutr Soc. 2006;65(4):403–411.
5. Pescatello LS, Franklin BA, Fagard R, et al. American College of Sports Medicine position stand. Exercise and hypertension. Med Sci Sports Exerc. 2004;36:533–553.
6. Pescatello LS, Franklin BA, Fagard R, et al. American College of Sports Medicine. American College of Sports Medicine position stand. Exercise and hypertension. Med Sci Sports Exerc. 2004;36(3):533–553.
7. Robergs RA, Ghiasvand F, Parker D. Biochemistry of exercise-induced metabolic acidosis. Am J Physiol Regul Integr Comp Physiol. 2004;287:R502–516.
8. Volek JS, Rawson ES. Scientific basis and practical aspects of creatine supplementation for athletes. Nutrition. 2004;20:609–614.

Suggested Readings

Dudley GA, Fleck SJ. Research—reading and understanding: the results section: major concepts and compounds. National Strength Coaches Association Journal 1982;4(5):22–22.

Kraemer WJ. Research—Reading and understanding the starter steps. Natl Strength Coaches Assoc J. 1982;4(3):49–49.

Sifft JM. Research—reading and understanding: guidelines for selecting a sample. Natl Strength Cond Assoc J. 1984;6(1):26–27.

Sifft JM. Research—reading and understanding: statistics for sport performance–basic inferential analysis. Natl Strength Cond Assoc J. 1986;8(6):46–48.

Sifft JM. Research—reading and understanding #4: statistics for sport performance—basic inferential analysis. Natl Strength Cond Assoc J. 1990;12(6):70–70.

Sifft JM. Research—reading and understanding: utilizing descriptive statistics in sport performance. Natl Strength Cond Assoc J. 1983;5(5):26–28.

Sifft JM. Research—reading and understanding #2: utilizing descriptive statistics in sport performance. Natl Strength Cond Assoc J. 1990;12(3):38–41.

Sifft JM, Kraemer WJ. Research—reading and understanding: introduction, review of literature and methods. Natl Strength Coaches Assoc J. 1982;4(4):24–25.

Starck A, Fleck S. Research—reading and Understanding: the discussion section. Natl Strength Coaches Assoc J. 1982;4(6):40–41.

Tipton CM. Publishing in peer-reviewed journals. Fundamentals for new investigators. Physiologist. 1991;34(5):275, 278–279.

Classic Reference

Cohen J. Statistical Power Analysis for the Behavioral Sciences. 2nd ed. Hillsdale, NJ: Lawrence Erlbaum Associates Publisher Inc, 1988.

2

Bioenergetics and Meeting the Metabolic Demand for Energy

After reading this chapter, you should be able to:

1. Determine which metabolic substrates predominate during periods of rest and exercise

2. Understand the production of energy from the adenosine triphosphate-phosphocreatine system, glycolysis, and aerobic systems

3. Explain adaptations of each energy system that accompany training

4. Determine which energy substrates predominate during different exercise protocols

5. Understand how anaerobic and aerobic metabolism interact during exercise

6. Differentiate between indirect and direct techniques of calorimetry

7. Explain the aerobic and anaerobic adaptations to exercise

8. Explain the metabolic role of recovery

Whether you are sleeping, awake but sedentary, or performing physical activity, energy is needed to maintain your bodily functions. In addition, when performing physical activity, energy is needed by your muscles to generate force and create bodily movement. The plant and animal products eaten as food are the fuel that provides the human body with energy. The chemical process of converting food into energy is termed **bioenergetics,** or **metabolism.** This process is similar in some ways to the burning of wood. Oxygen is needed for the burning of wood and for the conversion of food into useful energy by the human body. During both of these processes, chemical bonds are broken and energy is released. When wood burns, energy is released in the form of heat and light; steam or water, carbon dioxide (CO_2), and ash are produced. When food is metabolized, heat, energy, water, and CO_2 are also produced.

A thorough understanding of bioenergetics is necessary to understand how the human body meets its energy needs at rest and during physical activity, why some foods are preferentially used in metabolism during various physical tasks, and what some of the causes of fatigue are during a physical task. In addition, an understanding of bioenergetics is necessary for a complete understanding of long-term body weight control and why it is possible to gain body fat by eating too much of any type of food. The purpose of this chapter is to introduce basic and specific concepts related to bioenergetics and how bioenergetics affects physical performance.

...imate source of all energy on
...ess of photosynthesis utilize
...mical reactions that produce
...of simple sugars. Human be-
...s and other animals to obtain
...d to maintain bodily functions.
Energy exists in several forms, including chemical, electrical, heat, and mechanical, and one form of energy can be converted to another form of energy. If it were not possible to convert one form of energy to another, the conversion of food into useful bodily energy could not take place. For example, through the use of metabolic pathways, cells within the body convert chemical energy in the form of chemical bonds in fat, carbohydrate, and protein into mechanical energy, resulting in muscle contraction and bodily movement.

Before discussing metabolism, it is important to know some information about the organic substances you can metabolize. It is also important to understand why enzymes are necessary to obtain that energy, via aerobic or anaerobic mechanisms, function in the body.

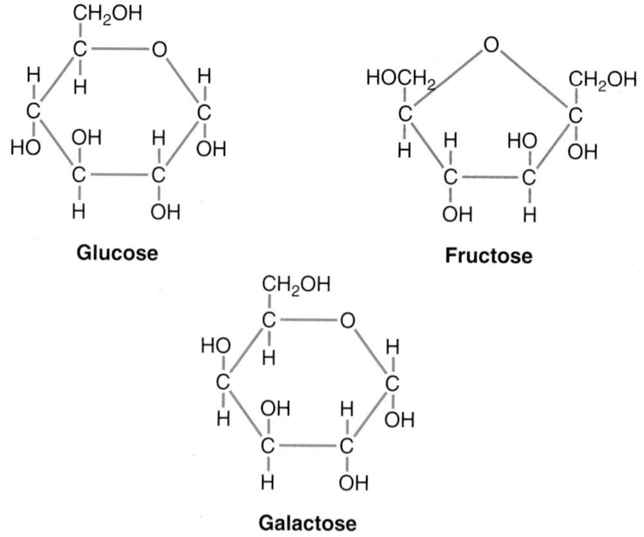

Carbohydrates

Carbohydrates stored within the body provide a rapid and readily available source of energy. These carbohydrates are found in three forms: monosaccharides, disaccharides, and polysaccharides. Monosaccharides are simple sugars such as glucose, fructose (fruit sugar), and galactose (milk sugar). All simple sugars contain six carbon molecules in a ring structure (Fig. 2-1). For metabolic purposes, glucose is the most important simple sugar and is the only form of carbohydrate that can be directly metabolized to obtain energy. Although the digestive tract can absorb monosaccharides after absorption, other simple sugars are converted by the liver into glucose. The term "blood sugar" refers to glucose.

Disaccharides are made up of two monosaccharides. For example, two glucose molecules can combine to form maltose, or glucose and fructose can combine to form

Figure 2-1. **Monosaccharides are composed of 6 carbon, 12 hydrogen, and 6 oxygen atoms in a six-carbon ring structure in different arrangements.** The monosaccharides glucose, fructose, and galactose are shown. Note the differences in the arrangement of the atoms of these monosaccharides. Each carbon molecule must have a total of four chemical bonds.

sucrose (table sugar) (Fig. 2-2). Although disaccharides are consumed in the foods we eat, they must be broken down into monosaccharides in the digestive tract before being absorbed into the bloodstream.

Polysaccharides are complex carbohydrates made up of three to many hundreds of monosaccharides. Two of the most common plant polysaccharides are starch and cellulose. Starch, which is found in grains and many other common plant foods, is digestible by humans, whereas cellulose is not digestible by humans and makes up part of the dietary fiber that is excreted as fecal matter. Because it is digestible, starch is absorbed by the digestive tract in the form of monosaccharides and can be used immediately for energy or stored in the form of glycogen.

Glycogen is not found in plants and is the polysaccharide form in which animals store carbohydrate. Glycogen is

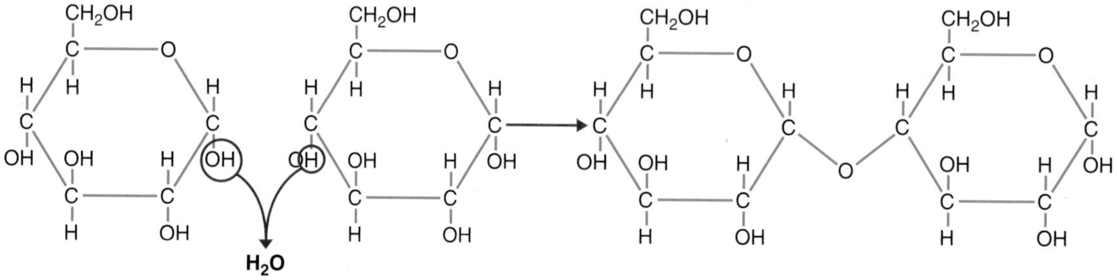

Figure 2-2. **The production of the disaccharide maltose from two glucose molecules is depicted.** This reaction is termed a *condensation reaction* because a water molecule is produced. This reaction can also take place in reverse, producing two glucose molecules. In the latter case, the reaction is a hydrolysis reaction because a water molecule is needed.

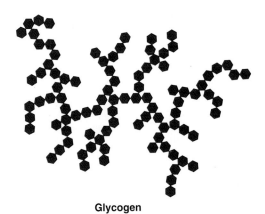

Glycogen

Figure 2-3. Glycogen is composed of the monosaccharide glucose bound together in long, highly branched chains. Each of the *red ring structures* (⬢) represents a glucose molecule.

composed of hundreds to thousands of glucose molecules bound together (Fig. 2-3). As mentioned earlier, after absorption by the digestive tract, all simple sugars are converted by the liver into glucose. The glucose can be released into the bloodstream as blood sugar, or glucose molecules can be combined within the liver or muscle tissue to form glycogen in a process termed **glycogenesis.** Cells within the body can metabolize the glucose released into the bloodstream or use it for glycogenesis and store the glycogen for later metabolic needs. During exercise, glucose molecules can be removed from glycogen in the liver, in a process called **glycogenolysis,** and released into the bloodstream to provide glucose as a metabolic substrate to other cells of the body.

Glucose and glycogen are the carbohydrates important for metabolism at rest and during exercise. During exercise, muscle cells can obtain glucose by absorbing it from the bloodstream or by glycogenolysis from intramuscular glycogen stores. In addition, glycogenolysis in the liver can maintain blood glucose levels during exercise and at times of rest between meals. However, there are relatively small amounts of glycogen stored within the liver and other cells of the body compared to skeletal muscle stores.

Fats

Fats found in the form of triglycerides are quite plentiful within the body and can be metabolized for energy production. Fats are contained in both plant and animal tissues. The two fats important for metabolism are fatty acids and triglycerides.

A **fatty acid** contains an even number of 4 to 24 carbon atoms bound together in a chain (Fig. 2-4). Fatty acids have an acidic group (COOH) and a methyl group (CH₃) at opposite

ends of the carbon chain. Fatty acids can be classified as saturated, unsaturated, monounsaturated, or polyunsaturated. Fats are saturated or unsaturated, and unsaturated fats can be further categorized as monounsaturated or polyunsaturated. A **saturated fatty acid** is a fatty acid containing the maximal number of hydrogen atoms and no double bonds. (see Fig. 2-4), whereas an **unsaturated fatty acid** does not contain the maximal number of hydrogen atoms and has at least one double bond between carbon molecules (Fig. 2-5). **Monounsaturated** and **polyunsaturated** fatty acids contain at least one and more than one, respectively, double bonds between carbon molecules and thus do not contain the maximal number of hydrogen atoms. Monounsaturated and polyunsaturated fatty acids compose a relatively large amount of the fats contained within vegetable oils, such as olive oil; numerous health benefits such as lowering total blood cholesterol, blood pressure, and blood clotting factors[45] have been attributed to these types of fatty acids within the diet.

Within the body, fatty acids are stored as triglycerides. A **triglyceride** is composed of a glycerol molecule plus three attached fatty acids (Fig. 2-6). Triglycerides are stored primarily in fat cells but can also be stored in other types of tissue, such as skeletal muscle. If needed for energy, triglycerides are broken apart into their component fatty acids and glycerol molecule, a process known as **lipolysis.** The fatty acids can then be metabolized to release usable energy. Glycerol cannot be metabolized by skeletal muscle directly; however, the liver can use glycerol to synthesize glucose, which can then be metabolized to provide energy. Fat stores are quite abundant, even in very lean individuals. Therefore, depletion of fat as an energy source during physical activity, even during long-term endurance events, does not occur, precluding fat depletion as a cause of fatigue.

Protein

Protein can be found in both animals and plants. Amino acids are the molecules that compose all proteins. The basic structure of all amino acids is similar, consisting of a central carbon molecule that has bonds with a hydrogen molecule, an amino group (NH₂), an acid group (COOH), and a side chain unique to each particular amino acid (Fig. 2-7). It is the side chain that distinguishes the approximately 20 amino acids from each other. **Essential amino acids** are those nine that must be ingested in the foods that we eat because they cannot be synthesized by the human body. **Nonessential amino acids,** which make up more than half of the amino acids, are those that the body can synthesize. Typically, only a small amount of protein or amino acids are metabolized to provide energy, largely due to nitrogen, which is not found in fat or carbohydrate.

Figure 2-4. Eighteen-carbon fatty acids are very common in the foods we eat. Stearic acid is the simplest of the 18-carbon fatty acids and is a saturated fatty acid.

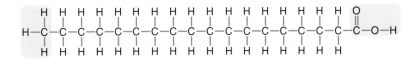

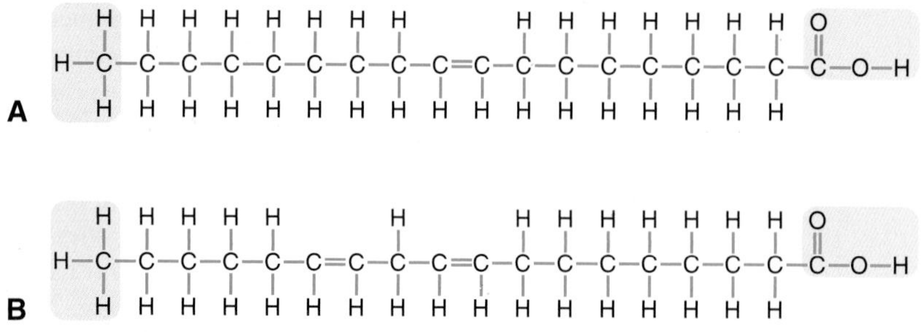

Figure 2-5. **Two 18-carbon unsaturated fatty acids are shown. (A)** Oleic acid is an 18-carbon monounsaturated fatty acid. **(B)** Linoleic acid is an 18-carbon polyunsaturated fatty acid.

Role of Enzymes

Enzymes are protein molecules that facilitate a chemical reaction, including metabolic ones, by lowering the energy needed for the reaction to take place. Although reactions can occur without an enzyme if there is sufficient energy, the enzyme lowers the energy necessary for the reaction to take place—which is termed the **energy of activation.** Note that the enzyme does not cause the reaction to take place but facilitates and increases the speed at which it takes place and, therefore, increases the rate at which the products resulting from the chemical reaction are produced.

Similar to all molecules, an enzyme has a unique, three-dimensional shape. The unique shape allows the molecule(s) or substrate(s) involved in the chemical reaction to adhere to the enzyme, in a fashion similar to a lock and its key (Fig. 2-8). The substrates fit into the indentations of an enzyme, forming an enzyme-substrate complex, which lowers the energy of activation so that the reaction can take place at a faster rate. After the reaction is completed, the product of the reaction disassociates from the enzyme.

Some enzymes can participate in either a **catabolic reaction,** in which a substrate is broken apart into two product molecules thus releasing energy, or an **anabolic reaction,** in which one product molecule is formed from two substrate molecules, which requires energy. The type of reaction that occurs depends on many physiological factors.

One major factor is what is termed the **mass action effect.** According to the mass action effect, if an enzyme regulates the production of a product molecule AB from the substrates A and B, the reaction can produce either AB or A and B, as shown in the equation below. The direction in which the reaction proceeds depends on whether there is more AB or A and B present. If there is more AB present, then the reaction will move in the direction to produce A and B; whereas, if there is more A and B present, the reaction will move in the direction to produce AB. The arrows pointing in both directions in the equation below indicate that the enzyme can facilitate the reaction to produce either AB or A and B.

$$AB \leftrightarrow A + B$$

The names of many enzymes end with the suffix "-ase" and give some indication of the chemical reaction they facilitate. For example, another term for fat is lipid, and lipase enzymes break triglycerides into glycerol and fatty acids so they can enter cells.

Several factors can affect the speed with which enzymes facilitate their respective reactions. Two very important factors during physical activity are temperature and acidity. The activity of an enzyme has an optimal temperature at which it facilitates chemical reactions. A slight increase in temperature generally increases the speed with which an enzyme facilitates its reactions. Thus, during physical

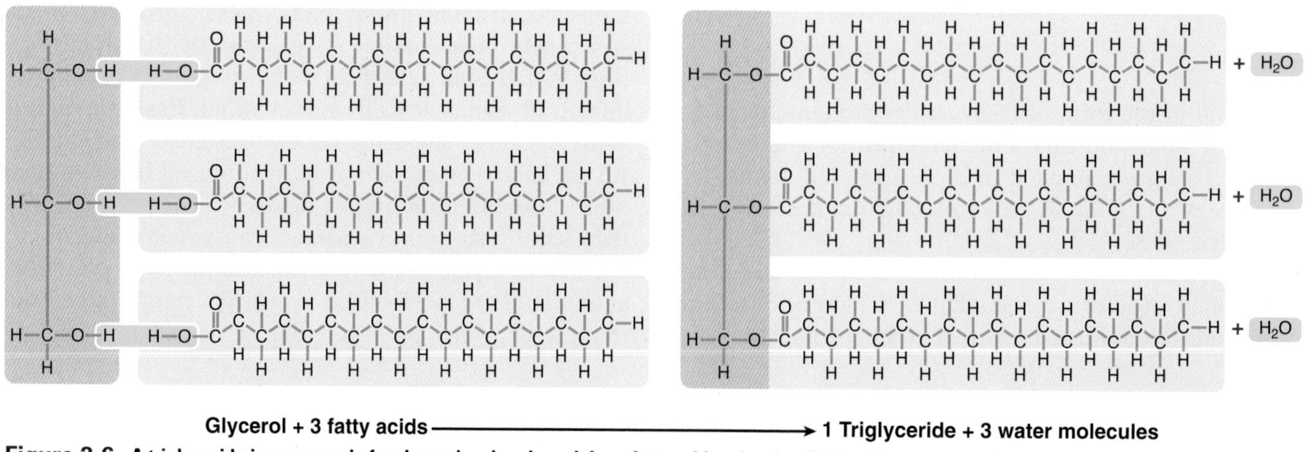

Glycerol + 3 fatty acids ⟶ 1 Triglyceride + 3 water molecules

Figure 2-6. A triglyceride is composed of a glycerol molecule and three fatty acid molecules. Triglycerides can be made during condensation reactions, yielding three water molecules. The depicted triglyceride is composed of a glycerol molecule and three stearic fatty acids, which are 18-carbon saturated fatty acids.

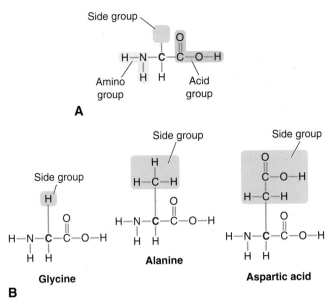

A

B

Glycine   Alanine   Aspartic acid

Figure 2-7. All amino acids have the same basic structure. (A) The basic structure of all amino acids is a central carbon molecule, an amino group, an acid group, and a unique side group. **(B)** Three amino acids are depicted with their unique side groups.

activity, the slight increase in body temperature generally increases the activity of enzymes involved in energy production, leading to a slight increase in the production of useful energy. Similarly, individual enzymes have an optimal pH or level of acidity at which they facilitate their respective reactions. During physical activity, intramuscular acidity can increase, meaning a decrease in pH occurs. The increase in acidity, especially if severe, decreases the activity

of some enzymes involved in bioenergetics. This slowing in enzymatic activity is one factor resulting in fatigue during some forms of physical activity.

Another factor related to enzymatic function is the need for coenzymes. Coenzymes are complex organic molecules, but not proteins, that associate closely with an enzyme. If an enzyme is dependent on a coenzyme, the enzyme will not function optimally without adequate amounts of that coenzyme. For example, the B vitamins serve as coenzymes for many of the enzymes involved in metabolism of carbohydrates, fatty acids, and amino acids. If the coenzymes are not present, energy metabolism ceases, and if there is an inadequate availability of those vitamins, the rate at which the metabolic reaction occurs will decline. Thus, both coenzymes and enzymes are necessary for bioenergetic mechanisms to take place.

AEROBIC AND ANAEROBIC METABOLISM

You are probably familiar with the term *aerobics* referring to the use of oxygen to obtain energy to perform an endurance type of activity. Similarly, **aerobic metabolism** refers to the use of oxygen to metabolize food. The products generated by aerobic metabolism are energy, CO_2, and water. The energy can be used to support bodily functions, the CO_2 can be transported in the blood and expired at the lungs, and the water molecules can be used by the body like any other water molecules. Thus, all products produced by aerobic metabolism can be readily used or expelled. Because of these factors, aerobic metabolism is used at rest and during long-duration, lower intensity physical activity to supply the vast majority of the needed energy. Although we typically think of aerobic metabolism as involving carbohydrate and triglyceride, protein can also be aerobically metabolized to supply energy if needed.

Anaerobic metabolism refers to producing energy without the use of oxygen. Only carbohydrate can be used to produce energy anaerobically. On the downside, anaerobic metabolism of carbohydrate results in the production

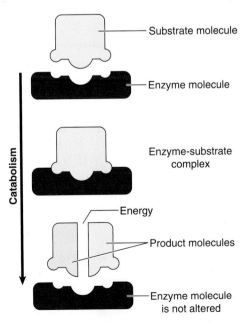

Figure 2-8. The lock-and-key concept helps to describe how enzymes facilitate catabolic and anabolic reactions. A catabolic reaction is depicted. However, many enzymes can also perform an anabolic reaction involving the products produced by the catabolic reaction to produce the substrates used in the catabolic reaction.

Quick Review

- Aerobic metabolism requires oxygen to produce energy and is the predominant energy source at rest and during low-intensity activity.
- Anaerobic metabolism does not need oxygen to produce energy and is used predominantly for short-duration, high-intensity activity.

Quick Review

- Adenosine triphosphate is the most important energy molecule produced, whether a metabolic process is aerobic or anaerobic.

of not only energy and CO_2, but also lactic acid, which is associated with an increase in blood and intramuscular acidity. An increase in acidity negatively affects the activity of some enzymes, which results in a decreased production of useful energy. If less useful energy is available, the intensity, speed, or pace at which the activity is being performed must decrease. Increased acidity also affects pain receptors within muscle. Both of these factors can result in an inability to maintain the intensity or speed at which an activity is being performed. The main advantage of anaerobic metabolism is that the energy it yields is made available quickly to the exercising muscle.

Energy from anaerobic metabolism of carbohydrate, along with that provided by the phosphagen system (ATP and PC), are the major energy sources during high-intensity, short-duration activity, such as sprinting and weight lifting. In contrast, aerobic metabolism is the predominant energy source for longer-duration, lower-intensity activity, such as road cycling or distance running.

ATP: THE ENERGY MOLECULE

Adenosine triphosphate (ATP) is not the only energy molecule in cells, but it is the most important one. Whether useful energy is produced anaerobically or aerobically, the energy molecule ATP is the result. ATP's molecular structure has three major components: adenine, ribose, and three phosphates (Fig. 2-9). The adenine and ribose mol-

ecules are also termed an *adenosine molecule*. ATP can be produced from **adenosine diphosphate** (ADP), inorganic phosphate (Pi), and a hydrogen ion (H^+) (Fig. 2-10). The energy needed to bond ADP to Pi can be obtained from either an anaerobic or aerobic reaction. ATP can then be broken down into ADP and Pi, releasing energy that can be used for processes in the cell, such as various muscle actions. The molecules ADP, ATP, and Pi are not destroyed during these reactions; rather, chemical bonds holding the phosphate groups together are broken to release energy, or energy is added to re-form the bond adhering the Pi to the remaining phosphate groups on the adenosine molecule, thus re-forming ATP. The production of a hydrogen ion when ATP is broken down is important because an increase in hydrogen ions results in an increase in acidity. The need for a hydrogen ion when ADP and Pi combine to produce ATP is also important because it results in a decrease in acidity. Thus, if more ATP is used than produced, there is an increase in intramuscular acidity, whereas if ATP use is balanced by an equivalent production of ATP, there is no change in intramuscular acidity. The following sections are a detailed discussion of the anaerobic and aerobic metabolic pathways resulting in the formation of ATP.

ATP-PC SYSTEM

The ATP-phosphocreatine (PC) energy system is important as an energy source for physical activities that require a lot of energy per second, such as sprinting or lifting a heavy weight. However, this energy source can only provide energy for a relatively short period of time. For example, if you start to jump vertically as high and as fast as possible you will notice in 10–15 seconds that you are not jumping nearly as high as in the first few jumps. This is in part because of the characteristics and limitations of the ATP-PC energy source. Understanding the ATP-PC

Adenine   +   Ribose   +   3 Phosphates

Figure 2-9. Adenosine triphosphate is composed of an adenine, ribose, and three inorganic phosphate groups. The wavy lines between the phosphate groups indicate a high-energy bond.

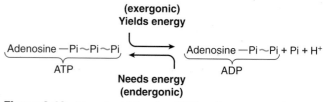

Figure 2-10. Adenosine triphosphate (ATP) produces energy when it is broken down into adenosine diphosphate (ADP) and an inorganic phosphate (Pi). ATP can be produced by combining ADP and a Pi, but this reaction requires energy.

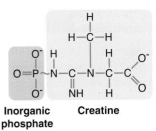

Figure 2-11. Phosphocreatine is composed of creatine and an inorganic phosphate. The wavy line between the creatine and the inorganic phosphate represents a high-energy bond.

energy source allows an understanding of performance in high-intensity, short-duration physical activity.

The intracellular ATP content of cells, including muscle cells, is relatively small. Thus, during physical activity, ATP concentrations within muscle cells decrease quite quickly, and if ATP levels were not rapidly replenished by energy coming from the various metabolic cycles there would be a concomitant decline in muscle force production. Intramuscular **phosphocreatine** (PC) (Fig. 2-11) provides a simple and thus rapid bioenergetic pathway to produce ATP. Within muscle cells, the enzyme ATPase facilitates the breakdown of ATP to ADP and Pi, resulting in useful energy for muscle actions. In a separate but coupled reaction, the enzyme **creatine kinase** facilitates the breakdown of PC to Pi and creatine, resulting in the donation of Pi to ADP to form ATP (Fig. 2-12).

The chemical structures and three dimensional shapes of ATP and PC are different; therefore, PC cannot be broken down by the enzyme ATPase located in muscle where energy is needed to cause muscle contraction. Thus, PC cannot be used to directly provide energy for muscle contraction. Intramuscular PC content is approximately four to five times greater than ATP content (3–8 nmol of ATP per kg of muscle). However, this is still a relatively low concentration of PC in the muscle and it decreases in parallel with ATP use due to the fact that PC is broken down during the resynthesis of ATP.

As the intramuscular concentration of PC decreases, so, too, does the production of ATP via the breakdown of PC. The bioenergetic pathway of ATP production by PC breakdown is termed the **ATP-PC system,** or the phosphagen system. As stated previously, intramuscular concentrations of ATP and PC are small; therefore, depletion of both phosphagens occurs rapidly during

high-intensity exercise. However, this anaerobic energy source can rapidly provide ATP in large quantities for a short period of time.

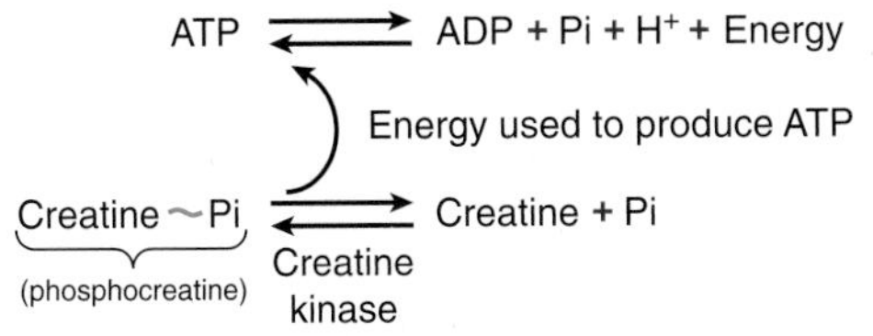

The ability to provide ATP rapidly for short periods of time makes the ATP-PC system important for performance in high-intensity, short-duration physical activities, such as short sprints, Olympic weightlifting, high jumping, and long jumping. It has been estimated that during maximal intensity activity ATP and PC intramuscular concentrations will be depleted in some muscle fibers (e.g., fast twitch) in approximately 4 seconds.[38] Although it is an attractive hypothesis to associate decreased intramuscular ATP and PC concentrations with the inability of muscle to generate force, several factors make a causal relationship unlikely.[16] For example, during high intensity exercise the intramuscular decrease in ATP does not show a correlation to the decline of muscular force, and the decrease in PC follows a different time course than the decrease in muscular force. This indicates that factors other than changes in intramuscular ATP and PC concentrations are responsible for decreases in muscular force. One such factor is an increase in intramuscular acidity or hydrogen ion concentration caused by anaerobic activity. Recall that the breakdown of ATP yields useful energy, but also a hydrogen ion. A second possible explanation is compartmentalization of ATP, meaning that even though total intramuscular levels of ATP are relatively high, there is a lack of ATP where it is needed within the muscle cell to provide energy for force production. More recently, it has also been shown that the accumulation of Pi that results from the rapid breakdown of ATP plays a role in muscle fatigue.

Ironically, the only means by which PC can be reformed from creatine and Pi is from energy released from the breakdown of ATP. During high-intensity activity, there will be little, if any, intramuscular ATP available for this purpose. However, during recovery from high-intensity activity, ATP can be obtained aerobically to replenish intramuscular PC as well as ATP content. Thus, after intramuscular PC and ATP are depleted during high-intensity activity, they cannot be effectively replenished until the intensity of the exercise is decreased or during postexercise recovery (discussed in "Metabolic Recovery After Exercise"). The ability to replenish intramuscular ATP and PC during recovery is an important consideration for sports and training activities involving repeated high-intensity, short-duration activity, such as basketball, weight training, and interval training. After a training program, the ability to perform high-intensity, short-duration physical activity improves as the capacity of muscle to re-establish phosphagen levels is enhanced.

As with all energy sources, an increase in the enzymes associated with that energy pathway, or an increase in substrate availability could potentially increase ATP production or replenishment. In doing so, performance in activities relying heavily on that particular energy pathway

$$\text{ATP} \rightleftharpoons \text{ADP} + \text{Pi} + \text{H}^+ + \text{Energy}$$

Energy used to produce ATP

Creatine ~ Pi $\rightleftharpoons$ Creatine + Pi
(phosphocreatine)   Creatine kinase

Figure 2-12. The energy released from the breakdown of phosphocreatine is used to produce adenosine triphosphate (ATP). Energy released from the breakdown of ATP can be used to resynthesize phosphocreatine if the intensity of activity is decreased or during recovery after exercise.

can also be expected to improve. Adaptations that could potentially increase performance in activities relying heavily upon the ATP-PC system include changes in the enzyme creatine kinase and resting intramuscular ATP and PC content.

Enzyme Adaptations to Exercise of the ATP-PC System

Increases in the activity of major enzymes involved in the ATP-PC system could result in faster regeneration of ATP, resulting in increased performance of short-duration, high-power activities. Creatine kinase is the main enzyme involved in regeneration of ATP from the breakdown of PC. Increases, decreases, and no change in this enzyme's activity have been noted after weight training and sprint-type training.[13,28,39,46] Although training-induced changes in creatine kinase activity have not been consistently reported, significant increases in the activity of this enzyme have been shown in some studies, including an increase of approximately 14% after isokinetic resistance training[13] and 44% after super maximal sprint cycle ergometer training.[39]

ATP and PC Adaptations to Exercise

Increases in intramuscular ATP and PC concentrations could increase performance in short-duration, high-intensity activity. Weight training[34,46] and sprint-type[14,42] training have resulted in significant increases as well as no change in intramuscular ATP and PC concentrations. In contrast, research has consistently demonstrated that endurance-type training has no significant effect on intramuscular ATP and PC concentrations.[1,31] After 5 months of resistance training, however, resting intramuscular concentrations of PC and ATP are elevated 22% and 18%, respectively, and maximal strength increased 28%.[34] In another study, it was shown that after 6 weeks of sprint-type training, resting concentrations of these phosphagens were unchanged, even though a decrease in 40-m sprint time and improved repeat sprint ability (total time for six 40-m sprints separated by 24 seconds) of approximately 2% occurred.[14] These results demonstrate that increased performance in short-term, high-intensity activity can occur with and without a significant increase in intramuscular ATP and PC.

Whether an increase in short-term, high-intensity performance can occur without a significant change in resting intramuscular ATP and PC may depend on whether or not depletion of these phosphagens occurs during activity. Estimations of ATP depletion during one-time sprints lasting 30 seconds and 10–12.5 seconds are approximately 45% and 14% to 32% of pre-exercise values, respectively.[14] Estimates of PC depletion after one-time sprints (10–30 seconds) and repeat sprints (30 seconds) indicate depletion ranges from 20–60% of pre-exercise values.[9] This indicates that complete depletion of ATP and PC may not occur in high-intensity activities of 30 seconds or less in duration.

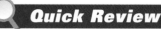

Quick Review

- Intramuscular adenosine triphosphate (ATP) and phosphocreatine (PC) are the predominant energy source for very short-term, high-intensity physical activity.
- Training adaptations to the ATP-PC energy source can include increases in some enzymes and increases in intramuscular stores of ATP and PC.

Thus, elevations in the content of resting intramuscular ATP and PC may not be necessary to enhance short-term, high-intensity performance.

GLYCOLYSIS

Glycolysis is a series of enzymatic reactions that metabolize glucose. Although this pathway does not need oxygen to function (so some refer to it as a nonoxidative process), it can result in a molecule called acetyl-CoA that can enter the mitochondria and participate in aerobic respiration if adequate amounts of oxygen are available in the cell. However, if enough oxygen is not available, glycolysis can instead result in the production of lactic acid, which cannot directly enter aerobic metabolism. So, glycolysis is important in producing energy for both aerobic and anaerobic activities.

Glycolysis results in ATP production from the breakdown of glucose through a series of 10 chemical reactions that take place in the sarcoplasm of muscle cells. The glucose can be obtained from either blood glucose or intramuscular stores of glycogen. There is only one difference between the production of ATP from glucose and that from glycogen. If glucose is used, an ATP is needed in a reaction to supply a phosphate to produce glucose-6-phosphate (Fig. 2-13). This step, like any involving the addition of a phosphate group to another molecule, is termed phosphorylation. Starting with glycogen, the chemical bond between one glucose molecule and the rest of the glycogen molecule is broken during a process called *glycogenolysis*. The glucose is phosphorylated by Pi already present, resulting in the formation of glucose-6-phosphate, thus sparing the cell the use of an ATP molecule that would be needed if blood-borne glucose were to be used. After the formation of glucose-6-phosphate, the remaining steps of glycolysis are identical whether starting with glucose or glycogen.

In addition to its first reaction, ATP is needed at the third reaction of glycolysis. So, early in the glycolytic pathway, it is an energy-consuming, rather than producing, process. In fact, if starting with glucose, two ATPs are needed, and if starting with glycogen, one ATP is needed to complete the first three reactions. Only during the later reactions does glycolysis produce energy by synthesizing two ATPs in two separate reactions, resulting in the total of four ATPs synthesized. So, the net gain in ATP is two molecules if

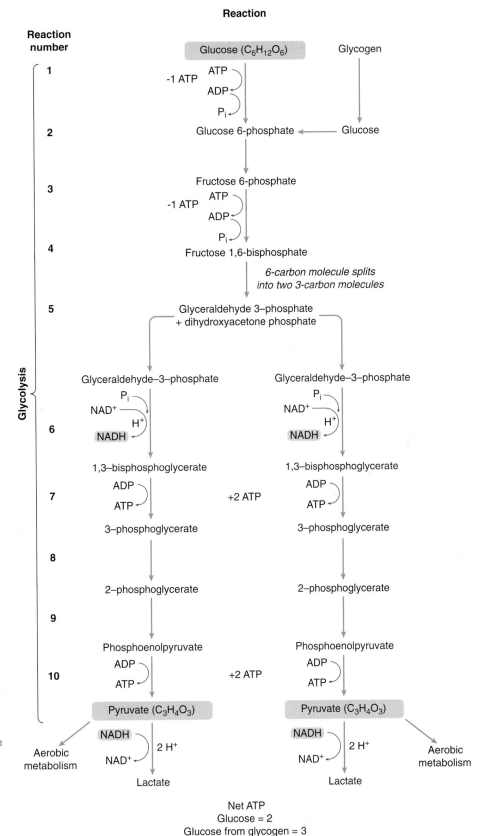

Figure 2-13. During glycolysis, glucose from the blood stream or a glucose obtained from glycogen is metabolized, resulting in pyruvate. Pyruvate can eventually enter aerobic metabolism or be transformed into lactate. A net gain of two and three adenosine triphosphates (ATP) occurs for each glucose and for each glucose obtained from glycogen, respectively, going through the reactions of glycolysis. There are enzymes associated with the various reactions. (Adapted from S.K. Powers and E.T. Howley. Exercise Physiology Theory and Application to Fitness and Performance. 5th ed. New York: McGraw Hill; 2004.)

starting with glucose and three if starting with glycogen as the substrate.

The fourth reaction splits the six-carbon chain of glucose into 2 three-carbon chains. The sixth reaction results in one hydrogen being removed from each of the three-carbon chains. The production of hydrogens is important because they are necessary to produce the majority of ATP aerobically (see "Aerobic Sources of ATP"). The hydrogens produced in glycolysis can be accepted by the hydrogen carrier molecule **nicotinamide adenine dinucleotide (NAD⁺),** resulting in NADH, a molecule that transports the hydrogens to the mitochondria for use in aerobic metabolism. NAD⁺ molecules, similar to other hydrogen carriers, are not destroyed as they transport hydrogens for use in aerobic metabolism. Once NADH has donated a hydrogen to the process of aerobic metabolism, NAD⁺ can again act as a hydrogen acceptor. NAD⁺ must accept hydrogens from glycolysis if the reactions of glycolysis are to continue. Thus, the continuation of glycolytic reactions in part depends on aerobic metabolism accepting hydrogens from NADH, and aerobic metabolism depends on sufficient oxygen being present. There is, however, another way by which NADH can donate its hydrogen, resulting in NAD⁺.

The last reaction of glycolysis results in pyruvic acid, a three-carbon molecule. If aerobic metabolism cannot accept hydrogens from NADH, pyruvic acid can accept a hydrogen and become lactic acid—also a three-carbon molecule. Formation of lactic acid is why glycolysis is also called the *lactic acid energy system.*

In summary, the first reactions of glycolysis need to consume ATP to proceed, and the later reactions produce ATP, as well as hydrogens, which can be used either in aerobic metabolism to produce ATP or to produce lactic acid from pyruvic acid. The net result is two ATPs if glycolysis starts with glucose and three ATPs if glycolysis starts with glycogen. The hydrogens carried by NADH will eventually result in an additional three ATPs being produced by aerobic metabolism and are not included in the calculation of net ATP produced directly by glycolysis (see "Aerobic Sources of ATP"). Now, let's examine several training adaptations that may enhance performance when glycolysis is the primary source of ATP during physical activity.

As with intramuscular ATP and PC, training adaptations occur in the enzymes of glycolysis and in substrate availability, in this case, intramuscular glycogen. Buffering capacity to offset the negative impact of lactic acid could also increase because of training. One or all of these adaptations could increase ATP production from glycolysis and, thus, performance. Whether these types of changes occur due to anaerobic or aerobic training and whether the change will positively affect performance appear to depend on several factors, including the particular glycolytic enzyme being examined, specifics (volume, intensity, duration) of a particular training program, and the definition of performance (one-time or repeat sprint ability, short- or long-sprint ability). Next, we will cover adaptations to exercise of the glycolytic enzymes, intramuscular glycogen, and buffering capacity.

Glycolytic Enzyme Adaptations to Exercise

Changes in glycolytic enzymes could improve performance in both aerobic and anaerobic activities by increasing ATP availability from glycolysis. Enzymes of glycolysis frequently studied are glycogen phosphorylase, phosphofructokinase (PFK), and lactate dehydrogenase (LDH). Glycogen phosphorylase catalyses the breakdown of intramuscular glycogen to glucose. PFK catalyses fructose-6-phosphate to fructose-1,6-bisphosphate and is the major rate-limiting enzyme of glycolysis. LDH catalyses the conversion of pyruvate into lactate. Increases in the levels of these enzymes have been shown due to weight training,[13,46] sprint training,[1,33,41,42] and endurance training.[1] However, changes in these enzymes are not always found with training. For example, endurance training programs lasting less than 12 weeks have generally failed to show an increase in PFK activity, whereas some programs 5 to 6 months in length have shown an increase in PFK activity.[1] Whether increases in a certain enzyme's activity will ultimately affect performance also depends on other factors. For example, an increase in LDH may not change glycolytic function because it is not a rate-limiting enzyme, whereas changes in PFK could increase overall glycolytic function because it is a rate-limiting enzyme. The effect of enzymatic changes is also made difficult to identify if muscle hypertrophy occurs because of training. Weight training that stimulates muscle hypertrophy has resulted in decreases in PFK activity[47] due to increased muscle size with no change in the total amount of PFK, resulting in dilution of PFK. Changes in key glycolytic enzymes could increase performance and have been shown with both aerobic and anaerobic training. But, an increase in enzymatic activity occurs may depend on the specific (training intensity, volume, duration, frequency) anaerobic or aerobic training program performed. Whether a change in an enzyme's activity results in a performance change may also depend on other factors. For example, weight training could increase muscular hypertrophy and maximal strength, but a decrease in a specific glycolytic enzyme's activity could occur simultaneously. Aerobic performance could be defined as either 5-km or marathon ability, and sprint ability could be defined as either one-time or repeat sprint ability. So, even though increases in glycolytic enzyme activities could improve performance, the effect of those increases on performance is unclear and dependent on numerous factors.

Intramuscular Glycogen Adaptations to Exercise

Increases in intramuscular glycogen could positively affect both glycolytic and aerobic production of ATP, because the end product of glycolysis—pyruvate—can either enter aerobic metabolism or become lactic acid. It is well accepted that endurance training increases intramuscular glycogen.[1,20] However, both increases and no change in intramuscular glycogen have been shown after weight[46] and sprint-type training.[9,42] As with glycolytic enzymatic changes, whether an increase in intramuscular glycogen occurs with weight and sprint-type training may depend on several factors such as the length of the training program and the specific type of training performed. For example, short-sprint repetitions (<10 seconds) and a combination of short- and long-sprint (>10 seconds) repetitions result in no change in intramuscular glycogen; however, long-sprint repetitions (>10 seconds) do result in an increase in intramuscular glycogen as glycolytic production of ATP becomes more important to performance.[42]

Buffering Capacity Adaptations

One way to increase performance in and recovery from any activity in which intramuscular acidity increases is to buffer the hydrogen ions produced. For example, one buffering system involves sodium bicarbonate. When a strong acid is present to release hydrogen ions, sodium bicarbonate ($NaHCO_3$) combines with the hydrogen ions, forming carbonic acid (H_2CO_3), a weaker acid. Skeletal muscle does have intracellular buffers. The most common intracellular buffers are proteins and phosphate groups (Table 2-1). However, intracellular bicarbonate can also act as a buffer. Both endurance and sprint-type training have been shown to increase buffering capabilities,[23,42] but not all studies show improved buffering potential. If buffering capabilities are increased, performance can be enhanced because more

ATP can be generated before increased acidity causes decreases in muscle force and power production.

AEROBIC ENZYMATIC SYSTEMS

Aerobic production of ATP is obviously very important for performance of endurance activities due to its ability to produce large amounts of ATP without generating fatiguing products. Aerobic production of ATP takes place in the mitochondria and involves two major enzymatic systems. The first of these enzymatic systems is the **Krebs cycle** (also termed the *citric acid cycle*). The function of the Krebs cycle is to oxidize (remove hydrogens and electrons) from substrates and produce some ATP. Carbohydrate, fat, and protein can all enter the Krebs cycle. The hydrogens removed from all substrates in the Krebs cycle are transported by hydrogen carrier molecules to the other major enzymatic system, the **electron transport chain** (ETC). You are already familiar with NAD^+, one of the hydrogen carrier molecules. Another hydrogen carrier molecule is **flavin adenine dinucleotide** (FAD). Both of these hydrogen carrier molecules transport hydrogens and electrons to the ETC. Transport of hydrogens and electrons to the ETC is important because it is the ETC that accounts for the vast majority of ATP production during aerobic metabolism. Oxygen originally taken into the body through the lungs is the final hydrogen and electron acceptor at the end of the ETC. Combining an oxygen atom with two hydrogens ($\frac{1}{2}O_2 + 2H^+ = H_2O$) results in the formation of water. The production of ATP by the ETC is termed **oxidative phosphorylation.** Oxygen does not participate in the reactions of the Krebs cycle, even though the Krebs cycle is typically thought of as part of aerobic metabolism. Regardless of whether carbohydrate, fat, or protein is aerobically metabolized, the process has three major components: reactions resulting in molecules that can enter the Krebs cycle, oxidation by the Krebs cycle of the molecules that enter it with the production of some ATP, and production of ATP in the ETC by oxidative phosphorylation. Alcohol can also be metabolized (Box 2-1), but it is not normally viewed as a nutrient because of its negative effects on health, such as increased risk of some types of cancer and cardiovascular disease.

Table 2-1. **Chemical Buffering Systems**

System	Component	Outcome
Bicarbonate	Sodium bicarbonate ($NaHCO_3$)	Converts strong acid to carbonic acid, a weak acid
Phosphate	Sodium phosphate (Na_2HPO_4)	Converts strong to weak acid
Protein	COO^- group of a protein	Combines with H^+ in the presence of excess acid
	Ammonia (NH_3^+) group of a protein	Combines with H^+ in the presence of excess acid

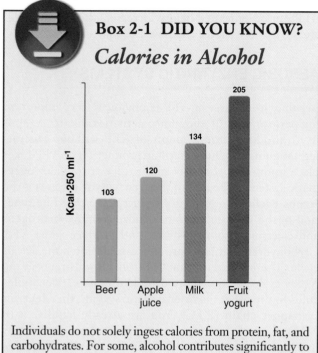

Individuals do not solely ingest calories from protein, fat, and carbohydrates. For some, alcohol contributes significantly to caloric intake. Alcohol contains 7 cal·g^{-1}. A single drink may contain approximately 15 g of ethanol, which equates to 105 calories from alcohol alone, not including any high-calorie mixers. Thus, those watching their weight should be aware of calories consumed from alcohol.

Krebs Cycle

We will now look at how the Krebs cycle and the ETC function in aerobic metabolism. Recall that glycolysis results in the formation of pyruvate, a three-carbon molecule. The pyruvate is broken down, forming a two-carbon molecule, acetyl-CoA, which can enter the Krebs cycle. In this process, one carbon and two oxygen atoms from pyruvate are given off as CO_2, which will eventually be expired at the lungs. The acetyl-CoA is combined with a four-carbon molecule, oxalo-acetate, resulting in citrate, a six-carbon molecule (Fig. 2-14). Note that oxaloacetate is the molecule with which acetyl-CoA combines to enter the Krebs cycle and is produced by the last reaction of the Krebs cycle. This is why the Krebs cycle is termed a cycle: oxaloacetate is used in the first reaction of this series of reactions and produced in the last reaction. Citrate then goes through the series of reactions making up the Krebs cycle, resulting in the formation of two CO_2 molecules and one ATP. At several points, hydrogens and their associated electrons are combined with the hydrogen carrier molecules NAD^+ and FAD to form NADH and $FADH_2$.

ATP formation during the Krebs cycle takes place at only one reaction (formation of guanosine triphosphate, GTP, which is immediately used to produce ATP). Only a small amount of ATP, then, is formed directly from the Krebs cycle. The vast majority of ATP is formed because of the transport of hydrogens and electrons to the ETC, where they are used to produce ATP. In summary, for each acetyl-CoA entering the Krebs cycle, two CO_2s, one ATP, three NADHs, and one $FADH_2$ are produced.

So, how are hydrogens and electrons transported to the ETC used to produce ATP by oxidative phosphorylation? Two processes take place simultaneously in the ETC, resulting in ATP production. One process involves electrons and the other hydrogens. In the ETC, pairs of electrons are passed from one cytochrome to another, and in doing so, sufficient energy is released at three points to phosphorylate ADP, resulting in ATP (Fig. 2-15). However, this does not totally describe how ATP is actually produced. Mitochondria have inner and outer membranes and inner and outer compartments (Fig. 2-16). Energy released as electrons are passed from one cytochrome to the next in the ETC, which is used to actively pump hydrogen ions from the inner to the outer compartment (i.e., inter-membrane space) of the mitochondria. This results in a concentration gradient, with more hydrogen ions in the outer compartment. This concentration gradient is the source of energy to produce ATP. Three pumps are within the inner membrane (Fig. 2-16). For every two electrons that move along the ETC, each of the three pumps moves electrons from the inner to the outer compartment (first and second pump move four hydrogen ions, third pump moves only two hydrogen ions). Hydrogen ions from NADH enter the ETC prior to the first pump while electrons carried by $FADH_2$ enter the ETC after the first pump. This results in more electrons being pumped from the inner to the outer compartment when hydrogens are carried to the ETC by NADH (10 vs. 6 electrons). This difference results in the ability to produce more ATPs when hydrogens are carried to the ETC by NADH compared with $FADH^2$.

The inner mitochondrial membrane is impermeable to hydrogen ions, so how can the existence of a hydrogen ion concentration gradient result in ATP formation? The hydrogen ion concentration gradient creates a kind of potential energy that can be used to phosphorylate ADP to ATP only if the hydrogen ions can move down their concentration gradient from the inner to the outer compartment. Although the inner membrane is impermeable to hydrogen ions, specialized hydrogen ion channels, termed **respiratory assemblies,** permit hydrogen ions to pass through the inner membrane. As the hydrogen ions pass through the membrane, they activate the enzyme ATP synthase, and sufficient energy is available to phosphorylate ADP to ATP. Although more ATP can be produced when electrons are carried to the ETC by NADH compared with $FADH_2$, the total amount of ATP produced by the ETC is an estimate, because the chemistry of hydrogen ion pumping, ATP synthesis, and hydrogen ion carrier molecules can vary slightly.[6]

Oxygen acts as the final acceptor of pairs of electrons passed down the ETC and, when combined with two hydrogens, results in the formation of water. Oxygen is needed to act as the final electron acceptor to keep the ETC functioning. In the next several sections, complete aerobic metabolism and ATP yield of carbohydrate, fats, and protein will be discussed in more detail.

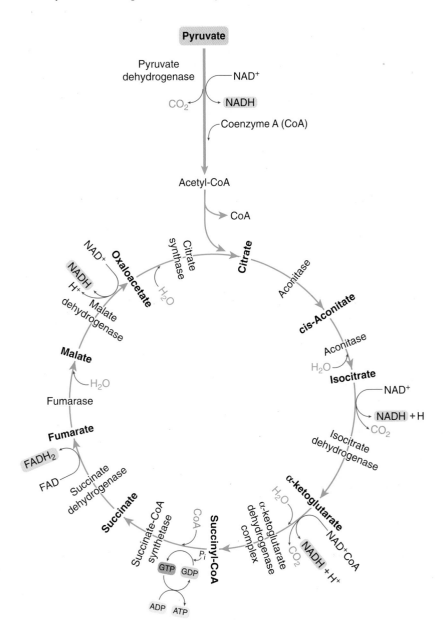

Figure 2-14. Acetyl-CoA obtained from the catabolism of pyruvate enters the Krebs cycle. Each acetyl-CoA in the Krebs cycle results in the production of one adenosine triphosphate (ATP), carbon dioxide, and hydrogen ions, which are carried to the electron transport system by electron carrier molecules, where the vast majority of ATP is produced by aerobic metabolism.

Carbohydrate Aerobic ATP Yield

The total ATP production from the oxidation of carbohydrate depends on the amount of ATP produced in glycolysis, the Krebs cycle, and the ETC (Table 2-2). Recall that the only difference between glycolytic metabolism of glucose derived from the bloodstream and a glucose molecule obtained from glycogen lies in the pathway's first reaction, which yields glucose-6-phosphate (see Fig. 2-13). If starting with glucose taken up from the blood, one ATP is required to produce glucose-6-phosphate, whereas starting with a glucose obtained from glycogen, this energy-consuming step is not needed. This difference results in the net production of one less ATP molecule when the original substrate is blood-borne glucose. So glycolysis results in the net gain of two ATPs from glucose and three ATPs from glycogen. The Krebs cycle results in the generation of two

ATPs per glucose molecule. In addition, glycolysis, the Krebs cycle, and the conversion of pyruvate to acetyl-CoA produce hydrogens that are carried to the ETC by either NADH or $FADH_2$ and the production of ATP by oxidative phosphorylation. The net result of the oxidation of glucose and glycogen is 38 and 39 molecules of ATP, respectively. However, these totals are estimates, because there can be slight variations in ATP production due to variations in hydrogen pumping in the ETC, ATP synthesis, and how hydrogen electrons are carried to the ETC.

Sources of Carbohydrate for Metabolism

Glucose for use in aerobic metabolism can be obtained from either blood glucose or intramuscular glycogen. If blood glucose concentration is low, such as between meals or due to the use of glucose in metabolism, the liver releases glucose

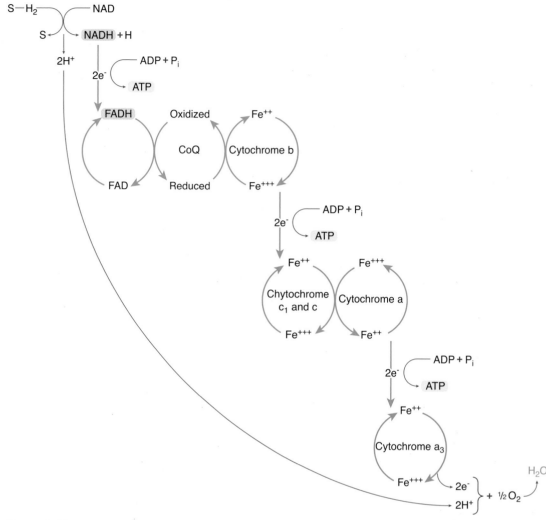

Figure 2-15. Simplified overview of the formation of adenosine triphosphate (ATP) at three places in the electron transport chain ETC. Note that electrons carried by FADH$_2$ enter the ETC after electrons carried by NADH, resulting in fewer ATP produced by electrons carried by FADH$_2$.

Table 2-2. **Total Adenosine Triphosphate (ATP) Formed from Carbohydrate during Aerobic Metabolism[a]**

Glycolysis	ATP From Glucose	ATP From Glycogen
Phosphorylation of glucose	−1	0
Phosphorylation of fructose-6-phosphate	−1	−1
Production at two steps in glycolysis	+4	+4
Two molecules of NADH to electron transport chain (ETC)	+6	+6
Pyruvate to Acetyl-CoA		
Two molecules of NADH to ETC	+6	+6
Krebs cycle		
Production from guanosine triphosphate	+2	+2
Six molecules of NADH to ETC	+18	+18
Two molecules of FADH$_2$ to ETC	+4	+4
Total	+38	+39

[a]Calculations assume 3 ATP per NADH and 2 ATP per FADH$_2$.

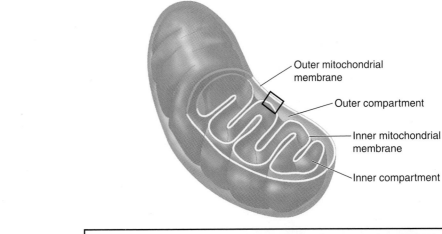

Figure 2-16. **Hydrogen ion (H⁺) pumps move H⁺ from the inner to the outer mitochondrial compartments.** The pumping results in a H⁺ concentration gradient, with a higher concentration of H⁺ in the outer compartment. This concentration gradient is used by respiratory assemblies to produce adenosine triphosphate (ATP).

into the bloodstream by breaking down its stores of glycogen. If blood glucose concentration is high, such as right after a carbohydrate-rich meal, the liver and other tissues, including skeletal muscle and the brain (see Box 2-2), remove glucose from the blood to be immediately used in metabolism or to be stored as glycogen. Maintaining blood glucose concentrations (see Chapter 7, Endocrine System) within normal ranges is the result of the interaction of the liver, muscle tissue, pancreas (secretion of the hormones glucagon and insulin), and the adrenal glands (secretion of the hormone epinephrine). For now, it is sufficient to know that during low-intensity activity, muscle tissue will mainly utilize blood glucose in aerobic metabolism, but during moderate-intensity exercise, muscle fibers will use both circulating glucose and intramuscular glycogen to supply aerobic metabolism. Normally, glucose metabolism is well controlled even during exercise; however, in McArdle disease, a genetic abnormality drastically impairs glucose metabolism (Box 2-3).

Besides intramuscular glycogen, liver glycogen, and blood glucose, there are indirect sources of carbohydrate available for metabolism. Some amino acids can be utilized to synthesize glucose (see the section on Protein Use in Aerobic Metabolism), and the glycerol portion of triglycerides (see the section on Triglyceride Aerobic Metabolism ATP Yield) can also be utilized to synthesize glucose. Normally, however, these gluconeogenic sources of glucose are utilized to a minimal extent. One source of carbohydrate metabolism that is utilized during exercise, and even at rest, is lactate. Use of lactate, or lactic acid, in aerobic metabolism can occur in two ways. The Cori cycle (Fig. 2-17) begins with the production of lactate by skeletal muscle or other tissues, which then enters the blood and is transported to the liver where it is used to synthesize glucose. The newly formed glucose can then be utilized to maintain blood glucose

Box 2-2 DID YOU KNOW?

Brain Power

Your brain represents only approximately 2% of your body weight. However, your brain is responsible for approximately 25% of total body glucose use. The brain uses glucose, which cannot be stored in the brain cells and must be provided through circulation, almost exclusively as its preferred energy source. In conditions such as starvation or diabetes, when only limited glucose is available, the brain has the specialized ability to also use ketones (products of fat metabolism in cases in which insulin and caloric intake are low) to produce energy.

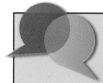

Box 2-3 AN EXPERT VIEW

McArdle Disease: A Genetic Problem Using Glycogen for Metabolism

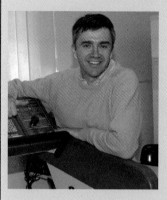

Alejandro Lucia, MD, PhD
European University of Madrid
Madrid, Spain

McArdle disease is a genetic disorder characterized by a total lack of activity of the enzyme responsible for glycogen breakdown in skeletal muscle fibers, that is, myophosphorylase. It is a relatively uncommon disease (frequency of 1:100,000 population in the United States) that has been described only in white and Japanese populations. Patients carry one of the approximately 90 genetic mutations. These mutations can produce different alterations (truncated protein, no mRNA, etc.), resulting in enzymatic inactivity and, thus, inability to breakdown stored glycogen in skeletal muscle fibers.

The disease was first described in a 30-year-old man by a British physician, Brian McArdle, in 1951. This young patient reported severe exercise intolerance in virtually all types of physical activities and myalgia (muscle pain) in any muscle involved in a given exercise.

There exists a large degree of individual variability in both the time of onset of the typical disease symptoms (childhood vs. adulthood) and the degree of exercise intolerance. The disease can be very incapacitating in many individuals, whereas in others it is more of an idiosyncrasy than a disease. Except in some cases, such as sudden infant death syndrome or fatal weakness respiratory failure, McArdle disease is a benign condition. Nonetheless, the patients' quality of life is commonly impaired, as virtually all of them have exercise intolerance and most have reduced functional capacity in most physical tasks of daily living. Most frequently, patients report premature muscle weakness, fatigue, and sometimes cramps after 10 to 20 seconds of short-term exercise involving predominantly anaerobic glycolysis, and during the first 5 to 10 minutes of endurance exercise involving large muscle groups (such as walking or cycling). In the latter case, patients experience very unpleasant myalgia, weakness, breathlessness, and tachycardia (e.g., up to 160 beats·min^{-1}) during the transition from rest to exercise due to substrate-limited oxidative phosphorylation and low availability of blood-borne fuels (glucose and free fatty acids). These symptoms are always attenuated in less than 10 minutes due to a blood glucose-mediated increase in oxidative phosphorylation, a phenomenon known as "the

second wind." Patients with McArdle disease are in fact the only humans who experience this phenomenon, which can be thus used to aid in the diagnosis of the disease. Ingestion of carbohydrates (75 g of sucrose) 30 to 40 minutes prior to the start of exercise completely removes the second wind phenomenon and alleviates patients' exercise intolerance, by increasing blood glucose availability to working muscles from the start of exercise.

The functional capacity of these patients is usually very low, that is, their peak oxygen uptake ($\dot{V}O_{2peak}$) is usually $^1/_2$ or $^1/_3$ ($\leq$20 mL·kg^{-1}·min^{-1}) of that of healthy individuals. They also exhibit a hyperkinetic cardiovascular response to dynamic exercise (increased cardiac output:$\dot{V}O_2$ ratio), which reflects the low ability of their muscles to consume oxygen due to blocked (aerobic) glycolysis. Except when fed glucose before exercise, their blood lactate levels gradually decrease from the start to the end of dynamic exercise that gradually increases in intensity due to lack of glucose for use in anaerobic glycolysis. Despite the lack of lactic acidosis, muscle weakness and fatigue rapidly occur in these patients. This indicates that lactic acidosis is not the main (or at least not the only) cause of muscle fatigue in humans.

Several interventions have been proposed to minimize the exercise intolerance of McArdle patients, such as the aforementioned preexercise carbohydrate ingestion, creatine loading, ketogenic diet, and endurance exercise training. Aerobic training for approximately 3 months has been shown to increase the peak work capacity of patients by as much as 36%. Although more research is needed, preliminary data suggest that the stimulus for muscle growth prompted by exercise training can to some degree counterbalance the increased susceptibility to muscle injury commonly observed in McArdle disease, as reflected by a marked decrease after exercise training in basal serum levels of creatine kinase, an accepted indicator of rhabdomyolysis.

Selected Readings

1. DiMauro S, Servidei S, Tsujino S. Disorders of carbohydrate metabolism: glycogen storage diseases. In: Rosenberg RN, Prusiner SB, DiMauro S, Barchi RL, eds. The Molecular and Genetic Basis of Neurological Disease. 2nd ed. Boston, MA: Butterworth-Heinemann, 1996:1067–1097.
2. Haller RG, Wyrick P, Taivassalo T, et al. Aerobic conditioning: an effective therapy in McArdle's disease. Ann Neurol. 2006;59:922–928.
3. Vorgerd M, Zange J, Kley R, et al. Effect of high-dose creatine therapy on symptoms of exercise intolerance in McArdle disease: double-blind, placebo-controlled crossover study. Arch Neurol. 2002;59:97–101.

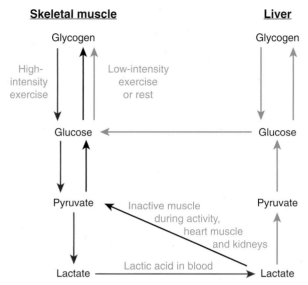

Figure 2-17. **A simplified version of the steps of the Cori cycle and lactate shuttle hypothesis is presented.** The *red arrows* indicate lactic acid production due to high intensity exercise. The *blue arrows* indicate lactic acid following the Cori cycle. The *black arrows* indicate lactic acid following the lactate shuttle hypothesis (other than the Cori cycle).

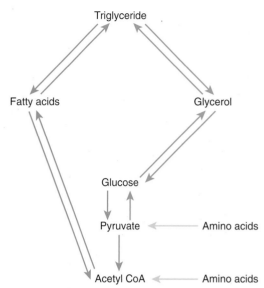

Figure 2-18. **A simplified version of the steps involved in the possible interactions of carbohydrate, amino acids, fatty acids, and glycerol in the synthesis of triglyceride.** Note that it is possible to transform both glucose and amino acids into glycerol and fatty acids and then combine them to synthesize a triglyceride.

levels or to synthesize liver glycogen. The "lactate shuttle hypothesis" is another way by which glucose can be utilized in metabolism.[18] According to this theory, once lactate leaves the muscle and enters the blood it can be utilized not only in the Cori cycle of the liver but also by other tissues, including skeletal muscle, to synthesize glycogen or be transformed into pyruvate and enter aerobic metabolism (Fig. 2-17). Lactate produced by skeletal muscle or other tissues can circulate in the blood and subsequently be used by inactive skeletal muscle, cardiac muscle, and the kidneys to synthesize glycogen or be transformed into pyruvate.[8] For example, if blood lactate levels rise above resting values, such as during anaerobic activity, inactive skeletal muscle can utilize lactate to synthesize glycogen or pyruvate, thus lowering blood lactate concentration. In addition, after an anaerobic activity, the same skeletal muscle that during activity produced lactate could convert lactate obtained from the blood into glycogen or pyruvate, thus lowering blood lactate concentration while concurrently replenishing intramuscular glycogen stores. Thus, the lactate shuttle hypothesis views lactate not as a waste product from anaerobic metabolism, but as a way to shuttle carbohydrate in the form of lactate around the body for use by different tissues.

Triglyceride Aerobic Metabolism

The total amount of ATP produced by aerobic metabolism of triglycerides is in large part dependent on the length of the three fatty acids that comprise a triglyceride and whether or not the fatty acid is saturated or unsaturated. However, both the fatty acid and glycerol portions of a triglyceride can be metabolized, since two glycerols (three-carbon molecules) can be transformed by the liver into glucose, a six-carbon molecule. The glucose can then be aerobically metabolized. Glycerol can also be transformed into pyruvate, another three-carbon molecule. The pyruvate can then be aerobically metabolized by entering the mitochondria, generating the same amount of ATP as described previously during the oxidative metabolism of a blood-borne glucose molecule, or pyruvate (Fig. 2-18). Fatty acids are composed of even numbers of carbon molecules of up to 24. Fatty acids can be broken down into two carbon subunits, which can be transformed into acetyl-CoA and then aerobically metabolized. The greater the length of the fatty acid, the greater the number of acetyl-CoAs that can be produced. Thus, the longer the fatty acid, the greater the ATP production.

Beta oxidation is a process during which fatty acids are broken down into two-carbon molecules (acetic acid), which can be transformed into acetyl-CoA and enter the Krebs cycle. Similar to glycolysis, ATP is needed to start the process of beta oxidation. Per fatty acid, two ATPs are needed to supply activation energy. The number of acetyl-CoAs resulting from a fatty acid depends on the length of the fatty acid's carbon chain. For example, from a 16-carbon fatty acid, eight acetyl-CoAs can be formed. For each round of beta oxidation resulting in an acetyl-CoA unit, (seven rounds for a 16-carbon chain), one NADH and one $FADH_2$ are formed. The NADH and $FADH_2$ eventually result in ATP production in the ETC. In the Krebs cycle, one ATP per acetyl-CoA is produced, along with some NADH and $FADH_2$. The net ATP production is a total of 17 ATPs produced per acetyl-CoA. However, the last two-carbon chain does not have to be broken off

Table 2-3. Total Adenosine Triphosphate (ATP) formed From a 16-Carbon Molecule Fatty Acid

Metabolic Process	ATP
Beta oxidation	
Activation energy per fatty acid	− 2
One molecule of NADH/acetyl-CoA to ETC	+3
One molecule of FADH$_2$/acetyl-CoA to ETC (no NADH or FADH$_2$ produced from the last acetyl-CoA formed)	+2
Total ATP/acetyl-CoA (ignoring activation energy and last acetyl CoA formed)	+5
Krebs cycle	
One ATP/acetyl-CoA	+1
Three NADH/acetyl-CoA to ETC	+9
One FADH$_2$/acetyl-CoA to ETC	+2
Total ATP/acetyl-CoA	+12
Total ATP/acetyl-CoA	
Beta oxidation 5 ATP/acetyl-CoA + Krebs cycle 12 ATP/acetyl-CoA (ignoring activation energy and last acetyl-CoA formed)	+17
Total ATP from a 16-carbon molecule fatty acid	
Beta oxidation and Krebs cycle for 7 acetyl-CoAs (7 × 17 ATP)	+119
Beta oxidation and Krebs cycle for last acetyl-CoA	+12
Activation energy per fatty acid	− 2
Total ATP	+129

of the fatty acid's carbon chain, resulting in no NADH or FADH$_2$ production during beta oxidation. ATP production from a typical 16-carbon molecule fatty acid is 129 ATPs (Table 2-3). Likewise, for an 18-carbon molecule fatty acid, an additional 17 ATPs would be produced, because an additional acetyl-CoA can be produced, resulting in a net gain of 146 ATPs during complete aerobic metabolism. Compared with carbohydrate, triglycerides or fatty acids result in substantially more ATP production because of the greater number of carbon and hydrogen molecules available for use in the Krebs cycle and the ETC for ATP production. The impressive amount of energy in triglyceride is in part what makes fat storage a good way to store large amounts of energy (Boxes 2-4 and 2-5).

Fatty acids used in aerobic metabolism can be obtained from triglyceride stores in adipose cells. The enzyme **hormone-sensitive lipase** inside the adipose cells breaks down the triglycerides into glycerol and fatty acids, which are released into the blood. When cells need these

substances as a substrate, they can remove them from the blood and aerobically metabolize them.

Fatty acids and glycerol can also be synthesized from both glucose and amino acids. Glucose can be transformed into glycerol, and the two-carbon molecule acetyl-CoA obtained from glucose or glycogen can be used to synthesize fatty acids. The fatty acids and glycerol can then be utilized by adipose cells to synthesize triglycerides (Fig. 2-18). Deaminated amino acids that can be used to synthesize pyruvate can either become glucose and then glycerol or acetyl-CoA and then utilized to synthesize fatty acids. Moreover, amino acids that can be directly converted to acetyl-CoA can also be utilized to synthesize fatty acids. Because of the ability to utilize both carbohydrate and protein to synthesize fatty acids and glycerol and then eventually triglycerides, it is possible to gain fat weight when ingesting excess protein and carbohydrate.

Metabolism of Protein

Proteins can provide energy through several different pathways. Many amino acids can be transformed to glucose, and are termed **gluconeogenic.** The glucose can then be utilized to produce energy. Some amino acids, such as alanine, leucine, and isoleucine, can be converted to metabolic intermediates or molecules that can enter the bioenergetic process at some point. Before any amino acid enters bioenergetic processes, it must first undergo **deamination,** or have its nitrogen group removed. When the nitrogen group is removed, it results in ammonia (NH$_3$). Ammonia is a base and can upset the acid-base balance of

Box 2-4 DID YOU KNOW?

How Much Energy is Available from Fat?

A 150-lb person with 15% body fat has approximately 22.5 lb of fat. Each pound of fat contains approximately 3,500 kcal. Assuming it requires approximately 100 kcal to run one mile, this individual theoretically contains the energy in body fat alone to run almost 800 miles!

Box 2-5 PRACTICAL QUESTIONS FROM STUDENTS

If the Body Prefers to Use Glucose as Energy during Exercise, Why is Most of the Body's Energy Stored as Fat?

The storage of fat does not require much additional water, whereas glycogen is stored with water due to its molecular properties. Each gram of glycogen is stored with approximately 2 g of water. Triglycerides, on the other hand, do not need to be stored with as much water. To put it into perspective, the amount of energy contained in 1 lb (0.45 kg) of fat would require approximately 6 lb (2.7 kg) of glycogen.

the body. To prevent this, the liver combines two ammonia molecules and CO_2 to produce urea (N_2H_4CO) and a water molecule. The urea is released into the bloodstream and is excreted in the urine.

Another bioenergetic pathway that amino acids can enter begins with their conversion to pyruvate, which can then be aerobically metabolized (Fig. 2-19). Other amino acids can be converted into acetyl-CoA and be metabolized, and still others can enter the Krebs cycle directly and be metabolized. Any metabolic substrate that can be converted into pyruvate can be either metabolized or used to synthesize glucose. So, the amino acids that can be converted into pyruvate can be used to produce glucose and are termed glucogenic.[21] However, amino acids that are converted into acetyl-CoA cannot be converted into glucose and, therefore, must be metabolized, as must the amino acids that enter the Krebs cycle directly. The amino acids that can enter the Krebs cycle directly are also glucogenic, but if they enter the Krebs cycle, they cannot be used to synthesize glucose.

Typically only a small amount of protein or amino acids are metabolized to provide energy. However, in some situations amino acids are far more likely to be metabolized. For example, during extreme dieting (ingestion of substantially fewer kilocalories than needed to support bodily function), amino acids are obtained from tissues, including skeletal muscle, to be metabolized to produce energy. This results in muscle tissue loss during extreme dieting. Also, diets featuring an unusually high protein intake may also result in greater use of proteins for energy production.

Quick Review

- Aerobic metabolism involves glycolysis for glucose, beta oxidation for fats, and the Krebs cycle and electron transport for both. The majority of ATP is produced during electron transport.
- Glucose taken up from the blood or from intramuscular glycogen can enter glycolysis. Pyruvate produced by glycolysis can be transformed into acetyl-CoA, which can enter Krebs cycle. Hydrogens and electrons from glycolysis and Krebs cycle are carried by $FADH_2$ and NADH to the electron transport chain to complete aerobic metabolism.
- Fatty acids enter beta oxidation. The two-carbon molecule (acetic acid) produced by beta oxidation is transformed into acetyl-CoA, which can enter Krebs cycle. Hydrogens and electrons from Krebs cycle are carried by $FADH_2$ and NADH to the electron transport system to complete aerobic metabolism.
- Glycerol can be transformed into pyruvate, which can be transformed into acetyl-CoA, which can enter Krebs cycle.
- Lactate can be converted into pyruvate and metabolized or used to synthesize glucose.
- All amino acids must be deaminated to enter aerobic metabolism.
- Some amino acids can be transformed into pyruvate, which can be transformed into acetyl-CoA, which can enter the Krebs cycle.
- Some amino acids can be transformed into acetyl-CoA, which can enter the Krebs cycle.
- Some amino acids can enter the Krebs cycle directly and be metabolized.

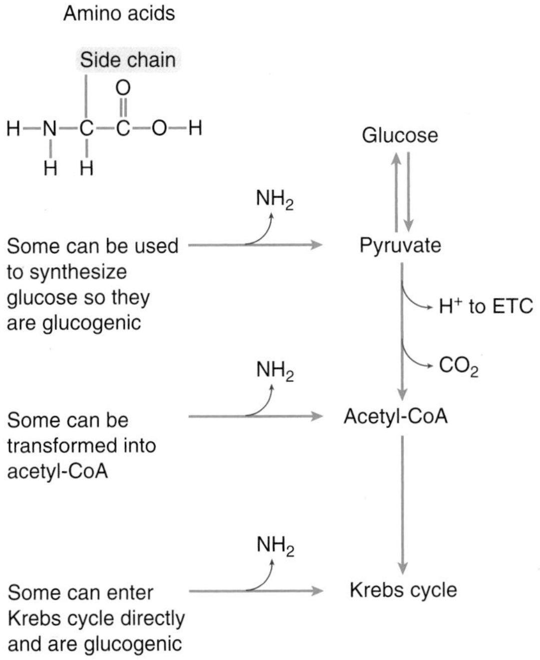

Figure 2-19. Amino acids after deamination can enter aerobic metabolism in three manners. Note that because some amino acids can become pyruvate, they can be used to synthesize glucose.

Assuming a typical, mixed diet of carbohydrates, fats, and proteins, only a small amount of those proteins are used for production of ATP during exercise, and this depends on the availability of the branch-chain amino acids and the amino acid alanine.[19] However, during long-term endurance activity, **proteases,** or enzymes capable of degrading protein, found within muscle are activated. This results in a small increase in amino acid metabolism.

Amino acid use in metabolism does increase when dieting, which results in muscle mass loss. To minimize the loss of muscle mass, exercise could be performed to create a stimulus that results in decreased protein metabolism. For example, the necessity of performing exercise while losing body weight was clearly demonstrated in a group of men who lost on average 19.8 to 21.1 pounds (9.0–9.6 kg) during 12 weeks of dieting or dieting and exercise.[30] Fat weight made up 69% of weight loss in men who only dieted but as much as 78% of weight loss in men who dieted and did aerobic training and 97% of weight loss in the men who dieted and did aerobic and weight training. These findings clearly show that exercise increased weight loss due to loss of fat and, in doing so, decreased protein metabolism, resulting in less loss of muscle mass.

METABOLIC SUBSTRATES FOR REST AND EXERCISE

Which substrate is metabolized at any particular time depends on many factors. Generally, if one substrate is available in large quantities, it will be preferentially metabolized. During physical activity, if a substrate is not available, such as when carbohydrate is depleted at the end of a long-distance race, there is a necessity to metabolize more triglycerides to continue with the race. The amount of energy produced by metabolizing each of the substrates also affects whether carbohydrate, triglycerides, or protein is metabolized. The intensity and duration of physical activity also affect which of the substrates will be preferentially metabolized. The factors affecting which substrate will be metabolized at rest or during exercise are explored in the following sections.

Interactions of Substrates

Several factors affect what substrate is preferentially metabolized at rest or during exercise. For a period of time after a mean high in either fat or carbohydrate, the substrate most available will be preferentially metabolized. When chronically ingesting either a high-fat or a high-carbohydrate diet, preferential metabolism of the substrate most readily available will also occur.

Protein is typically used in aerobic metabolism at rest or during exercise to a very small extent. Even though there are some enzymatic adaptations[1] due to endurance training that allow greater use of amino acids in aerobic metabolism, typically protein contributes less than 2% of the substrate utilized during exercise less than 60 minutes in duration. During longer-duration activity of 3 to 5 hours, protein metabolism may contribute up to 5% to 15% of the energy during the final minutes of activity. However, for most activities, a mixture of triglyceride and carbohydrate metabolism provides the vast majority of ATP needed for energy.

First, recall that anaerobic energy sources are intramuscular stores of ATP and PC and use of glucose from the bloodstream or glucose obtained from glycogen in glycolysis. Protein or triglyceride cannot be utilized to produce energy anaerobically. So during an anaerobic activity, proteins or triglycerides are not metabolized to any significant extent to provide the needed ATP. But during aerobic activities, the vast majority of needed ATP is obtained from the metabolism of either carbohydrates or triglycerides, depending on the exercise intensity and duration. The following sections discuss in more detail the effect of exercise intensity and duration on substrate use.

Exercise Intensity: Triglyceride or Carbohydrate Metabolism

At rest, approximately 33% of the needed ATP is derived from carbohydrate metabolism and 66% from fat or triglyceride metabolism. The figure of 66% of energy production from breakdown of triglycerides is the highest relative contribution that triglyceride metabolism will supply. As the exercise intensity increases, there is a gradual switch from predominantly relying upon triglycerides for energy production to the use of carbohydrates. In theory at least, this change continues until at maximal exercise intensity, when 100% of the energy needed by the working muscles is provided by carbohydrate metabolism (Fig. 2-20). The exclusive use of carbohydrate to supply energy at maximal exercise intensity is in part because anaerobic sources (remember triglycerides and proteins cannot be utilized in glycolysis) are supplying a portion of the needed ATP.

The amount of energy produced when metabolizing fat or carbohydrate explains, in part, why a switch to more carbohydrate metabolism is advantageous as exercise intensity

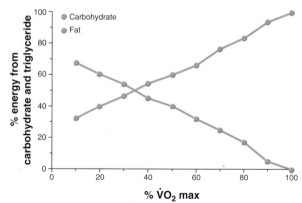

Figure 2-20. Percentage of energy from carbohydrate and triglyceride at different exercise intensities. As the exercise intensity (expressed as a percentage of maximal oxygen consumption) increases, the percentage of energy obtained from triglyceride decreases and that from carbohydrate increases.

increases. The amount of energy per gram of substrate is the highest in fat (9.4 kcal·g^{-1}) followed by both carbohydrate (4.1 kcal·g^{-1}) and protein (4.1 kcal·g^{-1}).[12] However, per liter of oxygen used in aerobic metabolism, more energy is produced when metabolizing carbohydrate (5.0 kcal·LO$_2$$^{-1}$) than fat (4.7 kcal·LO$_2$$^{-1}$) and protein (4.5 kcal·LO$_2$$^{-1}$). So, during near maximal or maximal activity, more energy can be obtained if more carbohydrate and less fat are aerobically metabolized.

Several other factors, however, result in the gradual switch from a predominant reliance on triglyceride metabolism at rest to an increasing dependence upon carbohydrate as energy demands increase during higher-intensity exercise. Perhaps the most important is that as the exercise intensity increases, more fast-twitch or type II muscle fibers are recruited (see Chapter 3 for a discussion of muscle fiber-type recruitment and characteristics). Type II muscle fibers possess a high level of glycolytic enzymes and a lower level of aerobic enzymes. Thus, type II fibers are well suited to perform anaerobic glycolysis to produce ATP. Greater recruitment of type II muscle fibers results in more carbohydrate metabolism to produce the needed ATP because triglycerides cannot be utilized to produce energy from glycolysis.

Hormonal changes (see Chapter 7 for a discussion of the hormonal impact on metabolism), in particular a greater release of epinephrine, also amplify carbohydrate metabolism as the exercise intensity increases. This is due to the stimulatory effect that epinephrine has on glycolytic enzymes. In addition, increased lactate concentrations resulting from rapid rates of glycolysis inhibit triglyceride metabolism by reducing triglyceride availability for use in aerobic metabolism.[48]

The gradual switch in substrate utilization from a greater dependence on fats at rest and during low-intensity exercise to carbohydrates as intensity is magnified raises an interesting question: At what exercise intensity is the rate of fat metabolism maximized? Typically the amount of triglyceride metabolism is maximized at approximately 65% to 75% of maximal heart rate. However, as explained in Box 2-6, this is only part of the answer.

Exercise Duration: Triglyceride or Carbohydrate Metabolism

During low-intensity, long-duration activity, such as jogging for 30 minutes or more, there is a gradual shift from carbohydrate to triglyceride metabolism, even if the same intensity is maintained throughout the session. This is related to a number of factors affecting the availability of triglyceride in the form of free fatty acids for use in aerobic metabolism.

Box 2-6 PRACTICAL QUESTIONS FROM STUDENTS

At What Aerobic Exercise Intensity Is the Most Fat Metabolized?

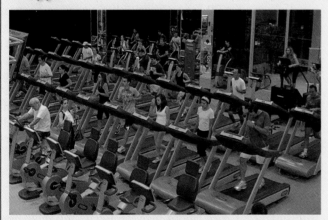

Many people perform aerobic exercise to help maintain a healthy body weight and percentage body fat. To help achieve both of these goals, exercising at the exercise intensity that maximizes lipid metabolism would be useful. As exercise intensity increases from rest to maximal levels, there is a gradual switch in the predominant energy substrate used, from lipid to carbohydrate, for the production of ATP. Fat metabolism is maximized at a mean exercise intensity of approximately 64% of maximal oxygen consumption, and 74% of maximal heart rate in well-conditioned cyclists performing cycling exercise. However, there is a zone of maximal fat metabolism on either side of these mean exercise intensities. So, lipid metabolism is actually near maximal between approximately 68% and 79% of maximal heart rate, or 55% to 72% of maximal oxygen consumption in well-conditioned cyclists. Above this zone, lipid metabolism decreases substantially and is negligible above 92% of maximal heart rate. The question of what exercise intensity maximizes lipid metabolism, however, is only partially answered by knowing at what exercise intensity fat metabolism is maximized. Maintaining that intensity for a sufficient duration so that a substantial amount of lipid metabolism takes place is also an important factor. For example, if your lipid metabolism, on a percentage basis of the needed energy, was maximized at 83% of maximal heart rate, but you could maintain this exercise intensity for only 3 minutes, the total amount of fat metabolized would be minimal. Using a maximal figure of approximately 0.6 g of lipid metabolized per minute, this would result in only 1.8 g (0.6 g·min^{-1} × 3 min) being metabolized. So, what must be considered in selecting proper exercise intensity is not only the rate of energy obtained from lipid metabolism but also the duration at which that intensity can be maintained. For most people, unless well-conditioned aerobically, this will be at the lower end of the maximal heart rate and maximal oxygen consumption zones given earlier.

(Data from Achten J, Gleeson M, Jeukendrup AE. Determination of the exercise intensity that elicits maximal fat oxidation. Med Sci Sports Exerc. 2002;34:92–97.)

One of these variables is the hormonal response, particularly that of epinephrine, norepinephrine, and glucagon, to exercise (see Chapter 7 for a discussion of the hormonal impact on metabolism). All of these hormones are elevated during exercise, and they increase the activity of lipases, which stimulates the breakdown of triglycerides into free fatty acids and glycerol, which can then be used in aerobic metabolism.

Conversely, the hormone insulin inhibits hormone-sensitive lipase activity, resulting in a decrease in the availability of free fatty acids for use in aerobic metabolism. In response to ingesting a high-carbohydrate meal or drink, blood insulin concentrations increase, resulting in inhibition of lipase activity and increased transport of glucose into skeletal muscle. The net result is an increase in carbohydrate metabolism and a decrease in triglyceride metabolism. The insulin response due to carbohydrate ingestion is one of the factors that increases use of the carbohydrate made available by a sports drink. However, during low-intensity, long-duration activity, in which carbohydrate is not ingested, blood insulin concentrations gradually decline, resulting in an increased use of triglyceride metabolism to supply the needed ATP to perform the activity.

Eventually, during long-duration, low-intensity activity, such as running a marathon, intramuscular and liver glycogen will be depleted. Depletion of glycogen stores to the point where carbohydrate metabolism is limited takes a minimum of approximately 60 minutes of continuous activity.[12] At this point, triglyceride metabolism will increase to supply the energy required to sustain activity. The above-mentioned factors indicate that in activities lasting less than approximately 60 minutes of continuous activity, ingestion of carbohydrate during activity will not necessarily improve endurance performance. So, whether ingestion of a carbohydrate sport drink during activity will improve performance due to an increase in carbohydrate metabolism in part depends on the duration of the activity. The depletion of glycogen stores in an endurance event is typically termed "hitting the wall," and is one aspect of fatigue during an endurance event. Accordingly, ingesting a carbohydrate sport drink during a long-term endurance event, such as a marathon, may postpone glycogen depletion in muscle fibers by maintaining high levels of blood-borne glucose available for rapid energy, resulting in improved performance.

Lactate Threshold

The terms **lactate threshold** and **onset of blood lactate accumulation** or **OBLA** are often used interchangeably. However, they have different meanings. *Lactate threshold* is defined as the exercise intensity at which blood lactic acid begins to accumulate above the resting concentration (Fig. 2-21). *OBLA* is the exercise intensity at which a specific (4.0 mM) blood lactic acid concentration occurs. In untrained individuals, lactate threshold occurs at approximately 50% to 60% of maximal oxygen consumption. Endurance-trained individuals' lactate threshold occurs at approximately 65% to 80% of maximal oxygen consumption, which allows performance of

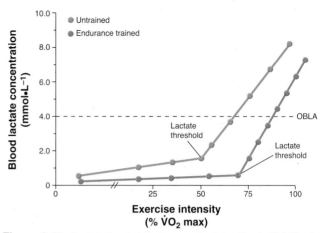

Figure 2-21. Lactate threshold is the exercise intensity at which blood lactate concentration substantially increases above rest; onset of blood lactic acid (OBLA) is when blood lactic acid level is 4.0 mM. The lactate threshold of an endurance athlete occurs at a higher exercise intensity than that of an untrained individual.

a higher exercise intensity without an increase in blood lactic acid concentration. This is important for endurance performances because lactate threshold represents the exercise intensity or race pace that can be maintained for a long period. It should be noted that the increased lactic acid concentration in blood and muscle may not be the direct cause of increased acidity (lowered pH). Rather, the increase in acidity may be more related to an inability to maintain ATP synthesis from ADP and Pi. Recall that ATP breakdown produces a hydrogen ion, whereas its synthesis consumes a hydrogen ion. As exercise intensity increases, so does acidity, because increasing amounts of ATP are hydrolyzed but exercising muscles experience difficulties in resynthesizing it, resulting in an accumulation of hydrogen ions.[11,32] Regardless of the cause, increased acidity affects the ability of muscle to generate force and power because, among other things, increased acidity affects the sarcoplasmic reticulum's ability to release and sequester calcium, impairs the binding of calcium to troponin, and decreases myosin ATPase activity (see Chapter 3).[11] All of these contribute to the muscle's inability to maintain a particular workload or pace.

Lactate threshold is of interest to endurance athletes because it has been shown that as lactate threshold increases, or occurs at a higher intensity, so does endurance performance, with significant correlations between lactate threshold and endurance performance being demonstrated.[25] For example, oxygen consumption at lactate threshold has shown significant correlations (r = 0.64–0.77) to 800-, 1500-, and 3000-m run times in male and female athletes.[49] Because of the correlation between lactate threshold and endurance performance, lactate threshold has been used to assign training intensity zones for runners, cyclists, and swimmers. Typically, training zones are established above, below, and at lactate threshold.

Aerobic Adaptations to Exercise

Aerobic adaptations to exercise can take place in both enzymatic activity and substrate availability. Increased enzymatic activity in both the Krebs cycle and the ETC could increase aerobic ATP production. Aerobic enzymes are located in the mitochondria, so an increased mitochondrial size and/or number results in an increase in aerobic enzymes. Increased availability of carbohydrate could increase the duration of exercise before carbohydrate availability limits aerobic production of ATP. Increased availability of triglyceride could increase aerobic triglyceride metabolism, resulting in less use of carbohydrate in aerobic metabolism, which would also increase the duration of exercise before reduced carbohydrate availability limits aerobic production of ATP.

Enzyme Adaptations to Aerobic Exercise

Increased mitochondrial density has long been observed in the muscles of endurance trained athletes. Thus, it is not surprising that increases in mitochondrial enzyme activity with endurance training range from 40% to 90%,[1] and that aerobic enzyme activity has been reported to be higher in "elite" than in "good" competitive endurance cyclists.[23] For example, succinic dehydrogenase (SDH) activity, one of the enzymes of Krebs cycle, has been shown to increase 95% with 5 months of endurance training, and 42% with 3 months of endurance training.[1] In contrast, increases in mitochondrial enzyme activity with sprint-type training are very inconsistent, with some studies showing increases and others showing no significant changes.[1,9] Whether an increase in mitochondrial enzymes occurs with sprint training may depend on the duration of the sprint. Short-term (less than 10 seconds) sprint training has resulted in a decrease in SDH activity, whereas long-term (greater than 10 seconds) sprint training has resulted in a significant increase in SDH activity.[42] So, as might be hypothesized, endurance-type training causes consistent increases in mitochondrial enzyme activity, whereas only long-term (greater than 10 seconds) sprint training appears to cause an increase in mitochondrial enzyme activity.

However, many factors contribute to a physical performance, and not all of them potentially limit or enhance the performance. In endurance cycling, or any endurance event, one important variable is blood supply, or capillary number and density, which determines the delivery of oxygen, blood glucose, and triglyceride to working muscle, and removal of CO_2 and lactate from working muscle. Maximal blood perfusion of muscle could potentially limit endurance performance. So, although endurance training does increase mitochondrial enzyme activity, other training adaptations must also occur to maximize improvements in endurance performance.

Substrate Adaptations to Aerobic Exercise

Availability of both carbohydrate and triglyceride for use as a substrate in aerobic metabolism could improve endurance exercise performance in several ways. If more substrate is available and used at the same rate, the duration of exercise could be increased before substrate depletion affects performance. Thus, it may be possible to run, swim, or cycle at the same pace after endurance training, but for a longer period of time. Most endurance events, however, are of a certain length. For example, a marathon is 26 miles and a stage in the Tour de France cycling race may be 100 miles (160 km). Thus, the goal of the race is to finish that distance in the least amount of time. So, to improve performance in most endurance events, not only must more substrate be available for use in aerobic metabolism but it also must be metabolized at a faster rate, so that more ATP per unit of time is obtained, and a faster race pace can be maintained for a longer period before substrate depletion. Adaptations that enable this faster rate of metabolism include, among others, increases in mitochondrial enzymes, increased capillary number and density, improved blood transport of oxygen, higher cardiac output, and faster removal of lactate.

Substrate Availability

As previously described, intramuscular glycogen does increase in response to endurance and long-duration (greater than 10 seconds) sprint training. This is important because glycogen can be used to produce ATP both aerobically and anaerobically, and significant intramuscular glycogen depletion (which can compromise performance) has been shown with endurance and sprint activities lasting as little as 6 seconds.[1] As intramuscular glycogen stores are depleted, there is an increased uptake of blood glucose by active muscle tissue. The increased blood glucose uptake appears to be controlled by local factors, with glycogen depletion stimulating increased uptake of blood glucose and lactate from the blood.[1] The increased uptake of blood glucose is in part related to an increased activity in a membrane-bound glucose transporter (GLUT-4).[20] As previously discussed, blood lactate is one means by which substrate can be moved around the body to be metabolized by different tissues, such as cardiac and inactive muscle tissue. Maintaining the availability of glucose or glycogen for use as a substrate for aerobic metabolism is important, as lack of carbohydrate is associated with fatigue[1] and "hitting the wall" in endurance events such as the marathon. Thus, the use of carbohydrate sport drinks during endurance events is not only to prevent dehydration but also to maintain blood glucose concentrations so that intramuscular glycogen depletion is delayed, along with fatigue. The need for carbohydrate use in metabolism is made apparent by dietary guidelines for athletes (Box 2-7).

Intramuscular triglyceride stores have been shown to increase with endurance training.[1] For example, with endurance training, lipid content of fast-twitch or type II muscle fibers increases 90% to 114%, and in slow-twitch or type I fibers, the lipid content increases 22%.[24] However, few studies have examined the intramuscular triglyceride response to sprint and resistance training, with the results of these studies being inconclusive.[1]

Fatty acids for use in aerobic metabolism by active tissue can also be obtained from the blood. Fatty acid concentration in the blood appears to be unchanged or even reduced after

Box 2-7 APPLYING RESEARCH

The Need for Carbohydrate during Aerobic Exercise

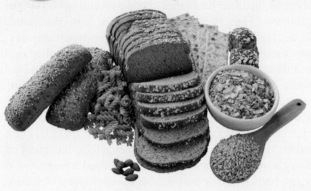

The need for carbohydrate during physical activity, especially endurance or aerobic athletic events, is clearly shown by the recommendations of the numerous governing bodies of sport nutrition, as detailed in the European Commission Report of the Scientific Committee on Food on composition and specification of food intended to meet the expenditure of intense muscular effort, especially for sportsmen (2001). The commission concluded that high pre-exercise muscle glycogen stores do not allow athletes to run faster; however, they do allow the athlete to maintain a given pace for a longer period, which results in improved endurance performance times. The improved performance is due, in part, to the decreased reliance of trained endurance athletes on the breakdown of muscle glycogen than less well-trained individuals during sub-maximal exercise at the same absolute intensity or pace. The increased aerobic capacity of the endurance athletes allows skeletal muscle to metabolize more fat at a given sub-maximal absolute intensity, therefore using less muscle glycogen. This results in "sparing" muscle and liver glycogen stores, which delays fatigue related to depletion of carbohydrate stores that are used to produce ATP.

Overall energy requirements are greater for athletes than the average person, with a significant amount often coming from carbohydrates. Keep in mind that there is a great difference between the average person exercising for a few hours each week and the competitive endurance athlete, as intake recommendations and needs are significantly increased for the latter individual. Elite endurance athletes attempting to maximize performance should consume a range of 55–65% of total daily energy from carbohydrates during periods of

heavy training, with the amount depending on the volume, intensity, type, and duration of activity. 60% of energy from carbohydrates during the training period, particularly the week before competition can result in improved muscle glycogen concentrations and improvements in performance, but again, that number varies based on the previously mentioned factors.

In absolute amounts, daily carbohydrate recommendations for athletes range from 6–10 g·kg body weight^{-1} and may reach as high as 10–12 g·kg·day^{-1} in elite endurance athletes, such as a competitive marathoner, during the finals days prior to competition. These recommendations allow for the maintenance of blood glucose levels during exercise and after exercise to maximize muscle glycogen levels. However, these intakes are highly individual based on the athlete's daily energy expenditure, type of sport, gender, and environmental factors.

During competition lasting longer than 1 hour, endurance athletes, such as road cyclists, long-distance canoeists, and triathletes, should consume easy-to-digest carbohydrate snacks. These are most often in the form of high-energy bars and carbohydrate-based sport drinks because they are easy to digest and carry throughout the race. For longer events, assuming the athlete has sufficiently pre-loaded glycogen stores, an hourly carbohydrate ingestion of 0.7 g·kg body weight^{-1} (30-60 g·hr^{-1}) helps to prolong athletic performance (Coggan and Coyle, 1991). Sport drinks should contain between 6 and 8% carbohydrate (Sawka et al., 2007) and should not exceed 10%, since higher carbohydrate concentrations slow intestinal absorption. The carbohydrate sources should be in the form of glucose, glucose polymers, sucrose, and other carbohydrates with similar properties (high glycemic index). It is clear from these recommendations that pre-exercise liver and intramuscular glycogen stores are important considerations in preparing for an endurance event and that adequate carbohydrate intake during an endurance event is vital to optimal performance, especially during the latter portions of endurance events.

References

Position of the American Dietetic Association, Dietitians of Canada, and the American College of Sports Medicine: Nutrition and Athletic Performance. *J Am Diet Assoc.* 2009;109:509–527.

Sawka MN, Burke LM, Eichner ER, Maughan RJ, Montain SJ, Stachenfeld NS. American College of Sports Medicine position stand. Exercise and fluid replacement. *Med Sci Sports Exerc.* 2007;39:377–390.

Coggan AR, Coyle EF. Carbohydrate ingestion during prolonged exercise: Effects on metabolism and performance. *Exerc Sport Sci Rev.* 1991;19:1–40.

aerobic training.[1] Although membrane-bound fatty acid transporters are increased after endurance training,[27] blood-borne fatty acid uptake by working muscles does not increase, suggesting that increased use of fatty acids following endurance training results from increased reliance on intramuscular triglycerides.[23] Substrate availability in part causes differences in the interaction of aerobic substrate use during exercise between an endurance-trained and an untrained individual. This topic will be discussed in the following section.

Substrate Use during Exercise

Recall that as exercise intensity increases, there is a gradual shift to metabolize more and more carbohydrate until at maximal workloads, in theory, 100% of aerobic metabolism occurs with carbohydrate. Evidence also shows that intramuscular glycogen depletion is associated with fatigue during endurance events. So, increased intramuscular glycogen stores brought about by training delays muscle fatigue. Another way to delay glycogen depletion and fatigue is to metabolize less glycogen and more triglyceride or fatty acids at the same absolute workload or race pace after training. In terms of substrate use, this is a major adaptation that occurs with endurance training. Endurance-trained individuals metabolize more triglyceride or fatty acids and less glycogen or glucose at the same absolute workload or race pace, resulting in a glycogen sparing effect and postponing fatigue.[1,23]

The ability to use more triglycerides and fatty acids in aerobic metabolism after training is associated with an increased aerobic capacity.[23] This means, for example, that endurance-trained individuals will metabolize a higher percentage of fat when running a 10-minute mile (1.6 km) compared with untrained individuals. As the intensity of exercise increases, trained individuals will still gradually start metabolizing more carbohydrate until, at maximal intensity, 100% carbohydrate will be metabolized. Trained individuals, however, will be at higher absolute workload or race pace than untrained individuals when they reach maximal intensity.

Quick Review

- Some amino acids can ente... metabolized.
- As the duration of activity i... triglyceride increases.
- As the intensity of activity... carbohydrate metabolism increases.
- Aerobic training adaptations include the following:
  - Increased activity of some enzymes of the Krebs cycle and electron transport chain
  - Increased intramuscular stores of glycogen and lipid
  - Increased reliance on fatty acid metabolism at the same intensity of aerobic activity after training compared with before training
  - Increased lactic acid threshold, which allows the performance of higher-intensity aerobic activity before increased blood and intramuscular acidity occurs
  - Increased density of mitochondria, number of capillaries, and myoglobin concentration

Lactate Threshold Adaptations to Exercise

The major training adaptation in lactate threshold is an increase in the relative exercise intensity (percentage of maximal oxygen consumption) at which an increase in blood lactate level occurs.[25] An increase in lactate threshold means that the trained individual is capable of performing a higher exercise intensity, predominantly using aerobic ATP production, and so can maintain a higher exercise intensity or race pace for a longer period (Fig. 2-21).

The increase in lactate threshold with training is rooted in numerous physiological adaptations, including increased ability to metabolize lipid, increased enzymes of Krebs cycle and ETC, and increased capillary density and number (see Chapter 4). All of these factors increase the workload at which the needed ATP is principally produced by aerobic metabolism, increasing the intensity or race pace that can be maintained before there is a need to rely on anaerobic metabolism.

Aerobic Metabolism at Its Best

Increases in enzyme concentrations of Krebs cycle and ETC increase the ability to perform aerobic metabolism. However, other physiological changes are also necessary to increase aerobic metabolism and lactate threshold. Mitochondrial density increases in response to aerobic training,[29] and by increasing mitochondrial volume within the cell, there is a concomitant increase in its aerobic enzyme concentration.[29] To increase the oxygen and blood glucose supply for use in aerobic metabolism and removal of CO_2, an increase in blood supply is necessary. This is accomplished by adaptations of the cardiovascular system, such as an increase in cardiac output, or the amount of blood pumped by

the heart per minute (see Chapter 5). Blood supply is also improved because of an increase in the number of capillaries surrounding each muscle fiber.[2] For example, with long periods of aerobic training, capillary number per muscle fiber increases approximately 15%.[40] This increases the surface area through which oxygen and glucose can move into and CO_2 can move out of the muscle fiber. Oxygen, once in the muscle fiber, needs to get to the mitochondria. Myoglobin, a molecule similar to hemoglobin, is found within the muscle fiber. Myoglobin not only stores small amounts of oxygen within the fiber but also assists the movement of oxygen taken up from the blood to the mitochondria, where aerobic metabolism occurs. Endurance training increases the amount of myoglobin within muscle fibers, and thus the transport of oxygen within muscle fibers.[22] It is obvious then, that training-induced improvements in the aerobic production of ATP rely upon more than just increases in the amount of aerobic enzymes.

METABOLIC RECOVERY AFTER EXERCISE

If you have ever sprinted as fast as possible for 200 m or lifted a heavy weight for 10 repetitions of the leg press, you know that your heart rate and breathing rate remain elevated for a period of time after the cessation of these activities In fact, heart rate, breathing rate, and metabolic rate remain elevated for a period of time after most types of physical activity. Metabolic recovery concerns what takes place following physical activity that allows recovery from

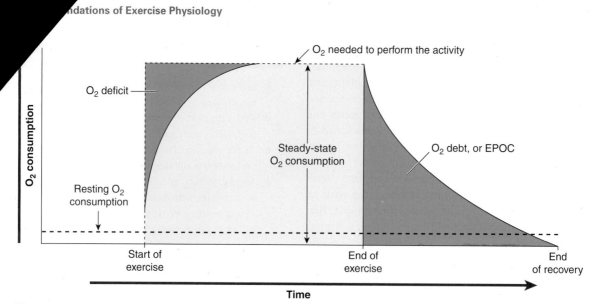

Figure 2-22. Representation of the oxygen deficit and excess postoxygen consumption (EPOC). Although oxygen consumed during the oxygen debt or EPOC is used to recover from exercise, it is greater than the oxygen deficit (see text for explanation).

the exercise just performed. After an exercise bout, especially exercise involving anaerobic metabolic processes, intramuscular PC needs to be resynthesized and intramuscular and blood acidity decreased if you are going to perform another anaerobic exercise bout soon after. Recall that energy to synthesize PC can be the obtained from the breakdown of ATP. The needed ATP for this process can be obtained from aerobic metabolism. Lactic acid concentration can be decreased if lactic acid is aerobically metabolized or used to synthesize glycogen. After an exercise bout, heart rate, breathing rate, and metabolic rate remain elevated because aerobic metabolism is used to recover from the preceding exercise bout. However, there are also other reasons why metabolic rate remains elevated for some time following an exercise bout.

Postexercise Oxygen Consumption

After an exercise bout, metabolic rate or oxygen consumption remains elevated (Fig. 2-22). Historically, the term **oxygen debt** has been used to describe the oxygen taken in above resting values after exercise. **Steady-state** oxygen consumption refers to the condition in which all the energy needed is provided by aerobic metabolism. **Oxygen deficit** describes the difference between the amount of oxygen actually consumed during exercise and that which would be consumed if energy demands could be met solely through aerobic metabolism. If the energy to perform a particular exercise intensity was not obtained aerobically, it must have been obtained anaerobically. Thus, indirectly, oxygen deficit refers to the anaerobic energy used to perform a particular workload.

Historically, oxygen debt has been divided into two major phases: the rapid phase and the slow phase. The rapid phase lasts approximately 2 to 3 minutes, during which it was thought the majority of intramuscular PC was

resynthesized. The slow phase lasts substantially longer (i.e., it may take up to several hours for the heart rate and breathing rate to return to true resting values) and was thought to involve aerobic metabolism of intramuscular and blood lactic acid and use of lactic acid in gluconeogenesis or synthesizing glucose. Approximately 70% of the lactic acid produced during exercise is aerobically metabolized, 20% is used to synthesize glucose, and 10% is used to synthesize gluconeogenic amino acids. However, substantially more oxygen is taken in during the oxygen debt than that required to perform these processes.

So, what else causes oxygen debt (Fig. 2-23)? Oxygen is needed to restore muscle and blood oxygen stores. Elevation of various hormone levels, increased body temperature, and increased heart rate and breathing rate all increase the metabolic rate slightly. As a result, oxygen debt does not

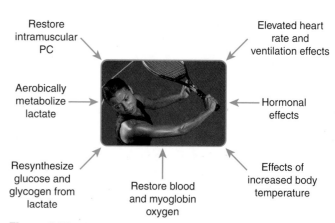

Figure 2-23. Excess postoxygen consumption is caused by several factors. Some of these factors directly result in recovery from exercise, whereas others are a result of the high metabolic rate during the exercise bout, which continues to exert an influence during recovery.

represent the same amount of oxygen as oxygen deficit, or the amount of oxygen representing the "borrowed" anaerobic energy used to perform the exercise. Therefore, the term **excess postoxygen consumption**, or **EPOC**, has been proposed to better describe the oxygen taken in above resting values after an exercise bout.

Exercise intensity has a greater impact than exercise duration on EPOC.[10,26,37] This is because at higher exercise intensities there is a greater reliance on anaerobic metabolic processes, resulting in greater PC depletion and higher lactic acid concentrations. In addition, higher-intensity exercise results in a greater increase in body temperature and hormonal response after exercise. With all these factors increasing EPOC, it might be hypothesized that performing activity during recovery could affect the recovery processes, which is discussed in the following section.

Maximizing Recovery

Maximizing the recovery processes after an anaerobic exercise bout is important, especially when repeat exercise bouts are performed, such as during interval training or running repeated sprints in any ball game. Performing **active recovery,** consisting of light-to-moderate aerobic exercise, decreases blood lactic acid concentrations significantly faster than performing no physical activity during recovery, or a **passive recovery** (Fig. 2-24). The faster decrease in lactic acid concentration with an active recovery is thought to be due to aerobic metabolism of lactic acid to provide ATP to meet the energy need of performing the light-to-moderate activity. The optimal light-to-moderate recovery aerobic exercise for cycling and running exercise are approximately 30% to 45% and 55% to 60% of maximal oxygen consumption, respectively.[35] The lower exercise intensity for cycling exercise reflects the more localized muscle involvement during this exercise mode, which

lowers the intensity at which lactate threshold occurs. No matter what type of exercise is performed during recovery, it is important that the exercise intensity is below the lactate threshold; otherwise, blood lactic acid concentration could actually increase.

Lactic acid can also be used by the liver and muscle tissue to synthesize glycogen. At 45 and 75 minutes after intense anaerobic cycling exercise, a passive recovery with no carbohydrate intake during recovery results in significantly higher muscle glycogen than does an active recovery.[15] This finding demonstrates that passive recovery results in more glycogen synthesis than active recovery because lactic acid is not metabolized to produce ATP when muscles are inactive after exercise. Activity during recovery also maintains circulation to the heart, liver, and inactive muscles, which are capable of metabolizing and using lactic acid to synthesize glycogen, thus enhancing the possibility that both of these processes take place during the recovery period.

If one way to reduce blood lactic acid concentrations is to aerobically metabolize it, you might hypothesize that individuals who are in better aerobic condition or have a higher maximal oxygen consumption might be able to decrease blood lactic acid concentrations more quickly than individuals with a lower maximal oxygen consumption. After cycling exercise, however, trained and untrained individuals show no difference in blood lactic acid concentration decreases.[5] There is, however, a positive correlation between blood lactic acid concentration decreases after weight training exercise and maximal oxygen consumption,[26] indicating that individuals with a higher maximal oxygen consumption demonstrate greater decreases in blood lactic acid concentration. This significant correlation was shown only after weight training, in which 15 repetitions were completed using 60% and 10 repetitions using 70% of one repetition maximum, but not after performing 4 repetitions using 90% of one repetition maximum. The blood lactic acid concentration was significantly lower after 90% of one repetition maximum compared with the other weight training protocols. Thus, a lack of a significant

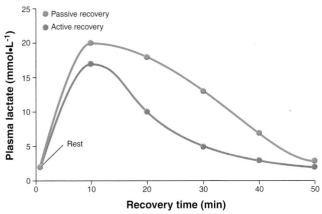

Figure 2-24. Plasma blood lactate removal occurs at a faster rate with an active recovery. Blood lactate concentrations in endurance-trained individuals with a passive and an active recovery after a cycling anaerobic work bout are shown. (Data from Fairchild TJ, Armstrong AA, Rao A, Liu H, Lawrence S, Fournier PA. Glycogen synthesis and muscle fibers during active recovery from intense exercise. Med Sci Sports Exerc. 2003;35:595–602.)

Quick Review

- Oxygen consumed above resting values during the oxygen debt or excess postoxygen consumption period following physical activity is used in recovery processes, including restoration of intramuscular PC and aerobic metabolism of lactic acid.
- An active recovery, during which light to moderate physical activity is performed, results in a quicker lowering of blood lactate than does a passive recovery.
- Increased aerobic ability is associated with quicker decreases of blood lactic acid after some, but not all, types of activity.

correlation with 90% of one repetition maximum protocol between maximal oxygen consumption and blood lactic acid concentration may be due to less lactic acid available for aerobic metabolism during recovery. The above-mentioned information demonstrates that aerobic condition or maximal oxygen consumption may help with quicker removal of blood lactic acid during recovery with some, but not all, types of activity.

MEASURING ENERGY PRODUCTION

The most accurate way to quantify any variable, including energy use or metabolic rate, during an activity is to do so directly. In the case of metabolic rate, this is achieved with a method called *direct calorimetry*. However, this technique is cumbersome and requires expensive equipment. Consequently, a less expensive and time-consuming method, termed *indirect calorimetry*, is more commonly used to determine metabolic rate. To completely understand indirect calorimetry, an understanding of direct calorimetry is needed.

Direct Calorimetry

All metabolic processes, whether aerobic or anaerobic, result in heat production and energy to perform cellular activities. In animals, including humans, the metabolic rate is directly proportional to the heat produced. Therefore, if heat production is accurately measured, metabolic rate is also directly determined. The procedure of measuring heat production to determine metabolic rate is termed **direct calorimetry.**

The most common unit used to measure metabolic rate is **kilocalorie (kcal),** which is also sometimes presented as a **Calorie** (note upper case C). A kilocalorie, as the name implies (kilo = 1,000), is actually 1,000 calories (1 kilocalorie = 4,186 joules). A calorie is defined as the heat required to raise the temperature of 1 g of water by 1°C. A calorie is a very small amount of heat; therefore, kilocalories are typically used when measuring metabolic rate.

Given the definitions of "calorie" and "kilocalorie," it is easy to calculate the number of calories or kilocalories produced if you know the temperature increase of a certain amount of water. For example, if 1.5 L (1,500 g) of water increased in temperature by 2°C, it would take 3,000 calories (1,500 g × 2°C) or 3 kcal of heat to do so. This is the basic calculation used to determine heat production or metabolic rate by direct calorimetry.

A calorimeter is an airtight chamber surrounded by a water jacket (Fig. 2-25). The heat produced because of the metabolic rate of the person in the calorimeter increases the temperature of the water jacket. Knowing the volume of water in the water jacket and the increase in temperature of the water, it is easy to calculate the number of kilocalories produced over a certain period.

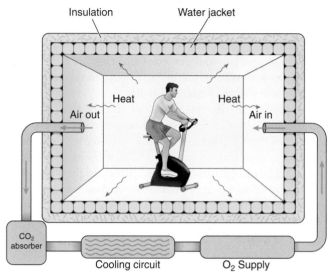

Figure 2-25. A calorimetric chamber measures heat produced. The heat produced by the person in the chamber can be calculated by measuring the temperature increase of the water jacket. Knowing the amount of heat produced allows direct calculation of the metabolic rate. Airflow through the chamber is allowed so that exchange of oxygen and carbon dioxide can take place and calculations can be corrected for evaporative cooling of sweat.

Direct calorimetry, although very accurate for determining metabolic rate, does require a calorimeter, which is an expensive piece of equipment. So, most laboratories estimate kilocalories expended at rest or during activity, or metabolic rate, by using a procedure referred to as *indirect calorimetry*.

Indirect Calorimetry

Aerobic metabolism of carbohydrate and fatty acid requires oxygen and produces CO_2 and water. The amount of oxygen used and CO_2 produced during aerobic metabolism typically is equivalent to the amounts exchanged at the lungs. So, by measuring the amounts of oxygen and CO_2 exchanged at the lungs, the amounts used and produced, respectively, in aerobic metabolism can be determined (Fig. 2-26). On the basis of the ratio of the oxygen used and CO_2 produced, which is different for carbohydrates and lipids, one can determine the percentage of carbohydrate and fatty acid being metabolized as well as the amount of energy produced. Using the amount of oxygen utilized, CO_2 produced, and their ratio to calculate energy production or metabolic rate is termed **indirect calorimetry.**

Oxygen Consumption

Oxygen consumption ($\dot{V}O_2$) can be expressed as either liters per minute of oxygen used ($L \cdot min^{-1}$) or milliliters per kilogram of body mass per minute ($mL \cdot kg^{-1} \cdot min^{-1}$). The unit $L \cdot min^{-1}$ may be most appropriate when evaluating aerobic fitness or athletic performance in situations in which you do not have to actually carry your own body weight, such as rowing or cycling on a flat surface. Alternatively,

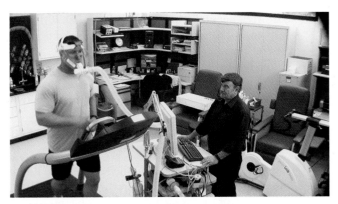

Figure 2-26. A metabolic cart determines all variables necessary to indirectly calculate metabolic rate. The variables necessary to calculate metabolic rate include oxygen consumed, carbon dioxide produced, and volume of air ventilated. (Courtesy of Bradley C. Nindl, PhD, Military Performance Division, US Army Research Institute of Environmental Medicine, Natick, Massachusetts.)

$mL \cdot kg^{-1} \cdot min^{-1}$ may be most appropriate when you have to actually carry your own body weight, such as running or cycling uphill. However, as we shall soon see, $\dot{V}O_2$ is only one part of the calculation used to determine energy expenditure when employing indirect calorimetry.

Respiratory Exchange Ratio

Respiratory exchange ratio (RER) refers to the ratio of oxygen used and CO_2 produced during metabolism. Energy expenditure and approximate percentages of lipid and carbohydrate used in aerobic metabolism can be calculated using the RER. This is possible because the amount of oxygen needed to metabolize carbohydrate and lipid and the amount of CO_2 produced are different and are in a specific ratio depending upon which substrate is being metabolized. The following equation shows the amount of oxygen needed and CO_2 produced when metabolizing a glucose ($C_6H_{12}O_6$) molecule:

$$6\ O_2 + C_6H_{12}O_6 \rightarrow 6\ CO_2 + 6\ H_2O + 30\ ATP$$

Note that six O_2 are needed and six CO_2 produced when completely aerobically metabolizing a glucose molecule. Thus,

the ratio (6 CO_2/6 O_2) of CO_2 produced and O_2 needed when aerobically metabolizing a glucose molecule is 1.0. This ratio will be the same whether calculated in the above-mentioned manner or by using the volume of CO_2 expelled ($\dot{V}CO_2$) and $\dot{V}O_2$ taken in at the lungs used, or $\dot{V}CO_2/\dot{V}O_2$.

The calculation of RER for a typical triglyceride ($C_{16}H_{32}O_2$) is shown by the following equation:

$$23\ O_2 + C_{16}H_{32}O_2 \rightarrow 16\ CO_2 + 16\ H_2O + 129\ ATP$$

Thus, the ratio of $\dot{V}CO_2/\dot{V}O_2$ will be approximately 0.70 (16 CO_2/23 O_2) when a fatty acid is aerobically metabolized. When the RER is 1.0, approximately 100% carbohydrate is being aerobically metabolized, and when the ratio is 0.7, approximately 100% triglyceride is being aerobically metabolized. When the RER is between 1.0 and 0.70, a mixture of carbohydrate and triglyceride is being metabolized (Table 2-4). Because the amount of ATP being produced is relatively constant when metabolizing either carbohydrate or triglyceride, it is also possible to approximate the number of kilocalories produced per liter of oxygen at a particular RER. At an RER of 0.85, approximately 50% carbohydrate and 50% triglyceride are being metabolized and approximately 4.86 $kcal \cdot LO_2^{-1}$ will be produced. At rest, the RER is approximately 0.80, so approximately 2/3 triglyceride and 1/3 carbohydrate are being metabolized and approximately 4.80 $kcal \cdot LO_2^{-1}$ will be produced. To obtain an estimate of energy expenditure in kilocalories used per minute, simply multiply $\dot{V}O_2$ in $LO_2 \cdot min^{-1}$ times the $kcal \cdot LO_2^{-1}$ produced at a certain RER.

Using the RER to calculate either the approximate kilocalories used per minute or the percentage of carbohydrate and triglyceride being metabolized is quite accurate during steady-state work or a workload at which the vast majority of needed energy can be obtained aerobically. The RER, however, does not account for anaerobic energy production, so if a substantial amount of energy is being obtained from anaerobic sources, the estimate of energy used is inaccurate.

Examining the above-mentioned information, you might think that the maximal value of RER is 1.0. However, at high-intensity workloads, when some of the energy required is being

Table 2-4.	The Respiratory Exchange Ratio (RER) Estimates of Percentage of Carbohydrate and Triglyceride Metabolized and Kilocalories Produced		
RER	**% Carbohydrate**	**% Triglyceride**	**kcal·LO$_2^{-1}$**
0.70	0.0	100.0	4.69
0.75	15.6	84.4	4.74
0.80	33.4	66.6	4.80
0.85	50.7	49.3	4.86
0.90	67.5	32.5	4.92
0.95	84.0	16.0	4.99
1.00	100.0	0.0	5.05

obtained anaerobically, the RER can reach values as high as 1.5 for short periods. This is due to the bicarbonate buffering system in the blood, resulting in the production of CO_2 ($H^+ + HCO_3 \rightarrow H_2CO_3^- \rightarrow CO_2 + H_2O$). This CO_2 produced by the bicarbonate buffering system can be expired at the lungs. This additional CO_2 did not come from aerobic metabolism, but it does result in an RER value greater than 1.0. However, if the RER is greater than 1.0, it is assumed that 100% carbohydrate is being metabolized (remember, only carbohydrate can be anaerobically metabolized). In addition, using RER to calculate kilocalories used when the RER is greater than 1.0 will result in an underestimation of the total energy used because anaerobic energy is not included in the calculation. The RER also does not account for protein metabolism and is more accurately termed *nonprotein RER*. In most situations, protein metabolism is minimal, so ignoring protein metabolism results in a relatively small amount of error. Despite these limitations, at steady-state exercise intensities, RER results in accurate estimates of the percentage of carbohydrate and triglyceride metabolized and total energy used.

Resting Energy Use

Basal metabolic rate (BMR) has a stringent definition. It is the metabolic rate determined in the supine position, 12 to 18 hours after a meal, immediately after waking up and in a thermoneutral environment. **Resting metabolic rate (RMR)**, on the other hand, has a less stringent definition: it is the metabolic rate approximately 4 hours after a light meal and after approximately 30 to 60 minutes of resting quietly. Most of us spend the majority of the day at or close to BMR, so it accounts for approximately 60% to 75% of the total number of calories metabolized during a day. Both RMR and BMR are affected by several factors, including the following:

- *Age:* As we get older, BMR gradually decreases because of a progressive decrease in fat-free mass.
- *Sex:* Men generally have a slightly higher BMR than women of the same body mass because of a greater fat-free mass.
- *Body temperature:* Increased body temperature results in an increase in BMR.
- *Stress:* Stress increases BMR due to increased activity of the sympathetic nervous system.
- *Body surface area:* The greater the body surface area available for heat loss, the greater the BMR.

In addition, $\dot{V}O_2$ indicates a time such as minutes. Energy expenditure at rest and during exercise can be estimated from the RER and the oxygen used in aerobic metabolism over a period of time. For example, at rest, you use approximately 3.5 $mL\cdot kg^{-1}\cdot min^{-1}$. Assuming a body mass of 100 kg (220 lbs), you would use in metabolism 350 $mLO_2\cdot min^{-1}$ (3.5 $mLO_2\cdot kg^{-1}\cdot min^{-1} \times 100$ kg) or 3.5 $LO_2\cdot min^{-1}$. This would result in 21,000 $mLO_2\cdot h^{-1}$ or 21 $LO_2\cdot h^{-1}$ and 504 $LO_2\cdot d^{-1}$. If we assume an average RER at rest of 0.8, this would result in approximately 4.80 $kcal\cdot LO_2^{-1}$. An estimate of energy expenditure in kilocalories over 1 day, assuming no strenuous physical activity, can be made by multiplying liters of O_2 used in metabolism and kilocalories obtained per liter of O_2. So, over 1 day, this individual would have a resting energy expenditure of 504 $LO_2\cdot d^{-1} \times$ 4.80 $kcal\cdot LO_2^{-1}$, or 2419.2 kcal. These same calculations can be used to estimate energy expenditure over any time frame, as well as during activity. However, the assumptions and limitations of RER as discussed earlier need to be considered and met if the estimate of energy use is to be as accurate as possible. Liters per minute and milliliters per kilogram per minute of oxygen used are the most common units for expressing oxygen consumption; however, oxygen consumption is also expressed in metabolic equivalents, or how much oxygen is being used relative to resting oxygen consumption (Box 2-8).

Box 2-8 PRACTICAL QUESTIONS FROM STUDENTS

When I Am on the Elliptical Machine at the Gym, the Computer Screen Tells Me That I Am at 9 METs. What Is a MET and What Does This Mean?

A MET is a metabolic equivalent of an individual's resting metabolic rate (RMR), used to express the energy cost of an activity. One MET is equivalent to RMR, and the number of METs is a multiple of RMR. As RMR differs for each individual based on such factors as age, weight, and body composition, a MET also differs. One MET is usually equivalent to 200 to 250 mL of oxygen, depending on the individual, or approximately 3.5 $mL\cdot kg^{-1}\cdot min^{-1}$ of oxygen per minute. Thus, if you are exercising at an intensity of 9 METs, you are working at an intensity equivalent to 9 times your resting metabolic rate. METs are also used to classify exercise intensity. An exercise that burns 3 to 6 METs is considered moderate intensity, and an exercise that burns more than 6 METs is considered vigorous intensity. Thus, at 9 METs, you would be exercising at a vigorous intensity.

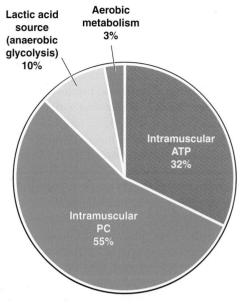

Figure 2-28. **Estimations of adenosine triphosphate (ATP) sources during a 3-second sprint show considerable interaction.** Even though a 3-second sprint is an anaerobic event, some of the needed ATP is generated aerobically. (Data from Spencer M, Bishop D, Dawson B, et al. Physiological and metabolic responses of repeated-sprint activities specific to field-based team sports. Sports Med. 2005;35:1025–1044.)

INTERACTIONS OF ANAEROBIC AND AEROBIC METABOLISM

Anaerobic energy sources provide the majority of needed ATP to perform high-intensity, short-duration maximal physical activity, and aerobic metabolism provides the majority of needed ATP to perform long-duration, low-intensity physical activity. This has led to estimates of the percentage of ATP obtained from anaerobic and aerobic sources to perform physical activity of varying lengths (Fig. 2-27), as well as for specific activities, such as Olympic weight lifting, the 200-m swim, soccer, and many other events. These estimates have been used by some coaches to estimate the percentage of training time that should be spent in various training activities in preparation for competing in a particular event. However, they must be viewed as guidelines concerning energy dependence on aerobic and anaerobic energy metabolism, because there will be individual variation. This variation may have as its basis the specific position played in a sport or differences in strategy or type of play that characterize many events. For example, the percentage of ATP derived aerobically and anaerobically will vary considerably in a soccer field player versus a goalie or in a fast-paced offense versus a slow-paced offense in basketball. In addition, no energy source of ATP is ever turned off, and all sources supply some ATP at all times. As will be discussed in the following sections, even though

aerobic or anaerobic metabolism supplies the majority of ATP for a particular type of activity, there is considerable interaction of aerobic and anaerobic metabolism that may not be readily apparent in many activities.

Anaerobic Event Metabolic Interactions

Activities such as Olympic weight lifting, shot-putting, high jumping, and diving, due to their high-intensity, very short-duration nature, rely predominantly on intramuscular ATP and PC as an energy source. Events requiring maximal power development lasting as short as approximately 3 seconds, however, start to derive a higher percentage of the needed ATP from other metabolic sources.[43] It has been estimated that a 3-second sprint, although still depending heavily on intramuscular ATP and PC, obtains considerable ATP from other metabolic sources (Fig. 2-28). Notice that glycolysis resulting in lactic acid provides approximately 10% of the needed ATP, and aerobic generation of ATP provides but a small percentage of the needed energy

Figure 2-27. **Anaerobic and aerobic energy contributions vary with the duration of activity.** The longer the duration of the activity, the greater the contribution of energy from aerobic metabolism. One assumption of these types of estimates is that the activity is performed at near maximal intensity for the duration of the activity. This means that the estimate of anaerobic and aerobic energy contributions for a 10-minute run assumes that the run is performed with the intent to run as far as possible in 10 minutes.

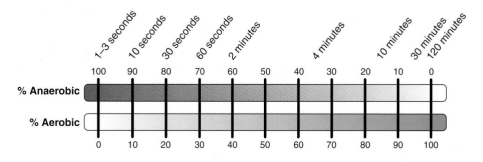

for a 3-second sprint. As the length of a sprint increases, an increasingly higher percentage of the needed ATP comes from sources other than intramuscular PC and ATP. In a 6-second cycling sprint, it has been estimated that approximately 44% and 50% of the needed ATP are derived from glycolysis, resulting in lactic acid production and intramuscular PC, respectively.[17] If a cycling sprint is 30 seconds in length, approximately 38%, 45%, and 17% of the needed ATP are provided by aerobic metabolism, glycolysis resulting in lactic acid, and intramuscular ATP-PC, respectively.[36] Even though short sprints are thought of as anaerobic events, notice that as the duration of the sprint increases, resulting in a decrease in maximal power development, a significant amount of the ATP needed is produced by aerobic metabolism. Thus, there is considerable interaction of the metabolic processes providing the needed ATP, even in high-intensity, short-duration sprints.

Short-duration repeated sprints interspersed with brief recovery periods are common occurrences in many sports, such as soccer and basketball, as well as during interval training. As might be expected, the percentage of needed ATP varies markedly depending on the duration of the sprint and length of the recovery period between successive sprints. During two 30-second cycle sprints separated by 4 minutes of recovery, there is approximately a 41% reduction in the amount of ATP generated anaerobically from the first to the second sprint.[7] The decrease in the amount of ATP generated anaerobically is partially offset by a 15% increase in oxygen consumption during the second sprint, resulting in only approximately an 18% decrease in the power during the second sprint. This indicates that a higher percentage of the needed ATP was generated aerobically during the second sprint compared with the first sprint. So, the interaction of the metabolic sources of ATP changes during successive sprints.

The duration of repeat sprints and the duration of the recovery period between sprints affect the interaction of the metabolic sources of ATP. After 15-, 30-, and 40-m repeat sprints, totaling a distance of 600 m, interspaced with 30-second passive recovery periods, EPOC was significantly higher after the 30- and 40-m sprints than the 15-m sprints.[4] However, postexercise blood lactic acid concentration was significantly lower after the 15-m sprints than the 30- and 40-m sprints, indicating that the longer repeat sprints depended more on aerobic metabolism and glycolysis, resulting in lactic acid production for the needed ATP.

The length of the recovery period between successive sprints also influences the interaction of the metabolic sources of ATP. Comparisons of performance during successive sprints of 15 and 40 m and blood lactic acid concentrations indicate that 30-, 60-, and 120-second recovery periods allowed sufficient resynthesis of intramuscular ATP and PC, so that these energy sources could be used to supply the needed ATP in successive 15-m sprints.[3] These data also demonstrated that a recovery

period of at least 120 seconds is needed between 40-m sprints to adequately replenish intramuscular ATP and PC to maintain sprint ability. The shorter recovery periods did not allow adequate resynthesis of intramuscular ATP and PC, so with the shorter recovery periods, more of the needed ATP was generated by glycolysis, resulting in lactic acid. So, both the duration of sprint intervals and the length of the recovery period separating repeat sprints affect the interaction of the metabolic processes. In general, as the length of repeat sprints increases, there will be a greater dependency on aerobic metabolism and glycolysis, resulting in greater production of lactic acid and resultant fatigue. Additionally, as the duration of recovery periods between repeat sprints shortens, there will be a greater dependency on glycolysis, resulting in lactic acid production, to supply the needed ATP. Note that sprint performance will decrease in successive sprints if the recovery periods are not of sufficient length to allow resynthesis of intramuscular ATP and PC and decreased intramuscular and blood acidity.

Endurance Event Metabolic Interactions

Long-duration, low-intensity activities, such as the marathon or road cycling, derive the majority of the needed ATP from aerobic metabolism. However, some of the needed energy is produced by anaerobic sources, and there is interaction of aerobic and anaerobic metabolism. If a road cyclist climbs a hill at a faster pace than that which can be maintained by using only aerobic metabolism, some of the needed ATP will be derived from anaerobic metabolism. If climbing the hill is followed by a downhill portion of the race, recovery, such as aerobic metabolism of lactic acid and decreasing intramuscular acidity, can take place because the downhill portion of the race does not require use of the maximal amount of ATP that can be obtained from aerobic metabolism. This type of interaction between aerobic metabolism, anaerobic metabolism, and recovery processes can occur in any long-duration, low-intensity activity.

Some activities that may appear to be predominantly anaerobic in nature actually obtain a substantial portion of the energy needed from aerobic metabolism. The relative contribution of aerobically synthesized ATP during 200-, 400-, 800-, and 1500-m runs performed by trained athletes is 29%, 43%, 66%, and 84%, respectively.[44] This demonstrates that the 800-m run derived the majority of the needed energy from aerobic metabolism and that sprinting 200 m also derived a significant portion of the needed ATP from aerobic metabolism. It also indicates the crossover to predominantly (>50%) ATP produced by aerobic metabolism occurs somewhere between 15 and 30 seconds into these running events (Fig. 2-29). In the longer events of 800 and 1,500 m, after the crossover to a predominant dependence on aerobic metabolism, there is a gradual increase in that dependence until virtually all

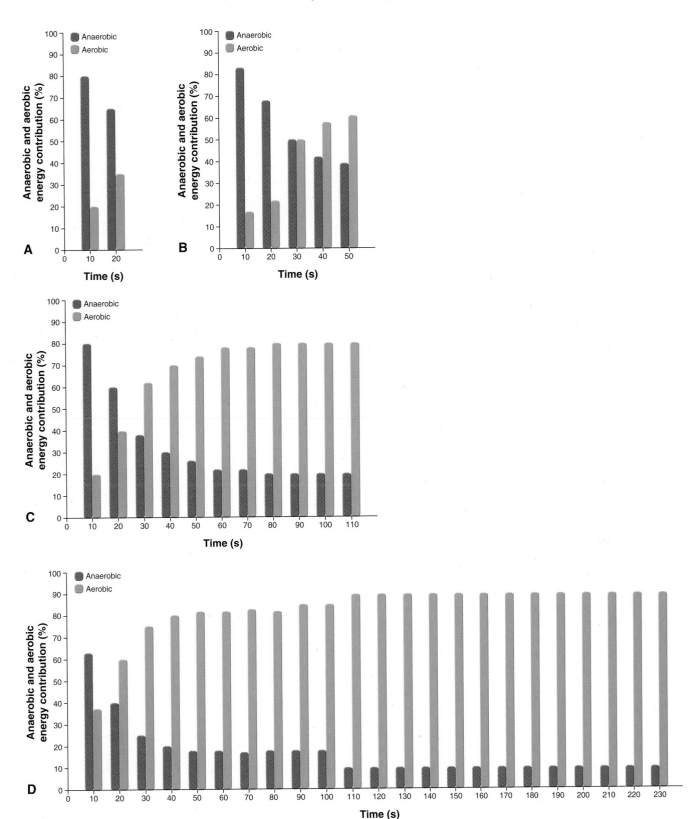

Figure 2-29. Percentages of anaerobic and aerobic energy contributions to running events 200 to 1,500 m vary during the event. During all of these events, there is initially a greater reliance on anaerobic sources of adenosine triphosphate (ATP). As the event continues, there is a greater reliance on aerobic metabolism to generate the needed ATP. **(A)** 200-m sprint. **(B)** 400-m. **(C)** 800-m. **(D)** 1,500-m. (Data from Spencer MR, Gastin B. Energy system contribution during 200- to 1500-m running in highly trained athletes. Med Sci Sports Exerc. 2001;33:157–162.)

the energy needed to sustain the activity for the duration of the race is provided by aerobic metabolism. As would be expected, as the duration of any particular activity increases, less ATP is obtained from anaerobic metabolism. However, some ATP is still obtained from anaerobic metabolism in the 1,500-m event.

There is considerable interaction of aerobic and anaerobic metabolism even in events or activities that are thought of as depending predominantly on a single metabolic pathway. For example, in a 3-second maximal sprint, approximately 3% of the needed ATP is derived from aerobic metabolism, whereas in a 1,500-m run, approximately 16% of the needed ATP is produced by anaerobic metabolism. Thus, even events or activities that are thought of as depending predominantly on aerobic metabolism do derive some energy from anaerobic metabolism, and vise versa.

Quick Review

- Anaerobic metabolism (intramuscular adenosine triphosphate [ATP] and phosphocreatine and glycolysis) provides the majority of ATP during short-duration, high-intensity physical activity.
- As the length of an anaerobic exercise bout increases, there is a greater dependence on glycolysis and aerobic metabolism for the needed ATP.
- As the duration of physical activity increases beyond approximately 3 minutes, exercise intensity decreases, and there is a greater reliance on aerobic than anaerobic metabolism.
- Even though some activities derive the majority of needed ATP from a particular source, there is a great deal of interaction among ATP sources in many activities.

CASE STUDY

Scenario

You are the director of the exercise physiology research team at the Olympic Training Center. An endurance athlete comes into your testing facility to have her maximal aerobic capacity evaluated. One of your exercise physiologist interns administers a graded maximal exertion treadmill exercise test. As the test is proceeding, he is monitoring heart rate, ventilation, ratings of perceived exertion, blood lactate, oxygen consumption, CO_2 production, and RER. The intern notices that as the test is progressing, heart rate is increasing, ventilation is increasing, and everything appears normal. However, the RER began at 0.80, was 0.85 at approximately 4 minutes into the test, was at 1.0 approximately 7 minutes into the test, and then surpassed 1.0 to achieve a maximum of 1.3 before volitional exhaustion was achieved. The intern was somewhat puzzled by how the RER could reach a number greater than 1.0 and insists that the oxygen analyzer was broken. He remembered learning in exercise physiology class that an RER of 0.85 indicates that approximately 50% carbohydrate and 50% triglyceride are being metabolized aerobically, and an RER of 1.0 indicates that 100% carbohydrate and 0% lipids are being metabolized. What do you do?

Options

You explain to the intern that he is partially correct; the RER is the ratio of $\dot{V}CO_2$ to $\dot{V}O_2$. When the RER is 1.0, approximately 100% carbohydrate is being aerobically metabolized, and when the ratio is 0.7, approximately 100% of the energy demand is being met by the aerobic metabolism of lipids. When the RER is between 1.0 and 0.70, a mixture of carbohydrate and triglyceride is being metabolized. At an RER of 0.85, approximately 50% carbohydrate and 50% triglyceride are being metabolized. Thus, it might be reasonable to think that the maximal value of RER is 1.0. However, at maximal exercise intensities, when energy is being obtained anaerobically, the RER can reach values as high as 1.5 for short periods. This is due to the bicarbonate

buffering system in the blood, which results in the production of CO_2 ($H^+ + HCO_3^- \rightarrow H_2CO_3^- \rightarrow CO_2 + H_2O$). This CO_2 produced by the bicarbonate buffering system can be expired at the lungs. This additional CO_2 did not come from aerobic metabolism but does result in an RER value greater than 1.0. However, if the RER is greater than 1.0, it is assumed that 100% carbohydrate is being metabolized (remember, only carbohydrate can be anaerobically metabolized).

Scenario

You are the coach of a track team. One of the athletes you are coaching insists on falling to the ground immediately after 150- to 200-m sprints during interval training sessions and stays lying flat on the ground until the next interval. He does this because he believes this will lower blood and muscle lactic acid between intervals and so allow a more rapid recovery between intervals. What do you do?

Options

First congratulate the athlete on knowing that blood lactic acid levels are related to fatigue during high-intensity activities such as interval training. Then explain that light to moderate activity such as slow jogging will lower the acidity faster than just lying on the ground between intervals, and that this is due to several reasons. First, the lactic acid can be metabolized by the muscle to provide energy (ATP) to perform the light activity. Second, the light activity keeps blood flowing to muscle, supplying it with lactic acid that can also be used to synthesize glucose that can be used for fuel in the next interval. Both of these factors help to reduce blood lactic acid at a faster rate than just lying on the ground between intervals. Ask the athlete to try slow jogging between intervals during the next interval training session. Tell him you are sure he will notice a quicker recovery between intervals and have a higher quality training session compared with just lying on the ground between intervals.

CHAPTER SUMMARY

Both the anaerobic and aerobic metabolic pathways provide cells with energy in the form of ATP for cellular activities and performing physical activity. Intramuscular ATP and PC, as well as glycolysis, resulting in production of lactic acid, are anaerobic sources of energy and are the predominant energy sources for short-duration, high-intensity physical activities. Carbohydrates, lipids, and proteins can all be aerobically metabolized in the mitochondria by the Krebs cycle and the electron transport system. Normally, carbohydrate and triglyceride are the predominant aerobic substrates, with protein in the form of amino acids being metabolized minimally. Aerobic metabolism is the dominant ATP source for long-duration, low-intensity physical activity. However, there is considerable interaction of aerobic and anaerobic metabolism during both short-duration, high-intensity and long-duration, low-intensity activities. Both aerobic and anaerobic metabolism adapt to training in various ways, such as increasing activity of various enzymes and increasing substrate availability, which increase physical performance capabilities. Effective recovery after an exercise bout is also in part dependent upon metabolic processes. During recovery, oxygen consumed above resting values (EPOC) is used by aerobic pathways to metabolize lactic acid and replenish intramuscular PC. An understanding of metabolic recovery processes, and of how ATP is generated both aerobically and anaerobically, is necessary to appreciate what limits performance and causes fatigue in various activities and sports. In turn, knowledge of these factors allows the development of training and competition strategies to optimize physical performance.

REVIEW QUESTIONS

Fill-in-the Blank

1. The process of converting the plant and animal products eaten as food into energy is termed _____.

2. _____ is a product of anaerobic metabolism, which is associated with an increase in blood and intramuscular acidity.

3. Anaerobic metabolism of carbohydrate produces more/less/the same energy per second than aerobic metabolism of carbohydrate, triglyceride, or protein.

4. Training adaptations to _____ include increased activity of some enzymes, increased intramuscular stores of glycogen, and increased intramuscular buffering ability.

5. At a respiratory exchange ratio of 1.00, approximately 100% _____ is being aerobically metabolized.

Multiple Choice

1. Which of the following is a factor in determining which energy substrate will be used during exercise?
   a. The duration of the exercise
   b. Whether energy is being supplied aerobically or anaerobically
   c. The intensity of the exercise
   d. Substrate availability
   e. All of the above

2. Which of the following energy substrates can be metabolized aerobically to supply energy?
   a. Carbohydrate
   b. Triglyceride
   c. Protein
   d. Fat
   e. All of the above

3. What bioenergetic adaptations occur with training to increase performance in short-duration, high-intensity activities such as weight training and short sprints?
   a. Changes in the level of enzyme creatine kinase
   b. Changes in the levels of enzymes of the Krebs cycle
   c. Changes in the levels of enzymes of electron transport chain
   d. Increased lipolysis
   e. Increased ability to utilize intramuscular triglycerides

4. Lactate threshold occurs at approximately _____of maximal oxygen consumption in **untrained** individuals and at approximately _____of maximal oxygen consumption in **endurance-trained** individuals, which allows endurance-trained individuals to perform a higher workload without an increase in blood lactic acid concentration.
   a. 100%; 100%
   b. 50% to 60%; 65% to 80%
   c. 80%; 50%
   d. 80% to 90%; 90% to 100%
   e. 30%; 50%

5. An endurance-trained individual will metabolize a higher percentage of fatty acids when running at the same absolute workload or race pace compared with an untrained individual due to what training adaptations?
   a. Increases in the level of enzyme creatine kinase
   b. Increases in the levels of enzymes of glycolysis
   c. Increases in the levels of enzymes of Krebs cycle and electron transport
   d. Increases in the levels of enzymes of beta oxidation
   e. c and d

True/False

1. Glucose is the predominant energy source for high-intensity physical activity lasting several seconds.
2. The net gain in ATP due to glycolysis is two, if starting with glucose, and three, if starting with glycogen as the substrate.
3. Lactic acid concentration in blood and muscle may not be the direct cause of increased acidity; however, its increase occurs at least coincidentally with factors associated with an inability to maintain a particular workload or pace.
4. The term oxygen deficit describes the oxygen taken in above resting values after exercise.
5. To determine metabolic rate, many laboratories estimate kilocalories expended during activity by using indirect calorimetry because direct calorimetry requires expensive equipment.

Short Answer

1. What determines whether glycolysis will produce pyruvic acid or lactic acid?
2. Describe the difference between ATP and ADP. How is each formed?
3. Why is it advantageous to gradually switch to carbohydrate metabolism as aerobic exercise intensity increases?

Matching

1. Match the following terms with their correct definitions:

Beta oxidation	A process in which an amino acid is metabolized and loses its nitrogen group
Electron transport chain	A process during which fatty acids are broken into two-carbon molecules that then are transformed into acetyl-CoA
Deamination	A series of chemical reactions taking place inside the mitochondria involved in metabolism of acetyl-CoA, resulting in production of adenosine triphosphate (ATP), carbon dioxide, and hydrogen ions
Cori cycle	A series of chemical reactions that takes place inside the mitochondria involving cytochromes that result in ATP and water being produced
Krebs cycle	A process that synthesizes liver glycogen from the lactic acid produced in skeletal muscle or other tissues

2. Match the following with what they are composed of:

Fatty acids and glycerol	Glycogen
Glucose	Protein
Amino acids	Triglycerides

Critical Thinking Questions

1. From a bioenergetics perspective, why is it possible to gain body fat if you eat excessive amounts of protein or carbohydrate?
2. What bioenergetic training adaptations bring about the ability to better perform an endurance event, such as running a marathon, after aerobic training?

KEY TERMS

active recovery: performance of light physical activity immediately after an exercise bout to aid recovery

adenosine triphosphate (ATP): a high-energy phosphate molecule synthesized and used by cells for energy to perform cellular activities

adenosine diphosphate (ADP): a molecule that combines with inorganic phosphate to form ATP

aerobic metabolism: a metabolic process needing oxygen

anabolic reaction: a process in which simple substances are synthesized into more complex substances

anaerobic metabolism: a metabolic process not needing oxygen

ATP-PC system: use of energy obtained from intramuscular ATP and phosphocreatine stores to perform cellular activities, normally utilized during short-duration, high-intensity physical activity

basal metabolic rate (BMR): metabolic rate determined in a thermal neutral environment, 12 to 18 hours after a meal, immediately after rising in a resting, supine position

beta oxidation: a series of reactions that breakdown fatty acids resulting in acetyl-CoA

bioenergetics: chemical processes involved in the production and breakdown of cellular ATP

catabolic reaction: a process in which complex substances are broken down into simpler substances, yielding energy

deamination: removal of the amino group (NH_2) from a molecule such as an amino acid

direct calorimetry: determination of the metabolic rate of an organism by direct measurement of the amount of heat produced

electron transport chain (ETC): a series of chemical reactions that takes place inside the mitochondria, involving cytochromes, that result in the production of ATP and water

enzyme: a protein molecule that lowers the energy of activation and in doing so facilitates a chemical reaction

essential amino acid: an amino acid that the human body cannot synthesize

excess post oxygen consumption (EPOC): the additional oxygen consumed above resting value after an exercise bout that is utilized to aid in many recovery processes a similar term is oxygen debt

fatty acid: a compound composed of a carbon chain and hydrogen atoms with an acid group (COOH) at one end and a methyl group (CH_3) at the other

flavin adenine dinucleotide (FAD): one of several molecules that serve as an electron and hydrogen carrier in bioenergetics

gluconeogenic: referring to synthesis of glucose from a noncarbohydrate precursor

glycogen: polysaccharide form in which animals store carbohydrate

glycogenolysis: breakdown of glycogen into glucose

glycogenesis: synthesis of glycogen from glucose molecules

glycolysis: series of chemical reactions breaking down glucose into pyruvic acid

hormone-sensitive lipase: enzyme found in adipose cells and muscle fibers that breaks down triglyceride into glycerol and fatty acids

indirect calorimetry: estimation of the metabolic rate of an organism from the amount of oxygen consumed and carbon dioxide produced

kilocalorie (kcal): amount of energy necessary to raise 1,000 g of water 1°C

Krebs cycle: series of chemical reactions taking place inside the mitochondria involved in metabolism of acetyl-CoA, resulting in production of ATP, carbon dioxide, and hydrogen ions

lactate threshold: workload at which blood lactate concentration increases significantly above the resting level

lipolysis: breakdown of triglyceride into glycerol and fatty acids

lipoprotein lipase: an enzyme that breaks down triglycerides in the bloodstream into glycerol and fatty acids

monounsaturated fatty acid: a fatty acid that has one double bond between its carbon molecules and so contains two less hydrogen atoms than it could maximally contain

nicotinamide adenine dinucleotide (NAD^+): one of several molecules that serve as an electron and hydrogen carrier in bioenergetics

nonessential amino acid: an amino acid that can be synthesized by the human body

passive recovery: performance of no physical activity immediately following an exercise bout

polyunsaturated fatty acid: fatty acid that has at least two double bonds between its carbon molecules and so contains at least four less hydrogen atoms than it could maximally contain

phosphocreatine (PC): a molecule stored intramuscularly that provides energy for the synthesis of ATP

onset of blood lactate accumulation (OBLA): the workload at which blood lactate concentration increases to more than 4.0 mM

oxidative phosphorylation: a process in which inorganic phosphate is bound to ADP, producing ATP during the ETC

oxygen debt: the additional oxygen consumed above resting value after an exercise bout that is used to aid in many recovery processes; a similar term is EPOC

oxygen deficit: the difference between the oxygen needed to perform a particular workload solely through aerobic metabolism and the oxygen actually consumed at the start of performing a work bout

protease: an enzyme that hydrolyzes a protein

respiratory assemblies: specialized hydrogen ion channels located in the mitochondrial inner membrane that are important in the production of ATP

respiratory exchange ratio (RER): the ratio of carbon dioxide production to oxygen consumed; this ratio is indicative of the percentage of carbohydrate and triglyceride being aerobically metabolized

resting metabolic rate (RMR): the metabolic rate determined 4 hours after a light meal and after approximately 30 to 60 minutes of resting quietly

saturated fatty acid: a fatty acid with no double bonds between its carbon molecules and thus containing the maximum number of hydrogen molecules

steady state: a workload during which aerobic metabolism supplies all of the needed energy

triglycerides: the major form of fat molecule composed of a glycerol and three fatty acid molecules

unsaturated fatty acid: a fatty acid that has at least one double bond between its carbon molecules and so contains at least two less hydrogen atoms than it could maximally contain

REFERENCES

1. Abernethy PJ, Thayer R, Taylor AW. Acute and chronic responses of skeletal muscle to endurance and sprint exercise: a review. Sports Med. 1990;10:365.
2. Andersen P, Henriksson J. Capillary supply of the quadriceps femoris muscle of man: adaptive response to exercise. J Physiol. 1977;270:677–690.
3. Balsom PD, Seger JY, Sjodin B, et al. Maximal-intensity intermittent exercise: effect of recovery duration. Int J Sports Med. 1992; 13:528.
4. Balsom PD, Seger JY, Sjodin B, et al. Physiological responses to maximal intensity intermittent exercise. Eur J Appl Physiol Occup Physiol. 1992;65:144.
5. Bassett DR Jr, Merrill PW, Nagle FJ, et al. Rate of decline in blood lactate after cycling exercise in endurance-trained and -untrained subjects. J Appl Physiol. 1991;70:1816.
6. Berg JM, Tymoczko JL, Stryer L. Biochemistry. WH Freeman and Co, 1991.
7. Bogdanis GC, Nevill ME, Boobis LH, et al. Contribution of phosphocreatine and aerobic metabolism to energy supply during repeated sprint exercise. J Appl Physiol. 1996;80:876.
8. Brooks GA. Intra- and extra-cellular lactate shuttles. Med Sci Sports Exerc. 2000;32:790.
9. Burgomaster KA, Heigenhauser GJ, Gibala MJ. Effect of short-term sprint interval training on human skeletal muscle carbohydrate metabolism during exercise and time-trial performance. J Appl Physiol. 2006;100:2041.
10. Burleson MA Jr, O'Bryant HS, Stone MH, et al. Effect of weight training exercise and treadmill exercise on post-exercise oxygen consumption. Med Sci Sports Exerc. 1998;30:518.
11. Cairns SP. Lactic acid and exercise performance: culprit or friend? Sports Med. 2006;36:279.
12. Convertino VA, Armstrong LE, Coyle EF, et al. American College of Sports Medicine position stand: exercise and fluid replacement. Med Sci Sports Exerc. 1996;28(1):i–vii.
13. Costill DL, Coyle EF, Fink WF, et al. Adaptations in skeletal muscle following strength training. J Appl Physiol. 1979;46:96.
14. Dawson B, Fitzsimons M, Green S, et al. Changes in performance, muscle metabolites, enzymes and fibre types after short sprint training. Eur J Appl Physiol Occup Physiol. 1998;78:163.
15. Fairchild TJ, Armstrong AA, Rao A, et al. Glycogen synthesis in muscle fibers during active recovery from intense exercise. Med Sci Sports Exerc. 2003;35:595.
16. Fitts R. Cellular, molecular, and metabolic basis of muscle fatigue In: Handbook of Physiology Exercise: Regulation and Integration of Multiple Systems. Bethesda, MD: American Physiological Society, 1996:1151.
17. Gaitanos GC, Williams C, Boobis LH, et al. Human muscle metabolism during intermittent maximal exercise. J Appl Physiol. 1993;75:712.
18. Gladden LB. The role of skeletal muscle in lactate exchange during exercise: introduction. Med Sci Sports Exerc. 2000;32:753.
19. Graham T. Skeletal muscle amino acid metabolism and ammonia production during exercise. In: Exercise Metabolism. Champaign, IL: Human Kinetics, 1995:131.
20. Greiwe JS, Hickner RC, Hansen PA, et al. Effects of endurance exercise training on muscle glycogen accumulation in humans. J Appl Physiol. 1999;87:222.
21. Groff J, Gropper S. Advanced Nutrition and Human Metabolism. Belmont, CA: Wadsworth/Thompson Learning, 2000.
22. Holloszy JO. Adaptation of skeletal muscle to endurance exercise. Med Sci Sports. 1975;7:155.
23. Hawley JA, Stepto NK. Adaptations to training in endurance cyclists: implications for performance. Sports Med. 2001;31:511.
24. Howald H, Hoppeler H, Claassen H, et al. Influences of endurance training on the ultrastructural composition of the different muscle fiber types in humans. Pflugers Arch. 1985;403:369.

25. Jones AM, Carter H. The effect of endurance training on parameters of aerobic fitness. Sports Med. 2000;29:373.

26. Kang J, Hoffman JR, Im J, et al. Evaluation of physiological responses during recovery following three resistance exercise programs. J Strength Cond Res. 2005;19:305.

27. Kiens B, Essen-Gustavsson B, Christensen NJ, et al. Skeletal muscle substrate utilization during submaximal exercise in man: effect of endurance training. J Physiol. 1993;469:459.

28. Komi P, Suominen H, Heikkinen E, et al. Effects of heavy resistance and explosive-type strength training methods on mechanical, functional, and metabolic aspects of performance. In: Komi PV, ed. Exercise and Sport Biology. Champaign, IL: Human Kinetics, 1982:90.

29. Koves TR, Noland RC, Bates AL, et al. Subsarcolemmal and intermyofibrillar mitochondria play distinct roles in regulating skeletal muscle fatty acid metabolism. Am J Physiol Cell Physiol. 2005;288:C1074.

30. Kraemer WJ, Volek JS, Clark KL, et al. Influence of exercise training on physiological and performance changes with weight loss in men. Med Sci Sports Exerc. 1999;31:1320.

31. Kubukeli ZN, Noakes TD, Dennis SC. Training techniques to improve endurance exercise performances. Sports Med. 2002;32:489.

32. Lamb GD, Stephenson DG. Point: lactic acid accumulation is an advantage during muscle activity. J Appl Physiol. 2006;100:1410.

33. MacDougall JD, Hicks AL, MacDonald JR, et al. Muscle performance and enzymatic adaptations to sprint interval training. J Appl Physiol. 1998;84:2138.

34. MacDougall JD, Ward GR, Sale DG, et al. Biochemical adaptation of human skeletal muscle to heavy resistance training and immobilization. J Appl Physiol. 1977;43:700.

35. McLellan TM, Skinner JS. Blood lactate removal during active recovery related to anaerobic threshold. Int J Sports Med. 1982;3:224.

36. Melbo J, Gramvik P, Jebens E. Aerobic and anaerobic energy released during 10 and 30s bicycle sprints. Acta Kinesiol Univ Tartuensis. 1999;4:122.

37. Melby CL, Tincknell T, Schmidt WD. Energy expenditure following a bout of non-steady state resistance exercise. J Sports Med Phys Fitness. 1992;32:128.

38. Meyer R, Wiseman R. The metabolic systems: control of atp synthesis in skeletal muscle. In: ACSM's Advanced Exercise Physiology. Philadelphia, PA: Lippincott Williams & Wilkins, 2006:370.

39. Parra J, Cadefau JA, Rodas G, et al. The distribution of rest periods affects performance and adaptations of energy metabolism induced by high-intensity training in human muscle. Acta Physiol Scand. 2000;169:157.

40. Rico-Sanz J, Rankinen T, Joanisse DR, et al. Familial resemblance for muscle phenotypes in the HERITAGE Family Study. Med Sci Sports Exerc. 2003;35:1360–1366.

41. Rodas G, Ventura JL, Cadefau JA, et al. A short training programme for the rapid improvement of both aerobic and anaerobic metabolism. Eur J Appl Physiol. 2000;82:480.

42. Ross A, Leveritt M. Long-term metabolic and skeletal muscle adaptations to short-sprint training: implications for sprint training and tapering. Sports Med. 2001;31:1063.

43. Spencer M, Bishop D, Dawson B, et al. Physiological and metabolic responses of repeated-sprint activities: specific to field-based team sports. Sports Med. 2005;35:1025.

44. Spencer MR, Gastin PB. Energy system contribution during 200- to 1500-m running in highly trained athletes. Med Sci Sports Exerc. 2001;33:157.

45. Stark AH, Madar Z. Olive oil as a functional food: epidemiology and nutritional approaches. Nutr Rev. 2002;60:170.

46. Tesch P, Alkner B. Acute and chronic muscle metabolic adaptations to strength training. In: Komi PV, ed. Strength and Power in Sport. 2nd ed. Oxford, England: Blackwell Scientific, 2002:265.

47. Tesch PA, Komi PV, Hakkinen K. Enzymatic adaptations consequent to long-term strength training. Int J Sports Med. 1987;(8)(suppl 1):66.

48. Turcotte L, Richter E, Kiens B. Lipid metabolism during exercise. In: Hargraves M, ed. Exercsie Metabolism. Champaign, IL: Human Kinetics, 1995:99.

49. Yoshida T, Udo M, Iwai K, et al. Significance of the contribution of aerobic and anaerobic components to several distance running performances in female athletes. Eur J Appl Physiol Occup Physiol. 1990;60:249.

Suggested Readings

Ardigo' LP, Goosey-Tolfrey VL, et al. Biomechanics and energetics of basketball wheelchairs evolution. Int J Sports Med. 2005;26(5):388–396.

Beneke R, Pollmann C, Bleif I, et al. How anaerobic is the Wingate Anaerobic Test for humans? Eur J Appl Physiol. 2002;87(4/5):388–392.

Billat VL, Lepretre PM, Heugas AM, et al. Energetics of middle-distance running performances in male and female junior using track measurements. Jpn J Physiol. 2004;54(2):125–135.

Capelli C, Pendergast DR, Termin B. Energetics of swimming at maximal speeds in humans. Eur J Appl Physiol Occup Physiol. 1998;78(5):385–393.

Cerretelli P, Veicsteinas A, Fumagalli M, et al. Energetics of isometric exercise in man. J Appl Physiol. 1976;41(2):136–141.

Chance B, Im J, Nioka S, et al. Skeletal muscle energetics with PNMR: personal views and historic perspectives. NMR Biomed. 2006;19(7):904–926.

Chasan-Taber L, Freedson PS, Roberts DE, et al. Energy expenditure of selected household activities during pregnancy. Res Q Exerc Sport. 2007;78(2):133–137.

Costill D. An overview of the 1976 New York academy of science meeting. Sports Med. 2007;37(4/5):281–283.

Da Silva ME, Fernandez JM, Castillo E, et al. Influence of vibration training on energy expenditure in active men. J Strength Cond Res. 2007;21(2):470–475.

Di Giulio C, Daniele F, Tipton CM. Angelo Mosso and muscular fatigue: 116 years after the first Congress of Physiologists: IUPS commemoration. Adv Physiol Educ. 2006;30(2):51–57.

Di Prampero PE, Capelli C, Pagliaro P, et al. Energetics of best performances in middle-distance running. J Appl Physiol. 1993;74(5):2318–2324.

Di Prampero PE, Francescato MP, Cettolo V. Energetics of muscular exercise at work onset: the steady-state approach. Pflugers Arch. 2003;445(6):741–746.

Formenti F, Minetti AE. Human locomotion on ice: the evolution of ice-skating energetics through history. J Exp Biol. 2007;210(pt 10):1825–1833.

Hagerman FC. Applied physiology of rowing. Sports Med. 1984;1(4):303–326.

Hunter GR, Byrne NM. Physical activity and muscle function but not resting energy expenditure impact on weight gain. J Strength Cond Res. 2005;19(1):225–230.

Iscoe KE, Campbell JE, Jamnik V, et al. Efficacy of continuous real-time blood glucose monitoring during and after prolonged high-intensity cycling exercise: spinning with a continuous glucose monitoring system. Diabetes Technol Ther. 2006;8(6):627–635.

Jones JH, Lindstedt SL. Limits to maximal performance. Annu Rev Physiol. 1993;55:547–569.

Kaneko M. Mechanics and energetics in running with special reference to efficiency. J Biomech. 1990;23(suppl 1):57–63.

Kaneko M, Miyatsuji K, Tanabe S. Energy expenditure while performing gymnastic-like motion in spacelab during spaceflight: case study. Appl Physiol Nutr Metab. 2006;31(5):631–634.

Lees A, Vanrenterghem J, De Clercq D. The energetics and benefit of an arm swing in submaximal and maximal vertical jump performance. J Sports Sci. 2006;24(1):51–57.

Lemmink KA, Visscher SH. Role of energy systems in two intermittent field tests in women field hockey players. J Strength Cond Res. 2006;20(3):682–688.

McCann DJ, Mole PA, Caton JR. Phosphocreatine kinetics in humans during exercise and recovery. Med Sci Sports Exerc. 1995;27(3):378–389.

McNeill AR. Energetics and optimization of human walking and running: the 2000 Raymond Pearl memorial lecture. Am J Hum Biol. 2002;14(5):641–648.

Scott CB. Contribution of blood lactate to the energy expenditure of weight training. J Strength Cond Res. 2006;20(2):404–411.

Tang JE, Hartman JW, Phillips SM. Increased muscle oxidative potential following resistance training induced fibre hypertrophy in young men. Appl Physiol Nutr Metab. 2006;31(5):495–501.

Yasuda N, Ruby BC, Gaskill SE. Substrate oxidation during incremental arm and leg exercise in men and women matched for ventilatory threshold. J Sports Sci. 2006;24(12):1281–1289.

Zamparo P, Capelli C, Guerrini G. Energetics of kayaking at submaximal and maximal speeds. Eur J Appl Physiol Occup Physiol. 1999;80(6):542–548.

Classic References

Dill DB, Folling A. Studies in muscular activity, II: a nomographic description of expired air. J Physiol. 1928;66(2):133–135.

Dill DB, Yousef MK, Vitez TS, et al. Metabolic observations on Caucasian men and women aged 17 to 88 years. J Gerontol. 1982;37(5):565–571.

Hill AV. Calorimetrical experiments on warm-blooded animals. J Physiol. 1913;46(2):81–103.

Hill AV. The absolute mechanical efficiency of the contraction of an isolated muscle. J Physiol. 1913;46(6):435–469.

Hill AV. The energy degraded in the recovery processes of stimulated muscles. J Physiol. 1913;46(1):28–80.

Robinson S, Dill DB, Robinson RD, et al. Physiological aging of champion runners. J Appl Physiol. 1976;41(1):46–51.

Whipp BJ, Bray GA, Koyal SN. Exercise energetics in normal man following acute weight gain. Am J Clin Nutr. 1973;26(12):1284–1286.

Exercise Physiology and Body Systems

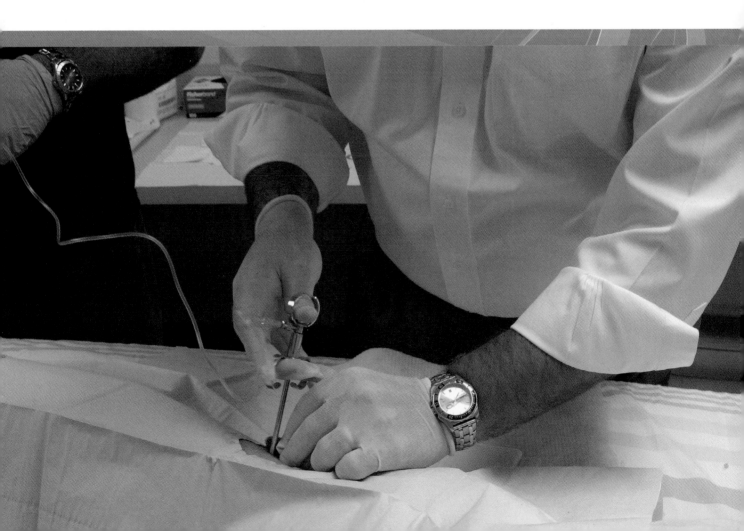

Chapter

3

Skeletal Muscle System

After reading this chapter, you should be able to:

1. Explain how skeletal muscle produces force and creates movement in the body

2. Describe the structural anatomy of skeletal muscle, including the different components of the sarcomere along with the phases of muscle action

3. List histochemical techniques that are used to identify muscle fiber types

4. List the different muscle fiber types using the myosin ATPase histochemical analysis scheme

5. Discuss the role of muscle fiber types as it relates to different types of athletic performances

6. Discuss the force production capabilities of muscle, including types of muscle actions

7. Explain proprioception in muscle and kinesthetic sense, including the roles of muscle spindles and Golgi tendon organs

8. List the practical applications for training-related changes in skeletal muscle, including specific training effects related to endurance and resistance exercise on muscle hypertrophy and muscle fiber subtype transition

9. Explain the effects of simultaneous high-intensity endurance and strength training on skeletal muscle fibers

From the ability to lift more than 1,000 pounds (453.5 kg) in the squat lift to the ability to run a marathon in less than 2 hours and 4 minutes, the human species demonstrates a dramatic range of physical performance capabilities (Fig. 3-1). We might ask, "How can such functional variability be possible in a single species?" As we will continue to discover throughout this textbook, there are many physiological functions that contribute to an exercise performance. One such contributor is the skeletal muscle system, which is covered in this chapter. The structure and function of **skeletal muscle**, which is muscle that is attached to a bone at both ends, profoundly affects the ability to perform exercise. Moreover, because of the very close functional relationship between skeletal muscles and nerves (covered in the next chapter), together they are known as the **neuromuscular system**, which profoundly influences athletic ability. Thus, different exercise training programs can be designed to favor neuromuscular adaptations for improving strength or endurance. Specifically, a combination of an individual's genetics and exercise training programs determines the performance capabilities of an individual.

To aid in understanding these concepts, this chapter presents the structure of skeletal muscle, sliding filament theory, muscular activity, and the types of muscle action. It also covers muscle fiber types, force production capabilities, and proprioception as applied to kinesthetic sense. Finally, it introduces the classical training adaptations in muscle to endurance and resistance exercise training.

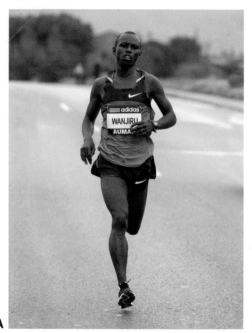

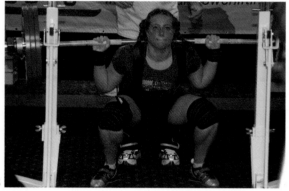

A   **B**

Figure 3-1. Examples of exceptional human performance. (A) The elite endurance runner. **(B)** The elite strength athlete. Each of these athletes brings a specific set of genetic capabilities to their sport. This includes the type and number of muscle fibers they have in their muscles. Elite competitive capabilities require an underlying neuromuscular system that can meet the physiological demands of the sport as evidenced by these two elite performances of running a marathon in just more than 2 hours or squatting several times one's body mass.

BASIC STRUCTURE OF SKELETAL MUSCLE

Despite the remarkable diversity in exercise performance abilities in humans, each person's neuromuscular system is similar in its basic structure and function. Every exercise training program will influence to some extent each of the components of muscle function (see Box 3-1). We will now examine the fundamental structures of skeletal muscle and gain some insight as to how they produce force and movement.

In order to understand the structure of skeletal muscle, we start with the intact muscle and continue to break it down to smaller and smaller organizational components. These basic organizational components of skeletal muscle structure are shown in Figure 3-2. The intact muscle is connected to bone at each end by **tendons**, which are bands of tough, fibrous connective tissue. The actions of muscle acting through the tendons to move the bones cause human

movement. The intact muscle is made up of many **fasciculi**. Each **fasciculus** is a small bundle of **muscle fibers**, which are long multinucleated cells that generate force when stimulated. Each muscle fiber is made up of **myofibrils** or the portion of muscle composed of the thin and thick myofilaments called **actin** and **myosin**, respectively, which are also known as the "contractile proteins" in muscle.

Connective Tissue

Connective tissue in muscle plays a very important role in helping to stabilize and support the various organizational components of skeletal muscle. When connective tissue is lost due to injury or exercise-induced damage (e.g., microtrauma to muscle resulting in overuse injuries), muscle strength and power are reduced. Connective tissue surrounds muscle at each of its organizational levels, with the **epimysium** covering the whole muscle, the **perimysium** covering the bundles of muscle fibers (fasciculi), and the **endomysium** covering the individual muscle fibers (see Fig. 3-3).

Box 3-1 APPLYING RESEARCH
Training Specificity

It is important to keep in mind that with exercise training each of the organizational components of muscle, from the myofibrils to the intact muscle, will undergo changes, or **adaptations**, to meet the specific exercise demands. Furthermore, the forces generated by the muscle will translate into adaptations in tendons and bones. Therefore, the development of optimal exercise training programs is not trivial, as the specificity of the demands placed on muscle results in very specific adaptations or training outcomes. This has become known as the principle of **training specificity**.

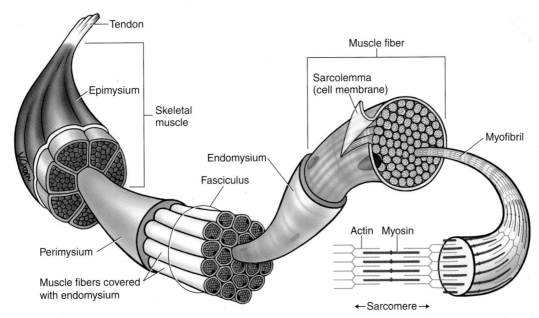

Figure 3-2. Basic organization of skeletal muscle. Muscle fibers are grouped together in a fasciculus, and many fasciculi form the intact muscle. Each muscle fiber contains a bundle of myofibrils. The myofibril proteins of actin (thin filaments) and myosin (thick filaments) make up the contractile unit, or sarcomere, which runs from Z line to Z line. Different bands exist on the basis of whether actin and/or myosin overlap in different stages of shortening or lengthening.

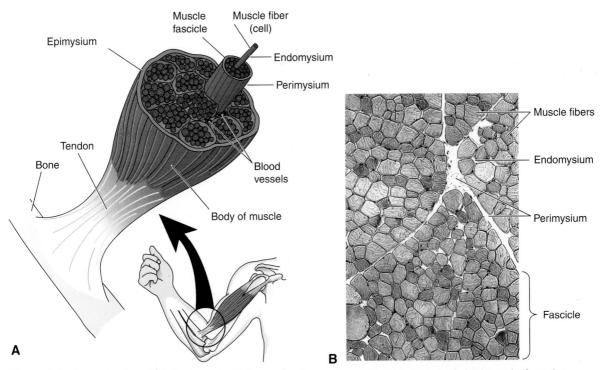

Figure 3-3. Connective tissue in skeletal muscle. (A) Connective tissue plays an important role in skeletal muscle, from the tendon attachments to the bone to the layers of connective tissue that tightly organize skeletal muscle into its different component parts from the whole muscle to the sarcomere. Muscle fibers are grouped together in a fasciculus, and many fasciculi form the intact muscle. Connective tissue surrounds each level of organization, including the epimysium, which covers the whole muscle, the perimysium, which covers each fasciculus, and the endomysium, which covers each muscle fiber. **(B)** The perimysium, endomysium. and individual muscle fibers can be seen in a cross-section of muscle.

Box 3-2 APPLYING RESEARCH
Think before You Stretch

A host of studies have demonstrated that stretching may be detrimental to force production.[6,30,43] It now appears that this loss of function is due to the fact that stretching may elongate the elastic component in muscle, thereby reducing the recoil forces of the muscle. This may be especially true if the stretching is performed immediately before an event (e.g., high jump). Thus, if maximal power, speed, and even strength can be reduced when stretching is performed immediately prior to the effort, we should carefully consider

when we should stretch. From a practical perspective, prior to an athletic event an individual should perform a dynamic warm-up with low-level cycling or jogging; static stretching right before an event requiring maximal force or power development should be eliminated. Flexibility training should be undertaken well before efforts requiring maximal force development in cool-down periods or at another time so that speed, strength, and power performances will not be negatively affected.

The connective tissue is vital for physical performance for several reasons. First, the muscle's connective tissue sheaths coalesce to form the tendons at each end of the muscle, helping to ensure that any force generated by the muscle will be transferred to the tendon and ultimately to the bone.[21] Second, the endomysium helps prevent the signal for muscle activation from spreading from one muscle fiber to an adjacent fiber. This is necessary to allow fine control of the activation of individual fibers, allowing the body to specifically control force generation and match it to the task at hand (see Chapter 4). Third, the muscle's connective tissue sheaths make up the **elastic component** of muscle, which contributes to force and power production. It has been shown that stretching right before a strength or power event may in fact reduce the elastic components' power capability (Box 3-2).

The elastic component of connective tissue is a vital contributor to the **stretch-shortening cycle**, which consists of controlled muscle elongation (**eccentric** action) followed by a rapid muscle shortening (**concentric** action). The force produced by the elastic component is analogous to the force involved with the recoil of a rubber band after being stretched and released. However, movements in which the prior eccentric action or elongation of the muscle is not followed immediately by the rapid shortening or concentric muscle action (e.g., starting a vertical jump from the squat position) do not take advantage of this added force production, resulting in a reduced level of performance (Box 3-3). Taking advantage of this connective tissue feature of muscle in a training program (e.g., plyometrics; Box 3-4) can contribute to improved force and power production.[29]

Box 3-3 APPLYING RESEARCH
Prove It to Yourself

You can see the effect of the stretch-shortening cycle by doing a simple experiment. Which movement allows you to jump the highest? First, get into a squat position, hold the position, and jump as high as you can. Next, begin from a standing position and drop into a downward

countermovement before you jump as high as you can. Try it. You will feel right away that a jump with a countermovement is higher, and in the laboratory, a difference in power on a force plate can be seen between the two types of jumps.

Box 3-4 APPLYING RESEARCH
Plyometric Exercise

Plyometrics is a popular form of exercise training that utilizes the stretch-shortening cycle to help in the development of muscular power. It has been shown that the stretch-shortening cycle can contribute up to 20% to 30% of the power in a stretch-shortening-type activity, such as a maximal vertical jump needed for high-jump performances.[23] By performing plyometric training, improvements in speed and power production can be achieved. Plyometrics range from low-intensity (standing hops) to high-intensity drills (drop or depth jumps from different heights).

Examples of plyometric exercises include the following:
- Standing vertical jumps
- Long jumps
- Hops and skips
- Standing hops
- Depth or drop jumps from different heights
- Push-ups with hand claps
- Medicine ball throwing drills

The Sarcomere

The **sarcomere** is the smallest or most basic contractile unit of skeletal muscle capable of force production and shortening. Skeletal muscle is also called **striated muscle** because the arrangement of protein filaments in the muscle's sarcomere gives it a striped or striated appearance under a microscope (Fig. 3-4).

At each end of a sarcomere are **Z lines**. At rest, there are two distinct light areas in each sarcomere: the **H zone**

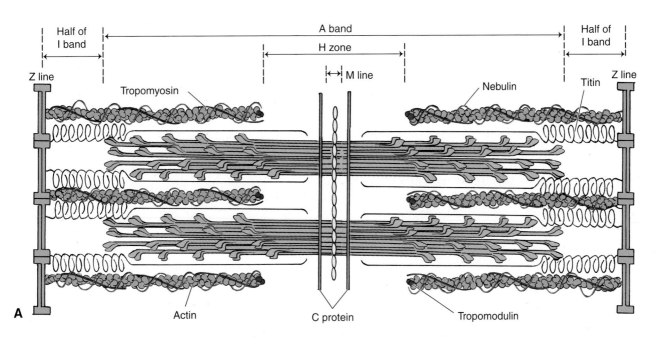

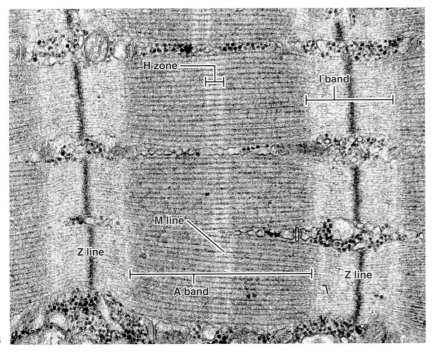

Figure 3-4. The sarcomere is the functional contractile unit of muscle. **(A)** A graphic depiction of a sarcomere. **(B)** An ATPase-stained micrograph. The myosin filaments (also called thick filaments) and the actin filaments (also called thin filaments) make up the sarcomere. One complete sarcomere runs from one Z line to the next Z line. When shortening occurs, the myosin and actin filaments slide over each other, causing the two Z lines of a sarcomere to come closer together.

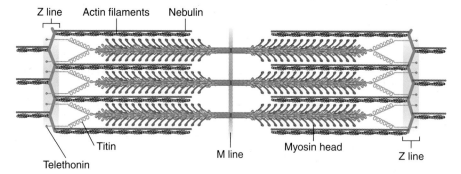

Figure 3-5. Noncontractile proteins. Noncontractile proteins are named such because they are not involved with the contraction process but hold the contractile proteins in place so that they are in close proximity with each other for optimal myosin–actin binding.

in the middle of the sarcomere, which contains myosin but not actin, and the **I bands** located at both ends of the sarcomere, which contain only actin filaments. These two areas appear light in comparison with the **A band**, which contains overlapping actin and myosin filaments. The A band represents the length of the myosin filaments. The **M line**, found in the middle of the H zone, is important as its proteins hold the myosin filaments in place.

As the sarcomere shortens, the actin filaments slide over the myosin filaments. This causes the H zone to disappear as actin filaments slide into it and give it a darker appearance. The I bands become shorter as the actin and myosin slide over each other, bringing myosin into the I band as the Z lines come closer to the ends of the myosin filaments. When the sarcomere relaxes and returns to its original length, the H zone and I bands return to their original size and appearance, as there is less overlap of myosin and actin. The A band does not change in length during either shortening or lengthening of the sarcomere, indicating that the length of the myosin filaments does not change during the process of shortening and returning to resting length when the fiber relaxes. This is also true of the actin filaments.

Noncontractile Proteins

As we have already discussed, the role of noncontractile proteins is vital for muscle function. Even at the level of the sarcomere, noncontractile proteins are needed to provide the lattice work or structure for the positioning of the actin and myosin protein filaments. The contractile proteins of actin and myosin are secured in a very close proximity by noncontractile proteins (Fig. 3-5). These noncontractile proteins in the sarcomere also contribute to the elastic component of the muscle fiber, as previously discussed. For example, **titin**, also known as **connectin**, connects the Z line to the M line in the sarcomere and stabilizes myosin in the longitudinal axis. Titin also limits the range of motion of the sarcomere and therefore contributes to the passive stiffness of muscle. Another noncontractile protein, **nebulin**, which extends from the Z line and is localized to the I-band, stabilizes actin by binding with the actin monomers (small molecules that can bond to other monomers and become a chain of molecules or a polymer, such as the actin filament).

Before we can explain how muscle contracts, it is important to understand the basic structures of the actin

and myosin filaments as they are found within muscle fibers.

Actin Filament

The **actin**, or thin filament, is composed of two helices of actin molecules intertwined. The actin filaments are attached to the Z lines and stick out from each Z line toward the middle of the sarcomere. Each actin molecule has an **active site** on it (Fig. 3-6). The active site is the place where the heads of the myosin crossbridges can bind to the actin filament that is needed to cause shortening of muscle. Wrapped around the actin filament are **tropomyosin** and **troponin**, two regulatory protein molecules. Tropomyosin is a tube-shaped molecule that wraps around the actin filament, fitting into a groove created by the intertwining of the actin molecule helices. Troponin protein complexes are found at regular intervals along the tropomyosin molecule. Troponin is made up of three regulatory protein subunits. Troponin I (I binds to actin) has an affinity for actin and holds the troponin–tropomyosin complex to the actin molecules. Troponin T (T for tropomyosin) has an affinity for tropomyosin and holds the troponin to the tropomyosin molecule. Troponin C (C for calcium) has an affinity for calcium ions, and this affinity is the stimulus within the muscle fiber that causes muscle activation, due to its role in causing the active site on the actin molecule to be exposed.

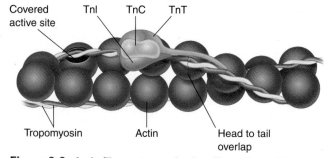

Figure 3-6. Actin filament organization. The actin, or thin filament, is made up of two helixes of actin molecules. Each actin molecule has a myosin binding site, or active site for interactions with the myosin heads. Wrapped around the actin filament are two other proteins, troponin and tropomyosin, which at rest cover the active sites on actin molecules, preventing the myosin heads from binding to the active sites. TnT, troponin T, binds to the tropomyosin strand; TnC, troponin C, binds to calcium; TnI, troponin I, binds to actin.

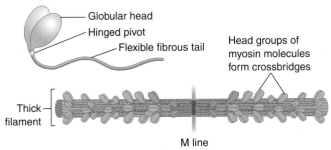

Figure 3-7. Myosin filament organization. The myosin filament (thick filament) is composed of myosin molecules. The fibrous tails of the myosin molecules intertwine to form the myosin filament. At regular intervals, two myosin molecule heads protrude from the myosin filament that can interact with actin molecules.

Myosin Filament

For the myosin and actin filaments to slide past each other, their molecular structure must allow them to interact in some way and develop a force that pulls them over each other. Each myosin molecule has a globular head, a hinged pivot point, and a fibrous tail (Fig. 3-7). **Crossbridges** are made up of two myosin molecules. Thus, when the myosin heads stick out from the myosin filament, notice that each crossbridge has two globular myosin heads. The dual heads of the myosin crossbridge are made up of the enzyme **myosin ATPase**. The fibrous tails of the myosin molecules making up the crossbridges intertwine to form the myosin filament. The crossbridge is the part of the myosin filament that will interact with actin and develop force to pull the actin filaments over the other myosin filaments. There are different isoforms, or kinds, of myosin ATPase found at the crossbridge. The specific isoform expressed by a fiber in many ways determines the type, and thus contractile characteristics, of that fiber.

Muscle Fiber Types

Skeletal muscle is a heterogeneous mixture of several types of muscle fibers, with each fiber type possessing different metabolic, force, and power capabilities. Several different fiber-type classification systems have been developed over the years (Table 3-1) on the basis of the different histochemical, biochemical, and physical characteristics of the muscle fiber.[34,35]

The major populations of **slow-twitch** (type I) and **fast-twitch** (type II) fibers are established shortly after birth; however, subtle changes take place within the two types of fibers over the entire life span. These changes are related to the types of activities performed, hormonal concentrations, and aging.[40] In fact, as we shall see later, exercise training acts as a potent stimulus for conversions in fiber type.

Common questions are, How does one determine an individual fiber type? and Have such conversions occurred? The first step is to obtain a biopsy sample from the muscle of interest (Box 3-5). After this, the sample must be sectioned into thin cross-sectional slices, which can then be stained to identify different fiber types. The most popular procedure used by exercise physiologists to classify muscle fiber types is the histochemical **myosin ATPase staining** method. Recall that ATPase is an enzyme that makes up the globular heads of the myosin crossbridges. From this assay method, type I and type II muscle fibers and their subtypes are classified on the basis of a histochemical reaction of ATPase with ATP supplied in the staining procedure. Each myosin isoform catalyzes this reaction at a unique rate, resulting in different staining intensities among the different fiber types. Using imaging software, the staining intensity can actually be quantified, and the range of staining intensity can be divided into different categories so that each fiber can be assigned to a specific fiber type based on its reaction with ATP.

Table 3-1. **The Primary Muscle Fiber Type Classification Systems**	
Classification System	**Theoretical Basis**
Red and White Fibers	Based on fiber color; the more myoglobin (oxygen carrier in a fiber), the darker or redder the color; used in early animal research; the oldest classification system.
Fast-Twitch and Slow-Twitch	Based on the speed and shape of the muscle twitch with stimulation; fast-twitch fibers have higher rates of force development and a greater fatigue rate.
Slow Oxidative, Fast Oxidative Glycolytic, Fast Glycolytic	Based on metabolic staining and characteristics of oxidative and glycolytic enzymes.
Type I and Type II	Stability of the enzyme myosin ATPase under different pH conditions; the enzyme myosin ATPase has different forms; some forms result in quicker enzymatic reactions for ATP hydrolysis and thus higher cycling rates for that fiber's actin–myosin interactions; most commonly used system to type muscle fibers today.

Box 3-5 PRACTICAL QUESTIONS FROM STUDENTS
Can You Explain What is Involved With a Muscle Biopsy Procedure?

In order to fiber type an individual, a biopsy sample must be obtained from the muscle. This has been called the **percutaneous muscle biopsy technique**. In this procedure, the skin area where the biopsy will be obtained is first bathed with a disinfectant. Then, several injections of a local anesthetic using a small-gauge needle and syringe are made around the biopsy site. A scalpel is then used to make a small incision through the skin and epimysium of the muscle from which the biopsy will be obtained. Then, a hollow, stainless steel needle is inserted through the incision and into the muscle and used to obtain about 100 to 400 mg of muscle tissue (typically from a thigh, calf, or arm muscle). A biopsy needle consists of a hollow needle and a plunger that fits inside the needle (see the figure below). The needle has a window that is closed when the plunger is pushed to the end of the needle but open when it is not. The needle is inserted with the window closed. The

plunger is then withdrawn slightly, opening the window, and suction is applied with a syringe attached to the back of the needle using plastic tubing. The suction creates a vacuum in the needle, pulling the muscle sample into the needle. The plunger is then pushed to the end of the needle, cutting off the muscle sample. The biopsy needle is withdrawn and the sample is removed from the needle, orientated, processed, and then frozen. After withdrawing the biopsy needle, the incision is dressed. The muscle sample is then cut (using a cryostat, which is a cutting device called a microtome set in a freezer case that keeps the temperature about −24°C) into consecutive (serial) sections and placed on cover slips for histochemical assay staining to determine the various muscle fiber types. Other variables (e.g., glycogen content of the fibers, receptor numbers, mitochondria, capillaries, other metabolic enzymes, etc.) can also be analyzed from serial sections of the biopsy sample.

A

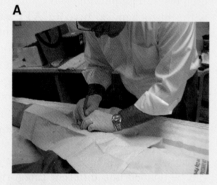

B

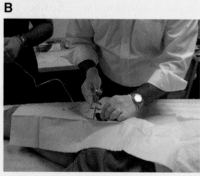

C

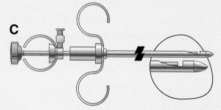

Muscle biopsy technique. The percutaneous muscle biopsy is the most common method of obtaining a small sample of muscle tissue with which to perform various assays on muscle, including histochemical analysis for the determination of muscle fiber types. **(A)** A small incision is made in an anesthetized area for entry of the muscle for the biopsy needle. Then the biopsy needle is introduced into the muscle to a measured depth in order to obtain a sample from the belly of the muscle. **(B)** Suction is provided, and a muscle sample is clipped off into the biopsy needle. **(C)** Example of a biopsy needle used to obtain the sample.

Myosin ATPase is an enzyme very specific to the speed with which the myosin heads bind to an actin filament's active site and swivels to generate force. Therefore, it provides a functional classification representative of a muscle fiber's shortening velocity. **Type I fibers** are also

termed slow-twitch fibers, meaning that not only do they reach peak force production at a slow rate, but also once achieved, their peak force is low. Yet type I muscle fibers possess a high capacity for oxidative metabolism since they receive a rich blood supply and are endowed with excellent mitochondrial density. As a result, type I fibers are fatigue-resistant and can continue to contract over long periods of time with little decrement in force production. Accordingly, these fibers are well suited for endurance performance.

Type II muscle fibers are also called fast-twitch fibers, as they develop force very rapidly and demonstrate high-force-production capability (Fig. 3-8). One can imagine that getting out of a starting block in the 100-m sprint or making a quick cut in soccer might be helped by having more type II muscle fibers (Box 3-6). But unlike type I fibers, fast-twitch (or type II) fibers do not display an abundance of mitochondria or a generous blood supply, resulting in a tendency to fatigue easily. Characteristics of type I and type II muscle fibers are overviewed in Table 3-2. In addition to those major characteristics, it has been shown that type I and type II muscle fibers have subtypes, so a continuum of muscle fiber types exists within each fiber

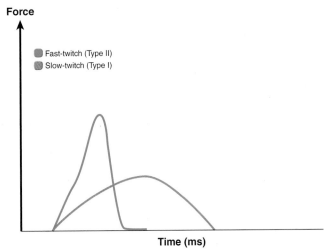

Figure 3-8. Muscle twitch characteristics. Fast-twitch (type II) fibers have a more rapid force production, produce higher amounts of force, and relax more rapidly than slow-twitch (type I) fibers.

Box 3-6 AN EXPERT VIEW
Muscle Fiber Types: Implications for Athletic Performance

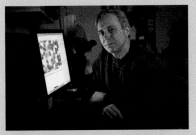

Dr. Robert S. Staron
Biomedical Sciences and Department of Biological Sciences, College of Osteopathic Medicine, Ohio University Athens, OH

Skeletal muscles of humans, like those of other mammals, contain two major fiber types (fast- and slow-twitch) which differ in their contractile and metabolic properties. As a general rule, the fast fibers are important for short-duration, high-intensity work bouts, whereas the slow fibers are better suited for submaximal, prolonged activities. As such, the slow fibers have the greatest aerobic capacity and are recruited first and, therefore, most often. As intensity and/or duration increases, the fast fibers are recruited as needed. If a maximal effort is required (e.g., attempting a maximal lift for one repetition), the nervous system will attempt to recruit all the muscle fibers (both fast and slow) in the working muscles.

The percentage of each of these major types in a given muscle appears to be genetically determined. Although a few muscles in everyone contain a predominance of either fast (e.g., triceps brachii) or slow (e.g., soleus), most muscles in the average person contain approximately a 50–50 mixture. Research has shown that the percentage of these two major fiber types and the percentage area occupied by each are two factors that have an impact on performance. The muscles of elite strength/power athletes have a high percentage of fast fibers, whereas elite endurance athletes have a predominance

of slow fibers. These two extremes demonstrate the importance of fiber composition in determining athletic excellence on the two ends of the strength–endurance continuum. Obviously, not everyone will be able to reach an elite level. Other factors such as motivation, pain tolerance, biomechanics, diet, rest, and skill all play a role in separating the very good from the very best.

Even though, as the research suggests, the percentages of the major fiber types are set early in life, significant adaptations to enhance performance can still occur. Regardless of the fiber-type composition, an individual can improve with training. Specific training regimens can increase force output (increase in the cross-sectional area of individual fibers) or aerobic capacity (quantitative and qualitative changes in metabolic enzyme activity levels) in specific muscles. For example, a strength/power athlete with a predominance of slow fibers is at a disadvantage compared with those individuals with a predominance of fast fibers. However, through training, significant increases in the cross-sectional areas of the fast fibers can help to overcome this disadvantage. As such, a muscle containing 40% to 50% fast fibers can undergo hypertrophic changes so that after training the fast fiber population makes up more than 60% to 70% of the total fiber area. Although under extreme conditions (e.g., paralysis, long-term electrical stimulation) muscle fibers do have the capability to induce transformations from slow-to-fast or fast-to-slow, exercise does not appear to be enough of a stimulus. Most research has shown that training is capable of eliciting transformations within the fast fiber population (fast subtype transitions), but not between fast and slow (i.e., a complete transition all the way from fast to slow or slow to fast).

Table 3-2.   Characteristics of Type I and Type II Muscle Fibers

Characteristic	Type I	Type II
Force per cross-sectional area	Low	High
Myofibrillar ATPase activity (pH 9.4)	Low	High
Intramuscular ATP stores	Low	High
Intramuscular phosphocreatine stores	Low	High
Contraction speed	Slow	Fast
Relaxation time	Slow	Fast
Glycolytic enzyme activity	Low	High
Endurance	High	Low
Intramuscular glycogen stores	No difference	No difference
Intramuscular triglyceride stores	High	Low
Myoglobin content	High	Low
Aerobic enzyme activity	High	Low
Capillary density	High	Low
Mitochondrial density	High	Low

type. This continuum, and how they are distinguished, will be described next.

Myosin ATPase Histochemical Analysis

The analysis used to differentiate among different muscle fiber subtypes involves a histochemical staining procedure that makes each subtype stain at a slightly different intensity, resulting in a unique shade of gray. To begin the process, a thin cross-section of muscle is obtained from the biopsy sample, and is placed into different pH conditions, with one alkaline bath (pH 10.0) and two acid baths (pH 4.6 and 4.3). When taken out, the fibers on the section can be classified according to each fiber's staining intensity under the various pH conditions, as shown in Figure 3-9.

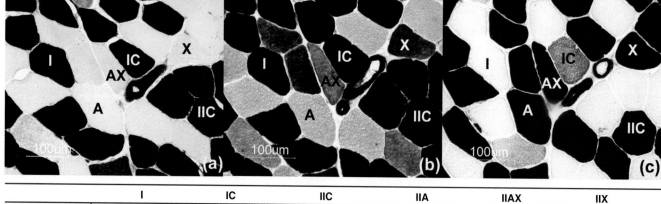

	I	IC	IIC	IIA	IIAX	IIX
pH 4.3	+++	+++	+/++	−	−	−
pH 4.6	+++	+++	++/+++	−	+/++	+++
pH 10.0	−	+/++	+++	+++	+++	+++

Figure 3-9. Myosin ATPase delineation of muscle fiber types. Histochemical assay used for the delineation of skeletal muscle fiber types. The separation of fiber types is based on differences in the pH stability of the ATPase molecule; i.e., the presence or absence of ATPase activity after exposure of the tissue to solutions of varying pH: **(a)** pH 4.3, **(b)** pH 4.6, and **(c)** pH 10.0. In human muscle, the array of fiber types that can be delineated includes type I, type IC, type IIC, type IIAC, type IIA, type IIAX, and type IIX. (Courtesy of Dr. Jenny Herman, Rocky Vista College of Osteopathic Medicine, Parker, CO).

Box 3-7 PRACTICAL QUESTIONS FROM STUDENTS

How Do the Muscle Fiber Types of Different Elite Athletes Compare?

Most muscles in the body contain a combination of fiber types, which is influenced by genetics, hormonal profile, training, and function of the muscle. In general, most untrained individuals have about 50% type I and 50% type II fibers. These proportions can be drastically different in elite athletes. For example, elite endurance athletes typically demonstrate a predominance of type I muscle fibers (e.g., 70–85%), whereas elite sprinters typically demonstrate a predominance of type II muscle fibers (65–70%). For elite performances, one must bring to the event a unique set of genetic predispositions including an optimal muscle fiber type. Although not the only factor needed for elite performances, fiber type is important.

The standard fiber types in humans span from the most oxidative fiber type to the least oxidative fiber type, or from type I, type IC, type IIC, type IIAC, type IIA, type IIAX, and type IIX. It should be noted that the oxidative capacity of a fiber is inversely proportional to its contractile velocity. That is, type I fibers, which are highly oxidative, are the slowest to develop peak force, while at the opposite extreme, type IIX fibers, which show the poorest oxidative potential, have the fastest contractile velocity. In animals (rat, mouse, cat, etc.) a greater array of muscle fiber types exist, again going from the most oxidative to the least oxidative types, from type I, type IC, type IIC, type IIAC, type IIA, type IIAX, type IIX, type IIXB, and type IIB. The greater array of muscle fiber types in lower mammals is thought to be due to a less sophisticated nervous system, requiring more adaptations at the level of the muscle fiber. Fiber type influences muscular performance in that type I fibers and its subtypes are conducive to endurance performance, while possessing a high percentage of type II fibers and related subtypes would be favorable to speed and power performance (Box 3-7).

Myosin Heavy Chains

The head of the myosin filament is made up of two **heavy chains** and two pairs of **light chains**. Each heavy chain has a molecular weight of about 230 kD and is associated with two light chains (the essential light chain and the regulatory light chain) (Fig. 3-10). Some investigators prefer using the myosin heavy chain (MHC) composition of muscle, which can be determined with electrophoresis to separate out proteins or by using protein-specific antibodies, to profile a muscle sample's fiber type composition. In the muscles of humans, three major types of myosin heavy chains exist: I, IIa, and IIx. In animals, four heavy chains have been identified: I, IIa, IIx, and IIb. If one collapses the multiple variations of fiber subtypes in humans into the three basic muscle fiber types of I, IIA, and IIX, and correlates them to the MHCs I, Ia, and IIx subtypes, a high correlation is found,[10] suggesting that the two procedures provide similar results concerning a muscle's fiber type profile. The muscle fiber subtyping discussed above, particularly as assessed by ATPase staining,

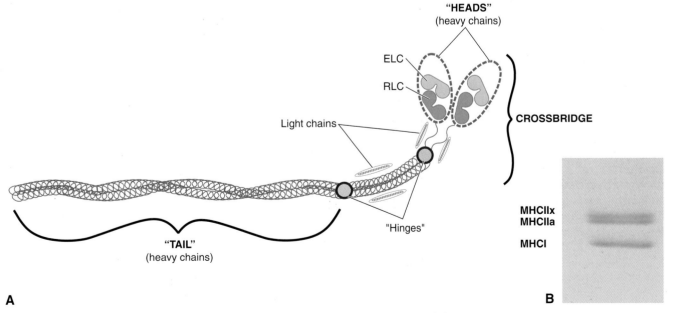

Figure 3-10. Myosin molecule. (A) The myosin molecule consists of two identical heavy chains and two pairs of light chains (regulatory light chains [RLC] and essential light chains [ELC]). **(B)** Myosin heavy chain electrophoresis gel representing the different heavy chains in humans.

allows greater detail as we attempt to better understand the adaptations of muscle to exercise training and the transitions of the major types, and their subtypes, to that stimulus.

SLIDING FILAMENT THEORY

Whether walking across campus, lifting a heavy weight, or running a marathon, movement is produced by the contracting muscle fibers. Exactly how muscle contracts to produce force remained a mystery until an interesting theory was proposed by two groups of scientists in the middle of the 20th century. This theory, referred to as the **sliding filament theory**, was proposed in two papers published in 1954 in *Nature*, one by Andrew Huxley and Rolf Niedergerke,[15] and another by Hugh Huxley (no relation to Andrew Huxley) and Jean Hansen.[17] These articles provided experimental evidence revealing how the muscle shortens and develops force. The sliding filament theory of muscle contraction remains the most insightful explanation of how muscle proteins interact to generate force.

The essence of the sliding filament theory requires changes in the length of the muscle to be caused by the **actin** filaments and the **myosin** filaments sliding over each other to produce force without these filaments themselves changing in length (think of opening the sliding doors leading onto the back deck of your home).[16] At rest, the arrangement of actin and myosin filaments results in a repeating pattern of light (actin or myosin filaments alone) and dark (overlapped actin and myosin filaments) areas. The change in the striated pattern in muscle indicates the interaction between the two myofilaments. In the contracted (fully shortened) state, there are still striations, but they have a different pattern. This change in the striation pattern occurs due to the sliding of the actin over the myosin.

But before this process can happen, Ca^{++} must be released into the cytosol of the muscle fiber so that it can interact with the regulatory protein troponin. The number of interactions between the actin and myosin filaments, or actomyosin complexes formed, dictates how much force is produced. In the next sections, we will learn in more detail how this shortening of muscle is accomplished at the molecular level of the muscle.

Steps Mediating the Contraction Process

At rest, the projections or crossbridges of the myosin filaments are near the actin filaments, but they cannot interact to cause shortening because the active sites on the actin filaments are covered by tropomyosin protein strands. To create an interaction with the actin filament, the heads of the myosin crossbridges must be able to bind to the active sites of the actin protein. This means that the tropomyosin protein strands, which cover actin's active sites under resting conditions, need to be moved to expose the active sites. This essential displacement of tropomyosin is triggered by an increase in the muscle fiber's cytosolic Ca^{++} concentration. To understand how this occurs, we must recognize that the initial excitement of the muscle fiber begins with an electrical impulse that is initiated at the neuromuscular junction, the synapse joining the motor neuron to the muscle fiber, when the neurotransmitter binds to its receptors on the muscle fiber's surface (This process is discussed in detail in chapter 4).

Spread of the Electrical Impulse

This electrical impulse, first detected at the neuromuscular junction, spreads across the muscle fiber's membrane, or sarcolemma, down into the transverse tubules (T-tubules), which penetrate into the core of the fiber, reaching the **sarcoplasmic reticulum**. The sarcoplasmic reticulum is a membrane-bound structure that surrounds each myofibril within the muscle fiber and acts as a depot that stores Ca^{++} (Fig. 3-11). When the electrical impulse travels down the T-tubules, it excites proteins called **DHP (dihydropyridine) receptors**, which act as voltage sensors. Upon this excitation, the voltage sensors interact with **ryanodine receptors** located in the membrane of the sarcoplasmic reticulum. These ryanodine receptors are actually channels that, when stimulated by the voltage sensors of the T-tubules, open to allow a sudden release of Ca^{++} from the sarcoplasmic reticulum into the cytosol of the muscle fiber.

Uncovering the Active Sites

The newly released Ca^{++} then binds to the troponin C subunit of the troponin protein complex, and this interaction is what triggers a conformational change in the tropomyosin, thus preventing it from covering the active sites on the actin filament, leaving them exposed. The process by which, under resting conditions, tropomyosin blocks the active sites on the actin filament is called the **steric blocking model** in muscle.[36] With the active sites of actin now exposed, the heads of the myosin crossbridges can start a binding process with actin that will ultimately result in

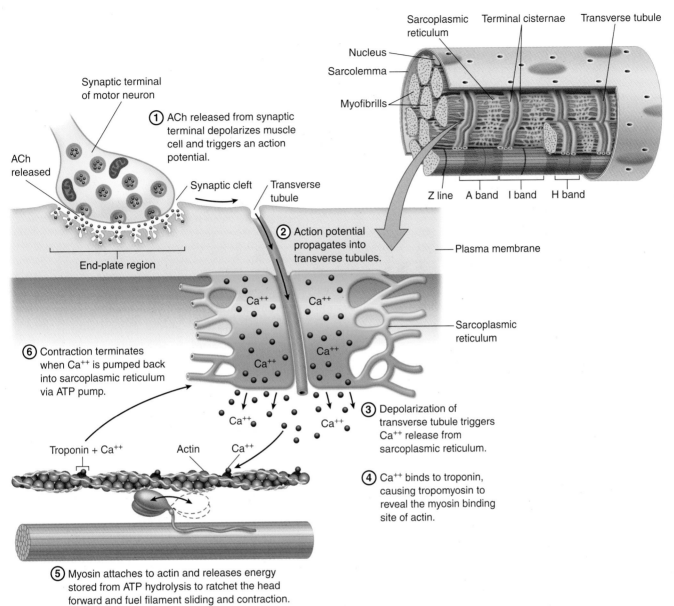

Synaptic terminal
of motor neuron

① ACh released from synaptic terminal depolarizes muscle cell and triggers an action potential.

ACh released

Synaptic cleft

Transverse tubule

End-plate region

② Action potential propagates into transverse tubules.

⑥ Contraction terminates when Ca⁺⁺ is pumped back into sarcoplasmic reticulum via ATP pump.

Ca⁺⁺

Ca⁺⁺

Ca⁺⁺

Ca⁺⁺

Ca⁺⁺

Ca⁺⁺

③ Depolarization of transverse tubule triggers Ca⁺⁺ release from sarcoplasmic reticulum.

④ Ca⁺⁺ binds to troponin, causing tropomyosin to reveal the myosin binding site of actin.

Troponin + Ca⁺⁺

Actin

Ca⁺⁺

⑤ Myosin attaches to actin and releases energy stored from ATP hydrolysis to ratchet the head forward and fuel filament sliding and contraction.

Sarcoplasmic reticulum

Terminal cisternae

Transverse tubule

Nucleus

Sarcolemma

Myofibrills

Z line A band I band H band

Plasma membrane

Sarcoplasmic reticulum

Figure 3-11. Sarcoplasmic reticulum. Muscular contraction is mediated by the electrical charge disruption of the calcium pump in the sarcoplasmic reticulum, which turns off the pump, allowing Ca⁺⁺ to be released. The release of Ca⁺⁺ from the sarcoplasmic reticulum into the cytosol results in the binding of Ca⁺⁺ with the troponin C component of the troponin molecule, which in turn initiates a conformational change of the troponin–tropomyosin complex, pulling the tropomyosin off the active site. This allows the heads of the myosin crossbridge to bind, and the ratcheting movement of the head inward pulls the the Z-lines toward each other.

muscle fiber shortening and force production. This binding process features two distinct phases. First there is a weak state, which under nonfatiguing conditions is followed by a phase of strong binding, which allows greater and faster force production. Under fatiguing conditions, however, the transition from the weak to the strong binding state does not occur, resulting in less, and slower, force production.

Interaction of Actin and Myosin Filaments

When the actin and myosin filaments combine, an acto-myosin complex is formed. Once this reaction occurs, the

myosin crossbridge heads pull actin toward the center of the sarcomere and force is produced. This movement of the myosin crossbridges is called the **power stroke**, which has been described as a type of ratchet movement.[25] In other words, the myosin head swivels at its hinged pivot point and pulls the actin filament over the myosin filament, causing the sarcomere to shorten, bringing the Z lines closer to each other (Fig. 3-12). Adenosine triphosphate (ATP), which is generated by the different energy pathways discussed in Chapter 2, is vital to the contraction process. The myosin head goes through the same cycle of events each time it binds to an active site. Let us start with the

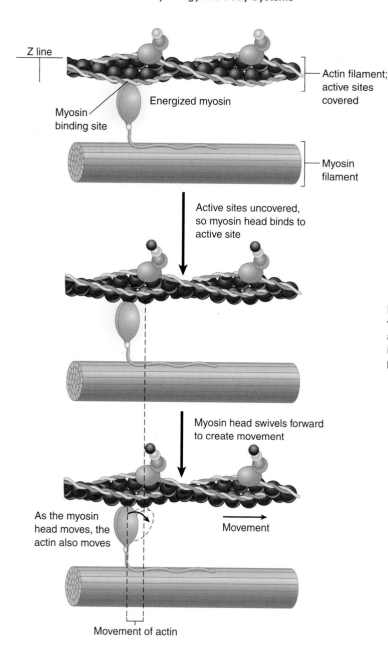

Z line

Myosin binding site

Energized myosin

Actin filament; active sites covered

Myosin filament

Active sites uncovered, so myosin head binds to active site

Figure 3-12. Ratchet movement of the head produces the power stroke of the myosin head. Successive binding and detachment of the myosin heads on active sites results in movement of the actin filament over the myosin filament, producing muscle contraction and force production.

Myosin head swivels forward to create movement

As the myosin head moves, the actin also moves

Movement

Movement of actin

myosin head bound to an active site after a power stroke has taken place. In order for the myosin head to be detached from the active site, an ATP molecule binds to the myosin head, breaking the actomyosin complex. Following this, the myosin ATPase found on the myosin crossbridge head hydrolyzes the ATP, and the energy is used to cock the myosin head back so it is over a new active site closer to the Z line. The ADP and inorganic phosphate (Pi) formed from the breakdown of ATP remain bonded to the myosin head. In this energized state, the crossbridge head is ready for its next interaction with another exposed active site closer to the Z line. After weakly binding to the new active site on actin to initiate the next power stroke, the Pi is released from the myosin head. At the end of the power stroke, the ADP is released from the myosin and the myosin head is again tightly bound to the active site.

This cycle is repeated, resulting in the ratcheting movement of repetitive power strokes described earlier. This crossbridge cycling sequence will continue to be repeated until the muscle fiber no longer is excited by the nervous system. At that point, no further release of Ca^{++} from the sarcoplasmic reticulum occurs, enabling the Ca^{++} pump located in the membrane of that organelle to return cytosolic Ca^{++} levels to those seen at rest by moving Ca^{++} back into the sarcoplasmic reticulum. Due to the drop in Ca^{++} concentration in the cytosol, the troponin C subunit is no longer bound to Ca^{++}, which causes the troponin to stop the tugging on the tropomyosin strand, allowing it to once again cover the active sites on the actin filament. As a result, the myosin crossbridge heads cannot bind to the active sites to form the actomyosin complexes necessary to execute the power stroke.

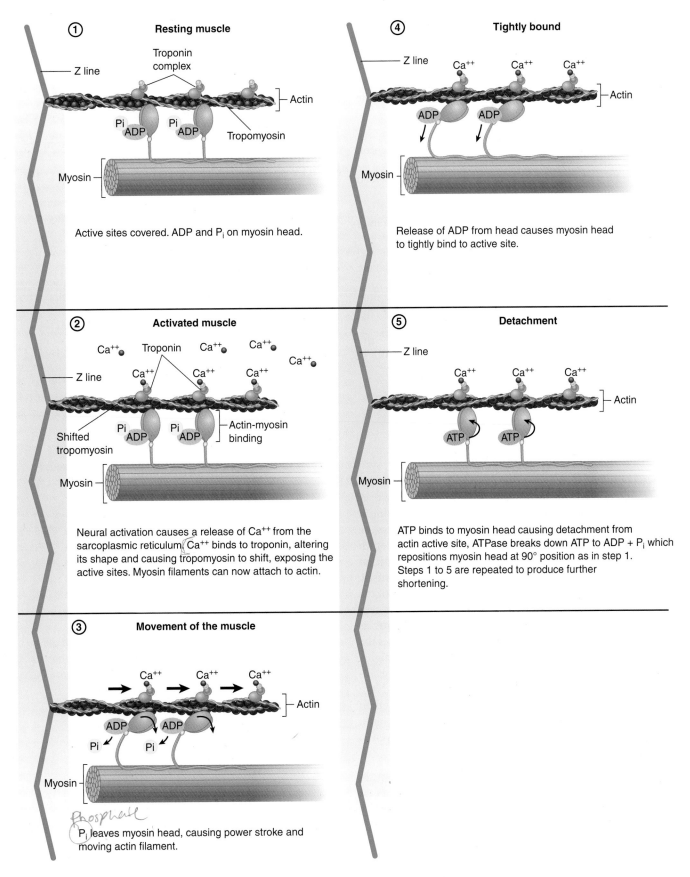

(1) Resting muscle

Z line — Troponin complex — Actin — Tropomyosin

Pi ADP   Pi ADP

Myosin

Active sites covered. ADP and P_i on myosin head.

(4) Tightly bound

Z line — Ca^{++} Ca^{++} Ca^{++} — Actin

ADP   ADP

Myosin

Release of ADP from head causes myosin head to tightly bind to active site.

(2) Activated muscle

Ca^{++} Troponin Ca^{++} Ca^{++} Ca^{++}

Ca^{++} Ca^{++} Ca^{++}

Z line

Shifted tropomyosin   Pi ADP   Pi ADP   Actin-myosin binding

Myosin

Neural activation causes a release of Ca^{++} from the sarcoplasmic reticulum. Ca^{++} binds to troponin, altering its shape and causing tropomyosin to shift, exposing the active sites. Myosin filaments can now attach to actin.

(5) Detachment

Z line — Ca^{++} Ca^{++} Ca^{++} — Actin

ATP   ATP

Myosin

ATP binds to myosin head causing detachment from actin active site, ATPase breaks down ATP to ADP + P_i which repositions myosin head at 90° position as in step 1. Steps 1 to 5 are repeated to produce further shortening.

(3) Movement of the muscle

Ca^{++} Ca^{++} Ca^{++} — Actin

ADP   ADP

Pi   Pi

Myosin

P_i leaves myosin head, causing power stroke and moving actin filament.

Figure 3-13. Muscle contraction steps. The contractile process is a series of steps leading to the shortening of the sarcomere. This is sometimes referred to as crossbridge cycling.

Box 3-8 APPLYING RESEARCH
Muscular Contraction

The basic steps in the contractile process of skeletal muscle are as follows:

Excitation

1. An action potential takes place in an alpha motor neuron axon.
2. The neurotransmiter acetylcholine (ACh) is released from the axon terminal.
3. ACh binds to receptors on the muscle fiber membrane.
4. Channels open on the muscle fiber membrane, generating an ionic current.
5. The ionic current sweeps through the T-tubules and stimulates the DHP receptors, which act as voltage sensors, in the T-tubules.
6. The stimulated voltage sensors activate the ryanodine receptors, which are Ca^{++} channels, located on the membrane of the sarcoplasmic reticulum.
7. Upon opening of the ryanodine receptors, the sarcoplasmic reticulum releases Ca^{++} into the cytosol.

Contraction or Shortening

1. Ca^{++} binds to the troponin C.
2. A conformational change in troponin causes the tropomyosin to move, exposing active sites on actin.

3. Myosin crossbridges bind to the exposed active sites.
4. Myosin heads swivel, pulling the actin filaments over the myosin filaments.
5. Myosin heads acquire a new ATP and release from the active site.
6. ATPase on myosin head hydrolyzes the ATP, energizing the crossbridge and "cocking" it back to its starting position so that it is ready to bind another active site.
7. As long as sufficient cytosolic calcium ions are present, the cycle continues.

Relaxation

1. Alpha motor neuron axon action potential stops.
2. Ca^{++} is actively pumped back into sarcoplasmic reticulum.
3. Ca^{++} is unbound from troponin C.
4. Active sites are covered by tropomyosin and troponin.
5. External force is needed to return the muscle to resting length.

Return to Resting Muscle Length

When bound to an active site, the crossbridges of the myosin molecule can swivel only in the direction that pulls actin over the myosin so that the Z lines come closer together, resulting in a shortening of the muscle. In short, they are designed to cause muscle shortening. So the muscle fiber cannot by itself return to its elongated resting length. To return to resting length, an outside force such as gravity or the work of an **antagonistic** muscle (i.e., one that performs the opposite movement of the agonist) must occur. For example, during an arm or biceps curl, the biceps causes flexion of the elbow when it contracts and the biceps muscle is considered the agonist as it causes the desired movement. The triceps causes extension, or straightening, of the elbow when it contracts, and would be considered the antagonistic muscle when doing an arm curl. Note that the action of the triceps, or antagonist, would lengthen during the return of the biceps, or agonist, to resting length. A summary of the steps causing muscle shortening is given in Figure 3-13 and Box 3-8.

Quick Review

- The proposed theory to explain muscular contraction is the sliding filament theory.
- This theory holds that changes in muscle length are caused by the actin and myosin filaments sliding over each other.

Steps of the sliding filament theory include:

- At rest, actin and myosin crossbridges are in near contact with each other, but no binding occurs.

- An electrical impulse crosses the neuromuscular junction and goes down the T-tubules where the impulse is detected by the DHP receptors (voltage sensors).
- When excited by the electrical impulse, DHP receptors activate ryanodine receptors located on the membrane of the sarcoplasmic reticulum.
- Ryanodine receptors are actually Ca^{++} channels embedded in the membrane of the sarcoplasmic reticulum, and upon activation, they open to release Ca^{++} stored in the sarcoplasmic reticulum into the cytosol of the muscle fiber.
- The released Ca^{++} can then bind to troponin, causing a shift in positioning of tropomyosin, thus exposing active sites on actin.
- This allows myosin crossbridge heads to bind to exposed actin active sites, forming actomyosin complexes.
- A swiveling movement of the myosin crossbridge head occurs, resulting in a power stroke, which creates a shortening of the sarcomere and, ultimately, the muscle.
- When electrical impulses are no longer delivered to the muscle fiber's surface, there is a cessation in the release of Ca^{++} from the sarcoplasmic reticulum, allowing the Ca^{++} pump of the sarcoplasmic reticulum to return cytosolic Ca^{++} back to resting concentrations.
- With no Ca^{++} to bind to the troponin, tropomyosin again blocks the active sites on actin, causing muscle contraction to stop.
- The intact muscle is returned to its resting length by an outside force such as gravity or an actively contracting antagonistic muscle.

PROPRIOCEPTION AND KINESTHETIC SENSE

For the body to optimally perform everyday activities (e.g., going down stairs) or sport skills (e.g., triple jump), feedback, or a constant flow of information about our body position, needs to occur within the neuromuscular system. We can appreciate how important this feedback is when we witness the complex skills exhibited by gymnasts, divers, figure skaters, basketball players, or almost any other athlete performing in his or her sport. The importance of this constant stream of neural feedback is highlighted during injury to the peripheral receptors and proprioceptive organs found in muscles and other tissues. Following this sort of injury, our sense of body position and orientation among different body segments is disturbed, making coordinated movements difficult to accomplish. How the body senses where it is in space is achieved through the neuromuscular system's proprioceptive capabilities.

This sense of the body's position is monitored by feedback as to the length of the muscle and force being produced. Such monitoring is achieved by **proprioceptors**, which are receptors located within the muscles and tendons. The information that proprioceptors gather is constantly being relayed to conscious and subconscious portions of the brain. Such information is also important for learning motor tasks, especially when repeated over and over again to create a **learning effect**, which is the ability to repeat a specific motor unit recruitment pattern that results in successful performance of a skill, such as making a jump shot in basketball. The reason coaches have athletes repeatedly practice their sport skills is to learn specific motor patterns that can be accurately reproduced during competition. Because of proprioceptive mechanisms, one can perform complex skills such as the pole vault, or a gymnastics maneuver, and just "feel it" as being right. Proprioceptors keep the central nervous system constantly informed as to what is going on with the body's movements, many times at the subconscious level. Many movements are conducted so quickly that the individual may not even think about the performance of the activity or skill except before it begins (e.g., visualizing a sport skill or seeing a long set of steps before descending them). Such continuous information is vital for normal human movement as well as any sport performance. This ability of knowing where the body's position is in space has been called **kinesthetic sense**.

Muscle Spindles

The proprioceptors in skeletal muscle are called the **muscle spindles**. The two functions of muscle spindles are to monitor stretch or length of the muscle in which they are embedded and to initiate a contraction when the muscle is stretched. The stretch reflex, in which a quickly stretched muscle initiates an almost immediate contraction in response to being stretched, is attributed to the response of the muscle spindles.[33]

Spindles are located in modified muscle fibers that are arranged parallel to the other fibers within the whole muscle (Fig. 3-14). The modified muscle fibers containing spindles are called **intrafusal fibers**. These intrafusal fibers are composed of a stretch-sensitive central area (or sensory area), embedded in a muscle fiber capable of contraction. If a muscle is stretched, as in picking up an unexpectedly heavy suitcase, the spindles are also stretched. The sensory nerve of the spindle carries an impulse to the spinal cord where the sensory neuron synapses with alpha motor neurons. The alpha motor neurons relay a reflex nerve impulse to the muscle, causing a contraction, or shortening, of the stretched muscle, relieving pressure on its spindles (more on reflexes in Chapter 4). Concurrently, other neurons inhibit activation of antagonistic muscles of the stretched muscle so that they do not interfere with the desired reflexive shortening of the agonist muscle. From a practical perspective, performing exercises with

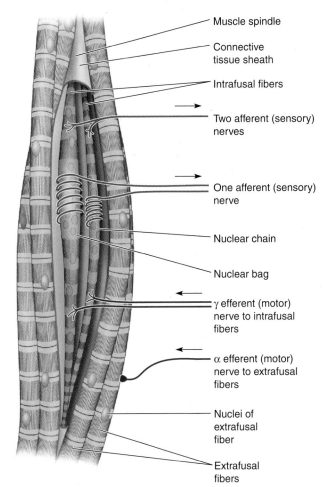

Muscle spindle

Connective tissue sheath

Intrafusal fibers

Two afferent (sensory) nerves

One afferent (sensory) nerve

Nuclear chain

Nuclear bag

γ efferent (motor) nerve to intrafusal fibers

α efferent (motor) nerve to extrafusal fibers

Nuclei of extrafusal fiber

Extrafusal fibers

Figure 3-14. Muscle spindles. Muscle spindles send information on the length and tension of the muscle fibers to the higher brain centers. This is very important to patterned skills, where position of the muscles and precise force development determines the effectiveness of the skill being performed (e.g., touch in a basketball jump shot).

prestretch (e.g., stretching your pectoral chest muscles in a bench press by taking a wide grip and pulling your clavicles together) takes advantage of this stretch reflex. This reflex is one explanation for the greater force output with a prestretch before an activity. For example, throw a ball as far as you can using a wind-up, which acts as a prestretch, and then throw a ball by stopping at the end of the wind-up for several seconds before throwing it. You will definitely throw the ball farther with a prestretch wind-up in part because of the reflex action of stretching the muscle spindles.

Alpha motor neurons innervate muscle fibers that do not contain spindles (called extrafusal fibers), and gamma motor neurons innervate the intrafusal fibers. Because muscle spindles are found in functioning muscle fibers, the nervous system can regulate the length and therefore the sensitivity of the spindles to changes in the length of the muscle fibers. Adjustments of the spindles in this fashion enable the spindle to more accurately monitor the length of the muscles in which they are embedded. Such adjustments appear to take place with trained athletes, making them more capable of performing highly complex, well-practiced movements.

Golgi Tendon Organs

The proprioceptor in the tendon that connects muscle to bone is called the **Golgi tendon organ**. The Golgi tendon organ's main function is to respond to tension (force) within the tendon (Fig. 3-15). If the forces exerted on the tendon are too high, injury might occur and the Golgi tendon organ is activated. Because of their location in the tendon, these proprioceptors are well positioned to monitor tension developed by the whole muscle and not just individual fibers.[37] The sensory neuron of each Golgi tendon organ travels to the spinal cord where it synapses with the alpha motor neurons of both the agonist and antagonist muscles. As an activated muscle develops force, the tension within the muscle's tendon increases and is monitored by the Golgi tendon organs. If the tension becomes great enough to damage the muscle or tendon, the Golgi tendon organ inhibits the activated muscle. The tension within the muscle is alleviated so that damage to the muscle and/or tendon can be avoided.

The proprioceptive sense of body position is affected by fatigue, demonstrating the importance of exercise training and conditioning to avoid, or at least reduce, fatigue during athletic competitions.[2] Interestingly, new methods of training are being added to many exercise programs with the goal of enhancing the flow of information from muscles to the central nervous system and back to the muscles. By effectively training these neuromuscular pathways of information flow, they can be expected to be more resistant to the onset of fatigue, allowing the performance of complex athletic movements to remain at their optimal level for a longer period of time. In some cases, the goal

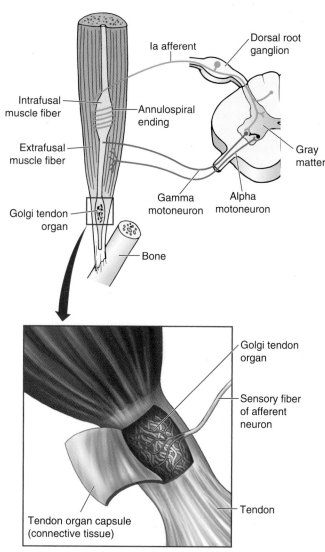

Figure 3-15. Golgi tendon organs. Golgi tendon organs function to protect the muscle and tendon by responding to the amount of tension in the tendons. If the tension is too great, the force development by the muscle is decreased.

is to increase the excitatory inflow from muscle spindles to the motor neuron pools and decrease inhibition by Golgi tendon organs, resulting in greater force production by the muscle(s).[18]

Quick Review

- Proprioceptors sense the body's position by monitoring the length of the muscle and force being produced.
- Proprioceptors relay important information regarding body position and orientation to the central nervous system.
- Muscle spindles monitor stretch and length of the muscle and initiate a contraction to reduce the stretch in the muscle.
- Golgi tendon organs respond to tension (force) within the tendon.

FORCE PRODUCTION CAPABILITIES

Because of its capacity to generate the force necessary to cause movement of limbs and the whole body, skeletal muscle plays, perhaps, the most important role in determining an individual's performance during exercise and sports. The muscle's capacity to generate force is critical not only to sports performance, but also to the ability to carry out the tasks of daily living. With this in mind, it is important to understand the different types of muscle actions, modes of exercise, and how force, power, and contractile velocity are related to each other.

Types of Muscle Actions

When muscle is activated and generates force, it can shorten, remain the same length, or resist elongation. These three types of muscle actions are typically referred to as concentric, **isometric**, and **eccentric**, respectively (Fig. 3-16). If we think about what occurs when lifting weights, we can easily see the differences among these muscle actions. Normally, when a weight is being lifted, the muscles involved are shortening (concentric muscle action), hence the term "contraction." During such concentric actions, the force produced by the muscle exceeds that imposed by the resistance, or load. So if one successfully completes a 200-lb (90.9-kg) bench press, it is because the muscles were able to generate more than 200 lb of force. In an isometric muscle action, the myosin heads keep attaching and detaching at the same or close to the same active site on the actin filament. Thus, no visible movement occurs, but force is developed by the attempt to shorten. In this case, the force produced by the active muscle is equal to the resistance opposing its

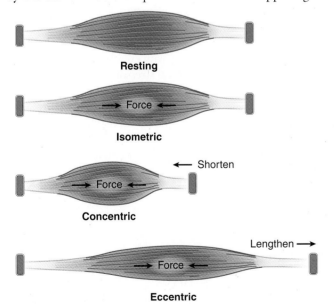

Figure 3-16. There are three basic muscle actions: concentric, eccentric, and isometric. Concentric, in which the muscle shortens; isometric, in which there is no change in muscle length (0 velocity); and eccentric, in which there is an elongation of the muscle while it produces force. (Adapted with permission from Knuttgen and Kraemer.[22])

movement. An example would be when in the middle of a repetition of a bench press, the weight is held stationary. An example of an eccentric action would be when a weight is being lowered in a controlled manner from the arms extended position to the chest touch position in the bench press. As the weight is lowered, the muscles involved are lengthening while producing force. During an eccentric muscle action, the load, or resistance, is greater than the force produced by the muscle. This can occur either when the muscle is exerting the maximal amount of force it is capable of, but it is inadequate to overcome the resistance, or when an individual deliberately reduces muscle force production to allow the muscle to gradually lengthen. In either case, the myosin heads interact with the actin filament's active site to slow the elongation of the muscle by binding, but do not complete the normal ratchet shortening movement discussed above.

Terms Used to Describe Resistance Exercise

The term **isotonic** is the most popular term used to describe types of resistance exercise and, often, any exercise movement. It infers that the muscle generates the same amount of force throughout the entire range of movement (*iso* meaning the same and *tonic* referring to tension, or force, produced by the muscle).[22] Since the amount of force produced over the muscle's range of motion varies (more on this later in the chapter), an isotonic muscle action would not typically occur unless using an advanced computerized resistance system that modulates the force and velocity of movement. Therefore, in place of the term isotonic, **dynamic constant external resistance** has been used to describe this typical type of muscle activity when exercising with external resistances such as free weights, or weight stacks on a machine, when the resistance remains the same throughout the range of motion.[8] **Isoinertial** is another term used in place of isotonic to describe an exercise movement with variable velocity and a constant resistance throughout a movement's range of motion. **Variable resistance** describes weight machines that produce a change in the resistance over the range of motion normally in an attempt to match the variation in the force produced by the muscle during an exercise. Hydraulic machines (concentric-only resistance) and pneumatic (concentric and eccentric resistances) machines using compressed fluids and air can also create external resistances that vary in attempts to match the resistance to the force production capabilities throughout the range of motion of an exercise.

The term **isokinetic** is used to describe muscular actions in which the velocity of the limb's movement throughout the range of motion is held constant using a specialized isokinetic dynamometer (*iso* again meaning the same and *kinetic* meaning motion). This type of sophisticated device (e.g., Biodex, Cybex, KinCom, Lido dynamometers) allows the speed of movement throughout a repetition to be set at a specific, constant rate and then measures the torque (i.e., rotational force) produced at that specific velocity.

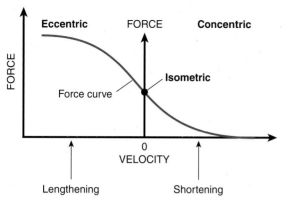

Figure 3-17. Force–velocity curve for the concentric and eccentric phases of movement. The force–velocity curve dictates the relationship of the muscle's ability to produce force with increasing velocity of movement concentrically and eccentrically. The force produced by a concentric muscle action decreases as the velocity increases; however, the force produced by the eccentric muscle action increases as the velocity increases.

Force–Velocity Curve

The **force–velocity curve** demonstrates the influence of changing the velocity of movement on the muscle's force production capabilities. This classic relationship was first described in experiments using isolated muscle by Nobel Laureate Professor Archibald Vivian (A. V.) Hill at University College in London. The relationship between the maximal force a muscle can produce and the velocity of movement depends on the type of muscle action used (i.e., eccentric, isometric, and concentric phases) and is shown in Figure 3-17.

As shown in the figure, there are distinct differences in the force–velocity relationships between concentric and eccentric muscle actions. As a starting point, we will use the maximal isometric force production, which by definition is at zero velocity. If we move with increasing velocity using a concentric muscle action, the force production declines at first very dramatically as movement velocity increases. As velocity continues to increase, the decline in force becomes more moderate. But at any velocity, the force produced by a concentric muscle action is *less than* that of a maximal isometric action. However, if we move with increasing velocity in an eccentric action, maximal force actually increases as the velocity increases; again, at first very markedly, but as velocity increases, elevations in eccentric force production become more moderate, eventually reaching a plateau. At any velocity of eccentric action, maximal force produced is always *greater than* that during maximal isometric actions. The increase in force production with increasing velocity during eccentric actions has been thought to be due to the elastic component of the muscle. However, complete understanding of the reasons of such a response remains unclear.

It is important to note that the high forces seen with maximal or near maximal eccentric muscle actions, which are much higher than those generated during maximal concentric or isometric actions, have been identified as one of the main contributors to muscle damage with exercise. Eccentric actions have been called the mechanical stressor of muscle. **Delayed onset muscle soreness (DOMS)** is one of the major symptoms of muscle damage due to high eccentric loads (Box 3-9). Untrained individuals are especially sensitive to such high mechanical stresses, and therefore exercise programs featuring eccentric actions (e.g., negative weight training or downhill

These types of machines are typically found in athletic training rooms and physical therapy clinics and are used for clinical assessments of joint function in a concentric and/or eccentric joint motion. An isokinetic action requires the use of a dynamometer to produce the desired effect of constant velocity because this type of joint action is not found in normal physical activity. Training with isokinetic dynamometers was initially attractive because it allowed training at high velocities of movement (e.g., 300°·sec⁻¹) that mimic power movements, and the devices automatically kept computerized records of the results of training sessions. But most isokinetic dynamometers allow only single muscle groups to be trained in simple or isolated movements (i.e., knee extension, calf extensions) that generally do not occur in sports activities. Thus, translation of training with isokinetic muscle actions to normal muscular activity in everyday life or sports may be minimal since most of those activities involve multiple muscle groups contracting in highly coordinated sequences. Although their use as effective training devices for competitive athletes may be limited, isokinetic dynamometers can be used effectively for accurately assessing, or testing, various parameters of muscle function, including strength, rate to peak force, and endurance.

Box 3-9 PRACTICAL QUESTIONS FROM STUDENTS
What Causes Delayed Onset Muscle Soreness?

Experts believe delayed onset muscle soreness (DOMS) is due to tissue injury caused by mechanical stress on the muscle and tendon. Microtears occur in the muscle fibers, causing disarrangement of the normally aligned sarcomere. This structural damage likely triggers an immune response involving the release of histamines and prostaglandins (specific agents involved in the immune regulatory process) and edema (fluid accumulation in the tissue), which results in the sensation of pain. DOMS is typically related to the eccentric component of muscular contraction, and appears 24 to 48 hours after strenuous exercise, and is more common in untrained people. One big coaching myth is that lactate causes DOMS; this is simply *not* the case, as no evidence has been presented to support this hypothesis.

running) must start out at lower intensities or volumes and gradually progress to higher intensities or volumes to allow for adaptations to occur that will minimize muscle damage and soreness. This approach of gradually increasing the resistance or load used during exercise sessions, especially with resistance training, is known as **progressive overload**.

Most training programs focus on the concentric phase of the force–velocity curve to increase muscular power. **Power** is defined as force times the vertical distance a mass moves divided by time or, alternatively, as force times velocity. Proper strength and power training can move the entire force–velocity curve upward and to the right (Fig. 3-18). This movement of the concentric force–velocity curve has positive benefits for both daily function and athletic performances, as power has increased. Improving power across the entire curve requires a training program that uses both heavy-strength training (loads > 80% of the 1-repetition maximum) and high-velocity ballistic training protocols (e.g., plyometrics). If only one training component, that is, either force or speed of contraction, is addressed, then changes will primarily occur over only part of the force–velocity curve. In other words, training heavy and slow will only improve force production at the slower velocities, whereas training light and fast results only in improvements at higher velocities of movement. From a practical perspective, many coaches use the term **speed-strength** to define training that is focused on force production at higher velocities and lighter resistances to improve power. Due to their interdependency in physical performance, optimal training should typically address the entire force–velocity curve.

Strength Curves

There are three basic types of **strength curves**, as shown in Figure 3-19. A strength curve is the amount of force that can be produced over a range of motion. For example, in a resistance exercise with an ascending strength curve, it is possible to lift more weight if only the final one-half or one-fourth of a concentric repetition is performed, rather than if the complete range of motion of a repetition is performed from the start of the concentric range of motion (e.g., squat exercise). If an exercise has a descending strength curve, such as with upright rowing, it is possible to produce less force near

the completion of the concentric phase of a repetition. An exercise, such as arm curls, in which it is possible to lift more resistance in the middle portion of the range of motion, and not the beginning or end portions, has a bell-shaped strength curve. Strength curves take on different patterns depending on the exercise movement and the individual's body structure, but all can be explained in part (biomechanics also affect measurable force in a movement) by the length–tension relationship, which dictates that the force that a muscle can generate is greatest when its length permits maximal overlap between the myosin and actin filaments. At any length beyond, or less than that, less force is developed because fewer actomyosin complexes can be formed (Fig. 3-20). Specific strength curves discussed above, where greater strength is manifested at different points within the range of motion, are due to the fact that different exercises begin and end at different levels of overlap between myosin and actin. For example, because of the biomechanics involved in doing the bench press, a greater number of actomyosin complexes can be formed early during the concentric phase of a repetition where the bar is close to the chest. In contrast, the biomechanics of doing repetitions of the upright row dictate that the length–tension relationship will be more favorable toward the completion of the concentric phase of a repetition, where the bar is pulled up under the chin, since it is at this point that a greater degree of overlap between myosin and actin exists.

Variable resistance weight training equipment has been designed to take advantage of the change in strength potential over a range of motion by varying the load during a repetition to help maximize strength development. Hypothetically, varying resistance at different points in the range of motion would allow the muscle to develop closer to its maximal strength throughout the range of motion, rather than be limited to what is possible when the muscle is at its weakest point in the

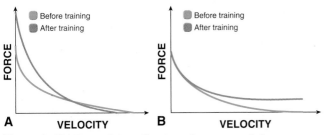

Figure 3-18. The training effects on the concentric force–velocity curve. (A) The change produced by heavy-strength training. **(B)** The change produced by low-load, high-velocity training. If one wants to affect the entire curve, both heavy-strength training and high-velocity power training are needed.

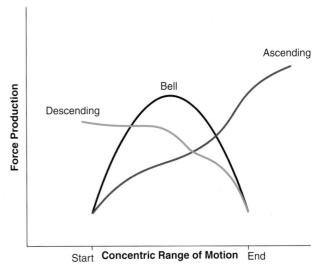

Figure 3-19. Strength Curves. There are three major strength curves: ascending (*red*), bell (*black*), and descending (*blue*) curves. Many standard exercises follow these basic strength curves. For example, a bench press has an ascending curve, a biceps curl has a bell curve, and a hamstring curl has a descending curve.

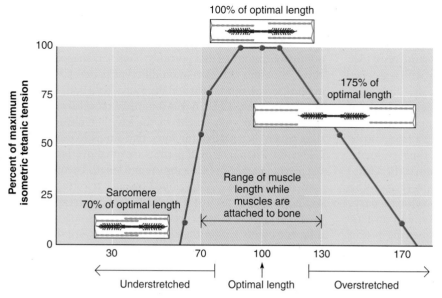

Figure 3-20. Length–tension relationship. The amount of force that a muscle fiber, and thus a muscle, can produce is related to the degree of overlap between myosin and actin. When the fiber is stretched too much or shortened too much, the number of actomyosin complexes that can be formed is limited, and, as a result, so is force generation.

strength curve. Although this type of training would seem to be desirable, individualizing the pattern of resistance variation would be essential, and many machines have not been very successful in the attempt to match the strength curve of a movement with the use of cams, rollers, or angle changes in the lever arm of the exercise machine. This is due to individual differences in limb length, point of attachment of the muscle's tendon to the bones, and body size. It is hard to conceive of one mechanical arrangement that would match the strength curve of all individuals for a particular exercise.

Force–Time Curves

Just as the force–velocity curve helps us visualize force production at different velocities of movement, the **force–time curve** helps us visualize force production over different

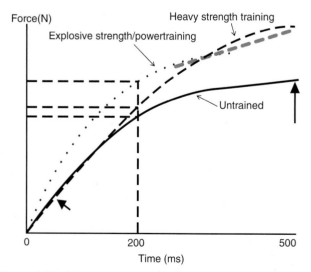

Figure 3-21. The force-time curve is affected differently by different types of strength training. Traditional heavy strength training increases maximal force ability. Explosive/strength power training increases maximal force and rate of force development.

segments of time. The ability to produce force quickly is an important quality of neuromuscular function, from an older person trying to prevent a fall after a momentary loss of balance, to a volleyball player spiking a ball over the net. The force–time curve also allows us to evaluate training programs directed at power development. In Figure 3-21, the amount of force produced over time is shown with three example curves, one normal curve for an untrained individual, one in which heavy strength and ballistic power training were included, and one in which only heavy-strength training was performed. Using both strength and power training components not only results in greater strength but also translates into a reduction in the time it takes to reach peak force production, that is, greater power. Since most physical performances require power for their performance, one can easily see that enhancing the ability to produce force very rapidly could be considered an important attribute of any conditioning program, whether it is for health and fitness or sports performance.

Quick Review

- The force–velocity curve describes the influence of changing the velocity of movement on the muscle's force production capabilities.
- The strength curve describes the amount of force that can be produced over a movement's range of motion.
- The force–time curve helps us visualize force production over different segments of time and allows us to evaluate training programs directed at power development.
- The ability to produce force quickly is an important quality of neuromuscular function.
- Proper strength and power training can improve power across the entire force–velocity curve.

SKELETAL MUSCLE TRAINING ADAPTATIONS THAT IMPROVE PERFORMANCE

Endurance and resistance training are the most prominent forms of exercise to enhance health and athletic performance. Understanding some of the basic adaptations of skeletal muscle to these two popular forms of exercise is essential if we are to appreciate how they can improve health and exercise performance. Each of these exercise modalities will be covered further in Chapter 12, but let us specifically look at skeletal muscle adaptations here. In addition, since few people perform one or the other training modalities exclusively, we will also take a closer look at exercise compatibility, or what happens when both forms of exercise are done concurrently with the same musculature.

Effects of Endurance Training

Looking at the effects of endurance training on skeletal muscle, we must remember that only those fibers that are recruited with the exercise will adapt to the exercise stimuli. The primary adaptations to endurance training are related to the need to better utilize oxygen and enhance muscular endurance. Motor units with type I muscle fibers are recruited first, and then, as the intensity of the endurance activity increases, type II motor units are recruited as needed. The more type II motor units that are recruited, the less efficient and effective the endurance performance will be, especially as the duration of activity increases. Perhaps this is presented best in the following sports scenario: It can be estimated that running a marathon race at about a 2:10:00 pace would require the athlete to run at a pace of about 4.84 m·s^{-1}. This would require the runner to recruit about 80% of the motor neuron pool. If motor units containing type I muscle fibers are better able to meet the aerobic demands of such a task, we can see the benefit of having a fiber-type profile of about 80% type I muscle fibers in the motor neuron pool in the muscles involved in running. In fact, many elite endurance runners actually have such a fiber-type composition of the thigh muscles. Although the above example may be a bit oversimplified, as many factors go into making an elite endurance performance, remember that motor units containing type I muscle fibers are better suited to endurance performance because of their high mitochondrial density and blood supply. Nevertheless, endurance adaptations will occur in all of the muscle fibers recruited to perform the endurance exercise. For many of us who have a more even distribution of fiber types (e.g., 45% type I and 55% type II), many motor units containing type II muscle fibers will be used to run a 10K race or even to go out for a noon time run with friends, and so they, too, undergo adaptations to improve their aerobic capacity. But if elite performance is the objective (e.g., running a marathon under 2 hours and 15 minutes), the runner needs to genetically have a predominance of type I motor units to optimize performance, because although type II fibers will show training-induced improvements in aerobic capacity, they will never match the aerobic capacity that is inherent in type I fibers.

So, what happens to the muscle fibers, both type I and type II, when they are recruited as a part of a motor unit to perform an endurance exercise workout? First, in order to enhance the delivery of oxygen to the muscles, an increase in the number of capillaries per muscle fiber will take place. This will enhance the delivery of oxygen to the exercising muscle, as will a training-induced increase in capillary density (i.e., number per unit size of muscle tissue). These adaptations appear to be fiber-type-specific, as type I fibers enjoy more pronounced improvements than type II fibers. In addition to these changes in capillarity, endurance training elicits an increase in the size and number of mitochondria within muscle fibers (see Chapter 2). Mitochondria are the organelles that produce ATP via the aerobic pathway, and the increase in a fiber's mitochondrial content is accompanied by an enhanced ability for aerobic metabolism. With the increase in mitochondrial content within the trained fiber comes a greater concentration of the enzymes of the Krebs cycle and of the cytochromes of the electron transport chain. Recall that these enzymes and cytochromes work together to synthesize ATP. As with changes in capillarity, gains in mitochondrial content stimulated by endurance training occur to a greater extent in type I muscle fibers, demonstrating the advantage of having more type I muscle fibers for optimal endurance performance. Keep in mind that capillaries are the vessels that exchange blood, oxygen, CO_2, nutrients, and waste products with the muscles, and mitochondria are the organelles inside the muscle cell where ATP is aerobically produced, thus linking increases in delivery of oxygen with greater capacity to use that oxygen to synthesize ATP (see Chapters 2 and 5). Additionally, the concentration of myoglobin, which facilitates the diffusion of oxygen from the muscle cell membrane to the mitochondria within the muscle fiber, is increased with endurance training. This means that the rate at which oxygen moves from the capillaries to the mitochondria is also increased.

In summary, with more capillaries surrounding each muscle fiber along with more myoglobin and mitochondria in each muscle fiber, the distance for diffusion to the mitochondria from the cell membrane or vice versa is shorter and the amount of time for the exchange of various substances to take place is reduced, which improves the efficiency and speed of the aerobic processes. This facilitates the exchange of oxygen, CO_2, nutrients, wastes, and heat between the muscle and the blood. With more oxygen and nutrients being delivered to the exercising muscle and more wastes and heat being removed, the muscle is better able to aerobically produce ATP to fuel the endurance energy demands, as well as remove potentially fatiguing metabolic byproducts. The overall result is improved endurance performance.

Box 3-10 DID YOU KNOW?

Can You Guess What the Largest Muscle in the Human Body Is?

Of the more than 600 muscles in the human body, which account for approximately 40% of body weight, the gluteus maximus (buttock muscle) is the largest (bulkiest). However, during pregnancy, the uterus (womb) can grow from about 1 oz (30 g) to more than 2 lb 3 oz (1 kg) in weight.

For your information, following are some additional interesting muscle facts: the smallest muscle in the human body is the stapedius, which controls the tiny vibrating stapes bones in the middle ear. The muscle is less than 0.05 in. (0.127 cm) long. The most active muscles in the human body are muscles controlling the eyes, which move more than 100,000 times a day. Many of these rapid eye movements take place during sleep in the dreaming phase. The longest muscle in the human body is the sartorius, which is a narrow, strap-like muscle extending from the pelvis, across the front of the thigh, to the top of the tibia. Its functions to abduct, rotate, and flex the leg into the cross-legged position.

Interestingly, changes in fiber size may also contribute to improved aerobic function. More specifically, type I (slow-twitch) muscle fibers typically experience a decrease in their size with endurance training resulting in a reduction in the distances from the capillaries to the mitochondria and expediting the rate at which gasses diffuse across the fiber.[12,24,42] The percentages of type I and type II fibers do not significantly change with endurance exercise training, but some changes may take place in the percentages of the subtypes to become more aerobic in nature (i.e., type IC to type I, type IIA to type IIC, and, if recruited, type IIX to type IIA).[24]

Effects of Resistance Training

Muscles come in different sizes and fiber-type distributions, both of which are related to a muscle's function (Box 3-10). Yet all muscles, regardless of fiber type, composition, or function, are capable of enlarging in response to a resistance training program. This growth in the size of the whole muscle is primarily due to the increase in the size of its individual muscle fibers.[24,27] In contrast, it has yet to be established whether muscles adapt to resistance training by increasing the number of their fibers, or what is referred to as **hyperplasia**. This may be because an increase in the number of muscle fibers would also result in an increase in total muscle size. Due to methodological difficulties (one cannot take out the whole muscle of a human for examination), the potential for hyperplasia in humans is debatable; however, it has been shown in response to various muscle overload protocols in birds and mammals.[3,4,11,28]

Hypertrophy

Hypertrophy is the increase in the size of the muscle, or its constituent fibers, which occurs as a result of participating in an exercise program. Myofibrillar protein (i.e., actin and myosin) is added, which results in the addition of newly formed myofibrils to existing fibers, thereby increasing fiber size. It does not, however, appear that the size of preexisting myofibrils is altered as a result of resistance training. Despite the increase in myofibrillar number, the myofibrillar packing distance (the distance between myosin filaments) and the length of the sarcomere appear to remain constant following 6 weeks to 6 months of resistance training.[8] Similarly, myofibrillar density, or the number of myofibrils within a given volume of muscle tissue, is unaltered by resistance training even though muscle fiber size is increased. And although increases in myofilament number take place, the spatial orientation of the contractile proteins in the sarcomere appears to remain unchanged following resistance training. To increase muscle cross-sectional area during resistance training, sarcomeres are added in parallel to each other, resulting in muscle fiber hypertrophy (Box 3-11).

The remodeling of muscle tissue with heavy resistance exercise is a function of the program and the sequential changes in contractile proteins. All fibers appear to hypertrophy but not to the same extent. Conventional

Box 3-11 DID YOU KNOW?

Largest Biceps

The world record, according to Guinness World Records, for the largest measured biceps is held by Denis Sester of the USA. The girth of his biceps measures 30 in. (77.8 cm). This frequently trained muscle of the upper arm that functions to flex the elbow, usually abbreviated as biceps, is actually named the biceps brachii, not to be confused with the biceps femoris, which lies in the posterior thigh and flexes the knee. The name biceps brachii is derived from the Latin words meaning two heads (biceps) and arm (brachii). The two heads of the biceps are called the long head and the short head. The tendon of the short head attaches to the coracoid process of the scapula, and the tendon of the long head attaches to the supraglenoid tubercle of the scapula.

weight training in humans and animals elicits a greater degree of hypertrophy in type II fibers compared to type I fibers. Also, type I and type II fibers appear to hypertrophy using different mechanisms. In type II muscle fibers, the process involves an increase in the rate of protein synthesis, and with type I muscle fibers, a decrease in the rate of protein degradation.

Recent research has added much to our understanding of the mechanism(s) involved in muscle fiber hypertrophy. It is now understood that the acquisition of additional **myonuclei** or nuclei located with the muscle fiber is required to support an increase in the size of the muscle fiber. The source of the extra myonuclei is the satellite cells, which are located between the muscle fiber's membrane and its thin, outer layer of connective tissue encasing the fiber, referred to as the basal lamina. Exercise stress, or other forms of damage to the connective tissue isolating these satellite cells, exposes them to agents called mitogens. As a result, the satellite cells undergo replication and newly produced satellite cells are fused into the muscle fiber. In this process, satellite cells contribute the needed increase in the number of myonuclei (i.e., DNA machinery). The added genetic machinery is necessary to manage the increased volume of protein and other cellular constituents (Box 3-12). A single myonucleus can only manage a specific volume of muscle protein, and therefore, without an appropriate increase in the number of myonuclei, increases in the amount of protein, which produce muscle fiber enlargement, would not be possible. The area within the fiber that each myonucleus is responsible for is called its **nuclear domain**.

With this in mind, Kadi and Thornell[20] showed that 10 weeks of strength training can induce changes in the number of myonuclei and satellite cells in women's trapezius muscles. These investigators found that their strength training program resulted in a 36% increase in the cross-sectional area of muscle fibers. This hypertrophy was accompanied by an approximately 70% increase in myonuclear number and a 46% increase in the number of satellite cells. Myonuclei number was positively correlated to satellite cell number, indicating that a muscle with an increased concentration of myonuclei will contain a correspondingly higher number of satellite cells.

Hyperplasia

Hyperplasia, or an increase in muscle fiber number, has been examined over the years as a possible mechanism for increasing the size of skeletal muscle. Interest in the viability of this concept was rekindled when several studies examining the muscles of body builders and power lifters

---

Box 3-12 AN EXPERT VIEW
Genes, Proteins, Exercise, and Growth

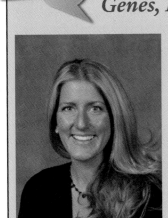

Maria L. Urso, PhD
Military Performance Division
United States Army Research Institute of Environmental Medicine
Natick, MA

Advances in molecular biology techniques have allowed us to evaluate alterations in gene expression and protein products in skeletal muscle during and following acute or multiple bouts of exercise. These advances have provided scientists with a better understanding of the molecular basis of skeletal muscle hypertrophy. This information is critical in the development of treatment interventions to promote hypertrophy, and possibly attenuate atrophy (see figure).

It is important to comprehend the role of genes and proteins in promoting hypertrophy. Fundamentally, each nucleus of every fiber (single muscle cell) contains combinations of four bases, known as nucleotides, which comprise deoxyribonucleic acid (DNA). These bases include

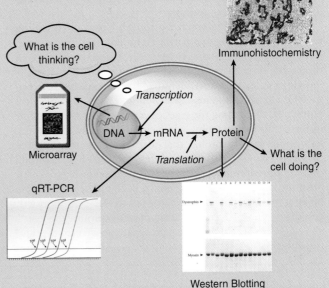

Basic genetic mechanisms mediate the production of protein and the development of muscular hypertrophy.

(Continued)

adenine (A), guanine (G), cytosine (C), and thymine (T). Unique combinations of these nucleotides provide the genetic code necessary to make messenger ribonucleic acid (mRNA) and proteins. The translation of the DNA code into a protein involves two processes: transcription (DNA to mRNA) and translation (mRNA to protein). In response to exercise, genes are up- or down-regulated. The extent and time course of these changes in gene expression are dependent on the duration, intensity, and frequency of exercise training. Depending on the magnitude and duration of increased or decreased gene expression, levels of mRNA can be affected to mirror those changes in DNA, resulting in a parallel change in the expression pattern of mRNA. Since the amount of mRNA dictates how much protein will be made, the magnitude of gene expression impacts the amount of protein made by each skeletal muscle fiber. Although the transcription:translation ratio is not 1:1, it is possible to modify stimuli to induce alterations in genes and gene products critical for hypertrophy.

Early research ventures to decode the molecular basis of hypertrophy were daunting due to the lack of technology allowing the analysis of global changes in mRNA. While it was clear that many genes were up- or down-regulated in response to a single bout of exercise, it was not possible to examine all of the genes simultaneously in a time- and cost-efficient manner. At the same time, investigators were suggesting that the molecular events that stimulate hypertrophy might be as unique as the stimuli because there was a lack of continuity between specific signaling pathways. In other words, molecular events that regulate adaptations in skeletal muscle mRNA and protein in response to resistance training were different than those that regulate adaptations to plyometric or sprint training. Furthermore, results from this work identified a unique time course of alterations, indicating that molecular adaptations that occur immediately after exercise differ from those that occur days to weeks following the onset of training.

Advances in gene transcription and protein profiling techniques, including microarray technology and proteomics, have allowed scientists to examine global changes in thousands of genes and proteins simultaneously in a single muscle sample. This work identified the relationship between specific changes in gene expression and their phenotypical outcomes, confirming the roles of certain genes and proteins in initiating hypertrophy, while simultaneously identifying new genes and proteins that also regulate the balance between protein synthesis and degradation. For example, there is a predominant increase in mitochondrial genes that promote mitochondrial biogenesis, such as the peroxisome proliferator receptor co-activator (PGC-1α), early growth response gene-1 (Egr-1), and nuclear respiratory factor-1 and -2 (NRF-1/2); metabolic genes that encode enzymes and transporters involved in carbohydrate and fat metabolism;

and satellite cell activators such as the myogenic regulatory factors, MyoD and MyoG (MyoD: differentiation; MyoG: myogenesis). However, these global screening tools only provide a snapshot of changes in gene expression, and it is not possible to identify specific biological processes involved in muscle protein synthesis.

Thus, investigators have taken a multifaceted approach to understanding molecular alterations in response to exercise. Recent investigations make use of several confirmational tools to measure what the cell is "thinking" at the DNA level, and also what the cell is "doing," by exploring alterations in the amount and location of gene products (proteins). Alterations in protein levels can be measured using Western blotting techniques. Western blotting is an assay that involves exposing an electrical current to a gel and separating proteins on the gel by their molecular weight. After transfer to a membrane, the membrane is exposed to an antibody, which recognizes the protein of interest, allowing the investigator to quantify the amount of protein in a sample. Immunohistochemistry is the technique used to identify the location of proteins in a muscle cell. Skeletal muscle samples are sectioned and probed with fluorescent-labeled antibodies that recognize proteins of interest or dyes that recognize specific structures, such as the nuclei. With these tools, investigators can visualize where a protein of interest is most active in a cell, revealing clues to its mechanism of action and relationship to other proteins.

The greatest challenge to date has been singling out the most critical genes and proteins involved in hypertrophy. Most recently, scientists have been employing sophisticated techniques to attenuate the activity of single genes to better understand their roles in complex pathways. RNA interference (RNAi) is one such tool that allows the study of single genes in cell culture and *in vivo* experiments. This tool uses double-stranded RNA that is synthesized with a sequence complementary to the target gene, and subsequently introduced into the cell or organism. Since this exogenous material is recognized as such by the cell or model system, the RNAi pathway is activated, causing a significant decrease in the expression level of the target gene. The effects of this decrease identify the physiological role of the protein product. By not completely abolishing the expression of target genes, RNAi is superior to knockout experiments, resulting in a more "physiologically accurate" system.

Great strides have been made in our understanding of the molecular basis of hypertrophy. However, with these advances, discoveries have been made that only add to the number of questions to be answered before we can fully understand signaling processes in skeletal muscle that has been stimulated by exercise, resulting in growth. Continued advances in technology that facilitate our understanding of this system will be critical in completing our quest to fully understand the complex interactions involved in promoting skeletal muscle growth in response to exercise.

concluded that the cross-sectional area of the body builders' individual muscle fibers was not significantly larger than normal; however, whole muscle size of these athletes was larger than normal.[26,41] About one decade later, a study reexamined the possibility of hyperplasia when McCall

et al.,[31] using both magnetic resonance imaging (MRI) and biopsy techniques, demonstrated an increase in muscle fiber number in the biceps after a typical heavy resistance training program, again presenting some evidence for hyperplasia; however, muscle fiber hypertrophy accounted for the greatest amount of whole muscle hypertrophy. It is possible that only high-intensity resistance training can cause hyperplasia and that type II muscle fibers may be targeted for this type of adaptation. Power lifters have been shown to have higher numbers of myonuclei, satellite cells, and small-diameter fibers expressing markers for early myogenesis, thereby indicating hyperplasia or the formation of new muscle fibers.[19] The effects appeared enhanced by anabolic steroid use, and thus one impact of anabolic drug use may be to increase the amount of hyperplasia that occurs.

Although limited data support hyperplasia in humans, there are indications that hyperplasia may occur as a consequence of resistance training. Due to these conflicting results, this topic continues to be controversial. Further research with elite competitive lifters and novel imaging techniques may help to resolve the controversy. Although hyperplasia in humans may not be the primary adaptational response to resistance training, it might represent one that is possible when certain muscle fibers reach a theoretical "upper limit" in cell size. It is possible that very intense long-term training may make some type II muscle fibers primary candidates for such an adaptational response. But even if hyperplasia does occur, it probably only accounts for a small portion (5–10%) of the increase in muscle size.[31]

Muscle Fiber Transition

The quality of protein refers to the type of proteins found in the contractile machinery and the muscle's ability to change its phenotype (i.e., actual protein expression) in response to resistance training, which, in turn, is based on the individual's genetic profile (i.e., inherited DNA).[35] Much of the resistance training research focuses on the myosin molecule and examination of fiber types based on the use of the histochemical myosin adenosine triphosphatase (mATPase) staining activities at different pHs. Changes in muscle mATPase fiber types also give an indication of associated changes that are taking place in the myosin heavy chain (MHC) content.[9] We now know that a continuum of muscle fiber subtypes exists, ranging from type I, to type IIA to type IIX fibers with interspersing subtypes. In addition, we know that transformation (e.g., type IIX to type IIA) within a particular muscle fiber type is a common adaptation to resistance training.[1,24,39] It appears that as soon as type IIX muscle fibers are recruited, they start a process of transformation toward the type IIA profile by changing the quality of proteins and expressing varying amounts of different types, or isoforms, of mATPase. For example, starting with type IIX, an initial transition might be to type IIXA, so that both types of mATPase are expressed in the muscle fiber. Minimal changes from type II to type I probably occur with exercise training unless mediated by damage and neural sprouting from another alpha motor neuron.[24] For example, sprouting of a type I motor neuron may result in

the innervation of a type II fiber that has been damaged with an exercise bout and has lost its neural connection to the fast motor neuron that had been innervating it. Thus, the fiber is said to have been re-innervated by a slow, or type I, neuron. However, the occurrence of such a phenomenon does not appear to be sufficiently frequent to alter absolute type I and type II fiber typing. Thus, a muscle's basic fiber type profile is determined by genetics, and although you are able to make transitions within the type I and type II fiber subtypes due to performance of strength or endurance training, one's fiber type distribution, as related to the broad categories of type I versus type II fibers, is pretty much set from birth.[24,38]

Compatibility of Exercise Training Programs

The topic of exercise compatibility first came to the attention of the sport and exercise science community when Hickson[14] showed that the development of dynamic strength may be compromised when both resistance training and high-intensity endurance training are included in a single training program. In contrast, improvements in cardiovascular fitness (VO_2max) and endurance performance (time to exhaustion at a given submaximal intensity) did not suffer as a result of a combined strength and aerobic training program. In short, a program that includes both strength and aerobic training may limit strength gains, but improvements in cardiovascular fitness and performance are as impressive as those observed when endurance training is performed alone. Subsequent studies seem to confirm Hickson's original results.[15,32]

The understanding of exercise training compatibility has focused on what is called concurrent training or simultaneous training of both aerobic performance and strength development. The effects of concurrent training on skeletal muscle are of interest to athletes and exercise scientists alike, as the body tries to adapt to both exercise stimuli. The challenge appears to be directed primarily to the motor units that are used in both training styles.

Studies examining concurrent training using high levels of training frequency and/or intensity for endurance and strength present the following conclusions (Box 3-13):

- Strength can be compromised, especially at high velocities of muscle actions, due to the performance of endurance training.
- Muscular power may be compromised more than strength by the performance of both strength and endurance training.
- Anaerobic performance may be negatively affected by endurance training.
- Development of maximal oxygen consumption is not compromised when a heavy resistance training and aerobic training program are performed.
- Endurance capabilities (i.e., time to exhaustion at a given submaximal intensity) are not negatively affected by strength training.

Box 3-13 APPLYING RESEARCH
Practical Applications

Exercise prescription must take into consideration the demands of the total program and make sure the volume of exercise does not become counterproductive to optimal physiological adaptations and performance. This requires the following steps:

1. Prioritize the training program and the goals of training. Do not attempt to perform high-intensity and high-volume strength and endurance training together.

Allow for adequate recovery from training sessions by using periodized training programs and planned rest phases.

2. If you are a strength/power athlete, limit your high-intensity aerobic training. One can perform lower intensity aerobic training, but high oxidative stress due to high-volume or high-intensity endurance training appears to negatively affect power development.

Few cellular data are available to provide insights into changes at the muscle fiber level with concurrent training. The muscle fibers that are recruited for both activities are faced with the dilemma of trying to adapt to the oxidative stimulus to improve their aerobic function, and at the same time, to the strength training stimulus by adding contractile proteins to increase their contractile force. Recall that endurance training alone typically decreases contractile protein content and fiber size to better enable diffusion of gasses across the muscle fiber. So, what happens to the muscle fiber population when it is exposed to a program of concurrent training? Kraemer et al.[24] examined changes in muscle fiber morphology over a 3-month training program in physically fit men. All training groups (endurance alone, strength alone, and combined endurance and strength) had a shift of muscle fiber types from type IIX to type IIA. In this study, the number of type IIX muscle fibers was lower after heavy strength training when compared with endurance training, which included both long-distance and interval training. The group completing a concurrent strength and endurance training program showed a sharp decrease in the percentage of type IIX fibers, much like the group performing strength training alone. This may be due to the greater recruitment of high-threshold motor units, those that contain type IIX fibers, with heavy resistance training performed by the strength only and the combined training groups.

Muscle fiber cross-sectional areas demonstrate that changes occur differentially across the continuum of exercise training modalities and are dictated by the type or combination of training stimuli to which the muscle is exposed. That is, when training only to develop strength, all muscle fiber types get larger. But when performing only cardiovascular endurance training, type I muscle fibers atrophy whereas no size changes are observed in the type II muscle fibers. And when training to concurrently develop strength and cardiovascular endurance, no changes are observed in the size of the type I muscle fibers, but increases are seen in the type II muscle fibers. Thus, attempting to train maximally for both muscle strength and cardiovascular endurance results in different size adaptations in the type I and type II muscle fibers, compared with just a single mode of training.

A multitude of factors (e.g., exercise prescriptions, pretraining fitness levels, exercise modalities, etc.) can affect the exercise stimulus and therefore the subsequent adaptational responses. Such factors will affect the muscle cell's signaling pathways for atrophy or hypertrophy.[5] The majority of studies in the literature have used relatively untrained subjects to examine the physiological effects of simultaneous strength and endurance training. Little data are available regarding the effects of simultaneous strength and endurance training using previously active or fit individuals, who are able to tolerate much higher intensity exercise training programs.[13] It appears that maximal simultaneous training may be particularly detrimental to

Quick Review

- Only muscle fibers that are recruited with the exercise will adapt to exercise stimuli.
- Adaptations to endurance training are related to the need to better deliver and utilize oxygen, in order to enhance muscular endurance.
- The growth in the absolute size of a muscle that results from resistance training is primarily due to the increase in the size of the individual muscle fibers rather than an increase in the number of fibers.
- When endurance and strength training programs are performed concurrently, the body tries to adapt to both of the exercise stimuli, but findings suggest that the body will experience greater improvements in endurance performance than strength.

optimal adaptations in muscle size, strength, and power, possibly due to overtraining with such high levels of work, volume of exercise, and intensity. Interestingly, aerobic capacity appears to be the least affected by such simultaneous training. If concurrent exercise training is properly designed, it may just require a longer time for the summation of physiological adaptations to occur; most of the studies to date have examined training programs lasting no more than 2 to 3 months. Based on the available data, it seems that one cannot have optimal adaptation to both modes of training. In addition to longer training program durations, other factors may be important to the successful concurrent development of strength and improved aerobic fitness. For example, both program **periodization** (varying the volume and intensity of the training) and **prioritization** (prioritizing what goals will be focused on in a training program) of training may allow individuals to adapt successfully.

CASE STUDY

Scenario

You are a strength and conditioning specialist working in the weight room at the Olympic Training Center in Colorado Springs, CO. You are trying to improve your strength and conditioning program for aspiring Olympic-level women figure skaters.

The coach has asked you what can be done to help the women better land their jumps in their routines. With the new scoring system requiring the skaters to perform triple and quad jumps to score high, more power training is needed.

Currently, you have each athlete on an individualized resistance training program. The program is periodized to complement each skater's on-ice training.

Questions

- What type of muscle action produces the force needed by skaters to perform jumps?
- What takes place in the muscle when a skater bends her knees in preparation for a jump?
- What provides the power for the upward movement in a jump?
- What type of muscle strength provides the skater with the braking system to absorb the load coming down on the leg during a landing?
- What types of training need to be included in the weight training program?

Options

Jumps are primarily a coordinated set of muscle actions that use the stretch-shortening cycle to produce the power output. The concentric action in the vertical jump that benefits from the stretch-shortening cycle propels the skater upward. Muscular power appears to be the primary muscular performance feature to propel the skater into the air, and the maximal eccentric strength determines the ability of the skater to brake upon landing on the ice. Thus, the training program needs to include stretch-shortening cycle or plyometric training to help with jump height, and eccentric training to assist in landing of jumps.

Scenario

You are a personal trainer for a triathlete getting ready for the ironman competition. In the past she has had trouble with stress fractures and you have added a heavy resistance training program to her total conditioning program in order to strengthen her connective tissue and prevent injuries. The other day she heard from a friend that lifting weights will hurt her endurance performance.

Questions

- Is it true that lifting weights will hurt endurance performance?
- What might be the expected adaptations in muscle when lifting weights and performing high volumes of endurance exercise?
- What are the benefits of combining both types of training protocols for this athlete?

Options

Although high-intensity endurance training has been shown to potentially interfere with power and strength development, few data are available to suggest that this will hurt endurance performances. This athlete is truly at a risk for connective tissue injury and resistance exercise will strengthen the connective tissue, making it better able to cope with the high volume of endurance training needed to compete and train for an ironman competition. The changes in the muscle would likely result in more protein in both the contractile and connective tissues with the type I fibers remaining unchanged in size but more resistant to protein loss. Overall the performance of resistance training will not decrease endurance performance and will help to decrease the chance of injury.

CHAPTER SUMMARY

Neural recruitment of skeletal muscle is what causes force production and movement in the human body. Several other systems of the body (e.g., skeletal, neural, immune) interact with skeletal muscle to sustain its health and assist it in force generation and movement. Skeletal muscle is highly organized, from the connective tissue that surrounds the intact whole muscle, to the connective tissue that keeps the contractile proteins of the sarcomere in place for optimal myofibril interactions. This connective tissue also contributes to the force and power production of muscle due to an elastic component, which upon stretch and recoil adds force to the muscle contraction. The elastic component in skeletal muscle provides the basis for plyometric training or for training using the stretch-shortening cycle. Skeletal muscle is a target of all training programs, whether for sport performance or health and fitness, and is highly plastic or adaptable to the exercise stimuli. Skeletal muscle is composed of different muscle fiber types, with each type being designed to accomplish different kinds of tasks, ranging from prolonged activities of low intensity (e.g., type I fibers are used during a marathon), to short, burst activities requiring tremendous force production (e.g., type II fibers used in sprint activities).

Resistance exercise typically results in muscle hypertrophy, whereas endurance training results in no change or even a decrease in muscle fiber size. Combining resistance training with endurance training will result in limited hypertrophy of the type I muscle fibers, with increases in size observed primarily in type II muscle fibers. Understanding skeletal muscle structure and function will allow a better understanding of the many methods of training and therapy that are used to enhance function, performance, and health. In the next chapter, we will examine how the nervous system controls muscle function and how it adapts to training.

REVIEW QUESTIONS

Fill-in-the-Blank

1. _____ proteins are those that are not involved with the contraction process, but hold contractile proteins in close proximity to each other for optimal myosin–actin binding interactions.

2. Tension receptors, called _____, which are located in the tendon of skeletal muscle, sense the amount of force in the tendon created by the skeletal muscle.

3. A form of exercise that utilizes the stretch-shortening cycle, termed _____, helps in the development of muscular power.

4. The acquisition of _____, formed from satellite cells which are found between the mature muscle

fiber's membrane and its basal lamina, is required to support muscle fiber hypertrophy.

5. With endurance exercise training only, the size of type I (slow-twitch) muscle fibers _____ to reduce the distance between the capillaries and the mitochondria.

Multiple Choice

1. Which protein of the sarcomere has the heads that bind to active sites?
   a. Actin
   b. Myosin
   c. Troponin
   d. Tropomyosin
   e. Titin

2. A marathon runner at the Olympic Games would have a high percentage of what type of fiber?
   a. Type II
   b. Type IIC
   c. Type I
   d. Type IC
   e. Both type I and type II fibers

3. What technique is used to obtain a small sample of muscle with a needle through the skin?
   a. Percutaneous muscle biopsy
   b. Subdermal musclectomy
   c. Myofibril biopsy
   d. Percutaneous sarcomere removal
   e. Incision musclectomy

4. What physiological adaptations occur when muscle fibers are recruited to perform an endurance exercise workout?
   a. The number of capillaries increase
   b. The capillary density in the type I fibers increases
   c. The number of mitochondria increases
   d. The concentration of myoglobin increases
   e. All of the above

5. Which of the following is an example of an isokinetic muscle action?
   a. Lifting a barbell in a biceps curl
   b. Lowering a barbell in a biceps curl
   c. Exerting force against an object that does not move
   d. A movement during which the velocity is held constant
   e. The action of the triceps during a biceps curl

True/False

1. At rest, the proteins troponin and tropomyosin cover the active sites on actin molecules, preventing the myosin heads from binding to the active sites.

2. When training for both strength and endurance at the same time, muscle fibers that are recruited improve their aerobic function as when training only for endurance.

3. Fast-twitch muscle fibers are characterized by the ability to resist fatigue and produce relatively small amounts of force.

4. The growth in the absolute size of a muscle due to resistance training is primarily due to the increase in the number of individual muscle fibers.

5. With endurance training, fiber types do not change from type I to type II.

Short Answer

1. Explain which adaptations are most affected by simultaneous strength and endurance training.

2. Explain the function of titin (connectin) and nebulin in the sarcomere.

3. Outline the steps during the contraction phase of the sliding filament theory.

Matching

Match the following terms with their correct definitions:

Eccentric	A movement characterized by maximal force exerted at a constant velocity of movement throughout a specific range of motion
Concentric	Muscle elongation while the muscle is activated and producing force
Isokinetic	Muscle action characterized by tension in the muscle with no change in muscle fiber length
Isometric	A muscle contraction characterized by muscle shortening against a constant load or tension throughout the entire range of movement
Isotonic	Muscle develops force and shortens

Critical Thinking

1. During a normal weight training back squat, what types of muscle actions take place during a repetition, and what type of muscle action will limit the maximal amount of weight that can be lifted for one complete repetition?

2. Describe the skeletal muscle adaptations to endurance training.

KEY TERMS

A band: the area in a sarcomere where actin and myosin overlap; it represents the length of the myosin filaments

actin: a thin myofilament that has active sites on it capable of interacting with the myosin protein to produce muscle force

active site: place on the actin filament where myosin heads can bind

antagonistic muscle: a muscle that contracts and acts in physiological opposition with the action of an agonist muscle

concentric (contraction): muscle activation characterized by muscle shortening

concurrent strength and endurance training: training for both strength and endurance at the same time

connectin (titin): a noncontractile protein of the sarcomere that connects the Z line to the M line, stabilizes myosin in the longitudinal axis, contributes to the elastic component of the muscle fiber, and limits the range of motion of the sarcomere

crossbridges: small projections on the myosin filament that interact with actin to cause muscle contraction and force production

cytosol: the liquid portion of the contents inside living cells, including muscle fibers

delayed onset muscle soreness (DOMS): pain several hours to several days after an exercise bout that is a symptom of muscle damage

DHP receptors: proteins found in the T-tubules that act as voltage sensors when the electrical impulse travels along the T-tubule

dynamic constant external resistance: isotonic muscle contraction; describes the type of muscle activity when exercising with external resistances in activities such as lifting weights

eccentric: muscle elongation while the muscle is activated and producing force

elastic component: the recoil force in the muscle after being stretched, due to noncontractile portions of muscle

endomysium: the connective tissue surrounding each individual muscle fiber

epimysium: the external layer of connective tissue surrounding the whole muscle

fasciculus (*pl.* fasciculi): a small bundle of muscle fibers

fast-twitch fibers: muscle fibers characterized by the ability to produce relatively large amounts of force quickly, a high glycolytic capacity, and a low oxidative capacity

force–time curve: a graph illustrating the force production over different lengths of time

force–velocity curve: a graph illustrating the influence of changing the velocity of movement on the muscle's force production capabilities

Golgi tendon organ: force receptors located in the tendon of skeletal muscle

H zone: the region in the middle of the sarcomere, which contains only myosin

heavy chains: protein components that form the myosin head and a portion of the tail of a myosin molecule

hyperplasia: an increase in the number of cells of a tissue

I bands: the light bands of the sarcomere that contain only actin

intrafusal fibers: modified muscle fibers arranged parallel to normal muscle fibers that contain muscle spindles

isoinertial: (isotonic) an exercise movement with a fixed resistance and variable velocity

isokinetic: a movement characterized by muscle force exerted at a constant velocity

isometric: a muscle contraction characterized by tension in the muscle with no change in muscle fiber length

isotonic: a muscle contraction characterized by muscle shortening against a constant external load, such as during the lifting of a barbell

kinesthetic sense: awareness of the body's position in space

learning effect: mastery of the motor unit recruitment pattern for a specific skill or movement due to repeatedly performing the skill or movement

light chains: protein components of the myosin filament that form the hinge portion of a myosin molecule

M line: proteins in the middle of the H zone that hold the myosin filaments in place

muscle fibers: long multinucleated cells that contain myofibrils that contract when stimulated

muscle spindle: a stretch receptor arranged in parallel to muscle fibers that monitors stretch and length of the muscle

myofibril: the portion of the muscle containing the thin and the thick contractile filaments

myonuclei: nuclei located beneath the sarcolemma of the muscle fiber

myosin: the contractile protein in the myofibril that has crossbridges that can bind to actin to cause tension development

myosin ATPase: an enzyme found on the globular heads of the myosin crossbridges, which breaks down ATP to release energy needed for muscle contraction

myosin ATPase staining: a method for distinguishing type I and type II human muscle fibers and their subtypes based on a staining for the enzyme that hydrolyzes ATP

nebulin: a noncontractile protein that stabilizes actin; it is localized to the I band and extends from the Z line

neuromuscular system: the close functional relationship between the nerves and skeletal muscle

nuclear domain: the area within a muscle fiber that each myonucleus controls

percutaneous muscle biopsy technique: a technique in which a hollow needle is inserted through the skin to obtain a sample of muscle

perimysium: the fibrous connective tissue surrounding each fasciculus of skeletal muscle fibers

plyometric exercise: a form of exercise that uses the stretch-shortening cycle to help in the development of muscular power

power: product of force exerted by the muscle and the vertical distance the load is displaced divided by time, or force times velocity

prioritization: a principle of prioritizing what goals will be focused on in a training program

periodization: varying the volume and intensity of training in a planned manner

progressive overload: a gradual increase in the intensity or volume of exercise

proprioceptors: sensory receptors located within the muscles, tendons, and joints that provide information about the body's position by monitoring the length of muscle, force produced by muscle, and joint position

ratchet movement: a movement in which the myosin head swivels at its hinged pivot point to a new angle, pulling the actin over the myosin filament and causing the sarcomere to shorten

ryanodine receptors: calcium channels located on the membrane of the sarcoplasmic reticulum, which open when activated by voltage sensors of the T-tubules

sarcomere: the smallest or most basic contractile unit of skeletal muscle capable of shortening

sarcoplasmic reticulum: membranous organelle found within the muscle fiber that stores the calcium needed for muscle force development

satellite cells: cells found under the basal lamina membrane of mature muscle fibers that are the source of new myonuclei

skeletal muscle: muscle that is connected at both ends to a bone

sliding filament theory: a theory of muscle contraction describing the sliding of the thin filaments (actin) past the thick filaments (myosin) by the attaching and detaching of the heads of myosin molecules to the actin filaments, drawing each end of a sarcomere toward each other

speed-strength: training that is focused on force production at higher velocities and lighter resistances to improve power

steric blocking model: the process of covering the active sites on the actin filament by tropomyosin preventing interaction with the myosin filament keeping the muscle fiber in a nonactivated condition

strength curve: a graph of the amount of force produced over a range of motion

stretch-shortening cycle: muscle elongation followed by a rapid muscle shortening

striated muscle: the striped appearance of muscle that is created by the arrangement of myofibrils in sarcomeres

T-tubules: a membrane-enclosed tunnel allowing electrical impulse to spread through the muscle fiber

tendons: a band of tough, inelastic fibrous tissue that connects a muscle with bone

titin (connectin): a noncontractile protein of the sarcomere that connects the Z line to the M line, stabilizes myosin in the longitudinal axis, contributes to the elastic component of the muscle fiber, and limits the range of motion of the sarcomere

tropomyosin: a protein covering the actin binding sites when muscle is at rest that prevents the myosin crossbridge from touching active sites on actin; when muscle is stimulated to contract, it moves, exposing the active sites so myosin and actin can interact to shorten

troponin: a protein, associated with actin and tropomyosin, that binds Ca^{++} and initiates the movement of tropomyosin on actin to allow the myosin crossbridge to touch active sites on actin and initiate contraction

type I muscle fibers (slow-twitch fibers): muscle fibers that contain large amounts of oxidative enzymes are highly fatigue-resistant and do not develop force as quickly as type II fibers

type II muscle fibers (fast-twitch fibers): muscle fibers that develop force very rapidly, demonstrate high force production capability, are less resistant to fatigue than slow fibers, have a relatively small number of mitochondria, and a limited capacity for aerobic metabolism

variable resistance: strength training equipment in which the resistance varies throughout the range of motion to better match the strength curve

Z line: a band delineating the ends of the sarcomere

REFERENCES

1. Adams GR, Hather BM, Baldwin KM, et al. Skeletal muscle myosin heavy chain composition and resistance training. J Appl Physiol. 1993;74:911–915.
2. Allen TJ, Proske U. Effect of muscle fatigue on the sense of limb position and movement. Exp Brain Res. 2006;170:30–38.
3. Alway SE, Winchester PK, Davis ME, et al. Regionalized adaptations and muscle fiber proliferation in stretch-induced enlargement. J Appl Physiol. 1989;66:771–781.
4. Antonio J, Gonyea WJ. Muscle fiber splitting in stretch-enlarged avian muscle. Med Sci Sports Exerc. 1994;26:973–977.
5. Coffey VG, Zhong Z, Shield A, et al. Early signaling responses to divergent exercise stimuli in skeletal muscle from well-trained humans. Faseb J. 2006;20:190–192.
6. Cramer JT, Housh TJ, Weir JP, et al. The acute effects of static stretching on peak torque, mean power output, electromyography, and mechanomyography. Eur J Appl Physiol. 2005;93:530–539.

7. Dudley GA, Djamil R. Incompatibility of endurance- and strength-training modes of exercise. J Appl Physiol. 1985;59:1446–1451.

8. Fleck SJ, Kraemer WJ. Designing Resistance Training Programs. 3rd ed. Champaign, IL: Human Kinetics Publishers Inc., 2004.

9. Fry AC, Allemeier CA, Staron RS. Correlation between percentage fiber type area and myosin heavy chain content in human skeletal muscle. Eur J Appl Physiol Occup Physiol. 1994;68:246–251.

10. Fry AC, Staron RS, James CB, et al. Differential titin isoform expression in human skeletal muscle. Acta Physiol Scand. 1997;161:473–479.

11. Gonyea WJ, Sale DG, Gonyea FB, et al. Exercise induced increases in muscle fiber number. Eur J Appl Physiol Occup Physiol. 1986;55:137–141.

12. Hawley JA. Adaptations of skeletal muscle to prolonged, intense endurance training. Clin Exp Pharmacol Physiol. 2002;29:218–222.

13. Hennessy LC, Watson AWS. The interference effects of training for strength and endurance simultaneously. J Strength Cond Res. 1994;8:12–19.

14. Hickson RC. Interference of strength development by simultaneously training for strength and endurance. Eur J Appl Physiol Occup Physiol. 1980;45:255–263.

15. Huxley AF, Niedergerke R. Structural changes in muscle during contraction. Nature. 1954;173:971–972.

16. Huxley AF. Cross-bridge action: present views, prospects, and unknowns. J Biomech. 2000;33:1189–1195.

17. Huxley HE, Hanson J. Changes in cross-striations of muscle during contraction and stretch and their structural interpretation. Nature. 1954;173:973–976.

18. Issurin VB. Vibrations and their applications in sport. A review. J Sports Med Phys Fitness. 2005;45:324–336.

19. Kadi F, Eriksson A, Holmner S, et al. Effects of anabolic steroids on the muscle cells of strength-trained athletes. Med Sci Sports Exerc. 1999;31:1528–1534.

20. Kadi F, Thornell LE. Concomitant increases in myonuclear and satellite cell content in female trapezius muscle following strength training. Histochem Cell Biol. 2000;113:99–103.

21. Kjaer M, Magnusson P, Krogsgaard M, et al. Extracellular matrix adaptation of tendon and skeletal muscle to exercise. J Anat. 2006;208:445–450.

22. Knuttgen HG, Kraemer WJ. Terminology and measurement in exercise performance. J Appl Sport Sci Res. 1987;1:1–10.

23. Komi PV. Stretch-shortening cycle: A powerful model to study normal and fatigued muscle. J Biomech. 2000;33:1197–1206.

24. Kraemer WJ, Patton JF, Gordon SE, et al. Compatibility of high-intensity strength and endurance training on hormonal and skeletal muscle adaptations. J Appl Physiol. 1995;78:976–989.

25. Kraft T, Mahlmann E, Mattei T, et al. Initiation of the power stroke in muscle: Insights from the phosphate analog AlF_4. Proc Natl Acad Sci U S A. 2005;102:13861–13866.

26. MacDougall JD, Sale DG, Elder GC, et al. Muscle ultrastructural characteristics of elite powerlifters and bodybuilders. Eur J Appl Physiol Occup Physiol. 1982;48:117–126.

27. MacDougall JD, Sale DG, Moroz JR, et al. Mitochondrial volume density in human skeletal muscle following heavy resistance training. Med Sci Sports. 1979;11:164–166.

28. MacDougall JD, Tarnopolsky MA, Chesley A, et al. Changes in muscle protein synthesis following heavy resistance exercise in humans: A pilot study. Acta Physiol Scand. 1992;146:403–404.

29. Malisoux L, Francaux M, Nielens H, et al. Stretch-shortening cycle exercises: An effective training paradigm to enhance power output of human single muscle fibers. J Appl Physiol. 2006;100:771–779.

30. Marek SM, Cramer JT, Fincher AL, et al. Acute effects of static and proprioceptive neuromuscular facilitation stretching on muscle strength and power output. J Athl Train. 2005;40:94–103.

31. McCall GE, Byrnes WC, Dickinson A, et al. Muscle fiber hypertrophy, hyperplasia, and capillary density in college men after resistance training. J Appl Physiol. 1996;81:2004–2012.

32. McCarthy JP, Agre JC, Graf BK, et al. Compatibility of adaptive responses with combining strength and endurance training. Med Sci Sports Exerc. 1995;27:429–436.

33. Mileusnic MP, Loeb GE. Mathematical models of proprioceptors: II. Structure and function of the Golgi tendon organ. J Neurophysiol. 2006;96:1789–1802.

34. Pette D, Staron RS. Myosin isoforms, muscle fiber types, and transitions. Microsc Res Tech. 2000;50:500–509.

35. Pette D, Staron RS. Transitions of muscle fiber phenotypic profiles. Histochem Cell Biol. 2001;115:359–372.

36. Pirani A, Vinogradova MV, Curmi PM, et al. An atomic model of the thin filament in the relaxed and Ca2+–activated states. J Mol Biol. 2006;357:707–717.

37. Potts JT. Inhibitory neurotransmission in the nucleus tractus solitarii: Implications for baroreflex resetting during exercise. Exp Physiol. 2006;91:59–72.

38. Staron RS, Johnson P. Myosin polymorphism and differential expression in adult human skeletal muscle. Comp Biochem Physiol B. 1993;106:463–475.

39. Staron RS, Leonardi MJ, Karapondo DL, et al. Strength and skeletal muscle adaptations in heavy-resistance-trained women after detraining and retraining. J Appl Physiol. 1991;70:631–640.

40. Staron RS. Human skeletal muscle fiber types: Delineation, development, and distribution. Can J Appl Physiol. 1997;22:307–327.

41. Tesch PA, Larsson L. Muscle hypertrophy in bodybuilders. Eur J Appl Physiol Occup Physiol. 1982;49:301–306.

42. Trappe S, Harber M, Creer A, et al. Single muscle fiber adaptations with marathon training. J Appl Physiol. 2006.

43. Young WB, Behm DG. Effects of running, static stretching and practice jumps on explosive force production and jumping performance. J Sports Med Phys Fitness. 2003;43:21–27.

Suggested Readings

Crepaldi G, Maggi S. Sarcopenia and osteoporosis: A hazardous duet. J Endocrinol Invest. 2005;28(10 Suppl):66–68.

French DN, Gomez AL, Volek JS, et al. Longitudinal tracking of muscular power changes of NCAA Division I collegiate women gymnasts. J Strength Cond Res. 2004;18(1):101–107.

Guillet C, Boirie Y. Insulin resistance: A contributing factor to age-related muscle mass loss? Diabetes Metab. 2005;31(Spec No 2):5S20–5S26.

Janssen I, Ross R. Linking age-related changes in skeletal muscle mass and composition with metabolism and disease. J Nutr Health Aging. 2005;9(6):408–419.

Narici MV, Reeves ND, Morse CI, et al. Muscular adaptations to resistance exercise in the elderly. J Musculoskelet Neuronal Interact. 2004;4(2):161–164.

Classic References

Costill DL. Physiology of marathon running. JAMA. 1972;221(9):1024–1049.

Costill DL. The relationship between selected physiological variables and distance running performance. J Sports Med Phys Fitness. 1967;7(2):61–66.

Costill DL, Winrow E. Maximal oxygen intake among marathon runners. Arch Phys Med Rehabil. 1970;51(6):317–320.

Fick A. Uber die messung des blutquantums in den hertzvent rikeln. (On the measurement of blood mass in the heart ventricles.) Sitz ber Physik-Med Ges Wurzburg 1870;2:16–28.

Gollnick PD. Armstrong RB, Saubert CW IV, et al. Enzyme activity and fiber composition in skeletal muscle of untrained and trained men. J Appl Physiol. 1972;33(3):312–319.

Hermansen L, Wachtlova M. Capillary density of skeletal muscle in well-trained and untrained men. J Appl Physiol. 1971;30(6):860–863.

Holloszy JO. Biochemical adaptations in muscle. Effects of exercise on mitochondrial oxygen uptake and respiratory enzyme activity in skeletal muscle. J Biol Chem. 1967;242:2278–2282.

Huxley AF, Niedergerke R. Structural changes in muscle during contraction. Nature. 1954;173:971–972.

Huxley HE, Hanson J. Changes in cross-striations of muscle during contraction and stretch and their structural interpretation. Nature. 1954;173:973–976.

Ingjer F, Brodal P. Capillary supply of skeletal muscle fibers in untrained and endurance-trained women. Eur J Appl Physiol Occup Physiol. 1978;38(4):291–299.

Saltin B. Physiological effects of physical conditioning. Med. Sci. Sports Exerc. 1969;1:50–56.

Saltin B. Oxygen uptake and cardiac output during maximal treadmill and bicycle exercise. Mal Cardiovasc. 1969;10(1):393–399.

Saltin B, Nazar K, Costill DL, et al. The nature of the training response; peripheral and central adaptations of one-legged exercise. Acta Physiol Scand. 1976;96(3):289–305.

4

The Nervous System

After reading this chapter, you should be able to:

1. Explain homeostasis and feedback systems
2. Describe the organization of the nervous system
3. Diagram the structure of a neuron
4. Differentiate the functions of the central nervous system, peripheral nervous system, autonomic nervous system, sympathetic nervous system, parasympathetic nervous system, and the sensory–somatic nervous system

5. Define a motor unit
6. Explain the conduction of nervous impulses
7. Apply the size principle of muscle fiber recruitment
8. Describe the nervous system in action
9. Consider practical applications of the nervous system
10. Explain neural adaptations to exercise

The nervous system is the basis of almost all communication in the body. It works intimately with other physiological systems, as is reflected in commonly used terms such as "neuro-muscular," "neuroendocrine," or "neurovascular." The basic functions of the nervous system are receiving, processing, integrating, and responding to information. More specifically, the nervous system receives input from both the internal and external environments. The nervous system must process and integrate such input and then properly respond to the different stimuli, thereby mediating effective outcomes. The nervous system is essential for rapid communication and co-ordination of many physiological functions critical in exercise performance. Thus, this chapter introduces you to primary functions and structures of the nervous system, the organization of the nervous system, the motor unit and the size principle, and practical applications of the nervous system to exercise.

FUNCTIONS OF THE NERVOUS SYSTEM

It is the nervous system, including the brain, that enables most of the characteristics that distinguish higher vertebrates from more primitive animals. The nervous system makes possible conscious awareness, memory, sensation, thought, perception, subconscious reflexes, and initiates bodily movements. In sum, the nervous system functions as the body's primary communication network that detects disturbances in the body's internal and external environment and elicits changes to properly respond to those disturbances. It is the nervous system, then, that is mainly responsible for maintaining the body's homeostasis and, accordingly, life itself.

Maintaining Homeostasis

In a term coined by the famous physiologist Walter B. Cannon of Harvard University in 1932, the nervous system is intimately involved with helping to maintain **homeostasis** of physiological systems. Homeostasis is the ability of an organism or cell to maintain internal equilibrium by adjusting its physiological processes to keep functions within physiological limits at rest or during exercise.[2] Exercise presents a formidable challenge to the body's homeostatic mechanisms as physical exertion results in a host of physiological perturbations, including increased body temperature, changes in acid–base balance, hypohydration, changes in blood pressure, and altered blood glucose. Proper function of the nervous system is essential for the body to both detect and respond to these exercise-related alterations.

Various types of feedback systems are used in the operational communication between the nervous system and almost every organ system throughout the body. The most common feedback systems are called "positive and negative feedback loops." In simple terms, a positive feedback loop can promote or even intensify a process. During exercise, for example, increased acidity produced by active muscle will cause an increase in blood flow to the affected tissue. As the activity level of muscle increases, resulting in even higher acidity, a greater increase in blood flow will occur. Conversely, negative feedback loops, which are even more common than positive ones, diminish or reduce the intensity of an ongoing process in an attempt to return to the initial status quo. A good example of a negative feedback loop is the sweating mechanism that is activated during exercise. Prolonged muscular activity increases the heat produced by skeletal muscle and elevates the body's temperature. To counter this and prevent the body from overheating, sweating occurs, which results in evaporative heat loss and a cooling effect. A variety of feedback systems are in place to regulate physiological function at rest, during exercise, and into recovery.

CELLS AND SUBCELLULAR COMPONENTS OF THE NERVOUS SYSTEM

Several different types of cells with specialized anatomy and physiology make up the nervous system. These specialized cells allow the nervous system to perform all of its functions related to control of the body and its physiological systems.

Neurons

Perhaps the most essential type of cell in the function of the nervous system is the **neuron**. The neuron is an electrically excitable cell that initiates, receives, and transmits information throughout the body. A typical neuron consists of three basic components: 1) **dendrites**, 2) a **cell body**, and 3) **axons** (Fig. 4-1A). The cell body of a neuron contains the nucleus, mitochondria, ribosomes, and other cellular constituents. Dendrites receive information (impulses) and send it to the cell body (also called the soma), which is the processing center for signal information received. Signals are then sent out from the cell body through the axon to another neuron or target tissue receptor (e.g., muscle). In order for an impulse to be sent out from the cell body through its axon, a threshold amount of stimulus must be received from dendrites. At the end of the axon that joins with the cell body lies the **axon hillock,** which is the site where the summation of incoming electrical signals takes place. At any given moment, a threshold amount of stimuli can be accumulated, causing the neuron to initiate and send an electrical charge, or "action potential," out from the cell body through its axon to continue information flow to the next neuron or target tissue. The collective influence of all neurons that conduct impulses via dendrites to a given neuron will determine whether an action potential will be initiated at the axon hillock and sent out from the neuron to the next neuron or target tissue.[30]

Structurally, neurons come in many different shapes and sizes (Fig. 4-1B). The three basic types are multipolar, pseudounipolar, and bipolar. A multipolar neuron has multiple processes that extend from the cell body, many dendrites, and a single axon. Pseudounipolar neurons are primarily sensory neurons. Early in their development, the axon and dendrite fuse to form a single process with a very short dendrite still existing and a long axon that conducts impulses to the central nervous system. Bipolar neurons have one axon and one dendrite and are primarily sensory; they can be found in the retina of the eye.

Axons vary in length due to the distance from the spinal cord to the target cells. Thus, the length of an axon can range from millimeters to more than a meter; think of an axon leaving a 7-foot-tall basketball player's spinal cord and extending all the way to the muscles of his foot. While there are many different types of neurons in the

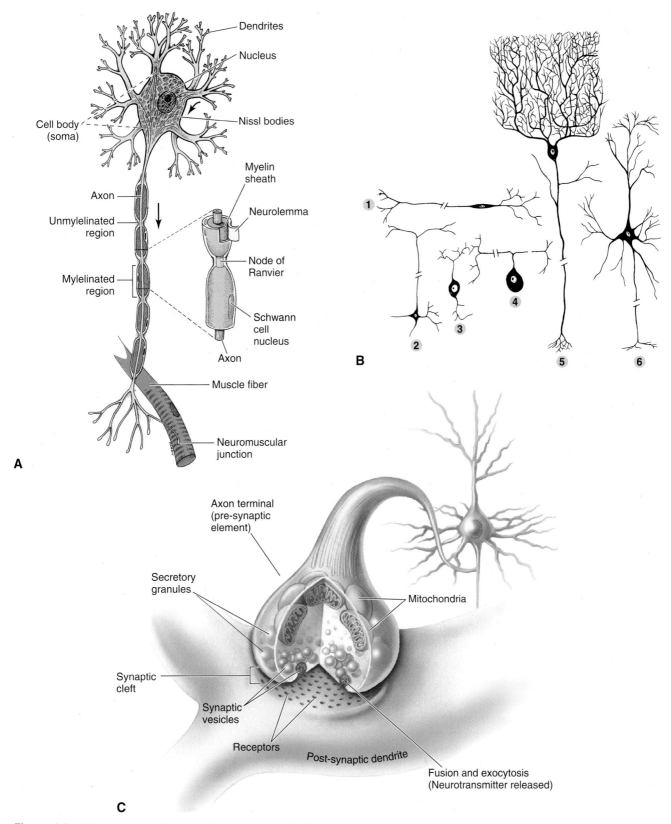

Figure 4-1. Different types of neurons found in the body. They come in all shapes and sizes, but fundamental to each is an axon and a dendrite. **A** shows the typical neuron; **B** shows the wide variety of neurons that make up the nervous system: 1. horizontal cell (of Cajal) from cerebral cortex; 2. Martinotti cell; 3. bipolar cell; 4. unipolar cell (posterior root ganglion); 5. Purkinje neurons; 6. pyramidal cell of motor area of cerebral cortex); and **C** shows a typical synapse made up of pre-synaptic and post-synaptic areas.

body, they all have the ability to generate and/or transmit information in the form of electrical impulses. Sensory neurons (also called afferent neurons) typically have a long dendrite, which carries information from peripheral cells (e.g., nose, eyes, finger tips) to its soma, found just outside the spinal cord in the dorsal root ganglia, where a short axon then relays the information into the central nervous system. Thus, **sensory neurons** carry messages from sensory receptors in the body's periphery to the central nervous system. **Motor neurons** (also referred to as efferent neurons) have their cell body in the spinal cord, so they have a long axon that innervates muscle fibers and short dendrites to receive impulses from other neurons. **Interneurons** are special neurons that are seen only in the central nervous system, where they account for more than 99% of all neurons. These cells function mainly to connect sensory and motor neurons, and to interact with each other to fine-tune motor control during muscle activity. These interneurons are obviously important in sports as they join sensory input, such as judgment of speed and location of a pitched baseball, with a desired response of the motor system, such as when to swing the bat in order to hit the pitched ball.

Neuroglia

Within the central nervous system, only about 10% of the cells are neurons (i.e., afferent, efferent, interneurons), and the rest are called neuroglia or glial cells. These cells are not able to initiate or conduct electrical signals, but they play vital roles by providing support and nourishment to neurons, and they also form myelin sheaths around the axons of some neurons. These myelin sheaths are important to sports and athletics as they increase the velocity with which an impulse is passed through the nervous system. A goalie in ice hockey must process information quickly if he is to have any success in stopping pucks fired at him at speeds of more than 100 miles·h^{-1}.

Synapses

The term **synapse** refers to the point of connection, and communication, between two excitable cells. (Neurons and muscle fibers are considered excitable cells.) The first neuron in this line of communication, or "pre-synaptic neuron," releases a chemical substance known as a **neurotransmitter**, which diffuses across a small gap and then binds to and activates specific specialized sites, called **receptors**, located on the target cell, which is sometimes called the "post-synaptic cell."[20] Thus, pre- and post-synaptic membranes are not in contact; as a result, the electrical impulse carried by the pre-synaptic neuron is transduced from one excitable cell to another by the release of the neurotransmitter specific to that neuron. The target cell may be another neuron, a

specialized region of a muscle cell, or a secretory cell (a cell that can make and secrete a chemical substance). The type of synapse described above, where a neurotransmitter is used to pass information from one excitable cell to another, is called a **chemical synapse**. Although rarely found in the nervous system of mammals, there is a second type of synapse, which joins excitable cells in heart muscle (myocardium) and smooth muscle cells found in glands and in the gastrointestinal tract. These are called **electrical synapses** and they communicate information from one cell to another by allowing ions or electrically charged particles to directly pass between them through specialized areas in the membranes of cells called gap junctions.

In chemical synapses, it is the neurotransmitter that is responsible for eliciting an electrical pulse in the post-synaptic cell, thus passing along, or transducing, information from one neuron to another, or to a muscle fiber. After crossing the synaptic cleft, or gap between the pre- and post-synaptic neurons, the neurotransmitter binds with receptors on the post-synaptic neuron. In turn, this event opens channels, allowing the movement of ions across the post-synaptic cell's membrane. If adequate amounts of ions cross the membrane, the charge created will be strong enough to cause a response of the post-synaptic membrane. If the synapse is between two neurons, the post-synaptic membrane is that of a dendrite, and the impulse is delivered by the pre-synaptic axon. If the synapse is between a neuron and a target cell, such as a muscle fiber, a response of the target cell is initiated, resulting in contraction of the muscle fiber. The neurotransmitter is quickly destroyed by an enzyme in the synaptic cleft; thus, the neurotransmitter is present and active only for a brief period of time at a synapse. For continued communication to occur, additional amounts of neurotransmitter must be released by the pre-synaptic neuron into the cleft so that it might bind to receptors on the post-synaptic cell, allowing more ions to enter it. More than 50 chemical neurotransmitter substances have been discovered, with the primary ones being acetylcholine, histamine, norepinephrine, dopamine, serotonin, glutamate, gamma-aminobutyric acid (GABA), glycine, substance P, enkephalins, and endorphins.

Receptors

There are many different types of receptors in the body, and all are involved in communication. Receptors are proteins designed to bind to a specific substance, such as a neurotransmitter, hormone, or other chemical substance that is called a **ligand**. Here we will focus on receptors that bind to neurotransmitters. Not only are these receptors specific for neurotransmitters as opposed to hormones or other chemical substances, but each neurotransmitter has its own unique receptor. This enables the communication among various neurons to maintain its fidelity or accuracy, so that target cells receive information only from the proper pre-synaptic cells. If different neurotransmitters shared receptors, the networks for communication would become confused, and post-synaptic target cells would receive unintended information from "wrong" pre-synaptic cells. As described above, upon binding a neurotransmitter, the receptor opens channels allowing ion flux, or movement, across the neuron's membrane, resulting in electrical charge. As a further example of the specificity of receptors, each kind allows only a single type of ion, be it Na^+, K^+, or Ca^{++}, to pass through its channels. The only exception to this rule is the acetylcholine receptor of the neuromuscular junction (NMJ). The channels embedded in this type of receptor allow both Na^+ and K^+ to concurrently cross the muscle fiber's membrane, albeit in different directions (Na^+ in and K^+ out). In sum then, the receptor is essential for communication from one neuron to another in that it binds the neurotransmitter released from the pre- to the post-synaptic neuron, and converts that chemical message into an electrical charge by allowing electrically charged ions to move across the post-synaptic cell's membrane. A typical synapse is displayed in Figure 4-2. Next we will examine how neurons are organized into the different divisions of the nervous system.

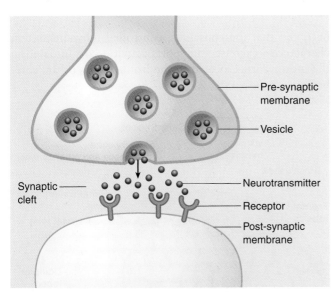

Figure 4-2. The basic structure of a synapse with its different components, including a receptor protein to receive the chemical signal from the neurotransmitter. An action potential arrives at the pre-synaptic terminal, and depolarization of the pre-synaptic terminal opens ion channels, allowing Ca^{2+} into the cell. The Ca^{2+} triggers the release of a neurotransmitter from the vesicles, and they bind to the receptors on the post-synaptic membrane, which results in the opening and closing of ion channels to cause a change in the post-synaptic membrane potential, and, when it reaches a threshold level, an action potential is produced, which propagates through to the next cell. (Modified from Bear M, Connors B, Paradiso M. Neuroscience, Exploring the Brain. 3rd ed. Baltimore: Lippincott Williams and Wilkins, 2000.)

Figure labels: Pre-synaptic membrane · Vesicle · Synaptic cleft · Neurotransmitter · Receptor · Post-synaptic membrane

Quick Review

- The nervous system helps maintain "homeostasis" of physiological systems.
- Positive and negative feedback systems regulate physiological function at rest, during exercise, and recovery.
- A typical neuron consists of three basic components: 1) dendrites, 2) a cell body, and 3) axons.
- Sensory neurons carry messages from sensory receptors to the central nervous system.
- Motor neurons have a long axon, to send impulses from the central nervous system to the muscle, and short dendrites.
- Interneurons are specialized neurons that are found only in the central nervous system and connect one neuron to another neuron.
- A synapse is the point of connection between two excitable cells.
- Neurons release neurotransmitters, which diffuse across a small gap and activate receptors on the target cell.
- Receptors receive chemical signals from a preceding neuron.

ORGANIZATION OF THE NERVOUS SYSTEM

The nervous system is divided into two major subdivisions: the central nervous system and the peripheral nervous system. The central nervous system is made up of the brain and spinal cord, whereas the peripheral nervous system is subdivided into a number of different divisions. Each subdivision has its own unique structural and functional capabilities, but all contribute to a highly integrated single nervous system. The basic organization of the nervous system is presented in Figure 4-3.

Central Nervous System

The **central nervous system** consists of the brain and the spinal cord and has more than 120 billion neurons processing information and managing many different physiological functions (e.g., pain perception, brain functions, sweating, etc.), including the activation or stimulation of skeletal muscles to contract and cause movement. The brain is protected by the skull and the spinal cord by the vertebrae. Both the spinal cord and the brain are bathed in cerebrospinal fluid (CSF) that protects the sensitive neural tissues and provides them with a constant internal environment (Fig. 4-4).

Brain

The brain contains more than 100 billion neurons that are organized into discrete regions and have specific functions associated with them (Fig. 4-4). The **cerebrum**, known as the "seat of consciousness," is the largest part of the human brain and is divided into left and right hemispheres, which are connected to each other by the *corpus callosum*. The two hemispheres are covered by a thin layer of gray matter

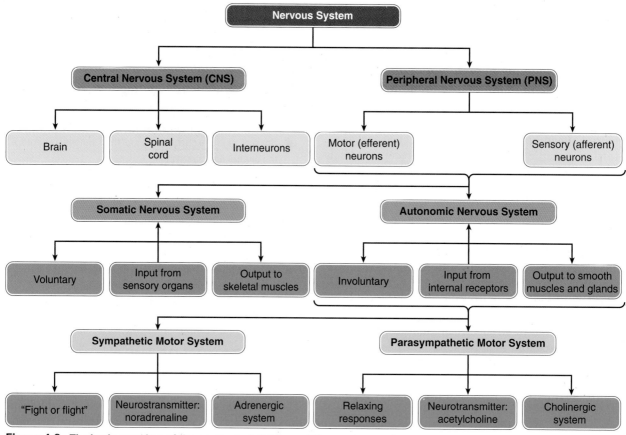

Figure 4-3. The basic overview of the anatomical divisions of the nervous system.

called the cerebral cortex. The cortex is divided into four regions, called the occipital, temporal, parietal, and frontal lobes. The functions that are regulated by these different regions of the brain are presented in Table 4-1. It should be noted that the conscious, controlled movements that characterize exercise and sports activities are initiated in the motor cortex located in the frontal lobes of the cerebrum.

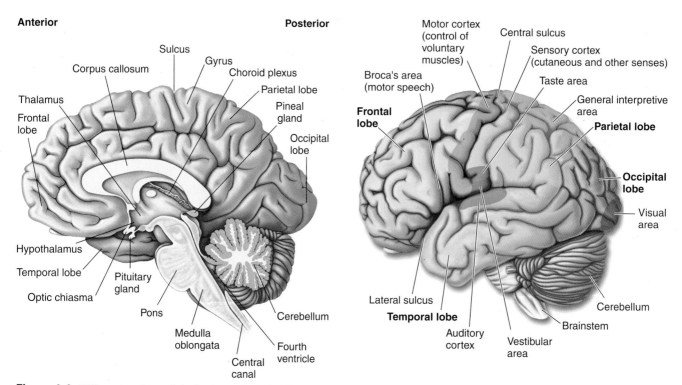

Figure 4-4. Different regions of the brain, each with different functions.

The **cerebellum** and the **medulla oblongata** are thought of as part of the unconscious brain, which also includes the midbrain and the pons. Regulation of the heart, breathing, blood pressure, and reflexes such as swallowing, hiccups, sneezing, and vomiting involve the medulla oblongata and the pons. The cerebellum is the second largest part of the brain. It is important in exercise and sports because it is involved in the regulation of muscle coordination during the execution of motor movements and also helps to coordinate balance and normal posture.

Table 4-1.	Functions Associated with the Lobes of the Brain
Lobe	**Function**
Occipital	Input and processing of visual information
Temporal	Input and processing of auditory signals, language
Parietal	Input and processing of information concerning touch, taste, heat, cold, pain, and pressure
Frontal	Input and processing of muscular activity, motor control, speech, and thought

Box 4-1 DID YOU KNOW?

Concussion and Sport

A blow to the head can cause injury and, in many cases, concussion. In sports, head trauma from contact is a distinct possibility. The effects of concussions on the function of the brain vary. Memory, reflexes, speech, coordination, and balance can all be affected. Interestingly, although a blow to the head usually initiates the concussion, not all concussions involve a loss of consciousness (a blackout), and many people have had concussions and were unaware of it. In addition, repeated concussions from a sport have been associated with many long-term potential health problems, some of them fatal.

Signs and symptoms can be delayed and can last for hours, days, months, or longer. Headache, dizziness, ringing in the ears, vomiting, nausea, speech problems, sleep disturbances, and mood and cognition problems can all be symptoms of concussion.

Concussion continues to be a major source of concern for sports with contact and collisions, most notably American football. Advances in equipment in American football, including the helmet, have actually amplified the severity of contact over the past 50 years.

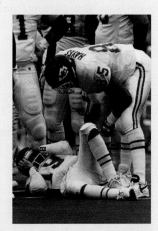

As discussed in this chapter, the CSF provides the cushioning that protects the brain from daily exposure to bumps and impacts, but violent blows to the head can cause the brain to hit the inner wall of the skull (see figure). Concussions occur most commonly in sports with extensive, direct contact between athletes, such as boxing, martial arts, judo, American football, and wrestling, despite rule changes designed to protect the athletes. Athletes who have a concussion are more prone to another concussion. Complications can occur if return to play occurs too quickly and further trauma is experienced. Many screening exams have been developed to set a baseline for each athlete to work from if a concussion occurs. The complications from concussion are called the postconcussion syndrome and are not well documented or understood. Concussions increase the risk for developing medical problems years after the injury, including epilepsy and (based on anecdotal evidence in NFL players) depression, Alzheimer disease, and Parkinson's disease. Prevention of concussions is something that cannot be taken lightly by sport governing bodies and medical committees.

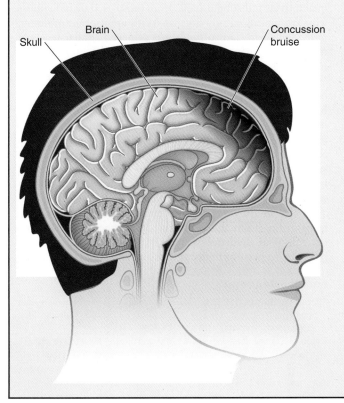

Skull — **Brain** — **Concussion bruise**

Further Readings

Boden BP, Tacchetti RL, Cantu RC, et al. Catastrophic head injuries in high school and college football players. Am J Sports Med. 2007;9: 1075–1081.

Omalu BI, DeKosky ST, Hamilton RL, et al. Chronic traumatic encephalopathy in a national football league player: Part II. Neurosurgery. 2006;59(5):1086–1092.

Omalu BI, DeKosky ST, Minster RL, et al. Chronic traumatic encephalopathy in a National Football League player. Neurosurgery. 2005;57(1):128–134.

The **hypothalamus** is one of the most important regulatory parts of the brain, influencing a host of different physiological functions involved in exercise, including thirst, body temperature, blood pressure, water balance, and endocrine function. It has been called the homeostatic center of the brain. The hypothalamus is vital as a relay center for incoming neural signaling. Because the brain controls bodily function, injury to the brain, such as concussion due to sports participation, has very serious ramifications (Box 4-1). Likewise developmental disabilities such as Down syndrome also affect mental and movement abilities (Box 4-2).

Spinal Cord

The spinal cord is a tubular bundle of nerves that is part of the central nervous system, arising from the brain. It is enclosed and protected by vertebra making up the vertebral column, and each level has nerves that come out of it to different target organs. Nerves related to muscle functions are shown in Figure 4-5. Information is passed from the higher brain centers to the peripheral target tissues, such as muscle. In addition, local circuits from a particular spinal cord level out to the periphery and back can also be operational for sensory (e.g., reflex to heat) and motor activities featuring local repetitive movements, such as running at a set speed.

The spinal cord is also the site of reflex actions. A reflex action is an involuntary response to a stimulus. Typically, a reflex involves a stimulation of a sensory neuron, which brings information to the spinal cord. In the spinal cord, it connects with an efferent neuron, which, in turn, causes a response in the periphery. Reflexes can be both simple and complex. The simplest reflex is the monosynaptic reflex, an example of which is the tendon jerk reflex or tendon tap reflex. Figure 4-6 shows the classical "knee-jerk" reflex when the patellar tendon is struck with a direct mechanical tap. We depend upon reflexes, not only during daily activities, but also during sports events, and even when sleeping, to respond to our environment without thinking about it. For example, the consequences of placing a hand on a hot stove could be severe if one had to take the time to consider the stimulus and consciously devise a response before pulling it off.

The patellar reflex is a bit different from other reflexes because it is mediated by what is called a monosynaptic reflex, and no interneuron connection is involved. Most

Box 4-2 APPLYING RESEARCH

Neurological and Motor Function: Movement Behaviors in Down Syndrome

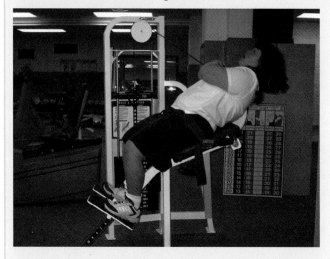

Down syndrome, or trisomy 21, is a genetic alteration caused by presence of an extra chromosome on the 21st human chromosome. It was named after the British physician who described it in 1866. The condition has been characterized by a combination of differences in body size and structure depending upon the penetration of the third chromosome on the phenotypic characteristic examined. Thus, a wide range of differences can occur even within people with Down syndrome.

Interestingly, for years it was thought that the careful movement and rigidity of locomotion was a result of this phenotypic penetration, or interference with normal motor neuron function. In 1994, Latash's research group concluded:

"This study supports the idea that subjects with Down syndrome can use patterns of muscle activation that are qualitatively indistinguishable from those used by individuals who are neurologically normal. With appropriate training, individuals with Down syndrome achieved similar levels of motor performance to that described in the literature for individuals who are neurologically normal."

Much of the movement inhibition was due to protective behaviors (e.g., limiting arm swing because such a movement had resulted in pain from hitting something in everyday movements) carefully reinforced to avoid injury. The importance of practicing new exercise and sport skills to reinforce the the idea that one could safely move in a new range of motion without the fear of pain or injury cannot be underestimated when working with people with Down syndrome, as seen with many athletes in "Special Olympics." This also might be very important in everyday movement tasks in the home and at work. Thus, what appeared as a neurological disorder was in fact a learned protective behavior to prevent injury and ensure survival.

Further Readings

Almeida GL, Corcos DM, Latash ML. Practice and transfer effects during fast single-joint elbow movements in individuals with Down syndrome. Phys Ther. 1994;74(11):1000–1012.

Latash ML, Anson JG. Synergies in health and disease: Relations to adaptive changes in motor coordination. Phys Ther. 2006;86(8):1151–1160.

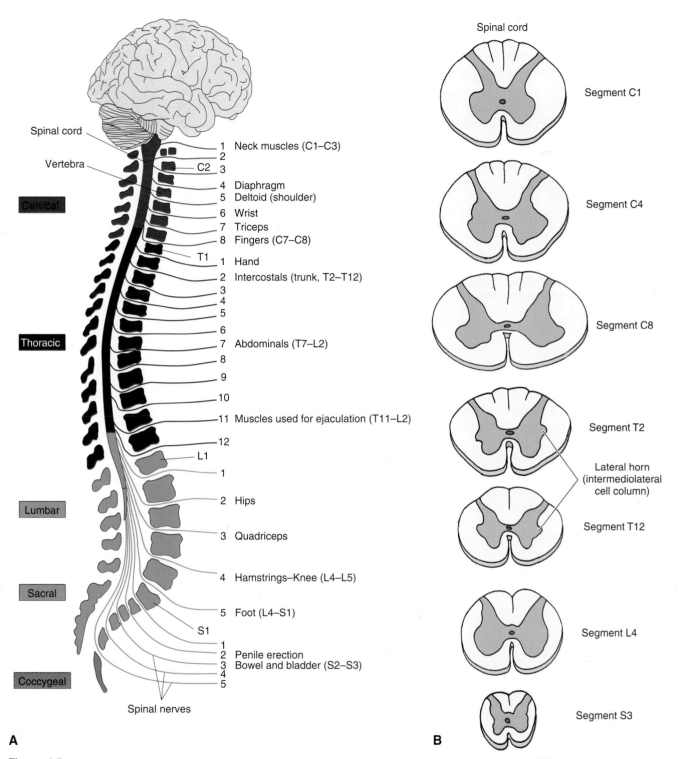

Figure 4-5. Example of nerves that come out of the spinal cord. A shows the nerves innervating muscles in different areas of the body. The view of each level in **B** shows the anatomical variety that exists over the course of the spinal cord length. It is important to understand that there are seven cervical vertebrae (C1–C7); however, there are actually eight cervical nerves (C1–C8); the nerves are shown in this figure. Note that all of the nerves except the C8 come out from above their corresponding vertebrae; the C8 nerve exits below the C7 vertebra. Interestingly, in the other areas of the spine, the nerve exits from below the vertebra with the same name.

reflexes have an interneuron connection between the afferent and efferent systems for potential modification of the reflex in the spinal cord. The patellar reflex is commonly used in clinical evaluations and there is a grading system of the response of the patellar reflex (Box 4-3).

Often in sports, learned responses and motor patterns are at the reflex level, allowing few, if any, higher brain impulses to impact rapid responses to stimuli. Continuous practice of neuromuscular movements trains the reflexes to automatically respond to sensory stimuli. Such athletic skills

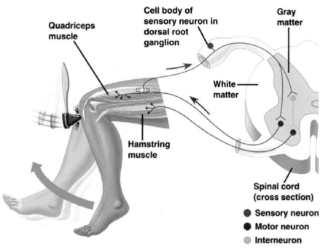

Figure 4-6. **The typical knee tap reflex is an interaction between the sensory neurons and motor neurons in response to stimulation of the patellar tendon.** The reflex causes contraction of the quadriceps and relaxation of the hamstring musculature.

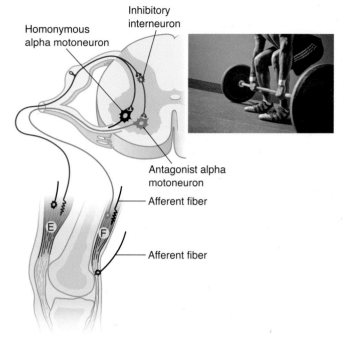

Figure 4-7. **Reciprocal innervation is depicted here.** *This is the type of reflex that can be affected by training.* An afferent fiber synapses with an inhibitory interneuron that synapses with a motoneuron of the antagonist muscle. F and E indicate flexor and extensor muscles, respectively. (Schadé JP, Ford DH: Basic Neurology. Amsterdam: Elsevier, 1965.)

as catching and hitting a baseball require amazing skills and reflexes. Due in part to reflexes, skilled players maintain movement patterns with very small positional errors and temporal errors of less than 2 or 3 milliseconds.[28]

Figure 4-7 shows the type of reflex that may be augmented by exercise training. In this type of reflex, called reciprocal innervation, an afferent nerve fiber synapses not only with the facilitatory interneuron to activate the primary muscle needed to contract for the movement to occur, but also on an inhibitor interneuron that prevents the contraction of the opposing, or antagonist, muscle to avoid the production of countering muscle forces. This is one of many different types of neural adaptations with exercise training.[10] Because the

spinal cord is involved, injury can have severe implications on the control of bodily functions (Box 4-4).

Peripheral Nervous System

The peripheral nervous system is made up of the neurons and ganglia (i.e., group of nerve cell bodies). These neurons extend out from the central nervous system into the periphery to interact with other tissues, such as muscles,

---

Box 4-3 PRACTICAL QUESTIONS FROM STUDENTS

How Can One Interpret the Response of the Knee Tap Test?

The response of the knee reflex is used in basic clinical examination of the body. The knee tendon reflex is a deep tendon reflex. It has been clinically graded so that a score can be attached to the response as follows:

- zero = absent
- 1+ = hypoactive (underactive)
- 2+ = "normal"
- 3+ = hyperactive (overactive) without clonus (extra jerks)
- 4+ = hyperactive with unsustained clonus (just one or two extra jerks)
- 5+ = hyperactive with sustained clonus (continued jerking)

Consistent responses in the 2 range are vital for normal neurological status. However, the normal knee-jerk reflex may range from hypoactive (1+) to brisk (3+).

If the response is different in each limb, it is called an asymmetric reflex. Absence of the knee jerk can be due to an abnormality in the reflex arc required for the reflex to occur. In patients with stroke and paralysis, the knee-jerk reflex may at first be absent, underactive, then recover and become hyperactive within a day or two. Medically, the knee-jerk reflex is also called the patellar reflex. It has also been called the knee reflex, the patellar tendon reflex, and the quadriceps reflex.

organs, and glands. The peripheral nervous system is further subdivided into the autonomic nervous system and the sensory–somatic nervous system.

Autonomic Nervous System

The autonomic nervous system controls physiological functions that are unconscious in nature. It is responsible for the regulation of a variety of the body's physiological functions, including regulation of heart rate, blood pressure, digestion, and breathing. Even though the autonomic nervous system is normally thought of as unconscious control of bodily functions, there may be some conscious control possible (Box 4-5). The autonomic nervous system is subdivided into two basic components: the sympathetic nervous system and the parasympathetic nervous system (Fig. 4-8).

Sympathetic Nervous System

The sympathetic nervous system is often times called the "fight-or-flight" nervous system, as it stimulates many of the physiological systems related to survival and stress. In response to stimulation of the sympathetic nervous system, there is an increase in heart rate and blood pressure, more blood flow to skeletal muscles, a release of glucose by the liver into the blood stream, and breakdown of glycogen in skeletal muscles to provide rich energy sources to exercising muscles. A variety of arousing situations might stimulate this system to elicit the fight-or-flight response, such as walking out to the center court for the finals of the U.S. Open or Wimbledon in tennis (Fig. 4-9), making the final push up "heartbreak hill" during the Boston Marathon, making a final lift in weightlifting at the Olympic Games, or wrestling in the finals of the NCAA tournament. Danger, thrills, excitement, exercise, and a host of different stressors can all elicit a dramatic response of the sympathetic nervous system. It is under these conditions that we experience the "adrenaline rush" associated with arousal and excitement prior to athletic events, allowing athletes to perform and tolerate intense exercise stress (Box 4-6).[9,14,22]

Box 4-4 DID YOU KNOW?
Spinal Cord Injury

More than 10,000 Americans experience spinal cord injuries each year due to automobile accidents (37%), violence (28%), or falling accidents (20%). Sports can also cause spinal cord injury (6%). This type of injury can have devastating effects on bodily functions, including control of skeletal muscle.

In the accompanying figure, one can easily see that injury to the spine from accident or sport can result in various levels of paralysis, depending on the site of the lesion or injury. These are noted as the numbers for each of the vertebra (e.g., C-1 to C-7 or T-1 to T-12).

Spinal cord injury is produced when an accident fractures or dislocates the vertebrae. It can also occur when the spinal cord is compressed or when vertebrae slip or slide out of line (called subluxation). If the blood supply to the spinal cord is cut off, injury also occurs.

The severity of the injury and how much of the cord has been damaged dictates how much loss of function there will be. Most injuries do not sever the spinal cord, but fractured pieces of vertebrae cut and damage nervous tissue, which decreases or eliminates nervous impulses traveling up and down the cord. Paralysis typically occurs below the level of the injury. Some spinal cord injuries allow partial movement and sensation depending on the severity of the injury to the spinal cord. The higher the spinal cord injury, the more severe and extensive the symptoms will be.

A complete injury in the thoracic area of the spine results in paralysis of the legs and is termed paraplegia. A complete injury at C-4 and C-7 (C = cervical) resulting in weakness in the arms and loss of leg function is known as quadriplegia. Injury between C-1 and C-3 results in no movement of the arms or legs and requires a respiratory device to breathe.

Another type of spinal cord injury is severing of a peripheral nerve, such as motor nerves coming out of the spine to innervate muscle. If a peripheral nerve is cut, often it can be reattached and will grow back or regenerate so that both movement function and sensations recover.

Recovery from this type of injury involves physical and occupational therapy to limit further injury. Although strengthening active muscle and teaching patients to care for themselves are important aspects of rehabilitation; counseling and support groups are also vital in helping patients cope with the effects of their injury.

There is no cure for spinal cord injuries, and prevention is the key to eliminating them. In sports, that means using proper techniques and safety practices as well as making practice and competitive venues clear of obstacles and barriers.

Further Readings

Gorgey AS, Dudley GA. Skeletal muscle atrophy and increased intramuscular fat after incomplete spinal cord injury. Spinal Cord. 2007;45(4):304–309.

Olive JL, Dudley GA, McCully KK. Vascular remodeling after spinal cord injury. Med Sci Sports Exerc. 2003;35(6):901–907.

Shah PK, Stevens JE, Gregory CM, et al. Lower-extremity muscle cross-sectional area after incomplete spinal cord injury. Arch Phys Med Rehabil. 2006;87(6):772–778.

Slade JM, Bickel CS, Modlesky CM, et al. Trabecular bone is more deteriorated in spinal cord injured versus estrogen-free postmenopausal women. Osteoporos Int. 2005;16(3):263–272.

Stoner L, Sabatier MJ, Mahoney ET, et al. Electrical stimulation-evoked resistance exercise therapy improves arterial health after chronic spinal cord injury. Spinal Cord. 2007;45(1):49–56.

(Continued)

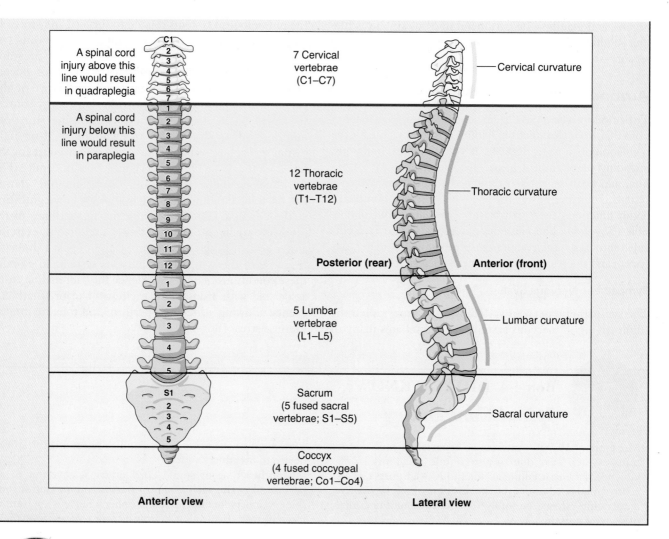

A spinal cord injury above this line would result in quadraplegia

A spinal cord injury below this line would result in paraplegia

7 Cervical vertebrae (C1–C7)

Cervical curvature

12 Thoracic vertebrae (T1–T12)

Thoracic curvature

Posterior (rear)   **Anterior (front)**

5 Lumbar vertebrae (L1–L5)

Lumbar curvature

Sacrum (5 fused sacral vertebrae; S1–S5)

Sacral curvature

Coccyx (4 fused coccygeal vertebrae; Co1–Co4)

Anterior view   **Lateral view**

Box 4-5 DID YOU KNOW?

Meditation and Yoga

Despite the common association of the autonomic nervous system with involuntary function, a certain amount of conscious control over this system seems to be possible, as demonstrated by the practice of yoga and Zen Buddhism. Studies have shown that people are capable of altering heart rate, blood oxygenation, blood pressure, and breathing rates below basal levels of function. In addition, yoga has been shown to reduce stress and anxiety. The fundamental basis of yoga is to increase your attention and awareness of your body. Research in the use of these techniques for health benefits is being undertaken in a variety of "alternative medicine" approaches, from addressing hypertension to reducing anxiety disorders. In sports, many athletes use yoga to help with recovery and the anxiety of competitive stress.

Further Readings

Bernardi L, Passino C, Spadacini G, et al. Reduced hypoxic ventilatory response with preserved blood oxygenation in yoga trainees and Himalayan Buddhist monks at altitude: Evidence of a different adaptive strategy? Eur J Appl Physiol. 2007;99(5):511–518.

Donohue B, Miller A, Beisecker M, et al. Effects of brief yoga exercises and motivational preparatory interventions in distance runners: Results of a controlled trial. Br J Sports Med. 2006;40(1):60–63.

Ernst E. Complementary or alternative therapies for osteoarthritis. Nat Clin Pract Rheumatol. 2006;2(2):74–80.

Telles S, Joshi M, Dash M, et al. An evaluation of the ability to voluntarily reduce the heart rate after a month of yoga practice. Integr Physiol Behav Sci. 2004;39(2):119–125.

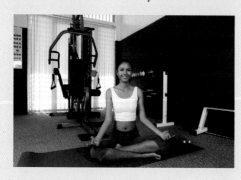

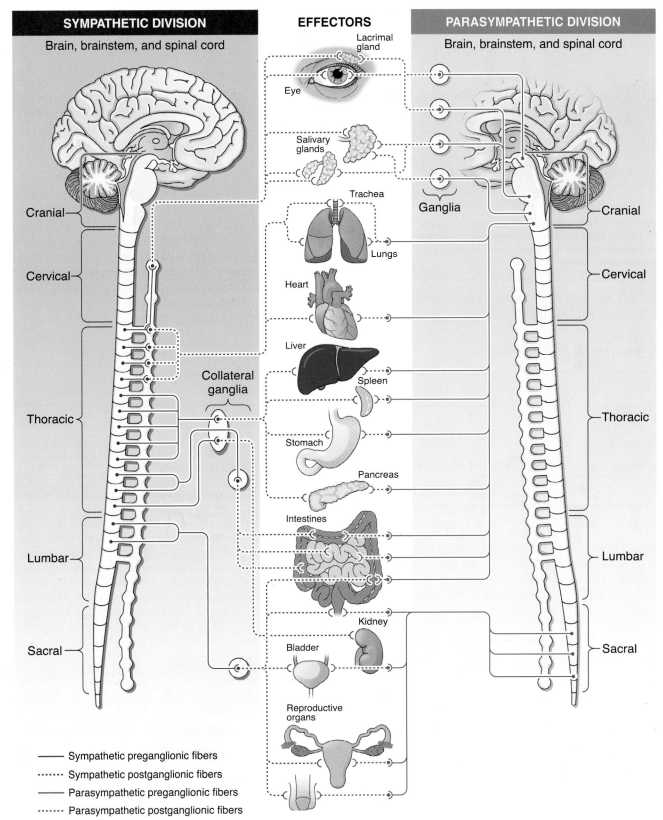

SYMPATHETIC DIVISION

Brain, brainstem, and spinal cord

EFFECTORS

PARASYMPATHETIC DIVISION

Brain, brainstem, and spinal cord

Cranial

Cervical

Thoracic

Lumbar

Sacral

Collateral ganglia

Lacrimal gland

Eye

Salivary glands

Ganglia

Trachea

Lungs

Heart

Liver

Spleen

Stomach

Pancreas

Intestines

Kidney

Bladder

Reproductive organs

Cranial

Cervical

Thoracic

Lumbar

Sacral

——— Sympathetic preganglionic fibers

······· Sympathetic postganglionic fibers

——— Parasympathetic preganglionic fibers

······· Parasympathetic postganglionic fibers

Figure 4-8. The sympathetic and parasympathetic nervous systems interact with many different target tissues and affect different types of physiological function. A ganglia is a mass of nerve tissue that forms a subsidiary nerve center, which receives and sends out nerve fibers.

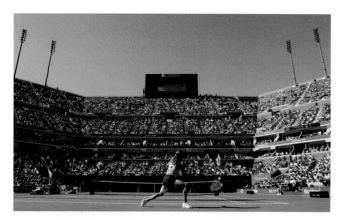

Figure 4-9. The excitement of playing on "Center Court" in a major world tennis tournament will create a host of sympathetic stimuli that many times must be controlled for optimal performance.

Table 4-2 lists some of the typical functions for the sympathetic nervous system.

Parasympathetic Nervous System

In contrast to the sympathetic branch of the autonomic nervous system, the parasympathetic branch is responsible for the body's constant or resting homeostatic state. It has been called the "rest and digest" system. Interestingly, most target tissues of the autonomic nervous system receive input from both the sympathetic and the parasympathetic nervous system. For example, sympathetic nerves stimulate heart rate to speed up whereas the parasympathetic nerves act to slow it down. The nature of the situation one is in (i.e., whether it is stressful or not) determines which branch of the autonomic system dominates at that time.

The parasympathetic nervous system has about 75% of its nerve fibers in the vagus nerves going to the thoracic and abdominal regions of the body. Parasympathetic stimulation helps the body maintain, or resume, normal resting function after sympathetic stimulation has occurred (Table 4-2). The primary role of the parasympathetic nervous system is to help the body "rest and digest," as it promotes normal functions of the digestive tract and secretions, including urination and defecation. Specifically, it elicits the following physiological functions:

- lowering of blood pressure
- slowing of heart rate
- constricting the pupils
- increasing blood flow to the skin and viscera

Box 4-6 APPLYING RESEARCH
Skin Receptors and Wrestling Performance

In the body, we have pain receptors, temperature receptors, chemical receptors, and—important to many sports—mechanoreceptors. The broad group of receptors that are sensitive to touch, pressure, and position are called "mechanoreceptors." A stimulus distorts their membrane structures and signals are sent to the central nervous system. The three basic mechanoreceptors are tactile, baroreceptors, and proprioceptors. The skin's six different tactile receptors are sensitive to touch, pressure, and vibration.

In sports, often skin receptors can play a role in the learned reflexes of movement needed for performance success. However, the fine touch and sensitive tactile receptors may not play as big of a role as the Pacinian corpuscles, which are large receptors sensitive to deep pressure and to pulsing or high-frequency vibrations. Of similar importance, Ruffini corpuscles, which are located in the dermis of the skin, are sensitive to slight pressure and distortions of the skin.

In the sport of wrestling, movements and responses to pressure are vital to success. If an opponent grabs an ankle in an attempt to lift it up and bring you down to the mat, you have to quickly respond to the touch by instinctively reaching back and picking the hand off your ankle in a matter of microseconds, or your opponent has the advantage. It has been said that elite wrestlers at the Olympic level are not separated by strength or power, but rather by the speed of movement and the appropriate trained reactions or reflexes to touch and pressure by an opponent.

Some wrestling coaches have used blindfolds during practice to take away the sense of sight and to force the wrestler to rely more on touch and pressure on their bodies to cue them in to responding appropriately with a defensive counter move to an opponent's offensive move. Some coaches have described this technique as "touch and response training." Neural sensations of touch and pressure play vital roles in this basic practice of wrestling techniques.

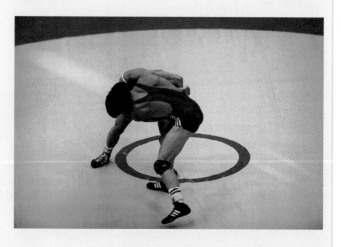

Table 4-2. Typical Functions of the Sympathetic and Parasympathetic Nervous Systems		
Target Organ	**Sympathetic Stimulation**	**Parasympathetic Stimulation**
Iris (eye muscle)	Pupil dilation	Pupil constriction
Salivary glands	Saliva production reduced	Saliva production increased
Oral/nasal mucosa	Mucus production reduced	Mucus production increased
Heart	Heart rate and force increased	Heart rate and force decreased
Lung	Bronchial muscle relaxed	Bronchial muscle contracted
Stomach	Peristalsis reduced	Gastric juice secreted; motility increased
Small intestine	Motility reduced	Digestion increased
Large intestine	Motility reduced	Secretions and motility increased
Liver	Increased conversion of glycogen to glucose	Influences relaxation of smooth muscle sphincters of blood vessels
Kidney	Decreased urine secretion	Increased urine secretion
Adrenal medulla	Increased secretion of norepinephrine and epinephrine	No effects
Bladder	Wall relaxed; sphincter closed	Wall contracted; sphincter relaxed

- peristalsis of the gastrointestinal tract
- stimulating the flow of saliva
- allowing normal bladder function

The parasympathetic nervous system is essential during the recovery period after exercise stress. The ability of the parasympathetic nervous system to respond in the modification of the sympathetic responses during exercise and into the recovery period is a trainable characteristic of the nervous system (e.g., quickly bringing blood pressure and heart rate back down to normal resting levels). This ability is essential for optimal health and fitness, especially with aging.

Sensory–Somatic Nervous System

In addition to the autonomic system, the peripheral nervous system is composed of the **sensory–somatic nervous system**. The interaction between the different components of the sensory–somatic system allows for coordinated actions and responses to the external environment, whether it is the last minute adjustments in throwing a football due to a gust of wind (Box 4-7) or a response to intense environmental heat, such as drinking water or toweling off sweat from the body.

The sensory division, often times called the afferent division, contains neurons that receive signals from the tendons, joints, skin, skeletal muscles, eyes, nose, ears, tongue, and many other tissues and organs. The motor division, also called the efferent division, contains pathways that go from the brain stem and spinal cord to the lower motor neurons of the cranial and spinal nerves. When these nerves are stimulated, they cause the contraction of skeletal muscles and limb movements. The interaction between sensory and motor neurons is depicted in Figure 4-10.

Quick Review

- The nervous system is divided into two major subdivisions: 1) central nervous system and 2) peripheral nervous system.
- The central nervous system is made up of the brain and spinal cord.
- The peripheral nervous system is made up of ganglia and neurons, which extend out from the central nervous system into the periphery to interact with other tissues, such as muscles, organs, and glands.
- The peripheral nervous system is subdivided into the autonomic nervous system and the sensory–somatic nervous system.
- The autonomic nervous system controls physiological functions that are unconscious in nature (heart rate, blood pressure, digestion, and breathing).
- The autonomic nervous system is subdivided into two basic components: the sympathetic nervous system and the parasympathetic nervous system.
- The sympathetic nervous system is active during physiological or psychological stress.
- The parasympathetic nervous system helps the body maintain, or resume, normal resting function after sympathetic stimulation has occurred.
- The sensory–somatic nervous system is the part of the peripheral nervous system that supplies information concerning the external environment (skin pressure, temperature) and allows the body to respond to changes in the environment.
- All our conscious awareness of the external environment and all our motor activity to cope with it operate through the sensory–somatic division of the peripheral nervous system.

Box 4-7 PRACTICAL QUESTIONS FROM STUDENTS

Can Your Nervous System Become Fatigued?

Fatigue may occur at several locations and have several causes (see figure). Additionally, the causes of fatigue may differ depending upon whether an activity is high-intensity and short-duration or low-intensity and long-duration in nature. **Central fatigue** refers to a decrease in force production due to an inability of the central nervous system to stimulate the motor neurons that activate muscle tissue. This results in a decrease in the ability to activate muscle fibers and therefore results in the loss of force production. **Peripheral fatigue** refers to fatigue due to a factor located within the muscle itself, such as lack of sufficient ATP and increased acidity, and includes inability to transmit the impulse for muscle activation from the motor neuron to the muscle fiber (NMJ).

Central fatigue could occur during high-intensity, short-duration activity predominantly relying on anaerobic energy or during low-intensity, long-duration activity relying predominantly on aerobic energy. Experiments have shown contradictory results concerning central fatigue. One study demonstrated that, after fatiguing, electrical stimulation could not restore maximal force development.[1] This indicated that the site of fatigue was in the periphery or muscle itself rather than an inability of the central nervous system to stimulate muscle. Another study indicated just the opposite: electrical stimulation of fatigued muscle resulted in an increase in force development,[2] indicating that central fatigue limited force output of muscle.

These previous studies utilized variations of what is termed the twitch interpolation technique. The twitch interpolation technique involves comparing maximal voluntary muscular force to maximal force developed by electrical stimulation of the muscle. If fatigued muscle develops greater maximal force with electrical stimulation compared to maximal voluntary force, central fatigue is indicated. If the opposite is true, then central fatigue is not indicated. Whether or not central fatigue occurs may be dependent upon the type of muscular activity. Using the twitch interpolation technique, shortening (concentric) muscle actions appear to result in peripheral fatigue first followed by central fatigue,[3] whereas static (isometric) muscle actions appear to result in the opposite fatigue pattern. When muscle is at a short length during a static muscle action, greater central fatigue results than peripheral fatigue, and when muscle is at a long length during a static muscle action, peripheral fatigue appears to predominate the fatigue process.[4] So central fatigue may or may not occur depending upon the type of muscle action performed.

Whether or not central fatigue occurs during endurance training is also unclear. During low-intensity, long-duration activity, serotonin, a neurotransmitter in the brain, may affect fatigue with increases in serotonin delaying fatigue. However, the relationship, if any, between serotonin and fatigue remains unclear.[5,6]

Whether central or peripheral fatigue occur during an activity or predominate during an activity may be dependent upon the type of muscle action predominantly utilized during the activity as well as other factors, such as the intensity, duration, and frequency of the activity. It seems that central fatigue does occur during some types of activity, although the exact mechanism explaining central fatigue is unclear.[7]

Potential Sites of Fatigue

```
"Psyche"/Will → Motor output → Motorneuron

              Central Fatigue
- - - - - - - - - - - - - - - - - - - - - - - -
              Peripheral Fatigue

T-tubule ← Sarcolemma

Sarcoplasmic reticulum–Ca²⁺ release      ATP availability

              Actin-myosin
              interaction
```

References

1. Babault N, Desbrosses K, Fabre MS, et al. Neuromuscular fatigue development during maximal concentric and isometric knee extensions. J Appl Physiol. 2006;100:780–785.
2. Davis JM, Bailey SP. Possible mechanisms of central nervous system fatigue during exercise. Med Sci Sports Exerc. 1997;29:45–57.
3. Desbrosses K, Babault N, Scaglioni G, et al. Neural activation after maximal isometric contractions at different muscle lengths. Med Sci Sports Exerc. 2006;38:937–944.
4. Ikai M, Steinhaus AH. Some factors modifying the expression of human strength. J Appl Physiol. 1961;16:157–163.
5. Merton PA. Voluntary strength and fatigue. J Physiol. 1954;123:553–564.
6. Struder HK, Weicker H. Physiology and pathophysiology of the serotonergic system and its implications on mental and physical performance. Part I. Int J Sports Med. 2001;22:467–481.
7. Struder HK, Weicker H. Physiology and pathophysiology of the serotonergic system and its implications on mental and physical performance. Part II. Int J Sports Med. 2001;22:482–497.

MOTOR UNIT

The key to any movement is the activation of motor units. The **motor unit** is the functional component of muscular activity under direct neural control. One challenge of exercise is to activate a very specific set of motor units that can generate just the needed amount of force to produce the desired movements (e.g., lifting a pencil vs. running up a set of stairs vs. lifting a heavy weight).[11]

A motor unit contains an alpha motor neuron and all the muscle fibers stimulated by that neuron, as shown in Figure 4-11. The alpha motor neuron has relatively short dendrites, which receive information and pass it along to the cell body, and long axons that carry impulses from

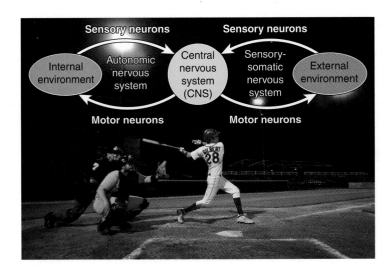

Figure 4-10. Relationship between the sensory and motor components of the nervous system play an important role in both exercise and sport performances.

the cell body to the NMJ, the synapse with the muscle fiber.

All motor units fall under one of three categories.[3] Slow (S) motor units include a motor neuron whose axon slowly conducts electrical impulses to its muscle fibers, which, in turn, twitch or reach peak force at a slow rate. The type I muscle fibers that are associated with slow motor units develop little force—they are small in size—but are difficult to fatigue due to their impressive aerobic capacity. Fast-fatigue resistant (FFR) motor units have larger axons and propagate electrical stimuli down to the muscle fibers more rapidly. The muscle fibers innervated by these axons are considered type IIA and, as such, are capable of developing considerable amounts of force—they are larger than type I fibers—and are only moderately fatigable. The third

category of motor units is referred to as fast-fatigable (FF). They have large motor axons that very quickly send electrical impulses down to their associated muscle fibers which, in turn, twitch very rapidly, developing high levels of force. However, because the muscle fibers comprising these motor units are type IIX (or type IIA if with training the type IIX is changed to all type IIA), they can maintain this high level of force, the highest among the three types of motor units, for only a very brief period of time.

Besides a difference in the type of muscle fibers making up slow and fast motor units, there is also a difference in the number of muscle fibers per motor unit. Muscles where fine control of force is needed have fewer muscle fibers per motor unit. While muscles where less control of force is needed have more muscle fibers per motor unit. For example, in muscles that stretch the lens of the eye, motor units may contain only 5 to 10 muscle fibers, whereas in the gastrocnemius, 1000 muscle fibers may be found in one motor unit. On average, for all of the muscles in the body, about 100 muscle fibers are in a motor unit.

Muscle function is controlled by the nervous system's ability to stimulate particular motor units. Understanding motor unit recruitment is paramount to understanding physical movement, the specificity of acute exercise stress, and the effects of chronic exercise training. The motor cortex activates different motor units to create different amounts of force by the different muscles around each joint during any movement.

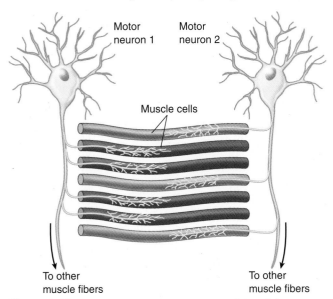

Figure 4-11. The basic motor unit consists of the alpha motor neuron and its associated muscle fibers. Notice that muscle fibers activated by one motor unit can be located side by side with muscle fibers activated by another motor unit. This allows for uniform muscle activation as well as gradations in force production.

CONDUCTION OF IMPULSES

As stated above, for a motor unit to be active, an impulse must originate from a neuron and travel down the axon to stimulate the muscle fibers to contract. A **nervous impulse** (i.e., **action potential**) in the form of electrical energy is the stimulus that causes muscle fibers to contract. When no impulse is being conducted, the inside of the neuron has a net negative charge, while the outside has a net positive charge. This arrangement of positive and negative charges (ions) accounts for what is termed the resting membrane potential. This resting membrane potential results not only from the separation of charged ions across the neuron's membrane, but also from the impermeability of that membrane to these ions under resting conditions, thus preventing their movement.

Sodium (Na^+) and potassium (K^+) ions are the major molecules responsible for the membrane potential. Na^+ ions are predominantly located outside the neuron's cell membrane, while K^+ ions are located mainly inside the neuron. There are, however, more Na^+ ions on the outside of the neuron than K^+ on the inside of the neuron. This, along with the preponderance of other negatively charged particles, such as phosphate groups, on the inside of the neuron, results in a net resting intracellular charge that is negative, about −65 to −70 mV, compared with the outside of the neuron.

When an impulse is being conducted down a dendrite or an axon, the cell membrane of the neuron becomes permeable to both Na^+ and K^+ ions (Fig. 4-12). Each ion has its own electrochemical gradient, which serves as its driving force across the membrane when channels on the membrane are open. If the resting membrane potential reaches threshold due to the summation of impulses reaching the neuron via its dendrites, a nervous impulse will occur (Fig. 4-13). Recall that the axon hillock summates impulses, and if threshold is reached, an impulse will be carried by the axon. When a nervous impulse occurs, channels in the membrane for Na^+ open and it enters the cell, resulting in **depolarization** of the membrane, or change from resting membrane potential to +30 mV. After a brief delay, K^+ channels open, allowing positively charged K^+ to leave the interior of the axon that, in conjunction with closing of Na^+ channels, results in the membrane potential becoming negative again during a process termed **repolarization**. This process of brief (channels remain open only for a few milliseconds) but rapid movements of Na^+ and K^+ across the membrane resulting in depolarization and repolarization is termed the **action potential**, which is sometimes referred to as a nervous impulse.

During repolarization, the membrane will become slightly more negative in charge than resting membrane potential, or hyperpolarized. After the repolarization phase of the action potential, the energy-dependent (needs ATP to function) Na^+–K^+ pump restores the separation of charge across the neuron's membrane by pumping out three Na^+ ions for every two K^+ ions that are returned to the interior of the neuron. This process is repeated each time a nervous impulse, or action potential, takes place.

The action potential traveling down an axon must initiate an impulse in a dendrite of another neuron or in the NMJ, the synapse connecting the motor neuron with the muscle fiber, to cause muscle fibers to contract. For

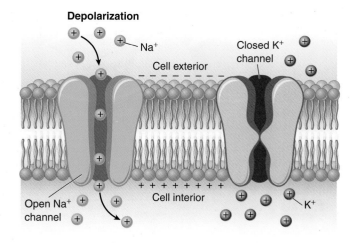

Depolarization

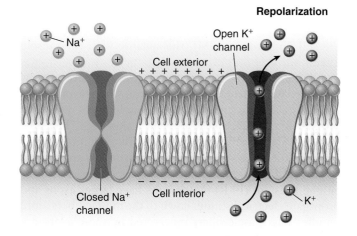

Repolarization

Figure 4-12. An action potential consists of both depolarization and repolarization. Both of these involve movement of ions through ionic channels in the membrane.

this to occur, an energy transformation takes place in the terminal portion of the axon. More specifically, electrical energy presented by the action potential is transformed into chemical energy when, upon the arrival of the action potential, neurotransmitters are released from the nerve terminal into the synapse. Upon crossing the synapse and binding to receptors on the target cell (either another neuron or a muscle fiber), the neurotransmitters cause channels to open, allowing ions to cross the target cell's membrane, thus initiating another electrical impulse.

There are two broad categories of neurotransmitters: 1) excitatory, which either make the membrane potential less negative or depolarize it by increasing the permeability of the membrane to Na^+, thus causing excitation of the post-synaptic membrane, and 2) inhibitory, which do the opposite and make the membrane more permeable to K^+ or Cl^-, making it even more negative and thus inhibiting the formation of an impulse. In some cases, inhibition might help performance, as seen when a batter makes a "check swing" at a pitch in baseball.

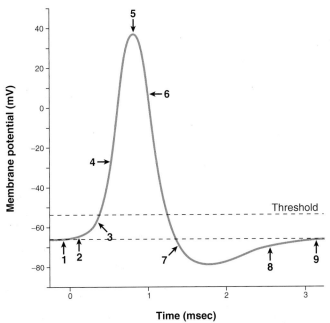

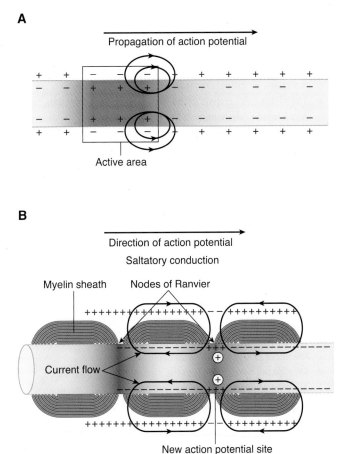

Figure 4-13. Depolarization and repolarization involve the movement of ions across the membrane. 1) Resting membrane potential; 2) stimulus to depolarize; 3) if threshold is reached, Na$^+$ channels open and Na$^+$ enters the cell; 4) Na$^+$ entering the cell causes depolarization; 5) Na$^+$ channels close and K$^+$ channels open; 6) K$^+$ moves from the interior to exterior of the cell; 7) K$^+$ channels remain open, causing hyperpolarization; 8) K$^+$ channels close, so less K$^+$ leaves the cell; 9) cell returns to resting membrane potential.

Role of Myelination

The rate of nervous system conduction down an axon is greatly affected by whether the nerve is myelinated or un-myelinated. Axons may be covered with a white substance high in lipid (fat) content called the **myelin sheath**, which is secreted by Schwann cells. The myelin sheath is sometimes even thicker than the axon itself and is composed of multiple, concentric layers of this lipid substance. Nerve fibers, or axons, possessing a myelin sheath are referred to as **myelinated** nerve fibers; those lacking a myelin sheath are said to be unmyelinated.

Myelinated nerves conduct their impulses using **saltatory** conduction and unmyelinated nerves use **local** conduction (Fig. 4-14). The movement of the ions producing an action potential remains the same as described above for either type of conduction. In myelinated nerves, the myelin sheath does not run continuously along the length of the axon, but is segmented by small gaps every 1 to 3 millimeters along the length of the axon. These small gaps are called the **nodes of Ranvier**. These nodes allow the action potential to jump from node to node along the axon (thus the term *saltatory*, meaning to jump) because although ions cannot readily cross the myelin sheath, they can easily cross the membrane at the nodes due to the presence of Na$^+$ and K$^+$ channels on the membrane. In essence, the action potential is re-charged at each node of Ranvier by movements of Na$^+$ and K$^+$ across the membrane at each node.

Figure 4-14. (A) Local conduction moves the electrical impulse via local changes in membrane charge. **(B)** Some neurons are myelinated and electrical impulses use saltatory conduction, jumping from one node of Ranvier to the next node of Ranvier. (From Bear M, Connors B, Paradiso M. Neuroscience, Exploring the Brain. 3rd ed. Baltimore: Lippincott Williams and Wilkins, 2000.)

Saltatory conduction has two advantages. First, it allows the action potential to make jumps down the axon, thereby increasing the velocity of neural conduction as much as 5- to 50-fold, or up to 100 m·s^{-1}. Second, it conserves energy, as only the nodes depolarize, reducing the energy needed by the Na$^+$–K$^+$ pump to reestablish the resting membrane potential between impulses.

Conversely, unmyelinated nerve fibers use a local circuit of ionic current flow to gradually conduct the action potential along the entire length of the nerve fiber. Thus, a small part of the nerve fiber membrane depolarizes and the continuation of local circuit ionic current flow causes nerve membrane depolarization to continue and the action potential travels down the entire length of the nerve fiber. The velocity of this type of nerve impulse conduction is much slower than myelinated nerve fibers, ranging from 0.5 to 10 m·s^{-1}.

In addition to the presence of myelination, the diameter of the neuron's axon affects impulse conduction velocity. In general, whether the nerve fiber is myelinated or unmyelinated, the larger its diameter, the faster the velocity of impulse conduction.[18] In addition to determining the speed at which action potentials are conducted along

Quick Review

- Alpha motor neurons control skeletal muscle activity.
- The myelin sheath on some axons provides insulation and maintains electrical signal strength.
- The motor unit consists of the alpha motor neuron and its associated skeletal muscle fibers.
- The motor cortex activates different motor units to create different amounts of force.
- A nervous impulse is conducted in the form of electrical energy.
- The resting membrane potential is created mainly by the distribution of positively charged molecules on either side of the cell membrane.
- The conductance of the nerve impulse or an action potential is achieved through a process of depolarization and repolarization, in which electrically charged ions move into and out of the neuron.
- Energy is transformed from electrical to chemical (neurotransmitters) to cross a synapse or NMJ.
- The type of nervous system conduction is related to whether the nerve is myelinated or unmyelinated.
- Myelinated nerves conduct their impulses using saltatory conduction, and unmyelinated nerves use local conduction.
- Larger diameter axons conduct impulses at faster velocities than smaller diameter axons.

the axon, the size of motor neurons also determines the recruitment threshold needed to fire the axon's initial action potential at the axon hillock, as described earlier in the chapter. Because type II, or fast-twitch, muscle fibers are innervated by larger motor neurons, they are more difficult to recruit (i.e., high threshold). In contrast, slow motor units feature not only smaller type I muscle fibers, but also smaller motor neurons, which are easier to recruit (i.e., low threshold). Thus, motor units made up of type I fibers are typically recruited first due to the lower recruitment thresholds of their neurons. Motor units made up of type II fibers are recruited after the type I fibers (type IIA followed by type IIX fibers) due to the larger cell size (axons and somas) of fast motor neurons, resulting in their higher recruitment thresholds. This is termed the "size principle of recruitment."

The Size Principle and Motor Unit Recruitment

One of the most important concepts related to neuromuscular function and exercise demands is called the **size principle**.[13,15–19] Put forth by the laboratory of Professor Henneman and colleagues in the Department of Physiology at the Harvard University School of Medicine in the 1960s, this principle helps explain how skeletal muscle is recruited and how gradations of muscle force can be produced during activity and exercise.

Henneman's research showed that the body uses different size criteria in the recruitment of individual motor units from the available pool of motor units that each muscle possesses. This selective recruitment can be accomplished by varying the strength of the electrical stimulus that is needed to stimulate individual motor units (recall that different sized motor units have specific threshold levels for recruitment). The electrical stimulus can also vary according to the number of motor units recruited or the size of the muscle fibers that make up the recruited motor units. Each of these is a type of sizing effect that helps to effectively produce the exact amount of force required for the task.

The size principle states that motor units are recruited from the smallest to the largest in terms of the size of the neuron found in that motor unit and, accordingly, the number of muscle fibers contained in that motor unit (large neurons have a greater number of axonal branches to innervate more muscle fibers). Accordingly, matching the force produced to the force demands placed on the muscle is accomplished by regulating the number and size of motor units recruited by the nervous system.[11] All of the muscle fibers contained within a single motor unit are of the same type since it is the motor neuron that determines the twitch characteristics of the muscle fibers it innervates. Slow motor units are composed of fewer muscle fibers and generally have a smaller axon innervating them than fast motor units. So slow motor units and their type I muscle fibers are normally recruited first in a muscle action, followed by the FFR and type IIA muscle fibers as force demands increase, with FF motor units and their associated type IIX (or all type IIA if all type IIX isoforms have been converted with training) muscle fibers being recruited only at maximal or near maximal efforts. Figure 4-15 depicts how this might occur. When greater

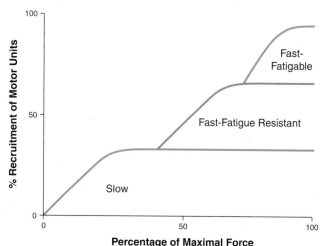

Figure 4-15. A general presentation of the size principle. As the demands of force production progress toward maximal, more motor units are recruited. At very low levels of force production, primarily slow motor units are recruited, and as more force is needed, more and more motor units are recruited, including the larger fast motor units.

force production is required, greater percentages of type II motor units are recruited since these fast-twitch units comprise not only more muscle fibers, but also larger and thus stronger ones. The absolute maximal force is dependent upon the number and type of motor units contributing to the movement. In practical terms, if one lifts light weights, not all of the muscle is recruited, as the force demands are not high enough to recruit the larger motor units containing the type II muscle fibers that have the greatest potential for hypertrophy. This is why lifting only light weights does not enhance muscle strength or size as much as lifting heavy weights[1] and why jogging, which predominately recruits type I muscle fibers, fails to result in muscle hypertrophy.

The total number of motor units in a particular muscle, as well as the relative composition of the different types of motor units, is largely determined by genetics. Accordingly, genetics has much impact on the type of neuromuscular performance in which one might excel. For example, a marathon runner may have been born with 80% type I fibers in the thigh muscles. Such a high percentage of slow motor units and type I fibers helps this athlete to be an elite endurance athlete (Fig. 4-16). This can be explained, in part, by the fact that when motor units are recruited, slow motor units featuring type I muscle fibers are recruited first, and they are better suited for aerobic activity than the type II muscle fibers included in fast motor units. Repeated activation of type II muscle fibers that are better suited for anaerobic activity results in higher acidity, which causes fatigue, reducing the ability to maintain a desired running pace. Thus, an individual's genetics will dictate what is available for motor unit recruitment to meet different types of exercise demands and thus the level of performance possible. So, can anyone be a gold medalist in the marathon race? No. Having the proper complement of motor units is a prerequisite.

Conversely, for a sprinter, a high percentage of fast motor units, with their associated type II muscle fibers, in the thigh musculature helps promote the explosive, high-power muscle actions needed for speed production over a short duration of time (Fig. 4-17). The recruitment of

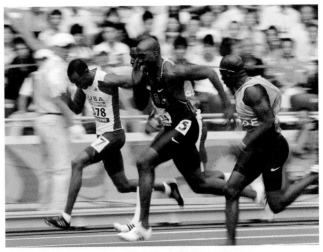

Figure 4-17. Type II motor units predominate in an elite sprinter's thigh and leg muscles.

type II muscle fibers that rely predominantly on anaerobic energy production will result in the high force and power output needed to sprint, but the type II motor units will also fatigue quickly (see Chapter 2). It is important to recall that due to the size principle of recruitment, the sprinter will still recruit his/her slow motor units prior to their fast motor units. So even slow motor units and their type I muscle fibers are recruited during the high-velocity muscle contractions that occur during sprinting. The marathon and short sprints represent two examples at the extreme ends of the motor unit recruitment spectrum.

The real physiological advantage of the size principle order of recruitment is that it ensures that low-threshold, or easily recruited motor units, composed of type I muscle fibers that are designed for aerobic metabolism and are fatigue resistant, are predominantly recruited to perform lower intensity, long-duration (endurance) activities, as well as normal daily activities. Higher threshold fast motor units, which are recruited only when there is a need for higher levels of force, quickly fatigue because they rely so much on anaerobic metabolism. As a result, the size principle order of recruitment helps to delay fatigue during submaximal muscle actions because the high-threshold, highly fatigable fast motor units are not recruited (Fig. 4-18). A positive feature of the higher threshold motor units, however, is that they recover more quickly than lower threshold motor units, which is of value during repeated high-force, short-duration-type activities, like interval training or repeat sprints in a game, such as soccer.

During endurance performances, those motor units that have good capacity for aerobic metabolism can be alternately recruited to meet the force demands of the active muscles (**asynchronous recruitment**). This means that within the pool of slow or type I motor units located in the exercising muscle, there is a cycling process of recruitment so that individual motor units take turns resting while others are active. This ability to rest motor units when submaximal

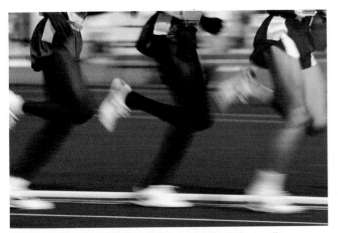

Figure 4-16. Type I motor units predominate in an elite distance runner's thigh and leg muscles.

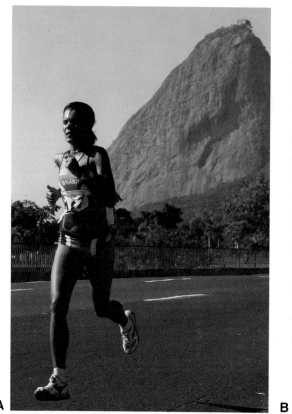
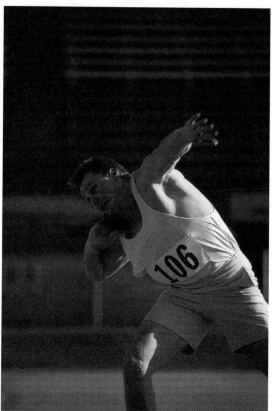

Figure 4-18. **(A)** An aspect of the size principle order of recruitment is that it ensures that low-threshold motor units are predominantly recruited to perform lower intensity, long-duration (endurance) activities. **(B)** Higher threshold motor units are recruited only when high force/power levels are needed.

force is needed also helps to delay fatigue. This strategy of rotating the recruitment of low-threshold motor units predominates during endurance performance, whether it is an activity such as distance running or lifting very light weights for a high number of repetitions. The greater the force required to perform an activity, the less this asynchronous recruitment strategy can be used, because a higher percentage of the total number of motor units is required to produce the needed force. The size principle and order of recruitment help to delay fatigue during tasks requiring submaximal force production by preventing the recruitment of the high-threshold motor units. However, one might ask the question, can fatigue occur within the nervous system (Box 4-7)?

Exceptions to the Size Principle and Dynamic Interactions

There are exceptions to the size principle. Such exceptions may occur when the time delay caused by first recruiting the smaller motor units that can only contribute small amounts of force may be detrimental to performance of a high-force activity. Exceptions to the size principle were first discovered in fish and mammals with the study of rapid escape movements (such as the tail flick in fish to change direction when pursued by a predator) or capture

movements (a cat's front paw flick to capture a prey), where even a minuscule time delay in going from the small to large motor unit recruitment order would be the difference between life and death.

In these exceptional circumstances, rather than starting with the recruitment of low-threshold, slow motor units, high-threshold, fast motor units are recruited first in order to allow faster movement velocity. This process appears to be facilitated by inhibiting activation of the slow motor units, making it easier to go directly to the fast motor units. In human performance, such situations may occur with very high velocity (ballistic) and high-power output movements using highly trained movement among well-trained athletes (e.g., Olympic weight lifters, baseball pitchers, sprinters, or sprint swimmers).

All-or-None Law and Gradations of Force

Another important concept in the regulation of muscle force production is the **all-or-none law**. This law states that when a threshold level for activation is reached by the motor neuron of a specific motor unit, all of the muscle fibers in that motor unit are activated. If the threshold is not reached, then none of the muscle fibers in that motor unit will be activated. Note, however, that this law holds true only for individual motor units within a muscle, and not for whole muscles, such as the biceps. The more motor units that are stimulated, the greater the amount of force that is developed. In other words, if one motor unit is activated, only a very small amount of force is developed. If several motor units are activated, more force is developed. If all of the motor units in a muscle are activated, then maximal force is produced by the muscle. This method of varying the force produced by a muscle is called **multiple motor unit summation**.

Gradations in the force developed by a muscle can also be achieved by controlling the force produced by its individual motor units. This is called **wave summation** and is defined as the product of the rapidity at which action potentials are generated by an alpha motor neuron to stimulate a motor unit's muscle fibers. A motor unit responds to a single nerve impulse (action potential) by producing a single muscle **twitch**. A twitch is a brief period of muscle activity producing force, which is followed by relaxation of the motor unit. When two impulses conducted by an axon reach the muscle fibers with only a brief interlude separating them, the second twitch occurs prior to complete relaxation following the first one. As a result, the second twitch summates with the force of the first twitch, producing more total force. The ability of neurons to vary the rate of generating action potentials is referred to as **rate coding**. At progressively higher rates of action potential firing, the rate of wave (twitch) summation increases until the impulses occur at a high enough frequency that the resultant muscle twitches are completely summated, or fused, and there is no evidence of relaxation between twitches (Fig. 4-19). The complete summation of twitches is called **tetanus** and is the maximal force a motor unit can develop. The ability to vary the force a muscle produces by multiple motor unit summation and rate coding results in an almost infinite variation of force produced by a muscle. The ability to vary force production is vital to the proper performance of athletic skills ranging from power events like the high jump, to those requiring minimal force, such as the drop shot in tennis that is intended to barely clear the net.

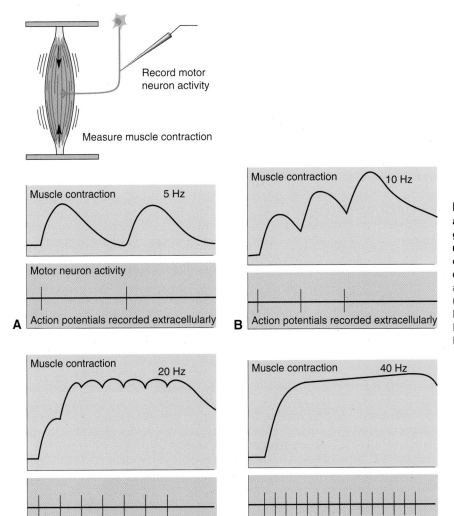

Figure 4-19. Wave summation (also known as frequency summation) occurs when a given set of motor units are stimulated repeatedly until the maximum amount of force is developed in a tetanic muscle contraction. (A) Complete relaxation between action potentials. **(B)** Wave summation. **(C)** Unfused tetanus. **(D)** Tetanus. (From Bear M, Connors B, Paradiso M. Neuroscience, Exploring the Brain. 3rd ed. Baltimore, MD: Lippincott Williams and Wilkins, 2000.)

Quick Review

- Motor units are recruited from the smallest to the largest on the basis of the force demands placed on the muscle.
- An individual's genetics determines the available number of the different types of motor units (i.e., slow, FFR, FF) that can be recruited to perform different types of exercise.
- Fast motor units are larger than slow ones in the diameter of the motor axon as well as in the size and number of the muscle fibers innervated.
- Recruiting the lower threshold motor units first helps to delay fatigue when high force or power is not needed.
- Asynchronous recruitment of motor units can occur when force production needs are low, delaying the onset of fatigue.
- An exception to the size principle, in which fast motor units are recruited first, may occur to allow faster movement velocity.
- The all-or-none law dictates that all muscle fibers of a motor unit will contract if that motor unit is recruited.
- Force produced by a muscle is varied by activating different amounts of motor units.
- Selective activation of motor units and the difference in size of motor units and rate coding of each motor unit allows for graded force production.
- Motor units respond to a single nerve impulse by producing a twitch.
- The complete summation of single nerve impulse twitches results in tetanus.

NEURAL ADAPTATIONS TO EXERCISE

Training adaptations to the nervous system can improve physical performance. Neural drive, a measure of the combined motor unit recruitment and rate coding of active motor units within a muscle, is one aspect of training adaptations. Neural drive, which is initiated within the central nervous system and then transmitted to the peripheral nervous system, can be quantified using integrated electromyography (EMG) surface electrode techniques (Box 4-8). EMG techniques measure the electrical activity within the muscle, including the activity within both the nerves and the muscle fibers, and indicate the amount of neural drive delivered to a muscle.

In a set of classic studies, 8 weeks of weight training resulted in a shift to a lower level of EMG activity to muscular force ratio.[24–26] In effect, the trained muscle produced a given amount of submaximal force with a lower amount of EMG activity, suggesting an increased contractile response to any amount of submaximal neural drive. This greater response to a given amount of electrical stimulus suggests that there is either an improved activation of the muscle during submaximal effort, or a more efficient recruitment pattern of the motor units. However, some studies have demonstrated that improved activation of the muscle does not occur after training,[23] indicating that more efficient recruitment order is probably responsible for much of the increased force.

Box 4-8 AN EXPERT VIEW
Electromyography

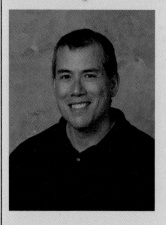

Joseph P. Weir, PhD, FACSM
Professor
Physical Therapy Program
Des Moines University
Osteopathic Medical Center
Des Moines, IA

EMG is a tool to measure the electrical signals created by muscles when they are stimulated to contract. Specifically, EMG records the action potentials that are generated on the muscle cell membrane (sarcolemma). Since the nervous system activates skeletal muscle at the level of motor units, and the muscle fibers in a motor unit will contract together, electromyographers often discuss EMG in terms of motor unit action potentials (MUAPs).

There are two general ways to make EMG recordings. First, surface electrodes can be placed over the belly of the muscle. The technology is similar to that used to

make recordings of the electrical activity of the heart (electrocardiogram [ECG]), although many systems incorporate small bioamplifiers that can be placed directly on the skin. Surface electrodes require some preparation of the skin at the recording site. This usually involves thoroughly cleaning the skin with alcohol and, in some cases, shaving and abrading the skin so that the electrical impedance is minimized. Traditional surface EMG recordings do not allow the visualization of individual MUAPs. Instead, many MUAPs exist under the recording site at any instant in time, and the resulting signal is referred to as an interference pattern. The interference pattern looks similar to an acoustic signal or a seismograph signal in geology. The second approach is needle EMG, where needle electrodes are inserted into the muscle belly. In the exercise sciences, needle electrodes are primarily used to make recordings from deep muscles that are not accessible with surface electrodes. Needle EMG is also used in clinical electrodiagnosis, since it allows for the examination of individual MUAPs. A variety of muscular and neurological disorders can often be identified on the basis of the shapes of MUAPs and other characteristics identified in the needle EMG examination. Recently, a new surface

EMG technology that uses an array of small surface EMG electrodes placed in a relatively small space has opened the potential to record individual MUAPs without using a needle. This is one of the frontiers in EMG research.

There are three general quantification approaches for surface EMG in the exercise sciences. First, EMG is used to examine the timing of activation of muscles. Here, the onset and ending of EMG bursts are quantified. If a variety of muscles are examined simultaneously, the timing of activation of agonists, antagonists, and synergists can be studied to give a picture of the pattern of muscle activation for tasks such as walking, running, and lifting. This type of information can also be used clinically. For example, clinical gait laboratories use surface EMG, along with kinematic and kinetic analyses, to help characterize gait dysfunction in individuals with conditions such as cerebral palsy. This information can be used to help guide orthopedic surgical interventions. Second, the amplitude of the EMG signal can be quantified. Generally, the larger the voltage changes

per unit of time, all else being equal, the greater the extent of the motor unit activation. Quantifying the amplitude of an EMG signal then allows the researcher or clinician to gauge the strength of a contraction. The amplitude of the EMG signal also varies during muscle fatigue, so changes in EMG amplitude are often used in studying muscle fatigue. Finally, frequency-domain analysis allows the researcher to characterize an EMG based on how much signal energy is located in various frequency bands. Typically, surface EMG signals contain almost all their signal energy at frequencies below 500 cycles per second (Hertz) and above 10 to 20 Hertz, depending on the characteristics of the recording system. Frequency-domain analysis is often used to study muscle fatigue. As a muscle fatigues, among a variety of changes that occur is that the action potential conduction velocity along the sarcolemma tends to slow down. This alters the frequency characteristics of the surface EMG signal, and these can be quantified using frequency-domain analysis.

In addition to this adaptation observed at submaximal efforts, resistance training was found to result in higher EMG recordings during maximal efforts, suggesting increased maximal neural drive to the muscle. In fact, although calculations predicted a 9% strength increase due to training-induced hypertrophy, strength actually increased by 30%. This and other research supports the idea that an increase in maximal neural drive increases muscular strength.[8] Moreover, it seems that such neural adaptations occur quite rapidly; it has been shown that the large increases in strength evident in the first few weeks of a resistance training program occur with little or no muscle hypertrophy and can be primarily attributed to greater neural activation of the trained muscles.[12] This early impact of the nervous system on strength gains can be observed in Figure 4-20. Interestingly, it has also been established that the early and more pronounced declines in strength that accompany muscle disuse can mainly be attributed to decreased neural drive to the maximally contracting muscle.[6]

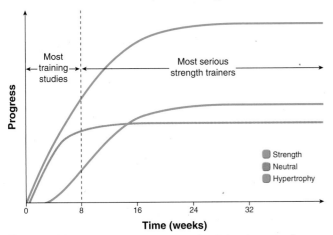

Figure 4-20. **During the first weeks of training, increased strength is initially due to neural adaptations.** As training continues, strength increases are also caused by increases in skeletal muscle hypertrophy.

Another neural adaptation that could improve muscle function is increased motor unit firing.[21] The greater the synchronization, the greater the number of motor units firing at any one time. Increased synchronization of motor unit firing has been observed after strength training, where it appears to have its greatest impact in improving power by decreasing the time it takes for the muscle to reach its peak force production. This would be of value during the performance of power sports such as the shot put or javelin throw.

There is additional evidence to support the belief that the impressive muscle power displayed by properly trained athletes is linked to alterations in neural recruitment patterns. For example, it has been demonstrated that sprint training not only increases the excitability of motor neurons, making high-threshold motor units easier to recruit, but it also enhances the nerve conduction velocity of motor axons, thereby improving rate coding and rate of muscle force production of those motor units.[29]

The greater excitability and nerve conduction velocity noted in the high-threshold motor units of power trained athletes increases force produced and the rate at which that peak force is generated, but by metabolic design, those motor units will fatigue rapidly. In comparing muscle performance between well-trained power athletes versus endurance ones, the former showed greater initial strength and power of the quadriceps muscles. But after a series of fatigue inducing maximal effort leg extensions, it was the power athletes who experienced the more severe decline in strength and power. This was accompanied by a greater decline in EMG activity among the power athletes, suggesting less participation of high-threshold motor units. These findings illustrate that while high-intensity power training may improve the ability to recruit high-threshold, fast motor units, they still remain more fatigable than the low-threshold, slow motor units.

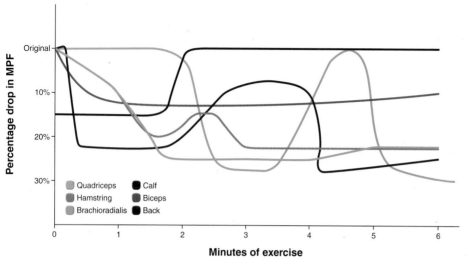

○ Quadriceps   ● Calf
○ Hamstring   ● Biceps
○ Brachioradialis ● Back

Figure 4-21. Relative mean power frequency (MPF) of different muscle groups in elite rowers during 6 minutes of rowing. A decrease in MPF indicates less use of a muscle group and fatigue. (Adapted with permission from National Strength and Conditioning Association, Colorado Springs, CO; from So RC, Tse MA, Wong SC. Application of surface electromyography in assessing muscle recruitment patterns in a six-minute continuous rowing effort. J Strength Cond Res. 2007;21(3):724–730.

In more complex athletic endeavors, such as rowing, where the fine coordination of numerous muscle groups is essential to optimal performance, training appears to elicit a type of adaptation in neural recruitment that is intermuscular in nature. In a recent study, it was determined that highly trained and accomplished rowers were more adept at recruiting among the various muscles used in the complex power stroke of rowing than less trained athletes who had not achieved prominence in their sport (Fig. 4-21).[27] Elite athletes were able to seamlessly rotate recruitment between muscle groups that participate in the power stroke of rowing during a 6-minute rowing bout. For example, they relied more on the quadriceps for the first 2 minutes, then more on the back for minutes 2 to 4, and then again more on the quadriceps for minute 5. In contrast, less accomplished rowers did not possess the ability to alternate use of different muscle groups during the 6 minutes of rowing.

Box 4-9 DID YOU KNOW?

The Neuromuscular Junction and Exercise

The NMJ is the gap between an axon and a muscle fiber where an excitatory signal generated by the motor neuron is transferred to the surface of the muscle fiber, ultimately leading to the contraction of that fiber. Interestingly, research studies have shown that the NMJ is at least one potential site of neuromuscular fatigue leading to diminished contractile force of skeletal muscle.

As with muscle fibers, the NMJ's structure and neurotransmitter concentrations that mediate their activation demonstrate an impressive adaptability to regular exercise training. For example, a program of treadmill running for several weeks results in significantly enlarged dimensions of both the pre-synaptic (nerve terminals) and post-synaptic (muscle fiber end plate) components of the NMJ. These adaptations are associated with a greater number of pre-synaptic vesicles containing neurotransmitters and post-synaptic receptors that bind a neurotransmitter upon its release. These structural modifications result in more efficient nerve-to-muscle communication—and thus, less fatigue—during prolonged activation of the neuromuscular system. Indeed, it has been documented that the decline in the amount of neurotransmitter released from the nerve terminals and bound at the muscle fiber's end plate that naturally occurs during a train of continuous neural stimulation is significantly attenuated in endurance-trained animals. This results in a reduced incidence of failure in neuromuscular transmission and the response of the involved muscle fibers to neural stimulation.

It is not only endurance training that impacts the NMJ, but a program of resistance training carried out for several weeks also has been found to produce similar, but less pronounced, NMJ remodeling. Whereas endurance training brought about an approximately 30% increase in the size of pre- and post-synaptic regions of the NMJ, resistance training expanded pre- and post-synaptic dimensions by about 15%. It is likely that this difference is due to the fact that the total amount of neuromuscular activity is greater during endurance training, which features continuous activity, than during resistance training, where the activity is more intermittent in nature. But in both modes of exercise training, it has been noted that pre- and post-synaptic adaptations are tightly coupled in order to maintain proper release/binding kinetics of neurotransmitters—and probability of muscle fiber contraction—during extended neuromuscular activity.

When considering the increased capacity of the neuromuscular system induced by exercise training, the vital role played by the NMJ in those improvements should not be overlooked. Remodeling of the NMJ is inextricably linked to enhanced neuromuscular performance.

Further Reading

Deschenes M, Judelson DA, Kraemer WJ, et al. Effects of resistance training on neuromuscular junction morphology. Muscle Nerve. 2000;23:1576.

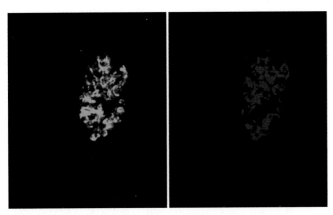

Figure 4-22. Micrograph of fluorescently stained NMJ. Green staining is of pre-synaptic vesicles containing acetylcholine. Red staining is of post-synaptic receptors for acetylcholine. (Courtesy Dr. Michael Deschenes, The College of William and Mary, Williamsburg, VA.)

Although strength and power training appear to elicit more modifications of the nervous system, one that has been shown following endurance training is improved asynchronous recruitment of low-threshold motor units. This improved rotation in the recruitment of low-threshold motor units within the same muscle during prolonged, submaximal exercise serves to provide rest intervals for individual motor units, reducing stress and fatigue among them, thus eliminating the need to recruit the higher threshold, more fatigable motor units.

An important component of the motor unit is the NMJ, which is the synapse that allows communication from the motor neuron to the muscle fibers it innervates. As part of both the nervous system and the muscle system, it too demonstrates adaptations to exercise training (Box 4-9). Principal characteristics of the NMJ are acetylcholine-containing vesicles, located at the terminal endings of the motor axon, and receptors for the neurotransmitter acetylcholine, on the endplate region of the muscle fiber's sarcolemma (Fig. 4-22). The NMJ has long been known as a site of neuromuscular fatigue.[31] However, it is now known that the NMJ is capable of undergoing positive adaptations to exercise training that serve to delay the onset of neuromuscular fatigue. For example, endurance training has been shown to increase the number of both acetylcholine pre-synaptic vesicles and post-synaptic receptors by about 30%, resulting in delayed fatigue and improved endurance performance.[5,7] Research has also shown that, like endurance training, resistance training can increase the size of the NMJ, but only by about 15%.[4] Thus, several types of training-induced adaptations result in improved sport performance.

PRACTICAL APPLICATIONS AND THE NERVOUS SYSTEM

So, how can we practically apply the information presented above on the nervous system to exercise? One application to keep in mind is that the type of activity that you use in a training session will dictate the type and amount of muscle fibers activated. Only muscle fibers activated by the nervous system can gain the benefits of a training program, due to the principle of specificity.

Quick Review

- EMG techniques measure the electrical activity within the muscle and nerves, indicating the amount of neural drive to a muscle.
- An increase in maximal neural drive to a muscle increases strength.
- After training, less neural drive is required to produce a given submaximal force due to either improved activation of motor units or a more efficient recruitment pattern of the motor units.
- The greater the synchronization, the greater the number of motor units firing at any one time.
- Exercise training can improve the synchronization of the firing patterns of the motor units within the muscle.
- Increased synchronization of motor unit firing can reduce the time needed to reach peak force production and improve power.
- Training may result in the ability to rotate the recruitment of the muscles involved in a task, helping to prevent fatigue and improve performance.
- The NMJ adapts to training with increases in both acetylcholine pre-synaptic vesicles and post-synaptic receptors.

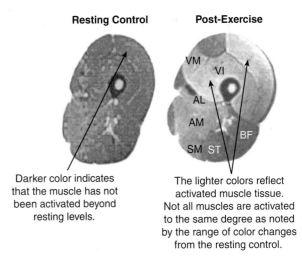

Resting Control   **Post-Exercise**

Darker color indicates that the muscle has not been activated beyond resting levels.

The lighter colors reflect activated muscle tissue. Not all muscles are activated to the same degree as noted by the range of color changes from the resting control.

Figure 4-23. Magnetic resonance imaging of the thigh muscles before and after a heavy squat exercise protocol of five sets of 10 repetitions to concentric failure (10 RM). A resting image is presented on the *left* and an image after exercise is on the *right*. The lighter the area the more the muscle tissue in that part of the thigh has been activated with the squat exercise protocol. Dramatic differences in activation among the different muscles of the thigh can be seen, which could be due to differences in the limb positions and squat mechanics of the exercise movement. RF, rectus femoris; VM, vastus medialis; VL, vastus lateralis; VI, vastus intermedius; BF, biceps femoris; ST, semitendinosus; SM, semimembranous; AM, adductor magnus; AL, adductor longus.

Another application to consider is that the motor units recruited in the muscle will depend on the exercise demands and the biomechanical positions used in an exercise or activity. For example, if you use different right- and left-foot positions in a squat exercise, the activation of the thigh musculature will not be the same due to the differences in the biomechanical movements of the right versus left limbs in the exercise movement (Fig. 4-23). Additionally, the magnitude of recruitment of different portions of the quadriceps is different for the performance of exercises that are biomechanically different despite exercising the same area of the body (e.g., leg press vs. a squat). Variation in the recruitment order and magnitude of recruitment of different muscles is one of the factors responsible for strength and power gains being specific to a particular weight training exercise and skills involving the same muscles. For example, one athlete may be a good sprinter and have a good vertical jump, but another athlete may have a higher vertical jump but not perform as well in the sprint. Perhaps the most important take-home lesson is that the design of the human neuromuscular system only allows muscles to contract, and adapt to exercise, if they are activated by the motor nervous system. And although we can consciously control the motor nervous system to regulate the amount, and type of muscle forces developed by skeletal muscle that moves our limbs, the autonomic nervous system, which regulates the rate and force at which the cardiac muscle contracts, is beyond our ability to consciously control.

CASE STUDY

Scenario

You are a new head track coach. The previous head coach had field athletes weight training and performing interval training prior to skill training for their specific events. You have decided to structure your training sessions beginning with a warm-up followed by technique training, performing interval or weight training at the end of the session. Several of the athletes have asked you why you are changing the sequence of the previous coach's training sessions. What is the physiological basis for the changes in the practice and training program? What other practice and training organizations could you use, and what are the rationales for them?

Options

You explain to the athletes that the sequence of your training sessions will result in more high-quality technique training than the previous coach's sequence of having weight or interval training prior to technique training. You explain to them that as field athletes they do not have to develop maximal force and power in their jumping and throwing events when fatigued. Technique for all of the field events involves coordination of muscle fibers within a specific muscle as well as coordination of many muscles within their bodies to generate maximal power. If they perform weight training and interval training prior to technique training, they will be fatigued when performing the technique training. This will change the recruitment of muscle fibers within the muscles utilized and coordination of the various muscles involved in their specific events. Practically this means that if they practice technique for their field events after other types of training that result in fatigue, they will be learning how to perform their specific events when fatigued, which means that they will recruit their muscle fibers within a muscle and various muscles involved in their event in a slightly different manner compared to performing the event when not fatigued. This means that they will be teaching themselves slightly different or improper technique for their events. You ask them to give your training sequence several weeks to prove itself, and state that you are confident they will see improvement in their event-specific technique.

Scenario

You are in charge of a beginning weight training class. You are aware that for general fitness typically one to three sets of each exercise are performed (see Chapter 12). However, you have a very limited amount of time in which to weight-train your class. Initially how many sets will you have your class perform? What is the physiological basis for the approach you choose to implement?

Options

Neural adaptations are a major reason for strength gains during the first several weeks of a weight training program. These adaptations include recruiting specific muscles at the correct time and in the proper order during the exercise movement and minimally recruiting antagonistic muscles to the desired movement. These neural adaptations occur to a large extent whether one, two, or three sets of an exercise are performed. To allow yourself more time during the initial training sessions to correct the exercise technique of students performing an exercise you had chosen, have your class perform only one set of each exercise. Due to neural adaptations, students will still see significant strength gains during the first several weeks of training. It has been shown that the eccentric phase of the repetition mediates the rapid gains made in strength early on in a resistance training program. After students have mastered proper exercise technique, you will increase the number of sets performed to two and then three per exercise as training adaptations allow the students to tolerate performing an increased number of sets per exercise. Additionally, one has to carefully examine the tolerance for the amount of work performed in a weight training workout.

CHAPTER SUMMARY

The nervous system interacts with every physiological system in the body. Neural signals, presented in the form of electrical activity, transmit information about the body's external and internal environments. These signals not only allow for normal resting homeostatic function of the body, they also allow the body to achieve an aroused physiological state or "fight-or-flight" response during intense exercise or physiological stress.

The brain and spinal cord make up the central nervous system, which functions as the primary controller of all of the body's actions. The peripheral nervous system includes nerves not in the brain or spinal cord and connects all parts of the body to the central nervous system. The peripheral (sensory) nervous system receives stimuli, the central nervous system interprets them, and then the peripheral (motor) nervous system initiates responses. The somatic nervous system controls functions that are under conscious voluntary control, such as skeletal muscles. The autonomic nervous system, mostly motor nerves, controls functions of involuntary smooth muscles and cardiac muscles and glands. The autonomic nervous system provides almost every organ with a double set of nerves—the sympathetic and parasympathetic nervous systems. These systems generally, but not always, work in opposition to each other (e.g., the sympathetic system increases the heart rate and the parasympathetic system decreases it). The sympathetic system activates and prepares the body for vigorous muscular activity, stress, and emergencies, whereas the parasympathetic system lowers arousal, and predominates during normal or resting situations. The nervous system controls movement by controlling muscle activity. To control the force produced by a muscle, the number of motor units recruited and rate coding of each motor unit can be varied. The performance of virtually all activities and sport skills requires the proper recruitment of motor units to develop the needed force in the correct order and at the right time. Training-induced adaptations of the nervous system are the basis of skill training for any physical activity, and serve to improve physical performance. In the next chapter, we will also see that the nervous system is important for cardiovascular function.

REVIEW QUESTIONS

Fill-in-the-Blank

1. The _____ nerves stimulate the heart rate to speed up while the _____ nerves stimulate it to slow down.

2. Motor units made up of _____ fibers are typically recruited first due to the _____ recruitment thresholds of their neurons.

3. When a threshold level of activation is reached in a motor unit, _____ of the muscle fibers in the motor unit will be activated; if the threshold level is not achieved, _____ of the muscle fibers in the motor unit will be activated.

4. The complete summation of nerve impulse twitches is called _____, which results in the maximal force a motor unit can develop.

5. The rapidity at which action potentials are fired down the motor axon helps control the force produced by a motor unit. This process is called _____.

Multiple Choice

1. Which of the following is true concerning a neuron?
   a. Dendrites carry impulses toward the cell body
   b. Axons carry impulses away from the cell body
   c. The axon hillock is between the axon and the cell body
   d. One neuron controls all the muscle fibers in a motor unit
   e. All of the above

2. Which of the following is true of a motor unit?
   a. Smaller and larger motor units are able to produce the same amount of maximal force.
   b. On average, for all of the muscles in the body, about 100 neurons control a muscle fiber.
   c. The number of muscle fibers in a motor unit depends on the amount of fine control required for its function.
   d. Motor units that stretch the lens of the eye contain 1000 muscle fibers.
   e. A motor unit consists of a beta motor neuron and its associated skeletal muscle fibers.

3. Which of the following is NOT true of saltatory conduction?
   a. It allows the action potential to "jump" from one Node of Ranvier to the next.
   b. It increases the velocity of nerve transmission.
   c. It conserves energy.
   d. It occurs only in unmyelinated nerves.
   e. It uses the movement of different ions.

4. Which of the following is, or are, exceptions to the size principle of recruitment?
   a. Recruit high-threshold type II motor units first
   b. Not recruiting low-threshold motor units first
   c. Recruiting slow prior to fast motor units
   d. None of the above
   e. a and b

5. Which of the following is NOT true of fast-fatigable motor units?

a. They have large motor axons

b. They feature type I muscle fibers

c. They feature type IIX muscle fibers

d. Of the three types of motor units, they develop the most force

True/False

1. The fight-or-flight response is brought about by the stimulation of the sympathetic branch of the autonomic nervous system.

2. All muscle fibers of a single motor unit are of the same type (i.e. I, IIA, or IIX).

3. During an action potential, repolarization occurs prior to depolarization.

4. An increase in maximal neural drive to a muscle increases force.

5. Slow motor units are made up of type I muscle fibers.

Short Answer

1. Provide and explain an example of a positive feedback loop during exercise.

2. Explain the different stages of the action potential, that is, depolarization and repolarization, and the movement of ions that occurs in each.

3. What is the advantage of the size principal of motor unit recruitment during an activity like jogging slowly?

4. Are all muscle fibers recruited when a light weight is lifted? Explain why or why not.

5. What contributes to training-induced changes in muscle strength with no significant hypertrophy of the muscle?

Critical Thinking

1. Describe what causes resting membrane potential in an axon or neuron, and then discuss how the movement of ions causes an action potential.

2. Discuss neural adaptations that could increase physical performance.

KEY TERMS

acetylcholine: a neurotransmitter released at motor synapses and neuromuscular junctions, active in the transmission of nerve impulses

action potential (nerve impulse): an impulse in the form of electrical energy that travels down a neuron as its membrane changes from -70 mV to $+30$ mV back to -70 mV due to the movement of electrically charged ions moving in and out of the cell

all-or-none law: when a threshold level for activation is reached, all of the muscle fibers in a motor unit are activated; if the threshold of activation is not met, none of the muscle fibers are activated

alpha (α) motor neuron: a neuron that controls skeletal muscle activity; it is composed of relatively short dendrites that receive the information, a cell body, and long axons that carry impulses from the cell body to the neuromuscular junction, which interfaces with the muscle fiber

asynchronous recruitment: alternating recruitment of motor units when force production needs are low

autonomic nerves (motor neurons): nerves of the autonomic nervous system, outside of the central nervous system

axon: part of a neuron that carries an impulse from the cell body to another neuron or target tissue receptor (e.g., muscle); it is sometimes referred to as a nerve fiber

axon hillock: the part of a neuron where the summation for incoming information is processed, if threshold is reached an impulse is transmitted down the axon

cell body (soma): the part of a neuron that contains the nucleus, mitochondria, ribosomes, and other cellular constituents

central nervous system: brain and spinal column

cerebellum: part of the unconscious brain; regulates muscle coordination and coordinates balance and normal posture

cerebrum: a region of the brain consisting of the left and right hemispheres that is important for control of conscious movements

dendrite: part of a neuron that receives information (impulses) and sends it to the cell body

depolarization: a reduction in the polarity from resting membrane potential (-70 mV) to a more positive value ($+30$ mV) of a neuron's membrane

energy transformation: the conversion of one form of energy to another; in the transmission of an action potential, electrical energy is transformed into chemical energy to cross a synapse or neuromuscular junction

excitability: ability of a neuron or muscle fiber to respond to an electrical impulse

homeostasis: the ability of an organism or cell to maintain internal equilibrium by adjusting its physiological processes to keep function within physiological limits at rest or during exercise

hypothalamus: the homeostatic center of the brain; regulates metabolic rate, body temperature, thirst, blood pressure, water balance, and endocrine function

interneurons: special neurons located only in the central nervous system that connect one neuron to another neuron

ligand: a neurotransmitter, hormone, or other chemical substance that interacts with a receptor protein

local conduction: conduction of nerve impulses in unmyelinated nerves in which the ionic current flows along the entire length of the axon

medulla oblongata: part of the unconscious brain; regulates the heart, breathing, and blood pressure and reflexes such as swallowing, hiccups, sneezing, and vomiting

motor cortex: an area in the frontal lobe of the brain responsible for primary motor control

motor (efferent) neurons: a neuron that carries impulses from the central nervous system to the muscle

motor unit: an alpha motor neuron and its associated muscle fibers

multiple motor unit summation: a method of varying the force produced by a muscle by activating different numbers of motor units within the same muscle

myelin sheath: white covering high in lipid (fat) content that surrounds axons, provides insulation, and maintains electrical signal strength of the action potential as it travels down the axon

myelinated: nerve axons possessing a myelin sheath

Na^+–K^+ pump: an energy-dependent pumping system that restores the resting membrane potential by actively removing Na^+ ions from the inside of the neuron and K+ ions from outside the neuron to the inside of the neuron

nervous impulse (action potential): the stimulus in the form of electrical energy that travels down an axon due to the movement of electrically charged ions moving in and out of the axon

neuron: a cell specialized to transmit electrical signals

neurotransmitter: a chemical substance released by a neuron that diffuses across a small gap and activates receptors on the target cell

nodes of Ranvier: small gaps in the myelin sheath occurring at regular intervals along the axon that allow the action potential to jump from node to node, which allows faster impulse conduction and conserves energy

receptor: a specialized site on the target cell that is activated by neurotransmitters; a protein that is found in a cell membrane or within the cytoplasm or cell nucleus that will bind with a ligand

peripheral nervous system: nerves that transmit information to and from the central nervous system

repolarization: restoration of a membrane back to its original resting membrane potential (–70 mV) after depolarizing (+30 mV)

saltatory conduction: conduction of nerve impulses in myelinated nerves in which the action potential "jumps" from node of Ranvier to node of Ranvier

Schwann cells: cells that create and maintain the myelin sheath

sensory (afferent) neurons: neurons that enter the spinal cord from the periphery and carry messages from sensory receptors to the central nervous system

sensory–somatic nervous system: a part of the peripheral nervous system that controls our conscious awareness of the external environment and motor responses

size principle: a principle that explains how the nervous system recruits individual motor units in an orderly, predictable fashion from smaller to larger motor units

soma (cell body): the part of a neuron that contains the nucleus, mitochondria, ribosomes, and other cellular constituents

synapse: the point of connection, and communication, between two excitable cells

tetanus: the summation of nerve impulse twitches, resulting in the maximal force a motor unit can develop

twitch: a brief period of muscle activity produced by the muscle in response to a single nerve impulse

REFERENCES

1. Anderson T, Kearney JT. Effects of three resistance training programs on muscular strength and absolute and relative endurance. Res Q Exerc Sport. 1982;53:1.
2. Blessing WW. The Lower Brainstem and Bodily Homeostasis. New York, NY: Oxford University Press, 1997.
3. Burke RE, Levine DN, Zajac FE, et al. Mammalian motor units: Physiological–histochemical correlations of three types in cat gastrocnemius. Science. 1971;174:709.
4. Deschenes M, Judelson DA, Kraemer WJ, et al. Effects of resistance training on neuromuscular junction morphology. Muscle and Nerve. 2000;23:1576.
5. Deschenes M, Maresh CM, Crivello JF, et al. The effects of exercise training of different intensities on neuromuscular junction morphology. J Neurocytol. 1993;22:603.
6. Deschenes MR, Giles JA, McCoy RW, et al. Neural factors account for strength decrements observed following short-term muscle unloading. Am J Physiol, Regul Integr Comp Physiol. 2002;282:R578–R583.
7. Dorlochter M, Irintchev A, Brinkers M, et al. Effects of enhanced activity on synaptic transmission in mouse extensor digitorum longus muscle. J Physiol. 1991;436:283.
8. Duchateau J, Semmler JG, Enoka RM. Training adaptations in the behavior of human motor units. J Appl Physiol. 2006;101:1766.
9. French DN, Kraemer WJ, catecholamines on muscle for
10. Gabriel DA, Kamen G, Fros Mechanisms and recommen 2006;36:133.
11. Gordon T, Thomas CK, Mu in the organization of motor skeletal muscles. Can J Physi
12. Hakkinen K, Kallinen M, Iz EMG, muscle CSA, and for older people. J Appl Physiol
13. Harris DA, Henneman E. Id in cat's plantaris pool. J Neurophysiol. 1977;40:16.
14. Harte JL, Eifert GH. The effects of running, environment, and attentional focus on athletes' catecholamine and cortisol levels and mood. Psychophysiology. 1995;32:49.
15. Henneman E, Clamann HP, Gillies JD, et al. Rank order of motoneurons within a pool: Law of combination. J Neurophysiol. 1974;37:1338.
16. Henneman E, Harris D. Identification of fast and slow firing types of motoneurons in the same pool. Prog Brain Res. 1976;44:377.
17. Henneman E, Olson CB. Relations between structure and function in the design of skeletal muscles. J Neurophysiol. 1965;28:581.
18. Henneman E, Somjen G, Carpenter DO. Excitability and inhibitability of motoneurons of different sizes. J Neurophysiol. 1965;28:599.
19. Henneman E, Somjen G, Carpenter DO. Functional significance of cell size in spinal motoneurons. J Neurophysiol. 1965;28:560.
20. Hucho F, ed. Neurotransmitter Receptors. Elsevier, 1993:3.
21. Kamen G, Roy A. Motor unit synchronization in young and elderly adults. Eur J Appl Physiol. 2000;81:403.
22. Krahenbuhl GS. Adrenaline, arousal and sport. J Sports Med. 1975;3:117.
23. McDonagh MJ, Hayward CM, Davies CT. Isometric training in human elbow flexor muscles. The effects on voluntary and electrically evoked forces. J Bone Joint Surg Br. 1983;65:355.
24. Moritani T, deVries HA. Neural factors versus hypertrophy in the time course of muscle strength gain. Am J Phys Med. 1979;58:115.
25. Moritani T, deVries HA. Potential for gross muscle hypertrophy in older men. J Gerontol. 1980;35:672.
26. Moritani T, deVries HA. Reexamination of the relationship between the surface integrated electromyogram (IEMG) and force of isometric contraction. Am J Phys Med. 1978;57:263.
27. Raymond CH, Tse MA, Wong SCW. Application of surface electromyography in assessing muscle recruitment patterns in a six-minute continuous rowing effort. J Strength Cond Res. 2007;21:724.
28. Regan D. Visual factors in hitting and catching. J Sports Sci. 1997;15:533.
29. Ross A, Leveritt M, Riek S. Neural influences on sprint running: Training adaptations and acute responses. Sports Med. 2001;31:409.
30. Scalettar B. How neurosecretory vesicles release their cargo. Neuroscientist. 2006;12:164.
31. Stephens JA, Taylor A. Fatigue of maintained voluntary muscle contraction in man. J Physiol. 1972;220:1.

Suggested Readings

Aagaard P, Simonsen EB, Andersen JL, et al. Neural adaptation to resistance training: Changes in evoked V-wave and H-reflex responses. J Appl Physiol. 2002;92:2309–2318.

Aagaard P, Simonsen EB, Andersen JL, et al. Neural inhibition during maximal eccentric and concentric quadriceps contraction: Effects of resistance training. J Appl Physiol. 2000;89:2249–2257.

Barry BK, Riek S, Carson RG. Muscle coordination during rapid force production by young and older adults. J Gerontol. 2005;60A:232–240.

Beaumont E, Gardiner PF. Endurance training alters the biophysical properties of hindlimb motoneurons in rats. Muscle Nerve. 2003;27:228–236.

Bellemare F, Woods JJ, Johansson R, et al. Motor-unit discharge rates in maximal voluntary contractions of three human muscles. J Neurophysiol. 1983;50:1380–1392.

Cha
Part II Exercise
134
Binder MD, Heckman
activity. In: Hand
of Multiple S
1996:1–53.
Carolan B,
train
Carro

, Powers RK. The physiological control of motoneuron
ook of Physiology. Exercise: Regulation and Integration
tems. Sect. 12, chapt. 1. Bethesda, MD: Am. Physiol. Soc.,

afarelli E. Adaptations in coactivation after isometric resistance
g. J Appl Physiol. 1992;73:911–917.

TJ, Riek S, Carson RG. The sites of neural adaptation induced by
resistance training in humans. J Physiol. 2002;544:641–652.

Datta AK, Stephens JA. Synchronization of motor unit activity during voluntary
contraction in man. J Physiol. 1990;422:397–419.

Davies CTM, Dooley P, McDonagh MJN, et al. Adaptation of mechanical properties
of muscle to high force training in man. J Physiol. 1985;365:277–284.

De Luca CJ, Erim Z. Common drive of motor units in regulation of muscle
force. Trends Neurosci. 1994;17:299–305.

De Luca CJ, LeFever RS, McCue MP, et al. Behavior of human motor units
in different muscles during linearly varying contractions. J Physiol.
1982;329:113–128.

De Luca CJ, Mambrito B. Voluntary control of motor units in human
antagonist muscles: Coactivation and reciprocal activation. J Neurophysiol.
1987;58:525–542.

Enoka RM, Christou EA, Hunter SK, et al. Mechanisms that contribute
to differences in motor performance between young and old adults.
J Electromyogr Kinesiol. 2003;13:1–12.

Enoka RM, Robinson GA, Kossev AR. Task and fatigue effects on low-threshold
motor units in human hand muscle. J Neurophysiol. 1989;62:1344–1359.

Fuglevand AJ, Winter DA, Patla AE. Models of recruitment and rate coding
organization in motor-unit pools. J Neurophysiol. 1993;70:2470–2488.

Gardiner PF. Changes in alpha-motoneuron properties with altered physical
activity levels. Exerc Sport Sci Rev. 2006;34:54–58.

Hainaut K, Duchateau J, Desmedt JE. Differential effects of slow and fast motor
units of different programs of brief daily muscle training in man. In: New
Developments in Electromyography and Clinical Neurophysiology. vol. 9.
Basel, Switzerland: Karger, 1981:241–249.

Jensen JL, Marstrand PC, Nielsen JB. Motor skill training and strength training
are associated with different plastic changes in the central nervous system. J
Appl Physiol. 2005;99:1558–1568.

Kent-Braun JA, Le Blanc R. Quantitation of central activation failure during
maximal voluntary contractions in humans. Muscle Nerve. 1996;19:861–869.

Knight CA, Kamen G. Enhanced motor unit rate coding with improvements in a
force-matching task. J Electromyogr Kinesiol. 2004;14:619–629.

Lévénez M, Kotzamanidis C, Carpentier A, et al. Spinal reflexes and coactivation
of ankle muscles during a submaximal fatiguing contraction. J Appl Physiol.
2005;99:1182–1188.

Luscher HR, Ruenzel P, Henneman E. How the size of motoneurones determines
their susceptibility to discharge. Nature. 1979;282(5741):859–861.

Mottram CJ, Jakobi JM, Semmler JG, et al. Motor unit activity differs with load
type during fatiguing contraction. J Neurophysiol. 2005;93:1381–1393.

Munn J, Herbert RD, Hancock MJ, et al. Training with unilateral resistance
exercise increases contralateral strength. J Appl Physiol. 2005;99:1880–1884.

Ploutz LL, Tesch PA, Biro RL, et al. Effect of resistance training on muscle use
during exercise. J Appl Physiol. 1994;7:1675–1681.

Semmler JG. Motor unit synchronization and neuromuscular performance.
Exerc Sport Sci Rev. 2002;30:8–14.

Stotz PJ, Bawa P. Motor unit recruitment during lengthening contractions of
human wrist flexors. Muscle Nerve. 2001;24:1535–1541.

Van Cutsem M, Duchateau J. Preceding muscle activity influences motor unit
discharge and rate of torque development during ballistic contractions in
humans. J Physiol. 2005;562:635–644.

Wilson GJ, Murphy AJ, Walshe A. The specificity of strength training: The
effect of posture. Eur J Appl Physiol. 1996;73:346–352.

Yue G, Fuglevand AJ, Nordstrom MA, et al. Limitations of the surface
electromyography technique for estimating motor unit synchronization. Biol
Cybern. 1995;73:223–233.

Zoghi M, Pearce SL, Nordstrom MA. Differential modulation of intracortical
inhibition in human motor cortex during selective activation of an intrinsic
hand muscle. J Physiol. 2003;550:933–946.

Classic References

Adrian E, Bronk D. The discharge of impulses in motor nerve fibres. II. The
frequency of discharges in reflex and voluntary contractions. J Physiol.
1929;204:231–257.

Andersson Y, Edstrom JE. Motor hyperactivity resulting in diameter decrease of
peripheral nerves. Acta Physiol Scand. 1957;39:240–245.

Burke RE, Levine DN, Zajac FE, et al. Mammalian motor units: Physiological–
histochemical correlations of three types in cat gastrocnemius. Science.
1971;174:709.

Cannon Walter B. The Wisdom of the Body. New York, NY: W. W. Norton,
1932.

Henneman E. Relation between size of neurons and their susceptibility to
discharge. Science. 1957;126:1345–1347.

Sherrington C. Remarks on some aspects of reflex inhibition. Proc R Soc Lond
B Biol Sci. 1925;B97:19–45.

Stalberg E. Macro EMG, a new recording technique. J Neurol Neurosurg
Psychiatry. 1980;43:475–482.

Chapter 5

Cardiovascular System

After reading this chapter, you should be able to:

1. Outline the basic structure and function of the entire cardiovascular system

2. Describe the cardiac cycle and how it is controlled

3. Explain and interpret an electrocardiogram

4. Identify factors contributing to cardiac output

5. Explain the regulation of blood pressure

6. Describe the composition of blood

7. Distinguish cardiovascular training adaptations due to endurance and strength training

8. Describe oxygen delivery to tissue

9. Describe redistribution of blood flow during exercise

10. Discuss mechanisms of increased venous return and oxygen delivery during exercise

Whether at rest or during maximal exercise, the cardiovascular system is responsible for delivering needed substances, such as oxygen, hormones, and nutrients, to every cell in your body and for removing metabolic products, such as carbon dioxide, from cells. In addition, the cardiovascular system aids in temperature regulation (Chapter 10) and buffering of acidity (Chapter 2), and also plays a role in the immune response by transporting platelets and white blood cells. The respiratory system (see Chapter 6), which is responsible for the exchange of oxygen and carbon dioxide with the atmosphere, and the cardiovascular system, which is responsible for the transport of these substances throughout your body, together form the "cardiorespiratory system."

The cardiovascular system is composed of a pump—the heart—and two major systems of vessels that transport blood to every cell within your body and to the lungs. The structure and organization of the cardiovascular system, and its ability to adapt to the acute and chronic stress of exercise, allow tremendous increases in its performance. For example, during heavy exercise, the demand for oxygen by exercising muscle tissue increases up to approximately 25 times more than the need for oxygen at rest. Understanding the structure, organization, function, and adaptation of the cardiovascular system to exercise allows for an understanding of how it is possible to increase oxygen delivery to exercising tissue so that an international-class marathon runner can complete slightly over 26 miles in a little over 2 hours. However, the cardiovascular system also undergoes adaptation to other types of training, which is important to the performance of anaerobic activities, such as sprint-type races. Thus, the purpose of this chapter is to explore not just the basic physiological function of the cardiovascular system but also its adaptations to exercise.

RE, FUNCTION, GANIZATION OF THE OVASCULAR SYSTEM

he cardiovascular system is comprised of the heart, the blood, and circulatory system which is divided into the peripheral and pulmonary branches (Fig. 5-1).

Pulmonary and Peripheral Circulations

The **pulmonary circulation** transports blood from the heart to the lungs and back to the heart. The **peripheral circulation** delivers blood from the heart to all parts of the body and back to the heart. The heart's pumping action, or contraction, creates pressure, forcing blood into either the pulmonary or the peripheral circulation. Large vessels, termed **arteries**, carry blood away from the heart toward either the lungs or the periphery. The arteries branch extensively, forming small arteries, or **arterioles**. The smallest of the arterioles branch and form **capillaries**, the smallest and most numerous of all blood vessels. Capillaries are the site of all oxygen and carbon dioxide exchange

within both the pulmonary and peripheral circulations, and all nutrient exchange between tissue and blood within the peripheral circulation. Each cell within all tissues must be within a distance of 0.1 mm of the nearest capillary so that exchange of oxygen, carbon dioxide, and nutrients can take place. After passing through the capillaries, the blood enters **venules**, which are the smallest **veins**—the blood vessels that carry blood toward the heart. Blood within venules first enters small veins and then large veins and eventually returns to the heart.

Venous blood is blood that is returning to the heart, while **arterial blood** is blood that is leaving the heart and traveling toward other bodily tissues. In peripheral circulation, oxygen is delivered to bodily tissues, and carbon dioxide—a product of aerobic metabolism—leaves bodily tissues and enters the blood. So venous blood from the peripheral circulation is deoxygenated and high in carbon dioxide content. Arterial blood going to the lungs has just returned to the heart from the peripheral circulation, and so arterial blood in the pulmonary arteries is deoxygenated, with a high carbon dioxide concentration. At the lungs, oxygen enters the blood, whereas carbon dioxide leaves the blood and enters the lungs to be expired. Thus, venous blood in the pulmonary veins returning to the heart from the lungs is oxygenated and has a low content of carbon dioxide. The blood that just returned to the heart from the lungs is then pumped to the peripheral circulation, and the cycle of oxygen and carbon dioxide exchange between tissues, blood, and lungs is repeated. Note that both peripheral arterial blood and pulmonary venous blood are high in oxygen and low in carbon dioxide content, while both peripheral venous blood and pulmonary arterial blood are low in oxygen and high in carbon dioxide content.

In order to maintain the separation of oxygenated and deoxygenated blood, the heart is divided into two distinct pumps. This is the subject of our next section.

The Heart

The heart, which serves as a blood pump, is the second major component in the cardiovascular system that we will consider. Here, we will cover the structure of the heart, the

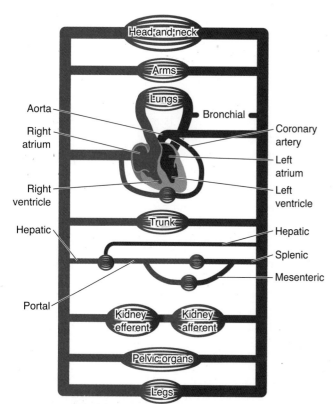

Figure 5-1. Schematic diagram of the cardiovascular system demonstrating the parallel arrangement of the vasculature. Each circulation to a body part or organ has a capillary bed where exchange of oxygen, carbon dioxide, and nutrients takes place. There are several circulations that, because of their specialized functions, are not arranged in a parallel fashion. Red indicates oxygenated blood, and blue indicates deoxygenated blood.

Quick Review

- The pulmonary circulation circulates blood from the heart to the lungs and back to the heart.
- The peripheral circulation circulates blood from the heart to all parts of the body and back to the heart.
- Arteries carry blood from the heart to the peripheral and pulmonary circulations.
- Veins carry blood from the pulmonary and peripheral circulations toward the heart.

blood supply of the heart, the cardiac cycle, cardiac muscle, and cardiac output.

Structure of the Heart

To keep the oxygenated blood returning to the heart from the pulmonary circulation and the deoxygenated blood returning to the heart from the peripheral circulation separate from each other, the heart is divided into two distinct sides. The right side of the heart receives blood from the peripheral circulation and pumps blood to the pulmonary circulation (see Fig. 5-1), whereas the left side of the heart receives blood from the pulmonary circulation and pumps blood to the peripheral circulation.

Blood returning to the heart from the peripheral circulation enters the right atrium, and blood from the pulmonary circulation enters the left atrium (Fig. 5-2). From the atria, blood passes through one-way valves into the ventricles, which are the strongest chambers of the heart. Blood leaving the ventricles also passes through a one-way valve into the aorta, which is the large artery leaving the left ventricle, and the pulmonary artery, which is the large artery leaving the right ventricle. The one-way valves are important because they allow blood flow only in the desired direction and so prevent backflow of blood in the wrong direction. This is important because if there is a backflow of blood, more blood would have to be pumped in order to pump out a certain amount of blood, which would increase the amount of work the heart must do. Another important structure of the heart is the **pericardium**—a tough, membranous sac that encases the heart. The space between the pericardium and the external surface of the heart is filled with pericardial fluid. This fluid is necessary to reduce the friction between the pericardial membrane and the heart as it beats.

The heart, like all tissue, needs to be supplied with oxygen and nutrients and needs to have carbon dioxide produced by aerobic metabolism removed. Although the heart pumps all the blood circulating throughout the pulmonary and peripheral circulations, it does not extract oxygen and nutrients from, or release carbon dioxide into, the blood it pumps. Instead, the heart has its own circulatory blood supply.

Blood Supply of the Heart

The coronary artery, which supplies the heart with its blood supply, branches off of the aorta immediately after the aortic valve (Fig. 5-3). This means the heart receives blood that has just returned from the pulmonary

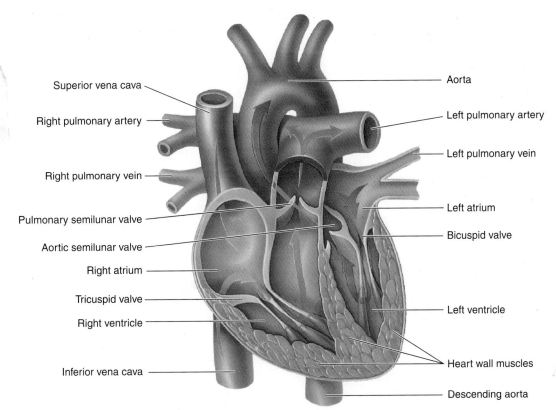

Figure 5-2. Circulation of blood through the heart, to and from the pulmonary and peripheral circulations.
The structure of the heart and circulatory system keeps oxygenated and deoxygenated blood separated in the heart as well as both the pulmonary and peripheral circulations. Red indicates oxygenated blood and blue indicates deoxygenated blood.

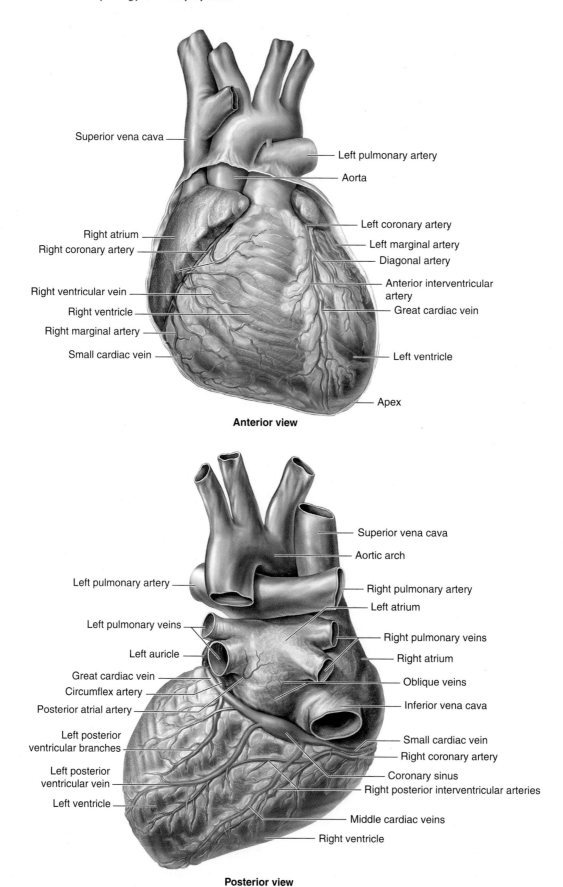

Anterior view

Posterior view

Figure 5-3. The coronary arteries and veins are located on the exterior surface of the heart. Being on the exterior surface of the heart prevents them from being compressed during contraction of the cardiac tissue.

circulation and therefore is fully oxygenated. Peripheral blood pressure (see "Blood Pressure") is the highest in the aorta. Therefore, blood pressure that causes perfusion of the arteries supplying the cardiac tissue is also quite high.

The major arteries supplying the right and left sides of the heart are the right coronary artery and the left coronary artery, respectively. There are several factors that help ensure a blood supply to the heart. An **anastomosis** is an intercommunication between two arteries that ensures blood flow to an area, even if an artery supplying an area is fully or partially blocked. For example, there is an anastomosis between the anterior intraventricular artery and the posterior intraventricular artery which ensures some blood flow through the anterior intraventricular artery even if it is blocked. The major arteries and veins of the heart are located on the outer surface of the heart, in effect, wrapping around the heart. This ensures they will not be compressed during cardiac contraction and so ensures blood flow throughout as much of the cardiac cycle as possible.

Cardiac Cycle

Each of the four chambers of the heart has a particular function during the cardiac cycle. **Systole** refers to the contraction phase of the cardiac cycle, whereas **diastole** refers to the relaxation phase of the cardiac cycle. When a chamber is contracting, blood is being pumped, and when a chamber is relaxing, it is being filled with blood for the next systolic phase of the cardiac cycle. During diastole, the right and left atria are filled with venous blood from the peripheral and pulmonary circulations, respectively. After filling, the atria contract approximately 1/10 of a second prior to the contraction of the ventricles. The contraction of the atria forces blood through the valves separating the atria and the ventricles and helps to fill the ventricles while they are still in diastole. The atria also allow venous blood to return to the heart during contraction of the ventricles, allowing continuous venous return to both

Quick Review

- The right ventricle pumps blood to the pulmonary circulation, and the left ventricle pumps blood to the peripheral circulation.
- One-way valves between the atria and the ventricles, and in the major arteries leaving the ventricles, help to maintain blood flow in the correct direction.
- The coronary artery is the first artery to leave the aorta and supplies the heart with blood.
- The coronary arteries and veins are found on the exterior surface of the heart so that they are not compressed during contraction of the heart.

the right and left sides of the heart. Thus, the atria serve several functions.

Once the right and left ventricles are filled, they contract and pump blood to the pulmonary circulation and peripheral circulation, respectively. The cardiac cycle is then repeated during each beat of the heart. In a normally functioning heart, all chambers of the heart go through a systolic phase during each and every heartbeat. This requires a constant supply of oxygen to cardiac musculature to perform aerobic metabolism, and therefore a constant oxygenated blood supply. As discussed earlier, the major coronary vessels are located on the outer surface of the heart to help ensure blood flow throughout as much of the cardiac cycle as possible. However, when a cardiac chamber goes through systole, the cardiac muscle, like all muscle, will expand in all directions, constricting blood vessels within the tissue and occluding, or partially occluding, blood flow. So, cardiac tissue receives the vast majority of its blood supply during diastole. One adaptation to aerobic or cardiovascular training is a slowing of the heart rate during rest as well as during submaximal exercise. With a slower heart rate, the diastolic phase of the cardiac cycle is longer. Thus, a slower heart rate during submaximal exercise helps ensure a sufficient blood supply to the cardiac tissue. This is one reason a lower heart rate is a positive adaptation to aerobic or cardiovascular training. Next we will examine control of the cardiac cycle.

Intrinsic Control of the Cardiac Cycle

Structures within the heart guarantee that the chambers of the heart contract in a specific order so that blood moves in the correct direction through the heart into the pulmonary and peripheral circulations. Specifically, anatomical and physiological mechanisms are needed to ensure that atrial systole will occur prior to ventricular systole. Cardiac muscle tissue, along with the specialized nervous tissue innervating cardiac muscle fibers, is capable of initiating its own impulse for contraction. The ability to initiate its own impulse for contraction at relatively regular time intervals is termed **autorhythmaticity**. The **sinoatrial node (SA node)** is an area of specialized nervous tissue in the upper portion of the right atrium that has the fastest rate of autorhythmaticity (Fig. 5-4). So, in a normally functioning heart, the SA node is the pacemaker of cardiac contraction. The stimulus to contract spreads throughout both atria, causing them to contract. The impulse also spreads to another area of specialized nervous tissue located in the lower portion of the right atrium, the **atrioventricular node (AV node)**. The AV node delays the impulse to contract approximately 1/10 of a second before spreading the impulse to the ventricles, allowing the atria to contract prior to the ventricles. From the AV node, the impulse is spread rapidly throughout the

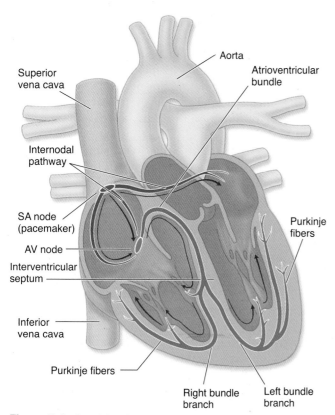

Figure 5-4. Specialized nervous tissues within the heart control the contraction sequence of the atria and the ventricles. The SA node is the pacemaker of the heart. The AV node delays the impulse to contract from the SA node by approximately 1/10 of a second, so the ventricles contract after the atria.

ventricles by first passing through the atrioventricular bundle, then right and left bundle branches, and finally the **Purkinje fibers**. These specialized nervous tissue fibers rapidly spread the impulse to contract throughout the ventricles so that all cardiac tissue is contracting with each and every beat of the heart, in a short time period, and in a very synchronized manner. This helps to guarantee that blood is pumped from the ventricles in a very efficient manner (i.e., using as little energy as possible).

Extrinsic Control of the Cardiac Cycle

In addition to the intrinsic control of the cardiac cycle, extrinsic control—or control from outside the heart—occurs and is responsible for adjustments in heart rate, such as a training-induced resting **bradycardia,** or slowing of the heart rate (less than 60 beats·min⁻¹), and an increase in heart rate because of the performance of physical activity. The two major factors that influence heart rate are the sympathetic and parasympathetic branches of the autonomic nervous system (Fig. 5-5).

The parasympathetic nerve fibers that innervate the SA and AV nodes arise from the cardiorespiratory

control center in the medulla oblongata and reach the heart as part of the vagus nerve. At the SA and AV nodes, **parasympathetic** nerve fibers release acetylcholine, which decreases the activity of both nodes, resulting in a decrease in heart rate. So, an increase in parasympathetic stimulation decreases heart rate, and removal of parasympathetic stimulation results in an increase in heart rate.

Sympathetic nerve fibers reach the SA node, AV node, and myocardium as part of the cardiac accelerator nerves. At the SA and AV nodes, **sympathetic** fibers release norepinephrine, which increases the activity of both nodes, resulting in an increase in heart rate. Norepinephrine also acts to increase the force of myocardial contraction, thus increasing the amount of blood pumped by the heart with each beat. In addition to direct neural influences, endocrine changes can alter heart rate. Specifically, epinephrine released by the adrenal gland into the bloodstream also acts to increase heart rate. This release of epinephrine occurs only when the adrenal gland is stimulated by the sympathetic system. So, an increase in sympathetic activity increases heart rate, and removal of sympathetic stimulation decreases heart rate. Heart rate, therefore, depends on the balance between parasympathetic and sympathetic stimulation.

The medulla oblongata receives information from various parts of the circulatory system (chemoreceptors, baroreceptors) concerning the functioning of the circulatory system, such as blood pressure and oxygen concentration within the blood (chemoreceptors and control of heart rate and breathing rate will be discussed in Chapter 6). For example, if at rest blood pressure within the aorta increases above normal, parasympathetic stimulation would increase and sympathetic stimulation would decrease, resulting in a decrease in heart rate and contractile force of the myocardium. This would result in less blood being pumped per beat of the heart and a decrease in blood pressure back toward normal resting values.

This information concerning sympathetic and parasympathetic stimulation may lead to the hypothesis that a decrease in resting heart rate because of aerobic activity is caused by an increase in parasympathetic stimulation and a decrease in sympathetic stimulation. However, data concerning sympathetic and parasympathetic stimulation of endurance-trained athletes are inconsistent, with indications of both increases and decreases in both sympathetic stimulation and parasympathetic stimulation.[44] At the onset of exercise, a consistent decrease in parasympathetic stimulation, resulting in an increase in heart rate, has been shown.[44] Although data concerning sympathetic stimulation at the onset of exercise are less consistent,[44] it is clear that an increase in sympathetic stimulation to the heart will increase heart rate and

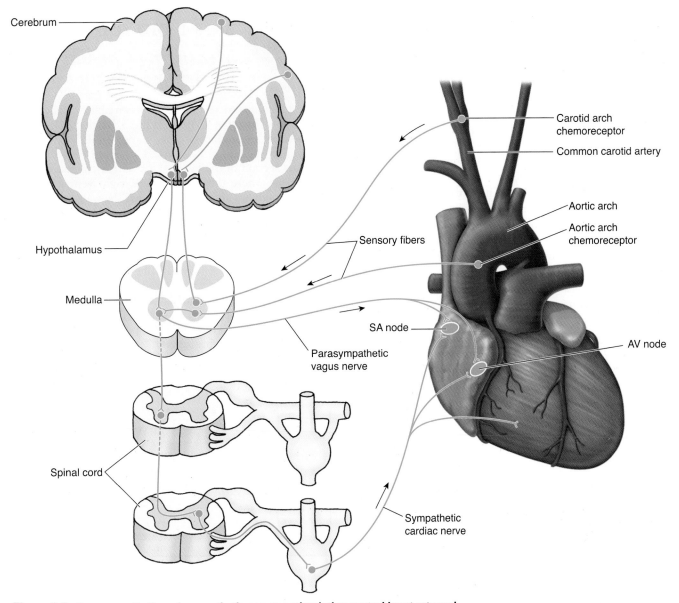

Figure 5-5. Parasympathetic and sympathetic nervous stimulation control heart rate and contraction force of the heart. Parasympathetic stimulation slows and sympathetic stimulation increases heart rate.

myocardial contractile force. Thus, whether at rest or during exercise, heart rate is controlled, in large part, by a balance between sympathetic and parasympathetic nervous stimulation.

Cardiac Muscle

Like skeletal muscle, cardiac muscle, or the **myocardium**, is capable of contraction and force generation. Although both skeletal muscle and cardiac muscle are capable of contraction, there are several differences between these two types of muscle. Autorhythmicity, as described earlier, is one such difference.

Quick Review

- Systole and diastole of the heart must be controlled in order for the heart to function efficiently.
- All cardiac tissue has autorhythmaticity, and the sinoatrial node—the pacemaker of the heart—has the fastest autorhythmaticity.
- The atrioventricular node delays the impulse for the ventricles to contract 1/10 of a second so that the ventricles contract after the atria.
- Extrinsic control of the cardiac cycle consists of parasympathetic stimulation, which decreases heart rate, and sympathetic stimulation, which increases heart rate.

Another major difference between skeletal muscle and the myocardium is the presence of intercalated discs in the myocardium. In skeletal muscle, the impulse to contract cannot spread from one muscle fiber to another, allowing for better control of the contraction of individual muscle fibers and thus the whole muscle. However, in the myocardium, the impulse to contract can spread from one muscle fiber to another by intercalated discs, which are leaky portions of the membranes separating individual muscle fibers. Thus, even if a cardiac muscle fiber is not stimulated by a nervous impulse to contract, it will contract during cardiac systole. It is because of these intercalated discs and the Purkinje fibers that the myocardium displays syncytial contraction. This means that the fibers contract simultaneously enhancing the heart's ability to act as an effective pump since individual myocardial fibers generate little force. Recall, however, that there is a delay in the spread of electrical activation from the atria to the ventricles, and in order to prevent spread of atrial contraction to the ventricles, there is a layer of connective tissue separating the atria from the ventricles.

Human myocardium, unlike skeletal muscle, cannot be divided into different types of muscle fibers, such as fast-twitch (type II) or slow-twitch (type I). Rather, the myocardium is composed of one primary muscle fiber type that exhibits a high mitochondrial density, has an extensive capillary network, and is capable of utilizing aerobic energy efficiently for contraction. The characteristics of the myocardium allow it to function efficiently and pump blood 24 hours a day for the lifespan of an individual.

Cardiac Wall Thickness

The thicker the wall of a cardiac chamber the greater the force that it can generate to eject blood. Because the left ventricle must pump blood to the entire body against a higher blood pressure (and thus resistance to flow) than that of the right ventricle, which pumps blood to the pulmonary circulation, the left ventricle has the greater wall thickness.

During any physical activity, peripheral blood pressure increases while performing the activity. Over time, perhaps weeks the regular performance of physical training results in a thickening of the wall of the left ventricle, allowing it to more easily overcome the greater blood pressure observed during activity (Box 5-1). Although not all studies support that physical activity results in an increase in left ventricular wall thickness, this is a possible outcome of endurance, sprint, and weight training.[14,30,31] Left ventricular wall thickness also increases with chronic hypertension. However, increases in left ventricular wall thickness because of physical training do not exceed the upper limit of what is considered normal (approximately 13 mm), whereas increased wall thickness due to chronic

Box 5-1 DID YOU KNOW?
Measuring Cardiac Wall Thickness

One method to determine cardiac variables is magnetic resonance imaging (MRI). With MRI technology, it is possible to produce a cross section of an anatomical structure, including the heart. The figure below shows a cross section of the heart of a strength-trained athlete at a level where the left ventricle, right ventricle, and right atrium are apparent. Note that the walls of the left ventricle are substantially thicker than those of either the right ventricle or the right atrium. The only place where the right ventricular wall is similar in thickness to the left ventricular wall is at the intraventricular septum; however, this is a shared wall between the ventricles. Thus, the intraventricular septum's increased wall thickness is related to the need of the left ventricle to eject blood against a high peripheral blood pressure and not to the need of the right ventricle to eject blood into the pulmonary circulation against a high blood pressure.

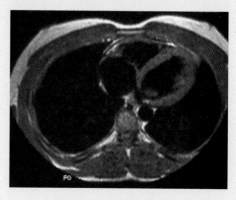

hypertension can. Thus, even though both physical training and chronic hypertension result in increases in left ventricular wall thickness, there is a difference in the magnitude of this response.

An increase in left ventricular wall thickness because of either physical training or chronic hypertension results in an increase in **left ventricular mass**, or the total amount of myocardium surrounding the left ventricle. As with left ventricular wall thickness, however, there are differences between increased left ventricular mass due to chronic hypertension and that due to physical training. For example, in highly trained Olympic weightlifters, left ventricular mass, when expressed relative to body mass or fat-free mass—a measure of total muscle mass—stays within normal limits.[11-13] This indicates that the increase in left ventricle mass because of Olympic weightlifting is a physiological adaptation to training as opposed to a pathological adaptation due to chronic hypertension. Another indication that the increase in left ventricular mass is a physiological adaptation is that the left ventricular mass has shown significant correlations to peak oxygen consumption in strength- and endurance-trained athletes.[12,42] These correlations are probably related to the need to pump blood against a higher peripheral blood pressure during activity, including a test to determine peak oxygen consumption.

It appears that the atria and right ventricle do not respond to physical training with a significant increase in wall thickness even in weight-trained individuals, in whom peripheral blood pressures during activity are extremely high.[11,13,24] In part, this may be true because these chambers do not have to eject blood against the extremely high peripheral blood pressures that must be overcome by the left ventricle during activity. Recall that the right ventricle pumps blood to the lungs which are in close proximity to the heart. So, it appears that the left ventricle is the only chamber that adapts to physical activity with a significant increase in wall thickness and mass.

If left ventricular mass increased without an increase in coronary vasculature, eventually delivery of oxygen to the myocardium would be insufficient. With exercise training causing physiological hypertrophy of the heart, coronary vasculature also adapts by increasing the size of the major arteries and capillarization of the myocardium.[37] However, when left ventricular mass increases because of a pathological adaptation to chronic hypertension, changes in the vasculature do not occur, again demonstrating that there is a difference between pathological and physiological adaptation of the myocardium. Next we will examine the electrical activity of the heart during a cardiac cycle.

Electrocardiogram

Contraction of the atria and ventricles occurs in a specific order because of the SA node, AV node, and other specialized nervous tissues within the heart that stimulate and control myocardial contraction. Within a normally functioning heart, the electrical activity that precedes the sequential contraction of the heart's chambers is graphically represented in the **electrocardiogram** or **ECG** (which is actually movement of ions occurring during muscle contraction and relaxation). Within the ECG, the height of a wave represents the amount of electrical activity, and indirectly represents the amount of cardiac muscle contracting or relaxing. The horizontal length of the wave represents time and, so, the shorter the length of the wave, the shorter the period of time for that wave to occur. The first deflection, or wave, is the P wave and represents atrial contraction (Fig. 5-6). There is then a period of time (approximately 1/10 of a second) during which no electrical activity is detected, followed by the QRS complex, representing contraction of the ventricles. The period of time between the P wave and the QRS complex is caused by the AV node holding the impulse for ventricular contraction before spreading the impulse to the AV bundle, bundle branches, and Purkinje fibers, stimulating ventricular contraction. Following the QRS complex is the T wave, which represents ventricular relaxation and repolarization. Relaxation of the atria occurs at the same time as the QRS complex, and, therefore, a wave representing atrial relaxation is normally not visible.

In addition to the P wave, QRS complex, and T wave, other portions of an ECG are named using the letters

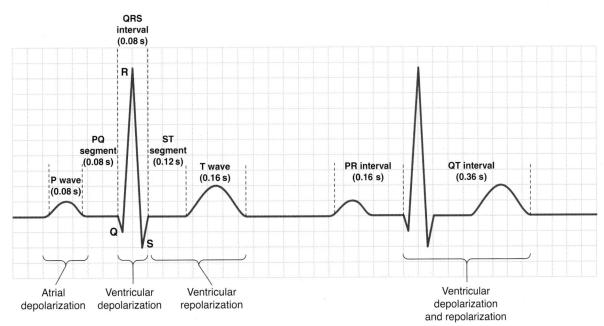

Figure 5-6. On an electrocardiogram, the height of a wave indirectly represents the amount of cardiac muscle contracting, whereas horizontal distance represents time. Various portions of the electrocardiogram are labeled with letters representing atrial contraction (P wave), ventricular contraction (QRS complex), and ventricular relaxation (T wave).

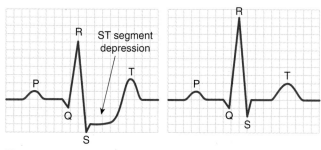

Figure 5-7. ST segment depression indicates an ischemic response of the heart (*left*). In a normal electrocardiogram, the ST segment is in line with the baseline of the electrocardiogram (*right*).

representing these waveforms. So, the ST segment represents the period of time after ventricular contraction until the start of ventricular relaxation. Likewise, the PR interval represents the period of time beginning with atrial contraction and ending with the start of ventricular contraction.

An ECG can be used to determine heart rate. However, it is also used to evaluate whether the heart is functioning normally or whether some abnormality exists. For example, during an exercise stress test, ST segment depression indicates myocardial ischemia (decreased blood flow, resulting in insufficient oxygen delivery to the myocardium) (Fig. 5-7). The most common cause of myocardial ischemia is a buildup of fatty plaque (termed atherosclerosis) on the inside of the coronary blood vessels, which reduces blood flow through the coronary vessels. If ST segment depression is apparent during a stress test, further diagnostic testing may be warranted. Other cardiac abnormalities can also be diagnosed using an ECG. For example, an increase or decrease in the PR segment indicates abnormal functioning of the AV node. So, there are many other factors besides heart rate that can be evaluated using an ECG.

Quick Review

- Intercalated discs allow the impulse to contract to spread from one cardiac muscle fiber to adjacent cardiac muscle fibers.
- The left ventricle has the greatest wall thickness of the cardiac chambers because it must pump blood into the peripheral circulation against the highest blood pressure.
- Both endurance training and strength training cause the left ventricular wall thickness to increase, resulting in an increase in left ventricular mass.
- An electrocardiogram is a recording of the movement of ions during a cardiac cycle, and can be used to determine whether the heart is functioning normally or if there is an abnormality within the cardiac cycle.

Cardiac Output

The function of the heart is to pump blood to both the pulmonary and peripheral circulatory branches of the cardiovascular system. The amount of blood pumped per minute by the heart is termed **cardiac output,** and is normally expressed in L·min⁻¹ or mL·min⁻¹. Cardiac output is determined by both the heart rate and the **stroke volume,** which is the amount of blood pumped per contraction of the ventricles, normally expressed in milliliters. Thus, cardiac output can be determined by the following equation:

$$\dot{Q} = HR \ (bpm) \times SV \ (mL) \tag{1}$$

Here $\dot{Q}$ is cardiac output in mL·min⁻¹ (1,000 mL = 1 L, so to obtain $\dot{Q}$ in L·min⁻¹, multiple by 1,000), HR is beats per minute (beats·min⁻¹), and SV is stroke volume in milliliters.

Typical values for heart rate and stroke volume at rest for a normal-sized untrained male (70 kg) and female (50 kg) are approximately 72 beats·min⁻¹ and 70 mL, and 75 beats·min⁻¹ and 60 mL, respectively. So, at rest an untrained male and an untrained female have a cardiac output of approximately 5 L·min⁻¹ and 4.5 L·min⁻¹, respectively. Trained males and females have approximately the same cardiac output at rest as their untrained counterparts. However, heart rate at rest is lower in trained (especially endurance-trained) individuals, and so to maintain the same cardiac output, trained individuals have a higher stroke volume at rest. The equation cited above dictates that an increase in stroke volume is the only manner in which cardiac output can be maintained at the same value with a decrease in heart rate. The above equation also makes it apparent that at rest, as well as during physical activity, changes in both heart rate and stroke volume can affect cardiac output. During physical activity, increases in stroke volume and heart rate can result in highly endurance-trained individuals having maximal cardiac outputs of approximately 35 L·min⁻¹. However, there may be some differences between how an endurance athlete increases cardiac output compared to an untrained person (Box 5-2), and between stroke volume when swimming compared to running (Box 5-3). Stroke volume, like heart rate, is controlled by several mechanisms. By controlling both heart rate and stroke volume, cardiac output can be adjusted to increase or decrease blood flow to oxygen-dependent tissues. This is the subject of the next section.

Regulation of Cardiac Output

If stroke volume remains unchanged, increases and decreases in heart rate would increase and decrease cardiac output, respectively. So, controlling heart rate is one mechanism by which cardiac output can be varied at rest as well as during physical activity. Likewise, increases and decreases in stroke volume, if heart rate remains the same, result in increases and decreases in cardiac output, respectively.

Stroke volume is affected by several major mechanisms. One mechanism involves how much blood is in the ventricles prior to contraction and how much blood is left in the

Box 5-2 APPLYING RESEARCH

Stroke Volume Plateau: Endurance Training Makes a Difference

Stroke volume gradually increases along with exercise intensity, up to approximately 40% to 50% of peak oxygen consumption in all individuals. However, at intensities higher than this point, stroke volume may only increase in endurance-trained athletes. Many studies reporting a plateau in stroke volume measured stroke volume during cycle ergometry. Compared with running exercise, more blood collects in the legs during cycle ergometry. This would limit venous return to the heart, resulting in a plateau in end-diastolic volume (EDV) and so stroke volume. Another explanation is that as workload increases, so does heart rate, and eventually there is not sufficient time during diastole to maintain EDV. These explanations, however, do not account for why highly trained cyclists do not show a plateau in stroke volume as workload

increases during cycle ergometry (Gledhill, Cox, and Jamnik 1994). Thus, the lack of a stroke volume plateau as workload increases in endurance athletes may be due to other training adaptations, such as increased plasma volume and increased contractility of the myocardium. The ability to continue to increase stroke volume as workload increases gives endurance athletes a substantial advantage in increasing cardiac output, and so oxygen delivery to the working muscles, compared to untrained individuals.

Further Reading

Gledhill N, Cox D, Jamnik R. Endurance athletes' stroke volume does not plateau: major advantage is diastolic function. Med Sci Sports Exerc. 1994;26:1116–1121.

Box 5-3 DID YOU KNOW?

Body Position and Stroke Volume

Body position has a substantial effect on stroke volume. This is in large part due to the effect of gravity and the pooling of blood in the legs when in an upright position. Accordingly, maintaining an upright position decreases venous return to the heart, which decreases end-diastolic volume and stroke volume (SV = EDV − ESV). In an upright position, such as that in running or cycling, stroke volume of endurance-trained athletes at rest is approximately 80 to 110 mL, and can increase to approximately 160 to 220 mL during maximal exercise. For untrained individuals, stroke volume can also more than double from resting values of 50 to 60 mL to maximal exercise values of 160 to 200 mL in an upright position. When one is in a supine position, however, such as in swimming, stroke volume only increases approximately 20% to 40% from resting to maximal exercise values. This is in large part because at rest, when in a supine position, EDV is elevated because of the increased venous return. Because of the increased EDV, stroke volume at rest is also elevated. EDV does have a maximal value no matter what body position you are in. So EDV and stroke volume are already quite high at rest when in the supine position, and when they increase to their maximal values the increases are smaller compared with an upright position, in which resting EDV and stroke volume are lower. Thus, differences in resting EDV and stroke volume account for differences in the increase from rest to maximal stroke volume between running and cycling compared to swimming.

ventricles after contraction (Fig. 5-8). **End-diastolic volume (EDV)** is the amount of blood in the ventricles at the end of the diastolic, or relaxation, phase of the ventricles. **End-systolic volume (ESV)** is the amount of blood left in the ventricles at the end of the systolic phase, or after contraction of the ventricles. The following equation demonstrates the relationship between stroke volume (SV), ESV, and EDV:

$$SV \text{ (mL)} = EDV \text{ (mL)} - ESV \text{ (mL)} \qquad (2)$$

Using typical values for an untrained individual at rest results in the following equation:

$$SV \text{ 70 mL} = EDV \text{ 110 mL} - ESV \text{ 40 mL} \qquad (3)$$

The above equation demonstrates that if EDV increases and ESV remains constant or decreases, SV will increase. At the onset of exercise, venous blood return to the heart increases (see "Muscle Pump and Respiratory Pump"). Increased venous return will increase EDV and stretch the ventricle slightly or increase the preload on the ventricle. Slightly stretching the ventricle results in increased contractile force, allowing the ventricle to achieve a lower ESV. This increase in contractile force in response to an increase in EDV is termed the Frank–Starling mechanism, which can be explained, in part, by the length–tension relationship[2] of ventricular muscle. This relationship reveals that at greater-than-resting length, muscle fibers contract with greater force resulting in a lower ESV. Both the increase in EDV and decrease in ESV result in an increase in SV. In addition, at increased muscle fiber lengths, the myocardium becomes more sensitive to changes in the concentration of Ca^{++},[28] and at increased fiber lengths, more Ca^{++} is released from the sarcoplasmic reticulum.[3] Both of these factors result in greater contractile force. Another factor increasing ventricular contractile force is increased

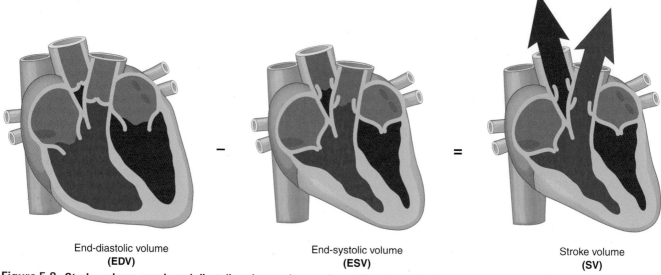

End-diastolic volume
(EDV)

End-systolic volume
(ESV)

Stroke volume
(SV)

Figure 5-8. Stroke volume equals end-diastolic volume minus end-systolic volume. Stroke volume can be increased by either increasing end-diastolic volume or decreasing end-systolic volume.

sympathetic stimulation of the myocardium,[37] which not only increases heart rate but also the force produced by the contracting myocardium (note in Fig. 5-5 that sympathetic cardiac nerves directly innervate the myocardium). All these factors increase ventricular contractile force, resulting in a lower ESV, thus increasing SV. So, several factors contribute to the increase in cardiac output that occurs during physical activity.

Blood pressure in the artery into which the ventricle is ejecting blood also affects the amount of blood pumped, as it reflects resistance to blood flow. For the left ventricle, if mean blood pressure in the aorta increases and contraction force of the ventricle does not change, SV will decrease. This is because the contraction force of the ventricle must exceed the mean blood pressure in the artery into which blood is being ejected. Thus, if mean blood pressure, or what is termed the afterload, increases, SV will decrease unless ventricular contractile force increases. It is important to note that during exercise the effect of afterload on the left ventricle is minimized in part because of arterial dilation, decreasing arterial blood pressure, and increasing venous return and EDV. As described above, a greater EDV increases ventricular contractile force because of Frank–Starling's law. The mechanisms increasing stroke volume during physical activity must take place if left ventricular contraction is to be powerful enough to overcome the higher blood pressure that occurs during physical activity.

Ejection fraction is a ratio of the amount of blood available to be pumped by a ventricle (EDV) to the amount of blood that is actually pumped (SV). The following equation represents ejection fraction and the calculation of a normal ejection fraction at rest:

$$\text{Ejection fraction (EF)} = \text{EDV/SV} \qquad (4)$$

where EF at rest = 100 mL/60 mL, so EF at rest = 0.60 or 60%.

An increase in EF (greater than 60%) would represent an increase in ventricular function, whereas a decrease in EF (less than 60%) would represent a decrease in ventricular function. One mechanism by which EF could decrease with all other factors of cardiac function remaining the same (i.e., no increase in cardiac contractility), is an increase in blood pressure within the vessel into which the ventricle ejects blood (i.e., greater afterload). This is one of the reasons an increase in resting blood pressure is typically deleterious to ventricular function. With an increase in blood pressure, the EF will decrease unless the ventricle develops more force, requiring more work and oxygen. If blood pressure increases too much, either at rest or during physical activity, the blood supply of the heart will not be able to supply sufficient oxygen for use in metabolism and an ischemic response will result. In a healthy heart and circulatory system (i.e., in which there is no significant buildup of plaque that narrows and hardens the coronary or peripheral vessels), such a mismatch of oxygen supply and demand does not occur. In addition, a decrease in resting blood pressure, one of the training outcomes of endurance or cardiovascular training, is important because it decreases the work the ventricles must perform to overcome afterload. Finally, training may also increase the volume of the ventricles.

Ventricular Volume and Training

With endurance training, ventricular EDV has been shown to increase both at rest and during physical activity.[18,30,31] This increase in EDV, and thus stroke volume, is responsible for the lower resting heart rates commonly observed among endurance-trained athletes. The increased EDV detected among the trained is also partly responsible for an increase in SV during submaximal and maximal work after endurance training (Fig. 5-9). Both resting left ventricular EDV and ESV have shown significant correlations to endurance performance (100 km ultramarathon) and peak oxygen consumption,[39,48] indicating that left ventricular volumes do affect endurance performance. The increase in EDV is in part caused by an increase in plasma volume,[19] which results in slightly greater filling of the ventricle prior to contraction, which increases the force of contraction by means of the Frank–Starling mechanism. After endurance training, SV at rest and during activity is also increased because of an increase in ventricular contractility, resulting in a lower ESV.[37] Thus, several factors result in an increase in SV at rest and during physical activity after endurance training.

In moderately trained or untrained individuals, SV increases along with exercise intensity up to approximately 40% to 50% of peak oxygen consumption. After this level of exercise intensity is achieved, SV does not increase further. However, heart rate has a good linear relationship to cardiac output and peak oxygen consumption up to maximal workloads. This nice linear relationship to $\dot{Q}$ and peak oxygen consumption, and the relative ease with which it can be accurately measured, is why heart rate is a good measure of intensity during endurance or cardiovascular training. Although SV of the right ventricle is not measured frequently, it is understood that if left ventricle SV increases, right ventricle SV must also increase to maintain equal cardiac output of the ventricles. Following a weight training program, resting left ventricular EDV changes very little, if at all.[14] Because of the relationship between heart rate, SV, and $\dot{Q}$, a lack of a change in EDV in part explains why resting heart rate typically changes very little with traditional strength (few repetitions with a heavy weight per set) training. Both endurance training and weight training can increase left ventricular wall thickness. However, with endurance training an increase in both EDV and wall thickness contribute to an increase in left ventricular mass. With strength training, however, the increase in left ventricular mass is due primarily to an increase in left ventricular wall thickness (Fig. 5-10). The

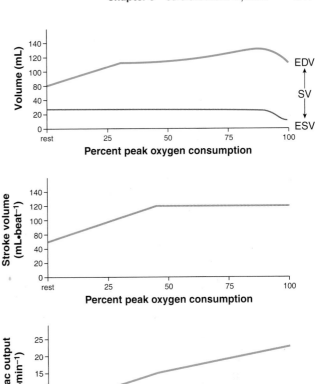

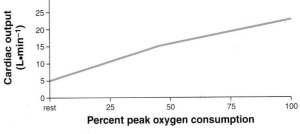

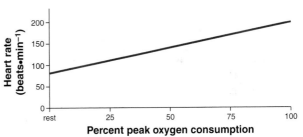

Figure 5-9. Increased end-diastolic volume and decreased end-systolic volume contribute to increased stroke volume and cardiac output during physical activity. In untrained or moderately trained individuals, after approximately 40% to 50% of peak oxygen consumption, stroke volume plateaus. Thus, after this work level, the only way to increase cardiac output is to increase heart rate.

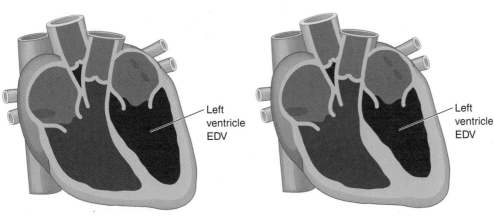

Endurance training   Weight training

Figure 5-10. Left ventricular mass increases with both endurance training and weight training. With endurance training, this increase is due in part to an increase in both end-diastolic volume and left ventricular wall thickness. With weight training, this increase is due predominantly to an increase in left ventricular wall thickness.

increase in left ventricular mass detected among resistance-trained athletes contributes to an improved ability to maintain SV and Q̇ during weight training activity[9] because it allows development of greater left ventricular forces to eject blood against the higher peripheral blood pressures encountered during weight training. Thus, both types of training can result in adaptations of the left ventricle.

Systolic and Diastolic Functions

EF is only one measure of systolic function. Average rate of blood flow out of a cardiac chamber, peak rate of flow out of a cardiac chamber, and muscle fiber shortening velocity are other measures of systolic function, all of which indicate greater or faster flow of blood out of the contracting ventricle. Measures of diastolic function are basically these same measures, except that they relate to the rate at which a chamber fills with blood during the relaxation phase of the cardiac cycle. Participation in a weight training program results in little or no change in resting left ventricular systolic or diastolic function,[14] whereas performance of endurance training, although not consistently shown, increases in systolic function can occur and increases in diastolic function are a consistent result of training.[30] Next we will look at a very important component of the cardiovascular system, the blood.

Blood

Blood is a major component of the cardiovascular system and is important for the performance of all the functions of the cardiovascular system. Covered in this section are blood pressure and the composition of blood, both of which are important for the movement of blood through the cardiovascular system, which in turn affects the overall function of the cardiovascular system.

Quick Review

- Cardiac output is the product of heart rate times stroke volume.
- Cardiac output can be increased or decreased by increasing or decreasing either heart rate or stroke volume.
- Stroke volume is the difference between end-diastolic volume and end-systolic volume.
- Aerobic training causes an increase in end-diastolic volume, resulting in an increase in stroke volume, whereas resistance training does not affect end-diastolic volume significantly.
- Aerobic training increases ventricular diastolic function, but changes in ventricular systolic function because of training are inconsistent.
- Weight training causes little or no change in either ventricular systolic or diastolic function.

Blood Pressure

Blood pressure within a specific blood vessel is vital to the functioning of the cardiovascular system because blood flows from an area of high pressure to an area of lower pressure. This principle is what determines the circulatory nature of blood flow as blood travels from the aorta (which is closest to the left ventricle and where pressure is greatest) through the arteries, then the capillaries, and finally through the veins, because blood pressure declines at each progressive step of this journey. The impact of blood pressure is also apparent in that it is the pressure within the blood vessels into which the left and right ventricles eject blood, which in part determines stroke volume and ejection fraction. A fundamental understanding of the effect of blood pressure on functioning of the cardiovascular system depends on knowledge of the laws governing the movement of any fluid, including blood.

Laws Governing Blood Flow

Like the flow of all fluids, blood flow in the circulatory system is governed by physical concepts. First, if allowed, blood will flow from an area of high pressure to an area of lower pressure. Not only will blood flow toward an area of lower pressure, but the rate of flow is proportional to the pressure difference between two ends of a blood vessel or between any two chambers within the cardiovascular system. Thus, one way to increase flow within the circulatory system is to increase the pressure difference between two areas, such as by increasing the force with which the ventricles contract.

Another way to increase flow is to decrease the resistance to flow. However, differences in pressure are directly proportional to an increase in flow, whereas resistance is inversely proportional to changes in flow. Thus, the following equation can be used to describe the effect of pressure and resistance on blood flow:

$$\text{Blood flow} = \text{Change in pressure}/\text{Resistance to flow} \qquad (5)$$

This equation demonstrates that flow can be increased by magnifying the difference in pressure between two areas or by decreasing the resistance to flow. However, a twofold increase in the pressure difference would increase flow twofold, whereas a twofold increase in resistance would decrease blood flow by one-half. So, it is possible to control changes in blood flow by simultaneously controlling changes in pressure and resistance to flow. Indeed, this is what occurs during exercise.

How can resistance to flow be changed? The longer the blood vessel, the greater the resistance to flow. However, the length of the vessel does not change except during normal growth. So, changing the length of the vessel is not really a mechanism by which resistance to flow can be changed. Second, the greater the viscosity of the blood, the greater the resistance to flow. Under normal conditions, blood viscosity may change slightly at rest or during physical activity. For example, dehydration would increase blood viscosity. However, controlling blood viscosity is not a mechanism by which the human body attempts to control blood flow. Another mechanism by which flow can be altered involves changing the radius of a blood vessel to affect resistance to flow.

It is possible to tremendously affect blood flow with relatively small changes in the radius of blood vessels, because reducing the radius of vessel by one-half increases the resistance to flow 16-fold. Controlling the radius of blood vessels is the major way in which blood flow to different areas of the body is controlled both during exercise and at rest. In addition, small changes in a vessel's radius because of the buildup of plaque on its interior walls also increases resistance to blood flow and so blood pressure must increase if flow is to be maintained. Changes in blood pressure during a cardiac cycle and differences in pressure in various portions of the circulatory system are discussed next.

Systolic and Diastolic Blood Pressures

Systolic and diastolic blood pressures refer to the highest pressure occurring during systole and the lowest pressure occurring during diastole, respectively. Typically, arterial blood pressure is measured within the brachial artery using a sphygmomanometer (blood pressure cuff) and stethoscope. Thus, the typical resting arterial blood pressure values of 120 and 80 mm Hg refer to blood pressure within the brachial artery. However, blood pressures within specific areas of the peripheral cardiovascular system are quite different from blood pressure within the brachial artery (Fig. 5-11). The highest pressures occur within the left ventri-

cle and then, because of the continuous decrease in vessel radius which increases resistance to flow, blood pressure decreases as blood passes through the large arteries, arterioles, and capillaries. The greatest pressure decrease occurs within the capillaries because the radius of these vessels is very small (approximately the radius of a red blood cell). Note that the pressures within the venous system are quite low compared with those in the arterial system largely because of the loss of pressure as the blood passes through the capillaries.

Pressure can also be affected by factors other than the radius of the vessel. If cardiac output is increased, pressure in the arterial system will increase because more blood will be ejected into the arteries (an increase in the amount of fluid in a container of fixed size increases pressure). Thus, blood pressure increases during physical activity because cardiac output is elevated. The increase in pressure as a result of a greater cardiac output is partially offset by the elasticity or capacitance—also termed compliance (change in volume per change in pressure)—of healthy peripheral arteries, allowing them to expand when more blood is ejected into them by the left ventricle. The ability of the major arteries to expand as more blood is ejected into them results in a smaller pressure increase with elevations of cardiac output.

Capacitance of arteries appears to increase with aerobic training,[16] whereas the effect of resistance training on capacitance is unclear, with decreases, increases, and no change shown after a period of resistance training.[4,16,22,34] An increase in capacitance with training would help counteract cardiovascular disease (arteriosclerosis or hardening of the arteries). Thus, any decrease in capacitance as a result of resistance training could have long-term negative consequences on cardiovascular health. Research indicates, however, that the performance of a training program featuring both resistance and endurance exercises (cross-training) results in an increase in compliance,[16] indicating that aerobic training may counteract any negative effect on compliance that may arise from resistance training alone. So resistance trainers interested in total fitness should also perform aerobic training.

Another important cardiovascular measure frequently determined is mean arterial pressure, which is viewed as the average pressure driving blood into the tissues throughout the cardiac cycle. Mean arterial pressure is defined as diastolic pressure plus 1/3 the difference between systolic and diastolic pressures. The following equation demonstrates the calculation of a typical mean arterial pressure at rest:

Mean arterial pressure (MAP) = Diastolic pressure + (0.33 × (Systolic pressure − Diastolic pressure))

MAP = 80 mm Hg + (0.33 × (120 − 80 mm Hg))

MAP = 93.2 mm Hg   (7)

Looking at this, you might wonder why mean arterial pressure is simply not the average of systolic and diastolic

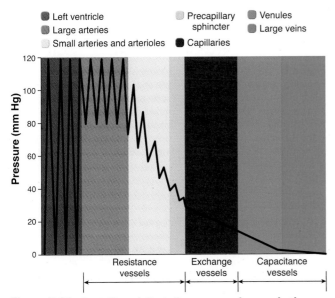

Figure 5-11. Systolic and diastolic pressure changes in the peripheral circulation. Pressure continually drops from the large arteries to large veins, resulting in blood flow through the peripheral circulation.

blood pressures, which would result in a pressure of 100 mm Hg. During the cardiac cycle, more time is spent at pressures closer to diastolic pressure than to systolic pressure, resulting in a mean arterial pressure less than the simple average of systolic and diastolic pressures.

Meta-analyses demonstrate that aerobic[8,21,27] and weight training[5,25,26] can significantly reduce resting systolic and diastolic blood pressures in individuals with normal blood pressure, that is, who are **normotensive**, and in individuals with **hypertension**, or increased resting blood pressure (see Chapter 12). Although these changes in resting blood pressure are significant, they are relatively small for both aerobic training (3–7 mm Hg) and weight training (3–4 mm Hg). Both types of training have been recommended

as effective in reducing resting blood pressure in both normotensive and hypertensive individuals.

During both aerobic and resistance training[32] exercises (Box 5-4) and with either arm or leg exercise (Box 5-5), peripheral blood pressure increases substantially. However, with long-term aerobic training, blood pressures at submaximal workloads are reduced,[1] and because after training the maximal workload attainable is increased, maximal systolic blood pressure may increase. With long-term resistance training, submaximal blood pressures during physical activity, such as treadmill walking and bicycle ergometry, and during weight training exercise [10,14] are also decreased. Generally, it appears that both aerobic training and resistance training can reduce

---

Box 5-4   PRACTICAL QUESTION FROM STUDENTS

How High Can Blood Pressure Get During Activity, and Do High Blood Pressures During Activity Present Any Danger?

During aerobic exercise, as the workload is increased, systolic blood pressures in normotensive individuals can reach values as high as 250 mm Hg[1] while diastolic pressure increases only slightly (Fig. A). During weight training, systolic and diastolic blood pressures in sets to failure of 320/250 mm Hg during leg press exercise[2] (Fig. B) and 198/160 mm Hg during knee extension exercise[3] have been shown. During weight training, blood pressure during repeated sets to failure progressively increases during each set performed. These increased blood pressures are in part responsible for the increase in left ventricular wall thickness brought about by long-term training, which could be viewed as a positive adaptation to training. High blood pressures during activity could precipitate a heart attack, but the reduction in blood pressure at rest and during submaximal activity, and other positive adaptations, like decreased low-density lipoprotein in the blood, result in an overall reduction in the risk of a heart attack (see Chapter 12).

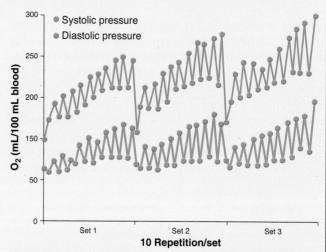

Figure B. During weight training, exercise blood pressure increases as a set is carried to failure and in successive sets. The blood pressure response during successive sets to failure in a leg press is shown. (Adapted from Gotshall RW, Gootman J, Byrnes WC, et al. Noninvasive characterization of the blood pressure response to the double-leg press exercise. J Exerc Physiol. online 2, www.css.edu/users/tboone2, 1999.)

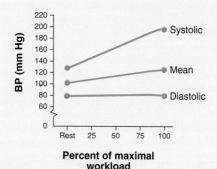

Figure A. During aerobic activity, systolic and mean arterial pressure increase. Diastolic blood pressure during aerobic activity normally increases very little.

References

1. ACSM's Guidelines for Exercise Testing and Prescription. Philadelphia, PA: Lippincott Williams & Wilkins, 2006.
2. MacDougall JD, Tuxen D, Sale DG, et al. Arterial blood pressure response to heavy resistance exercise. J Appl Physiol. 1985;58:785–790.
3. Fleck SJ, Dean LS. Resistance-training experience and the pressor response during resistance exercise. J Appl Physiol. 1987;63:116–120.

Box 5-5 PRACTICAL QUESTION FROM STUDENTS

My Grandfather Had a Heart Attack, and Initially the Doctors Wanted Him to Limit the Amount of Work He Did With His Arms. Why?

This relates to the blood pressure response to upper versus lower body exercise. You might hypothesize that blood pressure during dynamic leg exercise would be higher than during dynamic arm exercise because more muscle mass is active in leg than arm exercise. However, just the opposite is true. At the same percentage of peak oxygen consumption, blood pressure is higher during dynamic arm exercise compared with dynamic leg exercise (see the table to the right). The difference is related to the amount of muscle mass that is active during each of these activities. Because of the smaller muscle mass being active and, so, a smaller vascular bed undergoing vasodilation during arm exercise, there is greater resistance to blood flow, which results in a higher blood pressure. This is in part due to the increase in cardiac output during exercise being directed into a smaller vascular bed, which results in an increase in blood pressure. One practical application of this relates to cardiac rehabilitation programs. If upper body exercise is used to train coronary heart disease patients, the exercise prescription must be based on their blood pressure response to upper body exercise, and not on their response to lower body exercise, such as running or cycling. Basing their upper body exercise prescription on their response to lower body exercise could result in a blood pressure response that places them at risk for a cardiovascular event, such as a heart attack.

Systolic and Diastolic Blood Pressure in Dynamic Arm and Leg Exercise

% Peak Oxygen Consumption	Systolic Pressure (mm Hg)		Diastolic Pressure (mm Hg)	
	Arms	Legs	Arms	Legs
25	150	132	90	70
40	165	138	93	71
50	175	144	96	73
75	205	160	103	75

peripheral resting blood pressures and blood pressures during submaximal physical activity. Because of the positive effects of physical activity on blood pressure, guidelines for exercise prescription for those with hypertension have been established (Box 5-6). Next we will examine blood in more detail.

Composition of Blood

Blood can be divided into two major components (Fig. 5-12): plasma and formed components. **Plasma** is the "watery" or fluid component of blood and normally constitutes about 55% to 60% of the total blood volume. The total amount of plasma can decrease approximately 10% during intense physical activity, especially physical activity performed in hot and/or humid environments. However, plasma volume at rest can increase approximately 10% as an adaptation to aerobic training and/or because of acclimatization to hot, humid environments. Plasma is composed of approximately 90% water, 7% plasma proteins, and 3% nutrients, electrolytes, hormones, enzymes, antibodies, and other substances.

The formed elements normally make up about 40% to 45% of blood. Red blood cells (erythrocytes) comprise approximately 99% and white blood cells and platelets comprise 1% of the formed elements. Platelets are important for blood clotting, which prevents excessive blood loss after a wound. Platelets are also a factor in the formation of blood clots that result in a heart attack or

Quick Review

- Differences in blood pressure cause the movement of blood within the circulatory system.
- Differences in blood pressure are directly proportional to an increase in flow, whereas resistance is inversely proportional to changes in blood flow.
- Blood pressure is highest during systole and lowest during diastole of the ventricles.
- Capacitance of the major arteries helps to keep systolic pressure low.
- During both aerobic and weight training exercises, blood pressures increase substantially.
- Chronic performance of aerobic training decreases blood pressure at rest and when performing submaximal workloads.
- Chronic performance of weight training reduces resting blood pressure and decreases blood pressure during walking, riding a bicycle, and weight training activity.

Box 5-6   AN EXPERT VIEW
Exercise and Hypertension

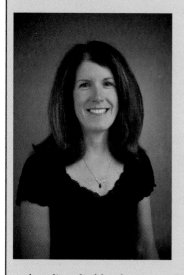

Linda S. Pescatello, PhD, FACSM

Professor
Human Performance Laboratory
Department of Kinesiology
Neag School of Education
University of Connecticut
Storrs, CT

Hypertension is a major public health problem. There are 65 million (31.3%) American adults who have hypertension. This condition may be defined as the following: having a systolic blood pressure (SBP) ≥140 and/or diastolic blood pressure (DBP) ≥90 mm Hg; requiring antihypertensive medication; and/or being told by a physician or other health professional on at least two occasions that an individual has high blood pressure (NHLBI 2004). Nearly 30% of American adults have "prehypertension" (SBP ≥ 120 to <140 and/or DBP ≥80 to <90 mm Hg) so more than 60% of adults in the United States have above optimal blood pressure, and nearly all will acquire hypertension if they live into old age. Aerobic exercise decreases blood pressure by 5 to 7 mm Hg (Pescatello 2004). For this reason, and because of its favorable effects on other cardiovascular disease risk factors, habitual physical activity is recommended as nonpharmacologic therapy to prevent, treat, and control hypertension (NHLBI 2004).

In order to effectively prescribe exercise for those with hypertension, the exercise dose, or *Frequency*, *Intensity*, *Time*, and *Type* (*FITT*), should be applied. The exercise prescription *FITT* recommendations for those with hypertension are as follows:

Frequency: on most, preferably all, days of the week

Aerobic exercise training performed between 3 and 7 days·wk^{-1} lowers blood pressure. A single bout of exercise results in immediate blood pressure reductions that persist for the remainder of the day, a physiologic response termed postexercise hypotension. Postexercise hypotension contributes to the blood pressure reductions resulting from more long-term aerobic exercise training. Many people with hypertension are overweight or obese. The guidelines for weight loss and successful weight loss maintenance recommend large amounts of energy expenditure (a minimum of 1,000 to over 2,000 kcal·wk^{-1}, to total from at least 2.5 hours to preferably more than 5 hours per week of aerobic, moderate-intensity activity) that can only be achieved with daily or near-daily exercise (Jakicic 2001). For these reasons, people with hypertension should engage in physical activity on most, preferably all, days of the week.

Intensity: moderate-intensity physical activity

Moderate-intensity (40% to <60% of $\dot{V}_{O_2}$ reserve [$\dot{V}_{O_2}R$]) aerobic exercise is as effective as vigorous intensity (≥60% $\dot{V}_{O_2}R$) aerobic exercise in lowering blood pressure. Thus, the recommended exercise intensity is moderate (40% to <60% $\dot{V}_{O_2}R$), corresponding to 64% to 84% of the age-predicted maximum heart rate or approximately 11 to 14 on the Borg Rating of Perceived Exertion (RPE) 6 to 20 scale.

Time: ≥30 minutes continuous or intermittent exercise per day

Aerobic exercise prescribed either as long continuous bouts (30 to 60 minutes per session), or shorter (10 to 15 minutes per session) bouts accumulated throughout the day, lower blood pressure. Thus, the recommendation is for 30 to 60 minutes of continuous or intermittent aerobic exercise per day (minimum of 10-minute intermittent bouts accumulated throughout the day to total 30 to 60 minutes of exercise). If overweight or obese, one should progress to a caloric energy expenditure of a minimum of 1,000 to over 2,000 kcal·wk^{-1} or from at least 2.5 hours to preferably more than 5 hours per week of moderate-intensity, aerobic exercise.

Type: primarily aerobic activity supplemented by resistance exercise

Aerobic exercise such as walking, jogging, running, or cycling lowers blood pressure. Resistance training reduces blood pressure, but the magnitude of the reduction is less than that for aerobic exercise. Thus, the recommendation is for the exercise type to be primarily aerobic, supplemented by resistance training and flexibility exercises.

More information and precautions concerning exercise prescription for hypertense individuals can be found in these references:

Jakicic JM, Clark K, Coleman E, et al. American College of Sports Medicine position stand. Appropriate intervention strategies for weight loss and prevention of weight regain for adults. Med Sci Sports Exerc. 2001;33:2145–2156.

National Heart Lung and Blood Institute. Seventh Report of the Joint National Committee on Prevention, Detection, Evaluation and Treatment of High Blood Pressure-JNC VII Bethesda, MD: U.S. Department of Health and Human Services, 2004:04–52302003.

Nelson ME, Rejeski WJ, Blair SN, et al. Physical activity and public health in older adults: recommendation from the American College of Sports Medicine and the American Heart Association. Circulation. 2007;1094–1105.

Pescatello LS, Franklin BA, Fagard R, et al. American College of Sports Medicine position stand. Exercise and hypertension. Med Sci Sports Exerc. 2004;25:533–553.

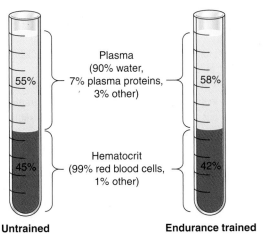

Figure 5-12. Hematocrit is the ratio of solids to liquid within the blood. With aerobic training, although both plasma and red blood cell number increase, hematocrit decreases slightly because of a greater increase in plasma than in red blood cell volume.

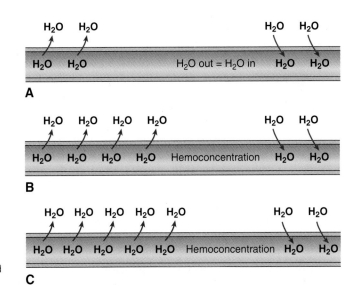

Figure 5-13. Hemoconcentration during exercise is caused by several factors. (A) At rest, water leaving the vascular compartment is equal to water entering the vascular compartment from the interstitial compartment, so there is no hemoconcentration. **(B)** At the start of exercise, because of an increase in blood pressure and buildup of metabolic wastes in the interstitial compartment, hemoconcentration occurs. **(C)** During long-term exercise, sweating also increases hemoconcentration.

stroke and in the formation of plaque on the interior of blood vessels (see Chapter 12). The percentage of the total blood volume composed of formed elements is referred to as **hematocrit**.

As an adaptation to aerobic training, the amount of red blood cells increases, which would increase the hematocrit. However, concomitantly, there is a greater increase in plasma volume, which results in a slight decrease in hematocrit (Fig. 5-12). Because of training-induced increases in both erythrocytes and plasma, the blood volume of endurance athletes is higher than the normal 5 to 6 L in men and 4 to 5 L in women. The increase in blood volume is important because it is one of the factors resulting in an increase in the total amount of oxygen that can be delivered to metabolically active tissue after aerobic training.

Red Blood Cells

The most familiar role of red blood cells (RBCs) is the transporting of oxygen. RBCs are capable of transporting oxygen because they contain **hemoglobin**, a substance composed of protein (globin) and an iron-containing pigment (heme) which is necessary for the binding of oxygen. Each gram of hemoglobin can combine with 1.33 mL of oxygen, so the greater the hemoglobin content within blood, the greater the oxygen-carrying ability.

In adults, RBCs are produced in the bone marrow of the long bones of the body. As one of the last steps in the production of RBCs, prior to being released into the blood, the nucleus is removed. Thus, RBCs cannot reproduce, like other tissues of the body, or repair themselves, resulting in a relatively short normal lifespan of approximately 4 months. Normally, the destruction and production of RBCs are balanced, resulting in no change in hematocrit or in the blood's oxygen-carrying ability.

Plasma Volume

With the onset of an aerobic or a weight training session, the acute effect on plasma volume is a substantial reduction. This can be mainly attributed to increased blood pressure which forces plasma, but not the cellular components of blood, out of the intravascular compartment. Reduction in plasma volume results in **hemoconcentration**, or a reduction in the fluid portion of blood relative to the formed element portion of blood. This results in a relative increase in hematocrit without a change in the actual amount of RBCs. The net effect of this is an increase in the number of RBCs and hemoglobin content per unit volume of blood (Fig. 5-13). This change increases the blood's oxygen-carrying capacity, which can be advantageous during exercise, especially aerobic exercise, at rest, and during submaximal exercise at altitude. Although hemoconcentration does increase blood's viscosity, it is unlikely that the increase in viscosity during normal exercise bouts would change resistance to blood flow to the point that blood flow is critically impaired.

During prolonged aerobic exercise, plasma volume can be decreased 10% to 20% or more.[45] The acute effect on plasma volume of weight training is a reduction in plasma volume of 0% to 22%.[6] The relatively wide range in acute changes in plasma volume is probably related to differences in exercise intensity and volume for both aerobic and weight training exercise bouts. In addition, if the exercise bout is of sufficient duration, sweat loss may also account for some of the plasma volume change.

The chronic effect of long-term aerobic training on plasma volume is an increase of 12% to 20%. Increases in plasma volume are noticed even 1 day after an aerobic exercise bout, with plasma volume increasing for up to several weeks at the start of an aerobic training program.[36,43,49] Initial changes in plasma because of training can result in a type of anemia but they are not detrimental to health (Box 5-7). Plasma volume increases are important because they aid in training-induced gains in ventricular EDV, stroke volume, and cardiac output, all of which serve to improve oxygen transport[17,20] and performance of aerobic activity. Increased plasma volume also aids in temperature regulation during exercise. Although fluid regulatory hormones (renin, angiotensin II) have been shown to be elevated after a single resistance training session,[29] the long-term effect of weight training on total plasma volume has not been investigated. It is unlikely, though, that a program of weight training results in any significant change in total plasma volume. Thus, although both aerobic and weight training activities result in an acute decrease in plasma volume, only aerobic training has been shown to elicit a chronic increase in the plasma volume.

Box 5-7 DID YOU KNOW?
Causes of Anemia

Low hemoglobin concentration resulting in lower-than-normal ability of blood to transport oxygen is termed **anemia**. Hemoglobin concentrations below 13 g·dL⁻¹ in males and 12 g·dL⁻¹ in females indicate anemia. Anemia can be caused by an acute loss of blood, such as when donating blood, and by a lack of sufficient vitamins and minerals in the diet. Most notably, a lack of iron or folate in the diet can cause anemia. Iron is necessary because of its role as part of the iron-containing pigment (heme) in hemoglobin molecules. Folate, also known as folic acid, is necessary for cell division and protein synthesis. One of the first functions affected by a folate deficiency is lack of replacement of red blood cells (RBCs), resulting in anemia. Folate deficiency slows DNA synthesis and the ability of cells to divide. This results in large, immature, oval-shaped RBCs that contain a nucleus. These abnormal RBCs do not carry oxygen or pass through capillaries as efficiently as normal RBCs. Good sources of folate include legumes, vegetables, and fortified grains and cereals. Another possible cause of short-term anemia is termed sports anemia. During the initial stages of an aerobic training program, plasma volume expands, resulting in a decrease in hemoglobin concentration. In addition, the increased aerobic activity shortens the lifespan of RBCs, also resulting in a decreased hemoglobin concentration. Both of these factors are, however, short-lived, and hemoglobin concentration returns to normal within several weeks.

Quick Review

- Red blood cells can reversibly bind oxygen because of the presence of hemoglobin.
- Chronic performance of aerobic training results in an increase in the number of red blood cells, but a greater increase occurs in plasma volume, resulting in a slight decrease in hematocrit.
- During the performance of both aerobic and weight training activities, hemoconcentration occurs.
- The increase in plasma volume caused by aerobic training aids to increase end-diastolic volume, and so an increase occurs in stroke volume, cardiac output, and oxygen transport.

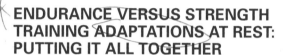

ENDURANCE VERSUS STRENGTH TRAINING ADAPTATIONS AT REST: PUTTING IT ALL TOGETHER

Adaptations to the cardiovascular system at rest are different between endurance- and strength-trained athletes (Table 5-1). Adaptations at rest due to endurance training carry over to increased cardiac output during endurance activity, which results in increased oxygen delivery to skeletal muscle and, consequently, to increased endurance performance. On the other hand, adaptations due to strength

Table 5-1. Resting Adaptations Due to Endurance and Strength Training

Adaptation	Endurance Training	Strength Training
Left ventricular mass	Increased	Increased
Left ventricular wall thickness	Increased	Increased
Left ventricular end-diastolic volume	Increased	Little change
Stroke volume	Increased	Little change
Cardiac output	Little change	Little change
Systolic blood pressure	Decreased	Decreased
Diastolic blood pressure	Decreased	Decreased
Plasma volume	Increased	Little change
Red blood cell mass	Increased	Little change
Hematocrit	Slight decrease	Little change
Blood volume	Increased	Little change
Large artery capacitance	Increased	Unclear

see page 139

see page 139

Quick Review

- Many of the cardiovascular changes at rest are interrelated.
- Some of the cardiovascular changes at rest set the stage for improved cardiovascular function during activity.

training result in increased ability to maintain cardiac output against the substantially increased blood pressures encountered during strength training.

Regardless of whether they are brought on by participating in aerobic or resistance exercise regimens, many of the training-induced cardiovascular adaptations observed under resting conditions are interrelated. For example, $\dot{Q}$ at rest is about 5 L·min^{-1} for the average male, but because of the decrease in resting blood pressure SV increases and heart rate decreases. Similarly, increased plasma volume due to endurance training increases EDV which results in an increase in SV because of the Frank–Starling mechanism, which, too, allows for a decline in heart rate (recall that training does not alter resting $\dot{Q}$). Some changes at rest also set the stage for changes during activity. For example, a decrease in resting blood pressure can result in having a decreased blood pressure during submaximal physical activity because the initial blood pressure is lower (i.e., any increase in blood pressure is added to a lower initial blood pressure). In addition, lower blood pressure during activity reduces resistance to blood flow, and, in doing so, increases cardiac output and oxygen delivery to the working muscles. Thus, the changes at rest set the stage for some of the cardiovascular changes occurring during activity (discussed at the end of this chapter).

CHANGES IN THE CARDIOVASCULAR SYSTEM DURING EXERCISE

During physical activity several changes take place to increase blood flow to active muscle. Greater blood flow to muscles increases delivery of things needed for metabolism to occur (oxygen, glucose, triglyceride) and expedites the removal of products generated during metabolism (carbon dioxide). The factors that result in increased blood flow to active muscle during activity are explored in the following sections.

Oxygen Delivery to Tissue

Oxygen delivery to tissue depends on two major factors: the amount of oxygen tissue takes out of a given amount of blood, and the amount of blood flowing through the tissue (Box 5-8). At rest both of these factors remain relatively constant for a given type of tissue, such as muscle. However, during exercise, both the amount of oxygen taken out of the blood by tissue and the amount of blood flowing through a given tissue increase substantially; as a result, the amount of oxygen delivered to tissue is amplified. The amount of oxygen delivered to tissue is explored in the following sections.

Arterial–Venous Oxygen Difference

Arterial–venous oxygen difference (a-v O$_2$ diff) is the difference between the amount of oxygen in 100 mL of arterial blood entering a tissue and the amount of oxygen in 100 mL of venous blood leaving a tissue (Fig. 5-14). During exercise, more oxygen is taken out of the blood by metabolically active muscle, which increases the a-v O$_2$ diff.[46]

Box 5-8 APPLYING RESEARCH

Fick Principle

The Fick principle and Fick equation are named after A. Fick, a cardiovascular physiologist who developed the principle in the 1870s. The Fick principle states that the amount of a substance removed from the blood passing through an organ per unit of time can be calculated by multiplying the blood flow through the organ times the arterial concentration minus the venous concentration of that substance. The Fick principle can be used to calculate oxygen consumption (see "Oxygen Delivery = Blood Flow × a-v O$_2$ diff") for the entire body or for a specific tissue or organ. In the case of oxygen consumption for the entire body, the Fick principle results in the following equation:

$$\dot{V}O_2 = \dot{Q} \times \text{a-v O}_2 \text{ diff}$$

where $\dot{Q}$ equals cardiac output and a-v O$_2$ diff equals arterial-mixed venous oxygen difference. This equation can be used to calculate oxygen consumption at rest, at submaximal workloads, and at maximal workloads. The Fick principle can also be used to calculate the uptake of any substance, such as glucose used in metabolism, by a tissue or organ. When a substance's concentration is greater in arterial than in venous blood, it indicates that tissue is removing that substance from blood (e.g., oxygen). When a substance's concentration is greater in venous blood compared with arterial blood, it indicates that the tissue is giving off that substance (e.g., carbon dioxide).

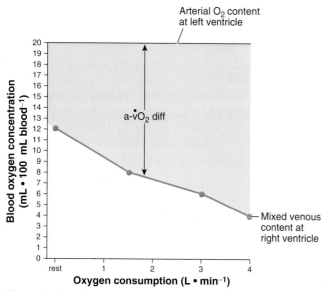

Figure 5-14. The arterial-venous oxygen difference (a-v O$_2$ diff) increases as oxygen consumption increases. Because of the mixing of venous blood from active tissue and inactive tissue, oxygen content of mixed venous blood is not zero.

In many cases, the a-v O$_2$ diff is expressed as the difference between arterial blood leaving the left ventricle and venous blood entering the right atrium and is termed arterial-mixed venous oxygen difference. The a-v O$_2$ diff represents the arterial venous difference for all of the body's tissues, including both active and inactive tissues. At rest, the a-v O$_2$ diff is approximately 8 mL O$_2$ per 100 mL of blood (Fig. 5-14). During exercise, the a-v O$_2$ diff increases to approximately 15 mL O$_2$ per 100 mL of blood, or more. So, changes in the a-v O$_2$ diff indicate that increasing the a-v O$_2$ diff can approximately double oxygen delivery. Note that the a-v O$_2$ diff does not indicate that all of the oxygen was taken out of the blood, as might be the case if measured only for very metabolically active tissue, in which case the a-v O$_2$ diff would be approximately 19 mL O$_2$ per 100 mL of blood. The definition of a-v O$_2$ diff is arterial blood leaving the left ventricle and venous blood entering the right atrium. The a-v O$_2$ diff of 16 mL per 100 mL of blood is caused by the mixing of all of the body's venous blood, which results in the mixing of venous blood from active muscle tissue with venous blood from inactive tissue. The a-v O$_2$ diff represents only one aspect of oxygen delivery to tissue because oxygen delivery to tissue is also affected by blood flow.

Oxygen Delivery = Blood Flow × a-v O$_2$ diff

Oxygen delivery or oxygen consumption ($\dot{V}O_2$) is a product of blood flow multiplied by a-v O$_2$ diff. This calculation is termed the Fick equation. To determine oxygen consumption for the entire body using the Fick equation, cardiac output ($\dot{Q}$) represents blood flow. So, the Fick equation

Quick Review

- Oxygen delivery to a tissue depends on total blood flow through the tissue and the arterial-venous oxygen difference.
- During activity, an increase in arterial-venous oxygen difference and blood flow can take place, resulting in an increase in oxygen delivery to tissue.

for the entire body becomes cardiac output times arterial-mixed venous O$_2$ diff:

$$\dot{V}O_2 = \dot{Q} \times \text{a-v } O_2 \text{ diff} \qquad (8)$$

The Fick equation clearly shows that increasing either $\dot{Q}$ or a-v O$_2$ diff, or a combination of the two, can increase $\dot{V}O_2$ for the entire body. An increase in both blood flow and a-v O$_2$ diff occurs during exercise to increase oxygen consumption from resting to maximal values. Blood flow to active tissue can be increased by increasing $\dot{Q}$ and by redistribution of $\dot{Q}$ so that the majority of $\dot{Q}$ is directed toward active muscle tissue, the subject of the next several sections.

Redistribution of Blood Flow During Exercise

At rest, 15% to 20% of cardiac output goes to skeletal muscle, but during maximal exercise, skeletal muscle receives up to 80% to 85% of cardiac output.[15] As exercise intensity increases, blood flow is diverted from tissues that can temporarily tolerate a decrease in flow, such as the kidneys, visceral organs, and splanchnic tissues,[38] and is instead directed toward active skeletal muscle (Fig. 5-15).[35] This combination of increased cardiac output and its redistribution during exercise results in substantial increases in total blood flow to skeletal muscle and so substantial increases in oxygen availability.

When examining tissue blood flow during exercise, note that several unique situations occur. During light and moderate exercise, blood flow to the skin increases to help moderate an elevation in body temperature.[23,50] However, during maximal exercise, skin blood flow decreases, resulting in a redirection of blood flow to active muscle.[41] During exercise, the heart, similar to skeletal muscle, performs more work than at rest and, therefore, requires more oxygen. Thus, myocardial blood flow increases approximately four to five times above rest during maximal exercise. However, the increase in myocardial blood flow is due to an increase in cardiac output rather than a redistribution of blood flow, because both at rest and during exercise the myocardium receives approximately 4% of cardiac output. The brain or cerebral area cannot tolerate a decrease in blood flow for more than several seconds without the result of fainting. However, greater

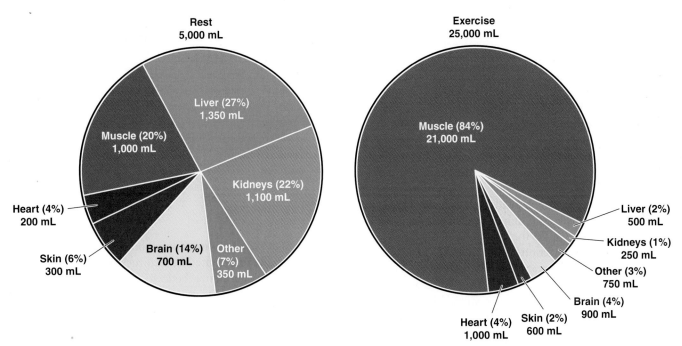

Figure 5-15. Absolute (mL) and relative (%) distribution of cardiac output at rest and during maximal exercise. During maximal exercise, the vast majority of cardiac output is redistributed to skeletal muscle. During maximal exercise, other organs, such as the kidney and liver, receive a smaller absolute and relative portion of cardiac output.

blood flow to the brain results in increased intracranial pressure. Accordingly, while blood flow increases to the brain during exercise, it does so only by about 200 mL or approximately 25%.[47]

Redistribution of blood flow during exercise is accomplished from several factors, but it would not be possible at all, if the circulatory system was not a parallel circuitry system (see Fig. 5-1). Parallel circuitry allows blood flow from the aorta to be distributed to all of the body's organs and tissues without the need to pass through another tissue or organ. Parallel circuitry will allow redistribution of blood flow only if it is possible to decrease and increase blood flow to different tissues or organs. The ability to change the flow to a particular organ or tissue is accomplished by increasing and decreasing vessel radius in specific tissues. **Vasodilation,** or an increase in radius, results in less resistance to flow, and so an increase in blood flow to the tissue. **Vasoconstriction,** or a decrease in radius, results in an increase in resistance to flow, and so a decrease in blood flow to the tissue, forcing flow toward other tissues where resistance to flow has been decreased. Flow into a capillary bed of a tissue depends on the vasoconstriction and vasodilation of the arteriole supplying the capillary bed and the contraction state of precapillary sphincters where present (Fig. 5-16). **Precapillary sphincters** are muscular rings at the entrance of a capillary bed that are capable of increasing and decreasing their internal diameter. Thus, they control flow into the capillary bed. Precapillary sphincters react to both local (intrinsic) changes, such as an increase in blood pressure, oxygen concentration, and

carbon dioxide concentration in the blood, and to neural (extrinsic) control. Extrinsic control and intrinsic control of vasoconstriction and vasodilation are discussed in the following sections.

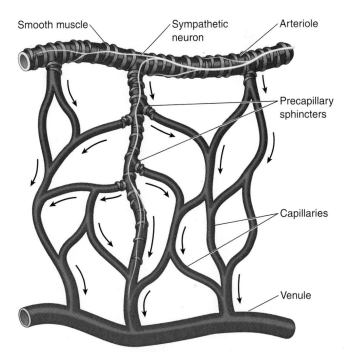

Figure 5-16. Flow into a capillary bed depends on vasoconstriction and vasodilation of the arteriole supplying the capillary bed and precapillary sphincters. Arterioles do receive sympathetic neural stimulation.

Extrinsic Control of Vasoconstriction and Vasodilation

Adrenergic sympathetic neural stimulation is the basis of extrinsic control of vasoconstriction and vasodilation. Sympathetic nerves release norepinephrine and epinephrine. Norepinephrine is the primary neurotransmitter released by sympathetic nerves innervating peripheral blood vessels, and affects primarily receptors (alpha receptors), causing vasoconstriction. On the other hand, epinephrine affects receptors, causing both vasoconstriction and vasodilation (beta 2 receptors). Thus, the amount of vasoconstriction and vasodilation depends on a balance of these two stimuli. At rest, there is a high degree of vasoconstriction within skeletal muscle. At the onset of exercise, there is an increase in vasoconstriction within inactive tissue, such as the intestinal tract, liver, and kidneys, which is due to sympathetic stimulation.[44] Also at the onset of exercise there is a change, possibly a decrease in stimulation by norepinephrine, in sympathetic stimulation to the vasculature of active muscle tissue, causing vasodilation.[44] The net result of these changes is a redistribution of blood flow toward active muscle and away from inactive tissues. Sympathetic neural stimulation to both active and inactive tissues starts to increase at exercise intensities ranging from approximately 25% to 50% of maximum capacity and becomes progressively greater, eventually reaching a maximum as exercise intensity increases.

It is also possible that release of epinephrine and norepinephrine into the bloodstream by the adrenal medulla as hormones affects vasoconstriction and vasodilation. However, these endocrine effects on vasoconstriction and vasodilation may be important only during relatively high-intensity submaximal and maximal exercise, or during the classic fight-or-flight response. Extrinsic control of vasoconstriction and vasodilation needs to be balanced with intrinsic, or local, control to bring about the desired increase in blood flow to active tissue.

Intrinsic Control of Vasoconstriction and Vasodilation

Changes within skeletal muscle during exercise stimulate muscle chemoreceptors, resulting in an increase in vasodilation because of a reflex change in neural sympathetic stimulation. This intrinsic control of vasoconstriction and vasodilation is termed **autoregulation**. Although not completely understood, the changes triggering these reflex actions are concentration increases in carbon dioxide, hydrogen ions, lactic acid, potassium, and other substances that occur in exercising muscle tissue.[33,44] The extent of vasodilation within active skeletal muscle during exercise is ultimately determined by a balance between adrenergic sympathetic neural stimulation and autoregulation. The vasoconstriction caused by sympathetic stimulation is thought to be an essential adjustment to exercise because it

Quick Review

- During exercise, blood is redistributed so that active skeletal muscle receives the vast majority of cardiac output, which increases oxygen delivery to the tissue.
- During activity, vasoconstriction, vasodilation, and precapillary sphincters are used to increase blood flow to active skeletal muscle and decrease blood flow to inactive tissue.
- Vasoconstriction and vasodilation are controlled by both extrinsic and intrinsic factors.

counteracts vasodilation brought about by autoregulation.[7] If the vasodilation elicited by autoregulation was not limited by adrenergic sympathetic stimulation, arterial blood pressure could decrease as a result of excessive blood flow entering active muscle. Potentially, this could result in a dangerous decrease in blood flow to other vital organs, such as the brain and heart. So, a balance between extrinsic and intrinsic control of blood flow is important, not just for redistribution of blood flow, but also to maintain blood pressure and blood flow to all vital organs.

Increasing Venous Return

At rest and during exercise, blood that does not return to the heart cannot be pumped to either the pulmonary or peripheral circulation. After blood has passed through a tissue's capillary bed, mean blood pressure is very low (10–20 mm Hg), and so although the pressure gradient is sufficient to move blood back toward the heart, it is quite small and by itself would only slowly drive blood flow. Several factors may aid venous return both at rest and during exercise, in order to help increase stroke volume and cardiac output and, thus, blood flow to tissue. These factors are venoconstriction, the muscle pump, and the respiratory pump.

Venoconstriction

At rest, venous vessels contain approximately 65% of the body's total blood volume. So, venous vessels can be viewed as storage reservoirs or **capacitance blood vessels** that contain a high volume of blood at a relatively low pressure. One way to mobilize the blood in venous vessels is through sympathetic stimulation causing venoconstriction, or constriction of veins, which would increase venous return to the heart. However, the veins of skeletal muscle may not receive sufficient sympathetic stimulation to substantially increase venous return. Thus, only the veins located in tissues other than skeletal muscle may contribute to an increase in venous return through venoconstriction. Within skeletal muscle, the majority of the increase in venous return probably occurs through the action of what is termed the muscle pump, which is examined in the next section.

Muscle Pump

The **muscle pump** is a mechanism through which rhythmic muscle contractions aid the venous return of blood to the heart. Large veins contain one-way valves that allow blood flow only toward the heart (Fig. 5-17). When muscle is active, it expands in all directions, compressing the veins. The compression forces blood back toward the heart because of the presence of the one-way valves. When the muscle relaxes, the one-way valves prevent blood from flowing away from the heart. This process of compression of the veins and relaxation of the muscle is repeated during rhythmic muscle actions, such as running, increasing venous return to the heart in a "milking" fashion. The muscle pump is active as soon as physical activity begins and remains in effect throughout the activity. Thus, venous return from muscle is enhanced as soon as activity begins and remains so throughout the activity, assisting in the increased cardiac output necessary to sustain exercise.

Respiratory Pump

The **respiratory pump** refers to the aiding of venous return to the heart by increases in intrathoracic pressure during expiration and decreases in intrathoracic pressure during inspiration. During inspiration, intrathoracic

Quick Review

● Venoconstriction of large veins caused by sympathetic stimulation may increase venous return to the heart, but this mechanism to increase venous return may not apply to skeletal muscle.
● The muscle pump increases venous return because of the compression of veins by the expansion of muscles during contraction and the presence of one-way valves in large veins.
● The respiratory pump increases venous return because of the increases and decreases in intrathoracic pressure during expiration and inspiration, respectively.

pressure decreases and intra-abdominal pressure increases, creating a pressure gradient for blood to move from the abdominal area to the thoracic area. During expiration, intrathoracic pressure increases, compressing the large veins contained within the thoracic cavity forcing blood toward the heart, and intra-abdominal pressure decreases, allowing the abdominal veins to fill with blood. This process is repeated during each inspiration and expiration cycle. The respiratory pump does aid venous return at rest but is enhanced during exercise because of the increased rate and depth of respiration.

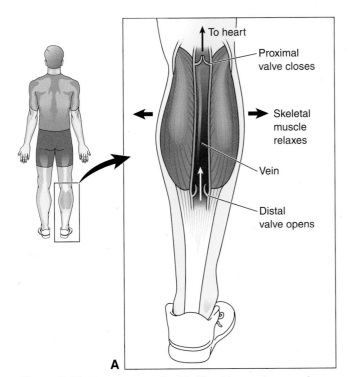

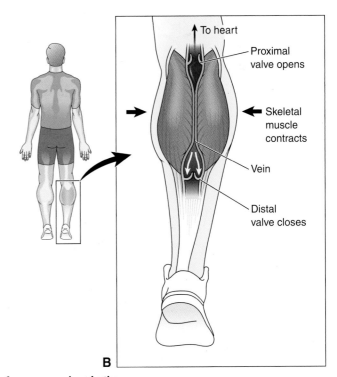

Figure 5-17. Venous return is aided by the muscle pump because of one-way valves in the veins. (A) When a muscle relaxes, the one-way valves do not allow blood flow back into the muscle from the direction of the heart. **(B)** When a muscle contracts, large veins are compressed, causing blood flow toward the heart because of the one-way valves.

Putting It All Together to Increase Oxygen Delivery During Exercise

Increasing oxygen delivery to active muscle tissue during exercise involves all of the factors previously described, including increased cardiac output, redistribution of blood flow, and increased arterial-venous oxygen difference. An adaptation to long-term endurance training is an increased capacity for each of these factors. During exercise, whether an individual is trained or untrained, there is a need to balance the effects of several factors on blood pressure to maintain sufficient pressure so blood flow occurs to all tissues and there is an increase in blood flow to active muscle tissue. These factors are an increase in cardiac output, which increases blood pressure throughout the entire arterial system, vasodilation within active tissue, which increases blood flow to active tissue but decreases arterial blood pressure, and vasoconstriction within inactive tissue, which decreases blood flow to inactive tissue but increases arterial blood pressure. Here we have focused on cardiovascular changes. It must be remembered, however, that other adaptations, such as increased aerobic enzyme concentrations and capillary density, must also take place in order for trained muscles to take advantage of the greater availability of oxygen made possible by cardiovascular changes to exercise and adaptations to long-term training.

As exercise intensity increases, so do heart rate and stroke volume, resulting in increased cardiac output (Fig. 5-18). The elevation in cardiac output with increased exercise intensity, coupled with a redistribution of blood flow to the active skeletal muscle, substantially increases its blood flow and oxygen delivery. In both trained and untrained individuals, cardiac output increases concomitantly with exercise intensity. However, an adaptation to long-term endurance training is increased stroke volume with little effect on maximal heart rate. So in endurance-trained individuals, the increase in maximal cardiac output is mostly dependent on increased stroke volume.

The increased maximal cardiac output in endurance-trained individuals allows them to achieve a greater blood flow to exercising muscle tissue, resulting in a higher peak oxygen consumption. The training adaptation of a decreased resting heart rate and increased stroke volume is also apparent during submaximal exercise where the endurance-trained athlete also demonstrates a lower heart rate, but a higher stroke volume than the untrained person.

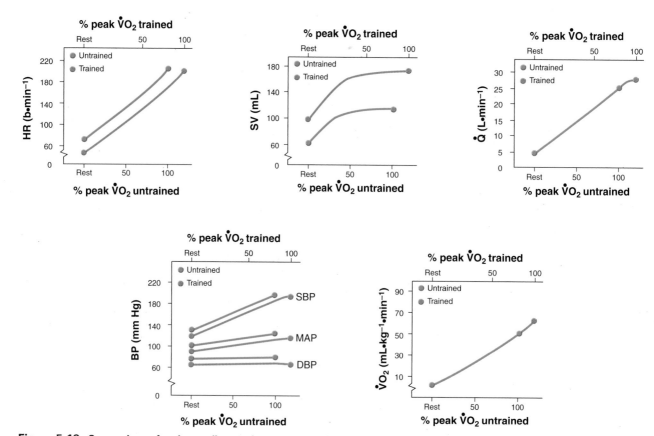

Figure 5-18. Comparison of major cardiovascular responses of an untrained individual and endurance-trained individual. Separate lines indicate that the variable (heart rate, stroke volume, and blood pressure) changes at rest and during activity because of training. One line for a variable with an extension of the line for the trained individual (cardiac output and peak oxygen consumption) indicates that the variable does not change substantially at rest or at submaximal workloads because of training.

CASE STUDY

Scenario

You are a personal trainer, and one of your clients who suffers from hypertension asks you why aerobic exercise makes the work of their heart easier. How would you explain this to your client?

Options

Long-term aerobic training decreases resting blood pressure. The decreased resting blood pressure makes it easier for your left ventricle to pump blood, because it must develop less force to eject blood into your peripheral circulation. Blood pressure during submaximal exercise at the same pace, such as jogging a 10-minute mile, is also lower after long-term training. So the work of your heart is also decreased during submaximal exercise. During maximal intensity work, blood pressure stays the same or increases slightly, which would increase the work of the left ventricle. However, most people, except athletes, spend little aerobic training time at maximal intensities, so if the work of the left ventricle increases at maximal intensities it is of little consequence to most people.

Scenario

You are a track coach, and one of your first-year male distance runners has a physical examination prior to the start of training indicating he has a hematocrit of 38%. Would you be concerned about this athlete's low hematocrit?

Options

A low hematocrit could indicate anemia. However, upon talking to the athlete you find out that he had started to train several weeks prior to the physical. Thus, because of a rapid training-induced increase in plasma volume, and a slower increase in RBC volume, a slightly lower than normal hematocrit could be expected in this situation. As a result, you are not overly concerned, but monitor the athlete for signs of fatigue which could indicate anemia. You may also want to have his hematocrit checked after several more weeks of training.

The relationship between heart rate, stroke volume, and cardiac output ($\dot{Q} = HR \times SV$) allows the endurance-trained individual to maintain the cardiac output needed to supply adequate amounts of blood to the muscles, but at a lower heart rate. This is why a typical marker of increased aerobic fitness is not only a decrease in resting heart rate, but also a decreased heart rate at any given submaximal workload (e.g., running a 10-minute mile pace).

Endurance training can also decrease peripheral blood pressure both at rest and during submaximal intensity exercise in normotensive individuals, but the decrease is relatively small.[1] This decrease in peripheral blood pressure is an important factor in explaining why stroke volume is higher among trained individuals than among untrained individuals under resting conditions and during submaximal intensity exercise. Recall that blood pressure represents resistance to blood flow. However, because the trained individual can perform more aerobic work, blood pressure at maximal workloads, especially systolic blood pressure, may be slightly higher in the trained versus the untrained individual. In addition to lower blood pressure, other adaptations to endurance training that account for increased stroke volume include increased EDV, increased total blood volume, increased left ventricular muscle mass, and, although not consistently shown, increased systolic function. In fact, because maximal blood pressure is either unaffected or even slightly increased as a result of aerobic training, the increase in stroke volume seen among the trained at maximal workloads is due primarily to these other adaptations to endurance training, particularly increased EDV. Thus, although stroke volume and, by extension, cardiac output are increased at submaximal and maximal workloads among endurance-trained athletes, the factors accounting for this improvement in stroke volume, and therefore cardiac output, can vary.

Quick Review

- During activity, there is a need to balance increased cardiac output, which increases blood pressure, vasodilation within active tissue, which decreases blood pressure, and vasoconstriction within inactive tissue so that blood pressure is maintained.
- With increased exercise intensity, increases in both heart rate and stroke volume occur, which increase cardiac output.
- Increased end-diastolic volume helps to increase stroke volume at rest and during submaximal and maximal workloads.
- With aerobic training, because maximal heart rate changes little with training, the training-induced increase in maximal cardiac output occurs primarily because of an increase in left ventricular end-diastolic volume, which causes an increase in stroke volume.
- Performance of endurance training causes a decrease in blood pressure at rest and during submaximal work, which is one factor that helps to increase stroke volume.

CHAPTER SUMMARY

The cardiovascular system can be divided into two major circulatory components: the peripheral and pulmonary circulations. The peripheral circulation delivers blood to all tissues of the body before returning it to the heart, whereas the pulmonary circulation sends blood to the lungs for oxygenation and removal of carbon dioxide before re-entering the heart. Similarly, the heart can be thought of as two separate pumps: the right and left atria and ventricles, which pump blood through the pulmonary and peripheral circulations, respectively.

A cardiac cycle consists of the systolic phase, or contraction of the myocardium, during which blood pressure is the highest, and the diastolic phase, or relaxation of the myocardium, during which blood pressure is the lowest. Blood flow is caused by differences in blood pressure in both the pulmonary and peripheral circulations. For blood flow to occur efficiently, the cardiac cycle needs to take place in a specific order and is controlled by specialized nervous tissue located within discrete segments of the heart, including the SA node, AV node, atrioventricular bundle, right and left bundle branches, and the Purkinje fibers. The cardiac cycle is also controlled by the extrinsic factors of sympathetic and parasympathetic nerve stimulation. During the various phases of the cardiac cycle, the electrical activity or movement of ions can be detected and result in the various electrocardiographic waveforms representing contraction and relaxation of the atria and ventricles.

Blood is composed of two major components: the plasma and the formed elements. The vast majority of formed elements are RBCs, which are responsible for transportation of oxygen.

Increasing blood flow to active tissue increases oxygen delivery to that tissue. Blood flow to a tissue can change because of several major factors, including alterations in cardiac output and redistribution of blood flow as a result of the vasodilation of blood vessels in active tissue, and vasoconstriction of vessels in inactive tissues.

Venous return to the heart at rest, but especially during physical activity, is aided by the respiratory pump and muscle pump. After training, blood flow to exercising muscles increases not only as a result of greater cardiac output and more efficient redistribution of blood flow, but also because of adaptations of the cardiovascular system. Combined, these adaptations act to increase blood flow (and oxygen delivery) to exercising muscles, enabling athletes to perform better at both submaximal and maximal efforts.

REVIEW QUESTIONS

Fill-in-the-Blank

1. If resting cardiac output is 5 L·min^{-1} and resting heart rate decreases, _____SV_____ must increase if cardiac output is to remain the same.

2. Parasympathetic nerve fibers at the SA and AV nodes release the neurotransmitter __Acetyl CoA__, which results in a decreased heart rate, whereas the sympathetic nerve fibers release __norepinephrine__, which results in an increased heart rate.

3. A major distinction between skeletal muscle and the myocardium is the presence of __intercalated discs__ in the myocardium to transmit the impulse to contract between cardiac muscle fibers.

4. If end-diastolic volume increases and end-systolic volume remains constant, stroke volume will _____.

5. The increase in systemic blood pressure because of an increase in cardiac output is partially offset by the elasticity or _____ (change in volume per change in pressure) of healthy peripheral arteries, allowing them to expand when more blood is ejected into them by the left ventricle.

Multiple Choice

1. Which artery is the first artery to leave the aorta and supplies the heart with its nutrients and blood supply?
   a. Pulmonary artery
   b. Coronary artery
   c. Brachial artery
   d. Radial artery
   e. Femoral artery

2. Which tissue of the heart has the fastest autorhythmaticity?
   a. Sinoatrial node
   b. Atrioventricular node
   c. Purkinje fibers
   d. Left bundle branch
   e. Bundle of His

3. Which of the following is (are) true of myocardial fibers?
   a. They contain a high number of mitochondria.
   b. They have an extensive capillary network.
   c. They are capable of using aerobic energy efficiently for contraction.
   d. They normally do not use anaerobic metabolism.
   e. All of the above

4. Which of the following factors most drastically affects the resistance to blood flow in the vessels in the human body?

a. The length of the blood vessel

b. The viscosity of the blood

c. Changes in hematocrit

d. The radius of the blood vessel

5. Which of the following composes the greatest part of hematocrit?

a. Proteins

b. Platelets

c. Hormones

d. Red blood cells

e. Electrolytes

True/False

1. A major distinction between skeletal and cardiac muscle is the autorhythmaticity of cardiac muscle.
2. The QRS complex in an electrocardiogram represents relaxation of the ventricles.
3. A typical stroke volume for a normal-sized untrained man at rest is about 5 L·min^{-1}.
4. According to the Frank–Starling mechanism, if end-diastolic volume of a ventricle increases, stroke volume will decrease.
5. An adaptation to long-term endurance training is a decrease in hematocrit.

Short Answer

1. If a blood cell was ejected from the left ventricle, what must it pass through in order to get to the left atrium?
2. Why are the major coronary arteries and veins found on the exterior surface of the heart?
3. What would happen if the atria and ventricles contracted at exactly the same time? Why?
4. What is the purpose of the specialized nervous tissue (i.e., bundle branches and Purkinje fibers) that cause the ventricles to contract?
5. How can we differentiate left ventricular hypertrophy due to a physiological adaptation from that due to a pathological adaptation?

Critical Thinking Questions

1. During exercise, how can blood flow be increased to active muscle tissue?
2. You are a track coach and one of your first-year distance runners has a physical prior to the start of training and has a low hematocrit. Would you be concerned about this athlete's low hematocrit?

KEY TERMS

anastomosis: an intercommunication between two arteries that ensures blood flow to an area, even if an artery supplying an area is fully or partially blocked

arterial blood: blood flowing away from the heart toward the peripheral or pulmonary circulations

arterial-venous oxygen difference (a-v O$_2$ diff): the difference between the amount of oxygen in 100 mL of arterial blood entering a tissue and the amount of oxygen in 100 mL of venous blood leaving a tissue

arteries: large vessels that carry blood away from the heart

arterioles: the smallest of the arteries

atrioventricular node (AV node): a node of cardiac muscle fibers located in the lower portion of the right atrium which delays the impulse to contract by 1/10 second so that the atria contract prior to the ventricles

autoregulation: intrinsic control of vasoconstriction and vasodilation

autorhythmaticity: the ability of cardiac tissue to initiate its own electrical impulse to stimulate contraction at regular time intervals

bradycardia: slower than normal resting heart rate (less than 60 beats·min^{-1})

capacitance blood vessels: blood vessels capable of containing a high volume of blood at relatively low pressures; typically referring to veins

capillaries: the smallest of the blood vessels, in which exchange of oxygen, other nutrients, and products of metabolism occur between the blood and other tissues

cardiac output: the amount of blood pumped per minute by the heart; normally expressed in L·min^{-1} or mL·min^{-1}

diastole: the relaxation phase of the cardiac cycle

electrocardiogram (ECG): a recording of the electrical activity of the heart during the cardiac cycle

end-diastolic volume (EDV): the amount of blood in a ventricle immediately prior to contraction

end-systolic volume (ESV): the amount of blood left in a ventricle after contraction

hematocrit: the percentage of total blood volume comprised by the cells or formed elements, most of which are red blood cells (erythrocytes)

hemoconcentration: reduction in the fluid portion of blood relative to the cells or formed element portion of blood

hemoglobin: substance composed of protein and an iron-containing pigment capable of reversibly binding oxygen

hypertension: higher-than-normal blood pressure

left ventricular mass: the myocardium surrounding the left ventricle

muscle pump: the aiding of venous return to the heart by the system of valves in veins and muscle contraction

myocardium: the muscle tissue comprising the heart

normotensive: having normal blood pressure

parasympathetic: nerve fibers using acetylcholine as a neurotransmitter, which decreases heart rate

pericardium: a tough, membranous sac that encloses the heart

peripheral circulation: the circulatory system that circulates blood from the heart to all parts of the body, except the lungs, and back to the heart

plasma: the fluid component of blood

precapillary sphincters: muscular rings at the entrance of the capillary bed, which are capable of increasing and decreasing their internal diameter

pulmonary circulation: the system that circulates blood from the heart to the lungs and back to the heart

Purkinje fibers: the network of nerve fibers that spreads the electrical impulse throughout the ventricles to cause their contraction

respiratory pump: the aiding of venous return to the heart by changes in intrathoracic pressure during inspiration and expiration

sinoatrial node (SA node): a node of cardiac muscle fibers located in the upper portion of the right atrium, which has the fastest autorhythmicity; it is also called the pacemaker of the heart

stroke volume: the amount of blood pumped per beat of the heart, normally expressed in milliliters

sympathetic: nerve fibers using the neurotransmitter norepinephrine, which increases heart rate and stroke volume

systole: the contraction phase of the cardiac cycle

vasoconstriction: a decrease in the interior radius of blood vessels

vasodilation: an increase in the interior radius of blood vessels

veins: large vessels carrying blood toward the heart

venous blood: blood returning to the heart from the peripheral and pulmonary circulations.

venules: the smallest of the veins

REFERENCES

1. ACSM's Guidelines for Exercise Testing and Prescription. Philadelphia, PA: Lippincott Williams & Wilkins, 2006.
2. Allen DG, Jewell BR, Murray JW. The contribution of activation processes to the length–tension relation of cardiac muscle. Nature. 1974;248:606–607.
3. Allen DG, Kurihara S. The effects of muscle length on intracellular calcium transients in mammalian cardiac muscle. J Physiol. 1982;327:79–94.
4. Arce Esquivel AA, Welsch MA. High and low volume resistance training and vascular function. Int J Sports Med. 2007;28:217–221.
5. Cornelissen VA, Fagard RH. Effect of resistance training on resting blood pressure: a meta-analysis of randomized controlled trials. J Hypertens. 2005;23:251–259.
6. Craig SK, Byrnes WC, Fleck SJ. Plasma volume responses during and after two distinct weight lifting protocols. Int J Sport Med. 2008;29:89–95.
7. Esler M, Jennings G, Lambert G, et al. Overflow of catecholamine neurotransmitters to the circulation: source, fate, and functions. Physiol Rev. 1990;70:963–985.
8. Fagard RH. Physical fitness and blood pressure. J Hypertens Suppl. 1993;11:S47–S52.
9. Falkel JE, Fleck SJ, Murray TF. Comparison of central hemodynamics between power lifters and body builders during resistance exercise. J Appl Sport Sci Res. 1992;6:24–35.
10. Fleck SJ, Dean LS. Resistance-training experience and the pressor response during resistance exercise. J Appl Physiol. 1987;63:116–120.
11. Fleck SJ, Henke C, Wilson W. Cardiac MRI of elite junior Olympic weight lifters. Int J Sports Med. 1989;10:329–333.
12. Fleck SJ, Pattany PM, Stone MH, et al. Magnetic resonance imaging determination of left ventricular mass: junior Olympic weightlifters. Med Sci Sports Exerc. 1993;25:522–527.
13. Fleck SJ. Cardiovascular adaptations to resistance training. Med Sci Sports Exerc. 1988;20:S146–S151.
14. Fleck SJ. Cardiovascular responses to strength training. In: PVK, ed. Strength and Power in Sport. Blackwell Science, 2003.
15. Fox S. Human Physiology. New York: McGraw-Hill Companies, 2002.
16. Gates P, Seals DR. Decline in large elastic artery compliance with age: a therapeutic target for habitual exercise. Br J Sports Med. 2006;40:879–899.
17. Goodman JM, Liu PP, Green HJ. Left ventricular adaptations following short-term endurance training. J Appl Physiol. 2005;98:454–460.
18. Goodman JM. The athletes heart. In: Shephard RJ, Astrand PO, eds. Endurance in Sport. Blackwell Publishing, Malden, MA. 2000.
19. Green HJ, Jones LL, Painter DC. Effects of short-term training on cardiac function during prolonged exercise. Med Sci Sports Exerc. 1990;22:488–493.
20. Hagberg JM, Goldberg AP, Lakatta L, et al. Expanded blood volumes contribute to the increased cardiovascular performance of endurance-trained older men. J Appl Physiol. 1998;85:484–489.
21. Halbert JA, Silagy CA, Finucane P, et al. The effectiveness of exercise training in lowering blood pressure: a meta-analysis of randomised controlled trials of 4 weeks or longer. J Hum Hypertens. 1997;11:641–649.
22. Heffernan KS, Rossow L, Jae SY, et al. Effect of single-leg resistance exercise on regional arterial stiffness. Eur J Appl Physiol. 2006;98:185–190.
23. Johnson JM. Physical training and the control of skin blood flow. Med Sci Sports Exerc. 1998;30:382–386.
24. Kasikcioglu E, Oflaz H, Akhan H, et al. Left atrial geometric and functional remodeling in athletes. Int J Sports Med. 2006;27:267–271.
25. Kelly G. Dynamic resistance exercise and resting blood pressure in adults: a meta-analysis. J Appl Physiol. 1997;82:1559–1565.
26. Kelly GA, Kelly KA. Progressive resistance exercise and resting blood pressure: a meta-analysis of randomized controlled trials. Hypertension. 2000;35:838–843.
27. Kelly M. Clinical snapshot: transient ischemic attack. Am J Nurs. 1995;95:42–43.
28. Kentish JC, ter Keurs HE, Ricciardi L, et al. Comparison between the sarcomere length–force relations of intact and skinned trabeculae from rat right ventricle. Influence of calcium concentrations on these relations. Circ Res. 1986;58:755–768.
29. Kraemer WJ, Fleck SJ, Maresh CM, et al. Acute hormonal responses to a single bout of heavy resistance exercise in trained power lifters and untrained men. Can J Appl Physiol. 1999;240:524–537.
30. Krieg A, Scharhag J, Kindermann W, et al. Cardiac tissue Doppler imaging in sports medicine. Sports Med. 2007;37:15–30.
31. Legaz-Arrese A, Gonzalez-Carretero M, Lacambra-Blasco I. Adaptation of left ventricular morphology to long-term training in sprint- and endurance-trained elite runners. Eur J Appl Physiol. 2006;96:740–746.
32. MacDougall JD, Tuxen D, Sale DG, et al. Arterial blood pressure response to heavy resistance exercise. J Appl Physiol. 1985;58:785–790.
33. MacLean DA, Vickery LM, Sinoway LI. Elevated interstitial adenosine concentrations do not activate the muscle reflex. Am J Physiol Heart Circ Physiol. 2001;280:H546–H553.
34. Maeda S, Otsuki T, Iemitsu M, et al. Effects of leg resistance training on arterial function in older men. Br J Sports Med. 2006;40:867–869.
35. McAllister RM. Adaptations in control of blood flow with training: splanchnic and renal blood flows. Med Sci Sports Exerc. 1998;30:375–381.
36. Mischler I, Boirie Y, Gachon P, et al. Human albumin synthesis is increased by an ultra-endurance trial. Med Sci Sports Exerc. 2003;35:75–81.
37. Moore L. The cardiovascular system: cardiac function. In: Tipton CM, ed. ACSM's Advanced Exercise Physiology. Philadelphia, PA: Lippincott Williams & Wilkins, 2006.
38. Mueller PJ, O'Hagan KP, Skogg KA, et al. Renal hemodynamic responses to dynamic exercise in rabbits. J Appl Physiol. 1998;85:1605–1614.
39. Nagashima J, Musha H, Takada H, et al. Left ventricular chamber size predicts the race time of Japanese participants in a 100 km ultramarathon. Br J Sports Med. 2006;40:331–333; discussion 333.
40. Ploutz-Snyder LL, Convertino VA, Dudley GA. Resistance exercise-induced fluid shifts: change in active muscle size and plasma volume. Am J Physiol. 1995;269:R536–R543.

41. Robergs RA, Icenogle MV, Hudson TL, et al. Temporal inhomogeneity in brachial artery blood flow during forearm exercise. Med Sci Sports Exerc. 1997;29:1021–1027.

42. Saito K, Matushita M. The contribution of left ventricular mass to maximal oxygen uptake in female college rowers. Int J Sports Med. 2004;25:27–31.

43. Sawka MN, Convertino VA, Eichner ER, et al. Blood volume: importance and adaptations to exercise training, environmental stresses, and trauma/sickness. Med Sci Sports Exerc. 2000;32:332–348.

44. Seals D. The autonomic nervous system. In: Tipton CM, ed. ACSM's Advanced Exercise Physiology. Philadelphia, PA: Lippincott Williams & Wilkins, 2006;197–245.

45. Senay LC Jr, Pivarnik JM. Fluid shifts during exercise. Exerc Sport Sci Rev. 1985;13:335–387.

46. Severinghaus JW. Exercise O_2 transport model assuming zero cytochrome PO_2 at VO_2 max. J Appl Physiol. 1994;77:671–678.

47. Thomas SN, Schroeder T, Secher NH, et al. Cerebral blood flow during submaximal and maximal dynamic exercise in humans. J Appl Physiol. 1989;67:744–748.

48. Wernstedt P, Sjostedt C, Ekman I, et al. Adaptation of cardiac morphology and function to endurance and strength training. A comparative study using MR imaging and echocardiography in males and females. Scand J Med Sci Sports. 2002;12:17–25.

49. Yang RC, Mack GW, Wolfe RR, et al. Albumin synthesis after intense intermittent exercise in human subjects. J Appl Physiol. 1998;84:584–592.

50. Yoshida T, Nagashima K, Nose H, et al. Relationship between aerobic power, blood volume, and thermoregulatory responses to exercise-heat stress. Med Sci Sports Exerc. 1997;29:867–873.

Suggested Readings

American College of Sports Medicine, American Heart Association. Exercise and acute cardiovascular events: placing the risks into perspective. Med Sci Sports Exerc. 2007;39(5):886–897.

Corrado D, Basso C, Schiavon M, et al. Does sports activity enhance the risk of sudden cardiac death? J Cardiovasc Med (Hagerstown). 2006;7(4):228–233.

Dodd KJ, Shields N. A systematic review of the outcomes of cardiovascular exercise programs for people with Down syndrome. Arch Phys Med Rehabil. 2005;86(10):2051–2058.

Gill JM. Physical activity, cardiorespiratory fitness and insulin resistance: a short update. Curr Opin Lipidol. 2007;18(1):47–52.

Hamer M. Exercise and psychobiological processes: implications for the primary prevention of coronary heart disease. Sports Med. 2006;36(10):829–838.

Kapetanopoulos A, Kluger J, Maron BJ, et al. The congenital long QT syndrome and implications for young athletes. Med Sci Sports Exerc. 2006;38(5):816–825.

Klabunde R. Cardiovascular Physiology Concepts. Baltimore, MD: Lippincott, Williams and Wilkins, 2004.

Lotan M. Quality physical intervention activity for persons with Down syndrome. Scientific World J. 2007;7:7–19.

Lucas SR, Platts-Mills TA. Physical activity and exercise in asthma: relevance to etiology and treatment. J Allergy Clin Immunol. 2005;115(5):928–934.

MacKay-Lyons MJ, Howlett J. ... aptations to aerobic training ... 2005;12(1):31–44.

Maughan RJ. The limits of hum ... 2005;10(4):52–54.

Mitzner W, Tyberg JV, Sticklan ... point series "Active venoco ... ing or raising end-diastolic ... and orthostasis." J Appl Ph ...

Plaisance EP, Taylor JK, Alhas ... cular inflammatory marke ... Nutr Exerc Metab. 2007;17(2):152–162.

Prior BM, Yang HT, Terjung RL. What makes vessels grow with exercise training? J Appl Physiol. 2004;97(3):1119–1128.

Rizvi AA, Thompson PD. Hypertrophic cardiomyopathy: who plays and who sits. Curr Sports Med Rep. 2002;1(2):93–99.

Rowell LB. Blood pressure regulation during exercise. Ann Med. 1991;23(3):329–333.

Rowell LB. Neural control of muscle blood flow: importance during dynamic exercise. Clin Exp Pharmacol Physiol. 1997;24(2):117–125.

Sui X, LaMonte MJ, Blair SN. Cardiorespiratory fitness and risk of non-fatal cardiovascular disease in women and men with hypertension. Am J Hypertens. 2007;20(6):608–615.

Thompson PD, Franklin BA, Balady GJ, et al. Exercise and acute cardiovascular events placing the risks into perspective: a scientific statement from the American Heart Association Council on Nutrition, Physical Activity, and Metabolism and the Council on Clinical Cardiology. Circulation. 2007;115(17):2358–2368.

Classic References

Astrand PO. J.B. Wolffe Memorial Lecture. "Why exercise?" Med Sci Sports Exerc. 1992;24(2):153–162.

Astrand PO, Saltin B. Maximal oxygen uptake and heart rate in various types of muscular activity. J Appl Physiol. 1961;16:977–981.

Austin WT, Harris EA. Measurement of heart rate in exercise. Q J Exp Physiol Cogn Med Sci. 1957;42(1):126–129.

Blomqvist CG, Saltin B. Cardiovascular adaptations to physical training. Annu Rev Physiol. 1983;45:169–189.

Boas EP. The heart rate of boys during and after exhausting exercise. J Clin Invest. 1931;10(1):145–152.

Drinkwater BL. Women and exercise: physiological aspects. Exerc Sport Sci Rev. 1984;12:21–51.

Hartley LH, Saltin B. Reduction of stroke volume and increase in heart rate after a previous heavier submaximal work load. Scand J Clin Lab Invest. 1968;22(3):217–223.

Robinson S, Pearcy M, Brueckman FR, et al. Effects of atropine on heart rate and oxygen intake in working man. J Appl Physiol. 1953;5(9):508–512.

Rose JC. The Fick principle and the cardiac output. GP. 1956;14(3):115–116.

Saltin B, Grimby G. Physiological analysis of middle-aged and old former athletes. Comparison with still active athletes of the same ages. Circulation. 1968;38(6):1104–1115.

Shephard RJ. For exercise testing, please. A review of procedures available to the clinician. Bull Physiopathol Respir. 1970;6(2):425–474.

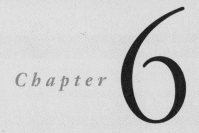

Chapter **6**

Respiratory System

After reading this chapter, you should be able to:

1. Explain the structure and function of the components of the respiratory system
2. Explain the mechanics of ventilation
3. Discuss gas diffusion at the lungs and tissue
4. Describe mechanisms of gas transport
5. Explain the oxyhemoglobin disassociation curve and the factors that cause it to shift
6. Describe the control of ventilation during rest and exercise
7. Identify and describe the receptors that control ventilation
8. Discuss the metabolic demands of ventilation
9. Describe ventilatory adaptations to exercise training

The respiratory system and the circulatory system are both necessary for the transport of oxygen to the body's tissues for use in aerobic metabolism and to remove carbon dioxide (a product of aerobic metabolism) from tissue and eventually from the body. The reason you breathe is to obtain oxygen from the atmosphere and to rid your body of carbon dioxide. The respiratory and circulatory systems combine to perform both of these functions, which involve several separate processes:

- **Pulmonary ventilation** or the movement of air into and out of the lungs, commonly referred to as breathing
- Movement of oxygen from air in the lungs into the blood and of carbon dioxide out of the blood to air in the lungs, or **pulmonary diffusion**
- Transport of oxygen and carbon dioxide in the blood
- The exchange of oxygen and carbon dioxide between the blood and the body's tissues or **capillary gas exchange**

Respiration can be divided into two major types. Pulmonary ventilation and pulmonary diffusion are referred to as **pulmonary respiration** because these two processes occur at the lungs. **Cellular respiration** refers to the use of oxygen in aerobic metabolism and production of carbon dioxide. Within this chapter, respiration will refer to pulmonary respiration. Cellular respiration or metabolism has already been discussed in Chapter 2. An understanding of pulmonary respiration, transport of oxygen and carbon dioxide in blood, and capillary gas exchange is necessary to understand not only the functioning of the body at rest, but also bodily function during exercise. Within this chapter the structure and function of the respiratory system at rest and during exercise is discussed.

STRUCTURE AND FUNCTION OF THE RESPIRATORY SYSTEM

The function of the lungs is to exchange gases between the air and the blood. To do this, there needs to be structures through which air can be moved into and out of the lungs, and there needs to be a place where capillary gas exchange can take place. Starting at the nose, air first moves through the nostrils and into the nasal cavity (Fig. 6-1). Air then travels through the pharynx, the larynx, and the trachea, which splits into two bronchi (one leading into each lung), with each then branching several times, forming bronchioles and finally terminal bronchioles. To this point, no gas exchange has taken place. The terminal bronchioles conduct air into the respiratory bronchioles, which in turn conduct air into the **alveoli** (the saclike structures surrounded by capillaries where gas exchange takes place). Some gas exchange also takes place at the level of the respiratory bronchioles. So, some structures within the respiratory system function mainly as conduits through which air travels, whereas others are where gas exchange takes place.

Humidifying, Warming, and Filtering of Air

Besides being conduits through which air travels, the structures prior to the respiratory bronchioles also humidify, warm, and filter the air. All three of these processes are necessary to protect the delicate membranes of the respiratory bronchioles and alveoli, where capillary gas exchange takes place. Humidifying the air prevents the membranes from damage due to drying out or desiccation. Increasing the water vapor content of the air is especially important in low-humidity or dry climates. Properly moistening the air as it travels into the lungs is also important in very cold climates, especially during the winter, since cold air is typically very dry.

Warming of the air helps to maintain body temperature of the lungs as well as the temperature of the structures where capillary gas exchange takes place. Warming of the air is probably most important in cold environments.

Filtering of the air occurs due to the presence of mucus secreted by the cells of the nasal passages to the bronchioles. Some of the mucus is expelled through the nostrils, some swallowed, and some expectorated. Movement of mucus so that it can be expelled is aided by small fingerlike projections, termed cilia, that collectively move in a wavelike fashion. The ciliary movement within the bronchi and bronchioles moves the mucus toward the oral cavity so that it can be expelled. Small airborne particles are present in virtually all air, but the filtering of air is especially important in polluted environments. Small airborne particles that escape being trapped in mucus and reach the alveoli are engulfed by macrophages (a type of immune system cell). The processes of humidifying, warming, and filtering of air are necessary to prevent damage to the alveoli.

🔍 **Quick Review**

- The major function of the pulmonary respiratory system is to exchange carbon dioxide and oxygen between the air within the lungs and the blood.
- Alveoli are saclike structures surrounded by capillaries where gas exchange takes place.
- The nasal passages and other structures prior to the respiratory bronchioles, besides being conduits through which air travels, also humidify, warm, and filter the air to protect the alveoli from damage.
- Pulmonary diffusion is aided by the large surface area created by the tremendous number of alveoli and the wrapping of alveoli by capillaries.

Alveoli

Exchange of oxygen and carbon dioxide takes place within the alveoli. The majority of alveoli are located after the respiratory bronchioles. However, the respiratory bronchioles do have a small number of alveolar clusters where some gas exchange does take place prior to terminating in the alveoli. There are approximately 300 million alveoli in the lungs. The large number of alveoli results in a tremendous surface area, approximately the size of a tennis court (70 m^2), where pulmonary diffusion can take place. This tremendous surface area is the major reason a person can live a relatively normal life even after the removal of one lung. Further aiding pulmonary diffusion are two cell membranes that compose the **respiratory membrane**, the membrane of the alveolar cells and the cells making up the wall of the capillary. It is through the respiratory membrane that gas must pass to move between the blood and the air within the alveoli (Fig. 6-2). Each alveolus is wrapped in capillaries, which aids in increasing the surface area available for pulmonary diffusion. Thus, the tremendous number of alveoli and their design results in a vast surface area available for pulmonary diffusion.

MECHANICS OF VENTILATION

One way in which lung volume could possibly be changed in order to move air in and out of the lungs would be to have lung tissue that is capable of contraction in a fashion similar to muscle tissue. However, lung tissue is not capable of contraction; therefore, there must be another means by which lung volume is changed. Each lung is encased by a double-layered pleural sac. The two membranes of the sac are referred to as the **pleura**. The visceral or pulmonary pleura lines the outer surface of the lungs, and the parietal pleura lines the inner surface of the thoracic cavity and diaphragm. Between these two membranes is a thin film of fluid that acts as a lubricant between the lungs

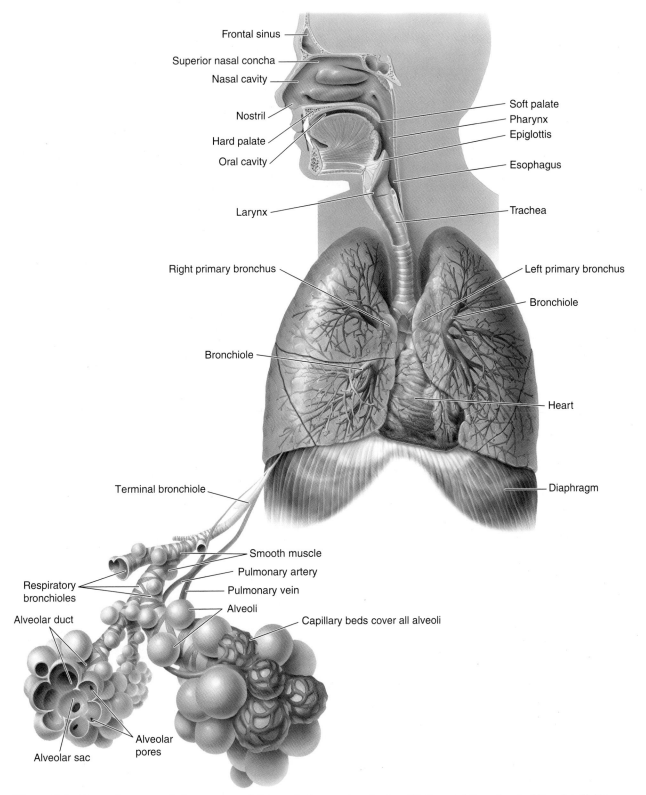

Figure 6-1. The major anatomical structures of the respiratory system begin with the nostrils and end at the alveoli. No gas exchange occurs from the nostrils to the terminal bronchiole. Some gas exchange does occur at the level of the respiratory bronchiole, but the majority of gas exchange takes place at the alveoli. (Asset provided by Anatomical Chart Co.)

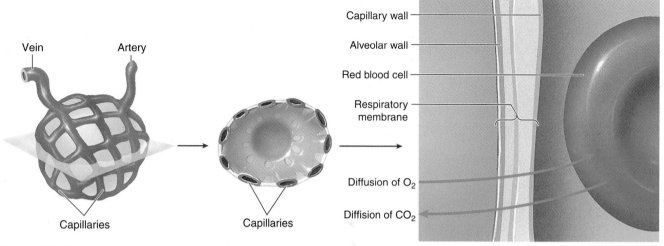

Figure 6-2. The respiratory membrane is composed of the capillary wall and the alveolar wall. The surface area available for gas exchange is increased by wrapping each alveolus with capillaries.

and the inner thoracic wall and diaphragm, as the lungs increase and decrease in volume during breathing. This fluid also results in **intrapleural pressure** or pressure in the space or pleural cavity between the visceral and parietal membranes being less than atmospheric pressure. The fact that the pressure within the pleural sac (intrapleural pressure) is less than that of the air in the alveoli causes the lungs to adhere to the inner surface of the thoracic cavity and the diaphragm. Additionally, if the ribs or diaphragm move such that the volume of the thoracic cavity changes, the lungs will remain in contact with the inner surface of the thoracic cavity and diaphragm, resulting in changes in lung volume. Thus, muscles external to the lung tissue must create a change in thoracic cavity volume for air to be moved in and out of the lungs. These muscles and other factors related to the movement of air into and out of lungs are discussed in the next sections.

Pressure Changes During Ventilation

Air is moved into and out of the lungs due to pressure changes within the lungs. If air pressure within the lungs, or **intrapulmonic pressure**, is greater than atmospheric pressure, air will move out of the lungs (expiration). If intrapulmonic pressure is less than atmospheric pressure, air will move into the lungs (inspiration). Between breaths, intrapulmonic pressure and atmospheric pressure are equivalent, and so no movement of air takes place (Fig. 6-3). During inspiration, the volume of the intrathoracic cavity increases. With an increase in the lung volume, intrapulmonic pressure decreases and air rushes into the lungs. During expiration, the volume of the intrathoracic cavity decreases, resulting in a decrease in the lung volume. The decrease in the lung volume results in an increase in intrapulmonic pressure and air rushes out of lungs. So, during inspiration and expiration, pressure gradients between atmospheric pressure

and intrapulmonic pressure are created by changing the volume of the intrathoracic cavity, resulting in movement of air into and out of the lungs. In the next section, the muscles responsible for changes in intrathoracic volume are discussed.

Inspiration

A muscle capable of increasing intrathoracic cavity volume is an inspiratory muscle. The **diaphragm** is the most important inspiratory muscle. As it contracts, it flattens (Fig. 6-3), resulting in an increase in intrathoracic volume and putting into motion the intrapulmonic pressure changes that cause inspiration. Additionally, contraction of the diaphragm causes movement of the abdominal contents forward and downward. At rest, the diaphragm performs most of the work of inspiration. During exercise, when greater changes in intrathoracic volume are needed in order to ventilate a greater volume of air, accessory inspiratory muscles also contract (Fig. 6-4). These muscles include the external intercostal muscles located between the ribs, which upon contraction elevate the ribs, increasing intrathoracic volume. Other accessory inspiratory muscles that elevate the ribs, increasing intrathoracic volume, include the scalene muscles, sternocleidomastoid, and pectoralis minor.

Expiration

At rest, no muscular effort is needed to cause expiration. The diaphragm and rib cage have elastic properties, and upon relaxation of the diaphragm and any accessory inspiratory muscles, intrathoracic volume decreases due to the passive recoil of those muscles. The decrease in intrathoracic volume puts into motion the changes in intrapulmonic pressure that cause expiration. However, during exercise or voluntary forced expiration, accessory muscles of expiration also contract. These muscles include the

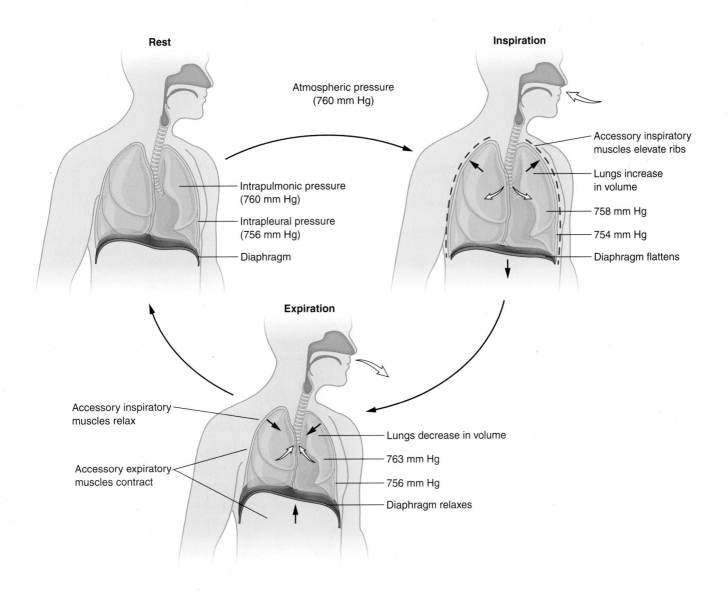

Figure 6-3. Inspiration and expiration are brought about by changes in intrapulmonic pressure. During inspiration, intrapulmonic pressure is less than atmospheric pressure, and during expiration, intrapulmonic pressure is greater than atmospheric pressure.

internal intercostals, the rectus abdominis, and the internal oblique muscles of the abdominal wall, which upon contraction pull the rib cage downward (Fig. 6-4). Contraction of the abdominal wall muscles also force abdominal contents upward against the diaphragm. Contraction of the accessory expiratory muscles decreases intrathoracic volume, resulting in an increase in intrapulmonic pressure and expiration. So the volume of air moved during inspiration and expiration can be increased due to the contraction of accessory muscles.

Airflow Resistance

As with blood flow, resistance to flow and the pressure difference between two areas within the respiratory system

affect airflow. These relationships are expressed by the following equation:

$$\text{Airflow} = P_1 - P_2 / \text{Resistance} \qquad (1)$$

where $P_1 - P_2$ is the pressure difference between two areas within the pulmonary system and resistance is the resistance to airflow between those two areas. Thus, airflow can be increased by amplifying the pressure difference between two areas and/or by decreasing the resistance to airflow. Under resting conditions, the diameter, or cross-sectional area, of an airway is the most important factor affecting airflow. As with blood flow, if the diameter of the airway is reduced by half, resistance increases 16 times. This relationship between resistance and airflow explains

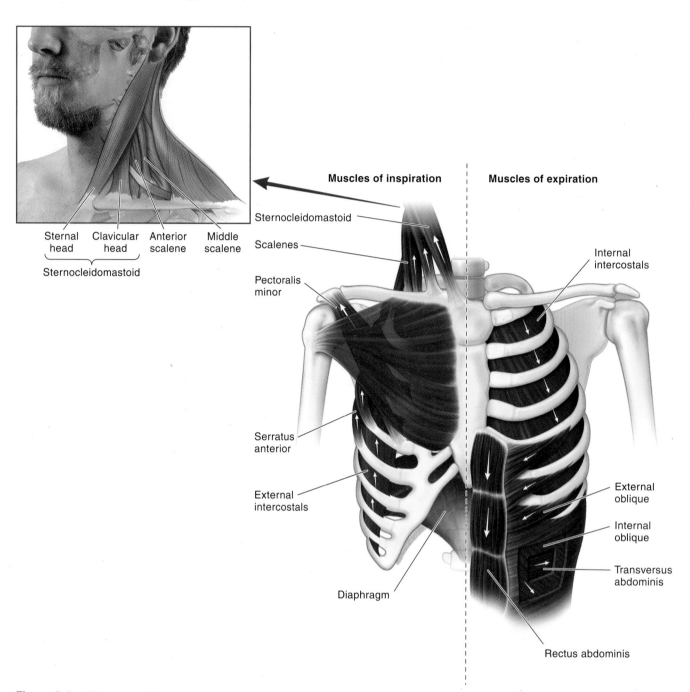

Muscles of inspiration

Muscles of expiration

Sternal head / Clavicular head / Anterior scalene / Middle scalene — Sternocleidomastoid

Sternocleidomastoid

Scalenes

Pectoralis minor

Serratus anterior

External intercostals

Diaphragm

Internal intercostals

External oblique

Internal oblique

Transversus abdominis

Rectus abdominis

Figure 6-4. Different muscles contract to cause inspiration and expiration. The diaphragm is the major muscle of inspiration. However, accessory muscles can contract to increase the volume of gas moved during both inspiration and expiration. (From Premkumar K. The Massage Connection Anatomy and Physiology. Baltimore, MD: Lippincott Williams & Wilkins, 2004. Inset adapted from an asset provided by Anatomical Chart Co.)

why disease states such as asthma and obstructive lung disease (COPD, asthma, emphysema, and chronic bronchitis) increase tremendously the force respiratory muscles must create and, so, the energy needs of the respiratory muscles in someone afflicted with one of these disease states. This relationship also explains why during exercise, when pulmonary ventilation increases up to 20 times, you start to breathe through your mouth (which has a larger diameter conduit compared with the nasal passages) as well as through your nose. Also, the stimulation of the sympathetic nervous system that occurs with exercise results in bronchodilation, decreasing resistance to airflow within the bronchial tubes. The effect on resistance to airflow due to disease states and nasal strips, an artificial means of possibly decreasing resistance to airflow, is further discussed in Boxes 6-1 and 6-2.

Box 6-1 APPLYING RESEARCH
Diseases That Increase Airway Resistance

Even small decreases in the pulmonary airways' cross-sectional area increase resistance to airflow dramatically. This increases the work of breathing and can result in dyspnea or shortness of breath. Several diseases cause increases in pulmonary resistance to airflow. Chronic obstructive pulmonary disease (COPD) comprises several different respiratory tract diseases that obstruct airflow (asthma, emphysema, and chronic bronchitis). Asthma is a reversible narrowing of the airways, termed a bronchospasm. If exercise triggers bronchospasms, the asthma is termed exercise-induced asthma. During an asthma attack, because resistance to airflow is increased, breathing becomes difficult for the patient. Asthma is typically treated with bronchodilator drugs that either relax pulmonary airways' smooth muscle, resulting in an increase in pulmonary airways' cross-sectional

area, or prevent bronchospasms. With COPD, the airways are always narrowed. Chronic bronchitis is a result of constant overproduction of mucus within the airways, resulting in airway blockage. Emphysema causes destruction of the alveolar walls, which decreases the elastic recoil of the alveoli and can result in their collapse, increasing airway resistance. With COPD, as a result of the increased airway resistance, breathing becomes difficult because the increased resistance means the workload on the respiratory muscles is increased. The narrowing of airways also traps air within the bronchioles and alveoli, increasing residual volume. Both of these factors result in increased work of breathing and decreased capacity for exercise, in part because more oxygen must be used by the respiratory muscles and so is not available for use by other muscles during exercise.

Pulmonary Ventilation

Pulmonary ventilation refers to the amount of air moved in and out of the lungs during a particular timeframe, such as 1 minute. Pulmonary ventilation per minute, similar to cardiac output (Chapter 5), can be calculated by multiplying breathing frequency per minute by the amount of air moved per breath, or **tidal volume**:

$$\dot{V}_E = V_T \times f \qquad (2)$$

where

$\dot{V}_E$ = volume of air expired per minute, or pulmonary ventilation (note that V with a dot over it indicates volume per unit of time, typically 1 minute)

V_T = tidal volume, or the amount of air moved per breath

f = breathing frequency per minute.

At rest, typical values for untrained young adults with a body mass of approximately 70 kg are $\dot{V}_E$ = 8.0 L·min⁻¹, V_T = 0.65 L, and f = 12·min⁻¹ (Table 6-1). With exercise,

Box 6-2 PRACTICAL QUESTIONS FROM STUDENTS
Do Nasal Strips Help with Performance?

Coaches and athletes are always looking for any advantage in competition or training. Many have turned to nasal strips as a source of potential advantage. Nasal strips or nasal dilator strips are worn externally on the nose. They have elastic qualities, which are supposed to increase the cross-sectional area of the nasal openings, reducing resistance to airflow into and out of the pulmonary system. If resistance to airflow is reduced, it could possibly result in decreased work for the inspiratory and expiratory muscles during physical activity, which could result in an increase in physical performance, especially during endurance or aerobic activities. However, it appears that for untrained and moderately trained individuals, nasal strips have little or no effect on the following parameters: oxygen consumption at a specified workload, peak oxygen consumption, maximal and submaximal pulmonary ventilation, maximal and submaximal frequency of breathing, maximal and submaximal tidal volume, maximal workload achieved, or perceived exertion, a psychological measure of how difficult it is to perform a specified workload.[1-3] Nasal strips have also been shown to be ineffective during recovery from an anaerobic work bout, with no significant change in recovery heart rate, oxygen consumption, or pulmonary

ventilation shown.[4] Nasal strips have also been shown to be ineffective during recovery from an aerobic work bout, with no significant change in pulmonary ventilation, frequency of breathing, oxygen consumption, and perceived exertion.[1]

The above results indicate that nasal strips have no physiological advantage during or after physical activity. However, it is possible that nasal strips result in a placebo or psychological advantage for some athletes during competition or training. So, some athletes will probably continue to use nasal strips because they believe that nasal strips do give them a competitive advantage.

References

1. Baker KM, Behm DG. The effectiveness of nasal dilator strips under aerobic exercise and recovery conditions. J Strength Cond Res. 1999;13:206–209.
2. O'Kroy JA. Oxygen uptake and ventilatory effects of an external nasal dilator during ergometry. Med Sci Sports Exerc. 2000;32:1491–1495.
3. O'Kroy JA, James T, Miller JM, et al. Effects of an external nasal dilator on the work of breathing during exercise. Med Sci Sports Exerc. 2001;33:454–458.
4. Thomas DQ, Larson BM, Rahija MR, et al. Nasal strips do not affect cardiorespiratory measures during recovery from anaerobic exercise. J Strength Cond Res. 2001;15:341–343.

Table 6-1. Typical Mean Values for Pulmonary Ventilation and Related Variables

	Rest	Mild Exercise	Moderate Exercise	Heavy Exercise	Maximal Exercise	Endurance Athlete Maximal Exercise
$\dot{V}_E$ (L·min⁻¹)	8.0	22	51	90	113	183
V_A (L·min⁻¹)	5	18	41	74	93	150
V_T (L·min⁻¹)	0.6	1.2	2.2	2.7	2.7	3.1
f per min	12	18	23	33	42	59

$\dot{V}_E$ = minute ventilation; V_A = alveolar ventilation; V_T = tidal volume; f = breathing frequency.

Data adapted from Dempsey JA, Miller JD, Romer LM. The respiratory system. In: ACSMs Advanced Exercise Physiology. Philadelphia, PA: Lippincott, Williams & Williams, 2006.

$\dot{V}_E$ increases to approximately 113 L·min⁻¹, with corresponding increases in V_T and f. These values for highly trained endurance athletes during maximal or near-maximal work are substantially higher, with $\dot{V}_E$ = 183 L·min⁻¹, V_T = 3.1 L, and f = 59·min⁻¹. The higher values in endurance athletes are probably due to both genetic factors and training.

There is always some air in the nasal cavity, larynx, trachea, and bronchi, so not all of the air inspired reaches the alveoli, where gas diffusion takes place. The air that never reaches the alveoli is termed **anatomical dead space**, whereas air that does reach the alveoli is termed **alveolar ventilation**. So, $\dot{V}_E$ can be divided into these two components:

$$\dot{V}_E = V_A + V_D \qquad (3)$$

where

V_D = anatomical dead space
V_A = alveolar ventilation.

Because of the tremendous surface area available for gas exchange within the lungs, it is not necessary to use all portions of the lungs for gas exchange at rest. The bottom or basal portions of the lungs receive more ventilation at rest than the apical or upper portions. During exercise, a greater proportion of the lung receives ventilation, with this being especially true for the apical portions of the lungs.[4] In the next section, the volumes of air within the lungs are explored.

Lung Capacities and Volumes

Lung capacities and volumes can be determined using spirometry equipment (Fig. 6-5). You are already familiar with tidal volume, which is one of several lung volumes (Fig. 6-6). All of the lung capacities and volumes have clinical significance in various disease states and situations. Here, however, only the major lung volumes and capacities important to the study of exercise are described.

At rest, there is a substantial reserve of tidal volume (V_T). This reserve allows V_T to increase during exercise by expanding into the inspiratory and the expiratory reserve

volumes. Voluntarily, it is possible to achieve the maximal V_T or vital capacity. If it were not for the reserve in V_T, it would be impossible to increase $\dot{V}_E$ to the extent possible during maximal exercise, because then the only means by which to increase $\dot{V}_E$ would be to increase frequency of breathing. **Residual volume** is the amount of air left in the lungs after a maximal exhalation. It is important because it means the lungs do not completely empty or collapse after a maximal exhalation, and because air remains within the lungs, it allows continuous exchange of gases at the alveoli between breaths.

Frequency and Depth of Breathing

During exercise, although both V_T and breathing frequency increase, it may be more energetically efficient to increase V_T first. That is, during the transition from rest to exercise, the first ventilatory response to occur is an increase in the depth of breathing. If this adjustment does not adequately meet increased ventilatory needs, an increase in breathing frequency will occur. In fact, during light to moderate exercise, $\dot{V}_E$ is increased due to an increase in both V_T and

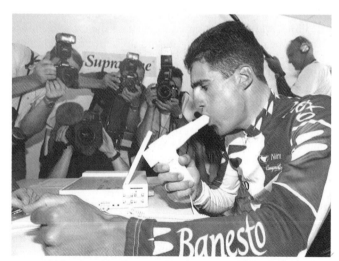

Figure 6-5. Spirometry refers to the determination of lung capacities and volumes. The use of a computerized spirometer is the most common way of determining lung capacities and volumes.

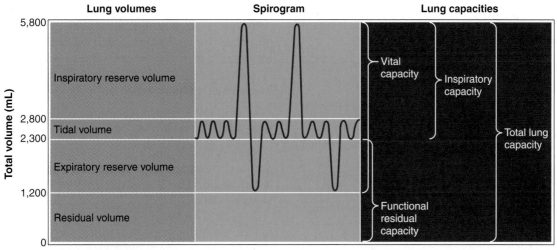

Figure 6-6. Lung volumes and capacities are important measures of the respiratory system's function. The various lung volumes and capacities are related to each other. For example, if tidal volume increases, functional residual capacity decreases. *Inspiratory reserve volume* is the greatest volume of air that can be inspired at the end of a normal resting inspiration. *Inspiratory capacity* is the greatest volume of air that can be inspired from a normal resting expiration (IC = IRV + V$_T$). *Tidal volume* is the volume of air that is inspired or expired during normal breathing at rest. *Expiratory reserve volume* is the greatest volume of air that can be expired after a normal resting expiration. *Residual volume* is the volume of air left in the lungs after a maximal exhalation. *Vital capacity* is the greatest volume of air that can be expired after a maximal inhalation (VC = IRV + V$_T$ + ERV). *Functional residual capacity* is the volume of air left in the lungs after a normal resting expiration (FRC = ERV + RV). *Lung capacity* is the greatest volume of air that can be contained in the lungs (TLC = VC + RV or IC + FRV or IRV + V$_T$ + ERV + RV). (From Cohen BJ, Taylor JJ. Memmler's the Human Body in Health and Disease, 10th ed. Baltimore, MD: Lippincott Williams & Wilkins, 2005.)

frequency of breathing.[5] However, at higher exercise intensities, V$_T$ tends to plateau, and the only way to increase pulmonary ventilation is to increase frequency of breathing. The increase in V$_T$ during exercise is brought about by higher activation levels of both the diaphragm and accessory inspiratory and expiratory muscles. Additionally, increased V$_T$, as opposed to only an increase in breathing frequency, means the increase in anatomical dead space ventilation is minimized, whereas alveolar ventilation is increased. The increase in alveolar ventilation is necessary in order to increase gas exchange.

Quick Review

- Expiratory and inspiratory muscles are needed to decrease and increase lung volume in order for expiration and inspiration to take place.
- Air moves into and out of the lungs due to pressure differences between the air within the lungs and atmospheric air.
- The diaphragm is the most important muscle of inspiration and expiration.
- Airflow between two areas of the ventilatory pathway depends on the pressure difference between the two areas and the resistance to flow between the two areas.
- Pulmonary ventilation can be changed due to a change in either tidal volume or frequency of breathing.

DIFFUSION AT THE LUNGS

Gas diffusion at the lungs or during capillary gas exchange is aided by the tremendous surface area of the alveoli and the respiratory membrane being only two cell membranes in thickness. Even with these aids to capillary gas exchange, there must be a force driving oxygen from the air within the alveoli into the blood and carbon dioxide from the blood into the air within the alveoli. The driving force is provided by a difference in the pressures of oxygen and carbon dioxide between the air in the alveoli and the blood. The respiratory membrane is permeable to both oxygen and carbon dioxide, so these gases will diffuse through the membrane from an area of high pressure to an area of low pressure. In order to determine the driving pressure of oxygen and carbon dioxide between the air within the alveoli and the blood, the **partial pressure,** or the portion of pressure due to a particular gas in a mixture of gases in both the blood and the alveoli, must be calculated. **Dalton's law** states that the total pressure of a gas mixture is equivalent to the sum of all the pressures of all the gases that compose the mixture. So, the partial pressure of a gas within a gas mixture can be calculated by multiplying the total pressure of the gas mixture by the percentage of a particular gas within the mixture. For example, at sea level, standard barometric pressure, or the total pressure of the gas mixture, is 760 mm Hg, and nitrogen, oxygen, and carbon dioxide compose certain percentages of the atmosphere. Thus, the partial pressure within the atmosphere of each of these gases can be calculated as follows:

$$\text{Nitrogen: } 760 \text{ mm Hg} \times 0.7904 = 600.7 \text{ mm Hg} \quad (4)$$

$$\text{Oxygen: } 760 \text{ mm Hg} \times 0.2093 = 159.1 \text{ mm Hg} \quad (5)$$

$$\text{Carbon dioxide: } 760 \text{ mm Hg} \times 0.0003 = 0.2 \text{ mm Hg} \quad (6)$$

Dalton's law also states that each gas in a mixture can move according to its own individual pressure gradient, rather than having all gases in the mixture move in unison by what is known as "bulk flow." Accordingly, it is possible for oxygen and carbon dioxide to move in different directions across the same membrane. The respiratory membrane is permeable to both oxygen and carbon dioxide, so diffusion across the membrane will take place according to Fick's law. This law states that the volume of gas that will diffuse is proportional to the surface area available for diffusion, the diffusion coefficient of the gas (which is the ease with which a gas will diffuse), and the difference in partial pressure of the gas on opposite sides of the membrane and inversely proportional to the thickness of the membrane:

$$V_{\text{gas diffused}} = \frac{A \times D \times (P_1 - P_2)}{T} \quad (7)$$

where
A = surface area
T = thickness of the membrane
D = diffusion coefficient of the gas
$P_1 - P_2$ = partial pressure difference on opposite sides of the membrane

The thin respiratory membrane and tremendous surface area, due to the large number of alveoli, make the lung an ideal place for gas exchange. The thickness of the respiratory membrane and diffusion coefficients of carbon dioxide and oxygen normally do not change. So the only ways to increase capillary gas exchange to approximately 30 times above resting values during intense exercise is to increase the surface area available for exchange or the partial pressures differences. Although alveoli surface area can increase during exercise due to the use of a greater portion of the lung receiving ventilation (see "Pulmonary Ventilation" section) at the respiratory membrane, the amount of oxygen and carbon dioxide that diffuses through the membrane is almost totally dependent on the partial pressure differences between the opposite sides of the membrane.

The amount of oxygen and carbon dioxide dissolved in blood is described by **Henry's law**. This law states that the amount of gas dissolved in any fluid depends on the temperature, partial pressure of the gas, and the solubility of the gas. The temperature of blood is relatively constant (although it elevates slightly during exercise), as is the solubility of oxygen and carbon dioxide within blood. Thus, similar to the amount of these gases that will diffuse through the respiratory membrane, the amount of these gases dissolved in blood is directly dependent on their partial pressures. The higher the partial pressure of the gas, the greater the amount of gas that will be dissolved in blood. In the next sections, the diffusion of oxygen and carbon dioxide across the respiratory and cellular membranes will be examined in more detail.

Oxygen Diffusion

Oxygen diffusion into the blood depends on the partial pressure of oxygen (P_{O_2}) being greater in the alveoli than in the blood. The P_{O_2} at the sea level is 159.1 mm Hg. However, within the alveoli this decreases to 105 mm Hg (Fig. 6-7). This decrease is due to the mixing of atmospheric air with a high P_{O_2}, with air left within the lungs after exhalation, which has a lower percentage of oxygen, approximately 14.5% compared to 20.9% in atmospheric air, because oxygen is diffusing from the air within the alveoli into the blood.

Additionally, as noted above, one function of the pulmonary system is to humidify the air entering the lungs. As the humidity of the air increases, the percentage of water vapor, which is a gas, and its partial pressure increases. According to Dalton's law the total pressure of a gas mixture is equivalent to the sum of all the pressures of all the gases that compose the mixture. Therefore, as the partial pressure of water vapor increases, the partial pressure of all other gases must decrease. These factors result in the P_{O_2} within the alveoli dropping to approximately 105 mm Hg.

The P_{O_2} within the arterial blood entering the lungs is 40 mm Hg. This results in a driving force for diffusion of 65 mm Hg between the air within the alveoli and the arterial blood entering the lungs. As blood flows through the pulmonary capillaries, it quickly equilibrates with the P_{O_2} within the alveoli and is oxygenated. This should result in a P_{O_2} within the venous blood leaving the lungs of 105 mm Hg. However, some blood circulating through the lungs passes through alveoli that are poorly ventilated (at rest, the basal portions of the lungs receive more ventilation than the apical portions), and the venous blood that supplies the lungs and cardiac circulations with oxygen and needed nutrients is added to the venous blood leaving the lungs within the pulmonary vein. Therefore, this added blood has a low P_{O_2} compared with the blood within the pulmonary vein that has just been oxygenated. These factors result in the blood leaving the lungs having a P_{O_2} of 100 mm Hg, which is a slightly lower P_{O_2} than that within the alveoli.

The blood within the pulmonary veins returns to the heart and is pumped by the left ventricle to the systemic circulation. The P_{O_2} within tissue is 40 mm Hg, resulting in a driving force for oxygen to diffuse from the blood into tissue. The blood quickly equilibrates to the P_{O_2} of 40 mm Hg within tissue or is deoxygenated. The deoxygenated blood returns to the right side of the heart and is pumped through the pulmonary artery back to the lungs, and the cycle of oxygenation and deoxygenation of blood repeats itself.

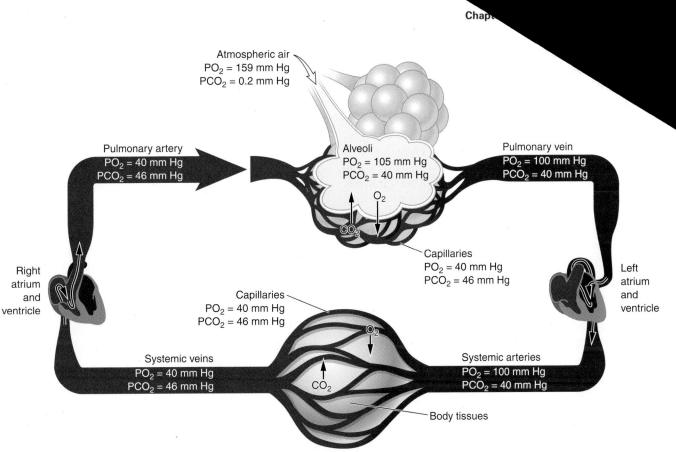

Figure 6-7. **Capillary gas exchange at the lungs and tissue takes place due to differences in the partial pressures of oxygen and carbon dioxide.** Carbon dioxide is more permeable to the membranes through which gas exchange takes place, so the difference in the carbon dioxide partial pressures between the opposite sides of a membrane can be less than the partial pressure difference of oxygen.

Carbon Dioxide Diffusion

Similar to oxygen diffusion, carbon dioxide diffusion at the lungs and tissue depends on differences in the partial pressure of carbon dioxide (P_{CO_2}). The P_{CO_2} within atmospheric air is 0.2 mm Hg and in the air within alveoli is 40 mm Hg (Fig. 6-7). The P_{CO_2} difference between atmospheric air and air within the alveoli is due to the same factors resulting in a change in P_{O_2} from atmospheric air to the air within the alveoli. In this case, however, the air within the alveoli has a high concentration of CO_2, resulting in an increase in P_{CO_2}. As blood returns from the body's tissues and enters the lungs, it has a P_{CO_2} of 46 mm Hg and then quickly equilibrates to the P_{CO_2} within the alveoli (P_{CO_2} of 40 mm Hg), before returning to the left side of the heart, and being pumped to the systemic circulation. Tissue has a P_{CO_2} of 46 mm Hg, and the blood quickly equilibrates to this P_{CO_2}, returns to the right side of the heart, and is pumped to the lungs. Then, the process of transporting carbon dioxide to the lungs for expiration repeats itself. The difference in P_{CO_2} on either side of the respiratory and cellular membranes to cause diffusion of carbon dioxide across the membrane can be substantially less than for oxygen because the membranes are much more permeable to carbon dioxide than to oxygen. For example, at the respiratory membrane,

there is only a 6 mm Hg driving force for the diffusion of carbon dioxide, but a 65 mm Hg driving force for oxygen to diffuse through the membrane.

Lung Blood Flow

Pulmonary blood flow determines the velocity at which blood passes through the pulmonary capillaries, and as blood flow increases and more blood flows through the lungs, such as during exercise, more total gas diffusion can take place. In an adult, cardiac output at rest of both the right and left ventricles is approximately 5 L·min^{-1}. Even though blood flow through the pulmonary and systemic circulations must be equivalent (see Chapter 5), one difference between these two circulatory networks is that blood pressure within the pulmonary circulation (25/10 mm Hg systolic/diastolic pressure) is very low compared with the systemic circulation. The low pulmonary circulation pressures are due to low vascular resistance within the pulmonary circulation, and this helps to protect the thin respiratory membrane from damage due to high blood pressure.

It takes approximately 0.25 seconds for the equilibration of oxygen between the air within alveoli and lung capillary blood to take place. As cardiac output increases during exercise, blood transit time through the capillaries

...is level, resulting in ...blood. Several factors, ...optimal conditions for ...use diffusion at the lungs ...g's alveoli (see "Pulmonary ...rcise as compared with rest, ...lable for gas exchange. The ..., resulting in a short diffusion ...ng exercise. P_{O_2} within the alveoli increa... ...d pulmonary ventilation, resulting in a greate... ...between P_{O_2} in the air within the alveoli and that w... ...the blood. Pulmonary capillary blood volume increases as capillaries expand and more capillaries are recruited, especially in the apex regions of lung, due to the increase in cardiac output as exercise intensity increases. The increased capillary blood volume results in a slowing of blood transit time through the capillaries surrounding alveoli, thus allowing more time for gas equilibration as well as for maintaining a low blood pressure within the pulmonary circulation.

The above factors maintain optimal or near-optimal gas exchange in untrained or moderately trained individuals. For example, if maximal cardiac output is 20 L·min^{-1}, mean transit time through the pulmonary capillaries (blood flow = pulmonary capillary volume divided by cardiac output) is 0.5 to 0.6 seconds, which permits sufficient gas equilibration.[5] However, aerobic training does not result in an increase in pulmonary capillaries and so training does not increase pulmonary capillary blood volume. This means that highly aerobically trained individuals, in whom cardiac outputs of 30 L·min^{-1} or higher are possible, transit time through the pulmonary capillaries can become less than that necessary for optimal gas exchange. This, along with possibly other factors, such as no hyperventilation response to intense exercise in aerobically trained athletes, results in a decrease in total gas exchange per volume of blood moving through the lungs. So, in highly trained individuals, gas exchange at the lungs can become inefficient at near-maximal exercise intensities.

Quick Review

- Capillary gas exchange at the lungs mainly is dependent on the partial pressure difference between air within the alveoli and blood.
- The amount of oxygen and carbon dioxide dissolved in the blood is directly dependent on the gas's partial pressure.
- The respiratory and cellular membranes are more permeable to carbon dioxide than oxygen, so the partial pressure differences on either side of these membranes can be less for carbon dioxide.
- Even at maximal exercise intensities, optimal pulmonary gas exchange is maintained in untrained or moderately trained individuals. However, for highly trained aerobic athletes, pulmonary gas exchange may become inefficient at maximal exercise intensities.

BLOOD GAS TRANSPORT

Once capillary gas exchange at the lungs has taken place, oxygen must be carried in the blood to the body's tissues. Similarly, carbon dioxide must be carried from the body's tissues to the lungs. Only approximately 3 mL of oxygen can be dissolved in a liter of blood plasma. Assuming a total plasma volume of 3 to 5 L, only approximately 9 to 15 mL of oxygen is carried dissolved in plasma, which is insufficient to meet the needs of the body's tissues even at rest. So, there needs to be another way to carry oxygen within the blood. Erythrocytes, or red blood cells containing **hemoglobin** (an iron-containing pigment capable of reversibly binding oxygen), increase the blood's ability to carry oxygen.

Similarly, only approximately 7% to 10% of the carbon dioxide found in blood is transported in a dissolved state. The remainder is transported as bicarbonate ions and bound to hemoglobin. In the next sections, gas transport is further explored.

Oxygen Transport

More than 98% of the oxygen transported in the blood is chemically bound to hemoglobin. Hemoglobin is composed of a protein (globin) and an iron molecule (heme) component. The iron is necessary in order to reversibly bind four oxygen molecules per hemoglobin molecule. When oxygen is bound to hemoglobin, **oxyhemoglobin** is formed, whereas hemoglobin not bound to oxygen is termed **deoxyhemoglobin**. Because the vast majority of oxygen is transported bound to hemoglobin, its concentration determines the amount of oxygen that can be transported by the blood. In men and women, hemoglobin concentration ranges from 14 to 18 g·100 mL^{-1} blood and 12 to 16 g·100 mL^{-1} blood, respectively. Each gram of hemoglobin can reversibly bind 1.34 mL of oxygen,[12] resulting in a range of oxygen-carrying ability in men and women of 16 to 24 mL of oxygen per 100 mL if the hemoglobin is 100% saturated with oxygen. When looking at hemoglobin concentration only, it would appear that maximal oxygen transport ability is greater in men. However, because the range of hemoglobin concentrations between the sexes overlaps, blood oxygen–carrying ability between the sexes also overlaps. Because of the importance of hemoglobin for the transport of oxygen, a decrease in hemoglobin is very detrimental to oxygen transport (see Box 6-3, "Common Types of Anemia").

Oxyhemoglobin Disassociation Curve

If hemoglobin is to transport oxygen from the lungs to the body's tissues, there has to be a stimulus for hemoglobin to reversibly bind oxygen at the lungs and release oxygen to the body's tissues. The ability of hemoglobin to bind and release oxygen at the correct sites within the body is explained by the oxyhemoglobin disassociation curve

Box 6-3 DID YOU KNOW?
Common Types of Anemia

Anemia is a deficiency in the number of red blood cells or of their hemoglobin content, or a combination of these two factors. Anemia results in a decrease in the ability to transport oxygen and so can affect endurance or aerobic capabilities. Symptoms of anemia include pallor, easy fatigue, breathlessness with exertion, heart palpitations, and loss of appetite. Iron deficiency can result in anemia and is the most common type of anemia. It most commonly occurs due to an insufficient intake of iron in the diet or impaired iron absorption. However, iron-deficient anemia can also occur because of hemorrhage or increased iron needs, such as during pregnancy.

Sports anemia refers to reduced hemoglobin concentrations that approach clinical anemia (12 and 14 g·dL^{-1} of blood in women and men, respectively) caused by the performance of physical training. Although physical training does result in a small loss of iron in sweat, loss of hemoglobin caused by increased destruction of red blood cells, and possibly gastrointestinal bleeding with distance running sports, anemia is typically not caused by these factors. Physical training, including both aerobic training

and weight training, results in a plasma volume increase of up to 20% during the first several days of training. This plasma volume increase parallels the decrease in hemoglobin concentration.[1,2] The total amount of hemoglobin within the blood does not significantly change, but due to the increase in plasma volume, hemoglobin concentration decreases. After several weeks of training, hemoglobin concentrations and hematocrit return toward normal. Thus, sports anemia is normally a transient event and less prevalent than once believed.[3]

References

1. Deruisseau KC, Roberts LM, Kushnick MR, et al. Iron status of young males and females performing weight training exercise. Med Sci Spots Exerc. 2004;36:241–248.
2. Schumacher YO, Schmid A, Grathwohl D, et al. Hematological indices of iron status of athletes in various sports and performances. Med Sci Spots Exerc. 2002;34:869–875.
3. Wright LM, Klein M, Noakes TD, et al. Sports anemia: a real or apparent phenomenon in endurance trained athletes. Int J Sports Med. 1992;13:344–347.

(Fig. 6-8). At the lungs, where there is a high P_{O_2}, hemoglobin binds oxygen, forming oxyhemoglobin, and becomes 100% saturated with oxygen. When hemoglobin is 100% saturated with oxygen, it is carrying the maximal amount of oxygen possible. At tissues where oxygen is used for aerobic metabolism, there is a low P_{O_2} and hemoglobin releases oxygen or becomes less than 100% saturated, with hemoglobin being converted to deoxyhemoglobin.

The oxyhemoglobin disassociation curve is sigmoidal, or has an "S" shape. This shape offers advantages to hemoglobin becoming both oxyhemoglobin at the lungs and deoxyhemoglobin at the tissue level. First, at a P_{O_2} ranging from 90 to 100 mm Hg, oxygen saturation is above 97% and the curve is quite flat, meaning there is only a small change in oxygen saturation when a change in P_{O_2} occurs. P_{O_2} at the lungs is approximately 105 mm Hg, ensuring that 100% oxygen saturation occurs, but even if P_{O_2} decreases to as low as 90 mm Hg, little change in oxygen saturation would occur. This is physiologically important because it ensures that close to 100% saturation takes place at the lungs even if P_{O_2} at the lungs decreases due to factors such as assent to moderate altitude.

The oxyhemoglobin disassociation curve has a very steep slope from 0 to 40 mm Hg P_{O_2}. At active tissue, where P_{O_2} is low, this portion of the curve ensures that for a small change in P_{O_2} a very large change in oxygen saturation will take place, meaning oxygen will be more readily released and available to the tissue. This portion of the curve is critical for the supply of oxygen to tissue during exercise, when P_{O_2} at the tissue level decreases. At rest, tissue needs little oxygen and approximately 75% of the oxygen remains bound to hemoglobin, meaning 25% of the oxygen is released to tissues. During exercise, only approximately 10% of the oxygen remains bound to hemoglobin, so 90% of the oxygen carried by hemoglobin is released to tissues. Other factors, in addition to the sigmoid shape of the oxyhemoglobin disassociation curve, help to ensure adequate oxygen delivery to tissue during exercise.

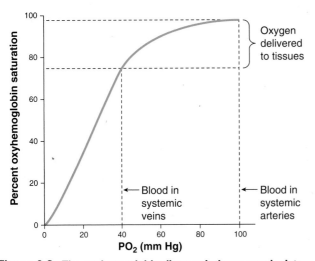

Figure 6-8. The oxyhemoglobin disassociation curve depicts the relationship between hemoglobin saturation with oxygen and the partial pressure of oxygen. The difference in oxygen saturation between the lungs and tissue is the amount of oxygen delivered to the tissue.

Temperature Effect

An increase or decrease in blood temperature shifts the oxyhemoglobin disassociation curve to the right and left, respectively (Fig. 6-9). This means that an increase in temperature, with other factors remaining constant, decreases the affinity of hemoglobin for oxygen, resulting in a lower percentage oxygen saturation at any given P_{O_2}. Conversely, a decrease in temperature increases the affinity of hemoglobin for oxygen, shifting the curve to the left. During exercise, the effect of temperature on the oxyhemoglobin disassociation curve helps in the delivery of oxygen to muscle tissue. This is because during exercise muscle tissue temperature increases, resulting in a shift to the right of the oxyhemoglobin disassociation curve, which in turn leads to more oxygen delivery to the active tissue.

pH Effect

The effect of pH or acidity on the oxyhemoglobin disassociation curve is termed the **Bohr effect**. An increase in

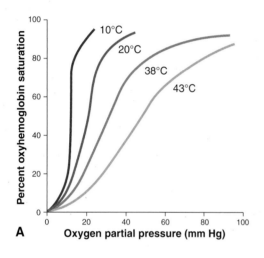

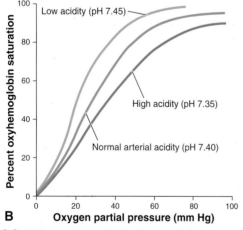

A

B

Figure 6-9. If the oxyhemoglobin disassociation curve moves to the right and left at any particular partial pressure of oxygen, saturation decreases and increases, respectively. Increased temperature and acidity move the oxyhemoglobin disassociation curve to the right. Decreased temperature and acidity move the oxyhemoglobin disassociation curve to the left.

acidity (decreased pH) shifts the curve to the right, whereas a decrease in acidity (increased pH) shifts the curve to the left (Fig. 6-9). During intense exercise, especially exercise that is anaerobic in nature, acidity or concentration of hydrogen ions (H^+) increases in the working muscle and in the blood circulating through the muscle (see Chapter 2). The H^+ reversibly binds to hemoglobin, reducing hemoglobin's affinity for oxygen and causing the oxyhemoglobin disassociation curve to shift to the right. This has the same effect as an increase in temperature at active muscle tissue, resulting in an increase in delivery of oxygen to the active tissue. So, in active muscle tissue, both an increase in temperature and increased H^+ shift the oxyhemoglobin disassociation curve to the right, resulting in increased oxygen delivery to the active muscle tissue.

2,3-Diphosphoglycerate Effect

Red blood cells contain no mitochondria and so derive energy only from the anaerobic reactions of glycolysis. A byproduct of these reactions is 2,3-diphosphoglycerate (2,3 DPG). 2,3 DPG can bind loosely to hemoglobin, reducing its affinity for oxygen, shifting the oxyhemoglobin disassociation curve to the right, and thus increasing oxygen delivery to tissue.[9] However, the effects of exercise training and acute bouts of exercise on 2,3 DPG are equivocal. For example, although it has been shown that resting levels of 2,3 DPG are higher in athletes than untrained individuals, it has also been reported that short-term moderate intensity exercise does not affect 2,3 DPG, but both high-intensity exercise and prolonged moderate-intensity activity increase 2,3 DPG levels in the blood.[13,15,17,18] So, the effect of exercise and training on 2,3 DPG concentrations and, therefore, any effect on the oxyhemoglobin disassociation curve is unclear. Higher levels of 2,3 DPG have been shown in people who live at altitude, which could represent a genetic factor or an adaptation to long-term exposure to altitude. So, although 2,3 DPG can affect the oxyhemoglobin disassociation curve, its physiological effect due to training is unclear.

Carbon Dioxide Transport

There are three methods by which carbon dioxide is transported in the blood: (1) 7% to 10% is dissolved in plasma, (2) approximately 20% is bound to hemoglobin, and (3) approximately 70% is transported as bicarbonate. All three methods of transport begin with carbon dioxide produced during metabolism, resulting in a high P_{CO_2} within the tissue, and the carbon dioxide diffusing into the plasma of blood. Some of the carbon dioxide remains in the dissolved state and is carried to the lungs. Red blood cells transport not only oxygen but also carbon dioxide. The transport of carbon dioxide bound to hemoglobin and as bicarbonate deserves some further explanation because these forms of carbon dioxide transport are linked to the transport of oxygen. The three methods of carbon dioxide transport and how they are linked to oxygen transport are depicted in Figure 6-10.

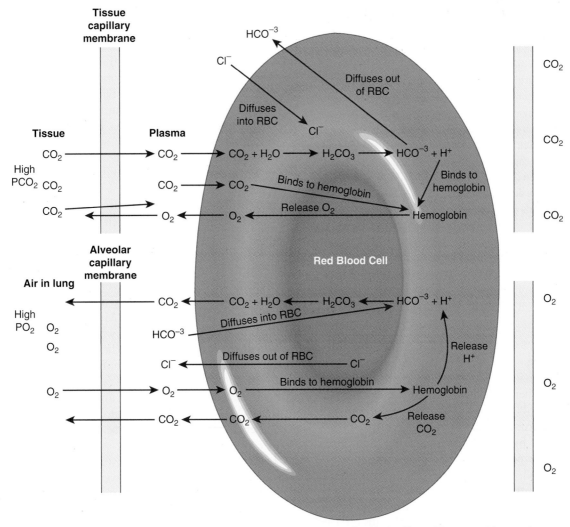

Figure 6-10. **The ability of hemoglobin to bind oxygen and carbon dioxide is affected by several factors in addition to the partial pressure of oxygen.** Changes in acidity, the chloride shift, and the noncompeting binding of carbon dioxide and oxygen by hemoglobin all effect hemoglobin's ability to bind oxygen.

Carbaminohemoglobin Transport of Carbon Dioxide

At tissue where P_{CO_2} is high, carbon dioxide can be bound to hemoglobin, forming **carbaminohemoglobin**. Carbon dioxide binds with amino acids that are part of the globin portion of hemoglobin. Because carbon dioxide binds to the globin and oxygen to the heme portion of hemoglobin, these two methods of transport do not compete. However, oxygenation of hemoglobin at the lungs reduces hemoglobin's ability to bind carbon dioxide by causing a conformational shift in the structure of the hemoglobin molecule. Thus, oxygenation and a low P_{CO_2} at the lungs both facilitate carbon dioxide being released from hemoglobin. Once released from hemoglobin, the carbon dioxide dissolves in plasma, diffuses into the air in the alveoli, and is expired.

Bicarbonate Transport of Carbon Dioxide

At tissues where a high P_{CO_2} exists, carbon dioxide is converted within the red blood cells to bicarbonate:

$$CO_2 + H_2O \rightleftarrows H_2CO_3 \rightleftarrows H^+ + HCO^{-3} \qquad (8)$$

Formation of carbonic acid (H_2CO_3) is facilitated by the enzyme carbonic anhydrase found in red blood cells. Once formed, carbonic acid disassociates, resulting in a hydrogen ion (H^+) and a bicarbonate ion (HCO^{-3}). The bicarbonate ion diffuses out of the red blood cell into the plasma. Note that the bicarbonate ion has a negative charge, and removal of the negative charge from any cell, including a red blood cell, results in an electrical imbalance across the cell's membrane. To prevent this electrical imbalance, a chloride ion (Cl^-) diffuses into the red blood cell. This exchange of the

Quick Review

- The reversible binding of oxygen to hemoglobin accounts for 98% of the oxygen transported by blood.
- The sigmoidal shape of the oxyhemoglobin disassociation curve ensures near-maximal formation of oxyhemoglobin at the lungs even when the atmospheric partial pressure of oxygen decreases. It also ensures that small changes in partial pressure result in release of oxygen at active tissue.
- Changes in temperature and acidity shift the oxyhemoglobin disassociation curve, causing greater delivery of oxygen to muscle tissue during exercise.
- Three methods are responsible for carbon dioxide transport, but 70% of carbon dioxide is transported in the form of bicarbonate.
- The transport of oxygen and that of carbon dioxide is linked by the formation of carbaminohemoglobin and the buffering of hydrogen ions by hemoglobin, which decrease hemoglobin's affinity for oxygen.

bicarbonate ion for a chloride ion is termed the **chloride shift**.

The hydrogen ion produced is bound to the globin part of hemoglobin. So, hemoglobin acts as a buffer and helps maintain normal acidity (pH) within the red blood cell. Hemoglobin's buffering of hydrogen ions reduces its affinity for oxygen. So, the buffering of hydrogen ions triggers the Bohr effect or moves the oxyhemoglobin disassociation curve to the right. At the tissue level, this results in the release of oxygen from hemoglobin so that it is available for metabolism.

The bicarbonate reaction can proceed in either direction. At the lungs, where P_{CO_2} is low within the alveoli, carbon dioxide diffuses out of solution, disturbing the balance of the bicarbonate reaction and causing this reaction to proceed in the direction of the production of carbon dioxide and water. Additionally, oxygenation of hemoglobin causes it to lose its affinity for hydrogen ions. Thus, they are available for the production of carbonic acid, which because of the low P_{CO_2}, disassociates into carbon dioxide and water. So, the release of oxygen by hemoglobin at tissue is linked to the transport of carbon dioxide by hemoglobin, and the release of carbon dioxide by hemoglobin at the lungs is linked to oxygenation of hemoglobin.

GAS EXCHANGE AT THE MUSCLE

Gas exchange at the muscle or any tissue occurs due to differences in P_{O_2} and P_{CO_2} between the tissue and capillary blood (Fig. 6-7). All of the factors previously described concerning partial pressure differences and blood transport of oxygen and carbon dioxide apply to capillary gas exchange at the tissue level. The amount of oxygen delivered to tissue can be calculated using the Fick principle and the arterial-venous oxygen difference (see "Oxygen Delivery

to Tissue" section in Chapter 5). Once oxygen has diffused into tissue, an oxygen carrier molecule (myoglobin) within muscle assists in its transport to the mitochondria.

Myoglobin is an oxygen transport molecule similar to hemoglobin except that it is found within skeletal and cardiac muscle. Myoglobin reversibly binds with oxygen, and its role is to assist in the passive diffusion of oxygen from the cell membrane to the mitochondria. Because the rate of diffusion slows exponentially as distance is increased, myoglobin located between the membrane and the mitochondria actually results in two smaller diffusion distances rather than a single long one. As a result, the transit time of oxygen across the muscle fiber to the mitochondria is significantly reduced.

Different from hemoglobin, myoglobin contains only one iron molecule, whereas hemoglobin contains four iron molecules. Muscle that appears reddish contains large amounts of myoglobin, whereas muscles that appear white contain small amounts of myoglobin. The concentration of myoglobin within a muscle fiber varies with the muscle fiber type (see Chapter 3). Myoglobin concentration is high in type I muscle fibers with a high aerobic capacity (slowtwitch), whereas type IIa (fast-twitch) and type IIx (fast-twitch) muscle fibers contain an intermediate and a limited amount of myoglobin, respectively.

In addition to speeding up the diffusion of oxygen across the muscle fiber, myoglobin functions as an oxygen "reserve" at the start of exercise. Even with the anticipatory rise (see "Effects of Exercise on Pulmonary Ventilation," below) in breathing rate prior to the beginning of exercise, there is a lag in oxygen delivery to muscle. During this period, the oxygen bound to myoglobin helps to maintain the oxygen requirements of muscle that is becoming active. Upon the cessation of exercise, myoglobin oxygen must be replenished and is a small component of the oxygen deficit (see Chapter 2).

Although myoglobin and hemoglobin are similar in chemical structure, one difference between these two molecules is that myoglobin has a much steeper oxygen disassociation curve and approaches 100% oxygen saturation at a much lower P_{O_2} (30 mm Hg). Because of these factors, myoglobin releases its oxygen at very low levels of P_{O_2}, which is important because within the mitochondria of active muscle, the P_{O_2} can be as low as 2 mm Hg. Thus, myoglobin's oxygen disassociation curve allows it to transport oxygen at the lower levels of P_{O_2} (40 mm Hg) found within skeletal muscle.

Quick Review

- Gas exchange at tissue occurs due to partial pressure differences in oxygen and carbon dioxide between the tissue and the blood.
- Myoglobin, a molecule similar to hemoglobin, transports oxygen from the cell membrane to the mitochondria for use in aerobic metabolism.

CONTROL OF VENTILATION

Control of ventilation and pulmonary gas exchange is necessary in order to maintain homeostasis at rest and to match the tissue needs for oxygen and removal of carbon dioxide during exercise. Much of this requisite control is met by involuntary regulation of pulmonary ventilation. Although the control of pulmonary ventilation has been studied by physiologists for many years, there is still much to learn. But what we do know is that there are several areas within the body and central nervous system that contribute to ventilatory control by monitoring P_{O_2}, P_{CO_2}, and H^+ concentrations within the blood and cerebral spinal fluid. As might be expected, a decrease in P_{O_2}, an increase in P_{CO_2}, and increased H^+ concentration, as would occur during exercise, increases pulmonary ventilation. In contrast, increased P_{O_2}, decreased P_{CO_2} and decreased H^+ concentrations result in decreased pulmonary ventilation. The next sections explore pulmonary ventilation control.

Respiratory Control Center

Although not completely elucidated, a portion of the medulla oblongata (ventral lateral medulla) and pons make up the respiratory control center, serving as a "pacemaker" capable of generating a rhythmical breathing pattern.[5] The rate and depth of breathing can be modified by input from higher brain centers, chemoreceptors in the medulla itself, and other peripheral inputs to change pulmonary ventilation so that it meets the gas exchange needs at rest and during exercise (Fig. 6-11). The breathing pattern generated by the respiratory control center is then passed down the spinal cord to the respiratory muscles. Control of pulmonary ventilation is involuntary. However, it is possible to voluntarily change pulmonary ventilation, such as holding your breath, but even in this situation involuntary control will normally override your voluntary effort to control pulmonary ventilation. The various inputs to control inspiration and expiration are discussed in the next sections.

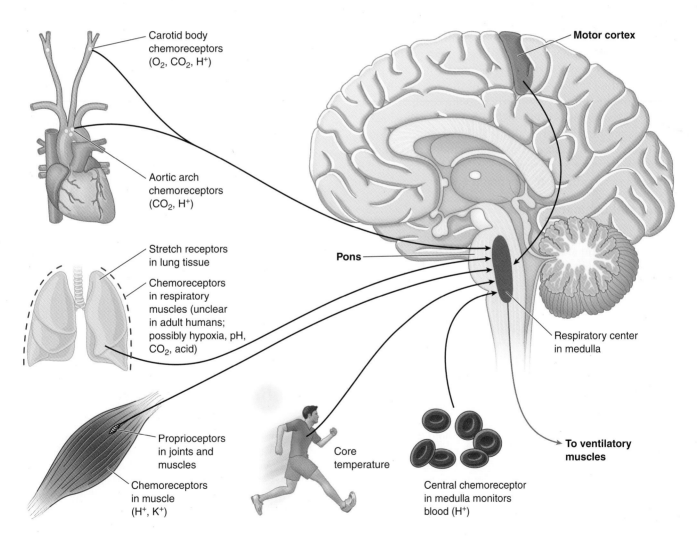

Figure 6-11. The respiratory control center is located within the medulla. The respiratory control center adjusts pulmonary ventilation to meet the body's needs due to feedback from chemoreceptors and proprioceptors.

Central Chemoreceptors

Chemoreceptors are receptors that respond to chemical changes. The **central chemoreceptors** are located within the medulla, but are anatomically separate from the respiratory control center. These chemoreceptors respond to changes within the cerebral spinal fluid and are especially sensitive to changes of H^+ concentration or pH.[5] The capillary membranes of cerebral blood vessels are very permeable to carbon dioxide, so carbon dioxide readily and quickly diffuses into the cerebral spinal fluid when blood P_{CO_2} increases, such as during exercise. Increased carbon dioxide concentration within the cerebral spinal fluid quickly increases the hydrogen ion concentration due to the bicarbonate reaction as described above. The increased H^+ concentration of the cerebral spinal fluid stimulates an increase in pulmonary ventilation to increase the elimination of carbon dioxide from the body. So, changes in H^+ concentration, not P_{CO_2}, are the stimulus for central chemoreceptors to change pulmonary ventilation. During exercise, hydrogen ion concentration in the blood could increase indirectly due to greater carbon dioxide concentrations, as mentioned earlier, or due to an increased reliance on anaerobic metabolism and lactic acid production (see Chapter 2). However, hydrogen ions are not very permeable to the capillary membranes of the cerebral blood vessels, so they diffuse very slowly into the cerebral spinal fluid from the blood. So, although either carbon dioxide or H^+ diffusion into the cerebral spinal fluid from the blood would increase H^+ concentration and so pulmonary ventilation, the response to an increased carbon dioxide concentration and the bicarbonate reaction is quicker.

Peripheral Chemoreceptors

Peripheral chemoreceptors are chemoreceptors located within the carotid arteries and the aortic arch. The receptors located within the aortic arch are termed the aortic bodies, and those within the carotid arteries are termed the carotid bodies. Both the aortic and carotid bodies respond to changes in blood P_{CO_2} and H^+ concentration, with carotid bodies also responding to changes in blood P_{O_2}.[5] However, these receptors would only be stimulated by severe (>40%) decreases in P_{O_2}, and they typically affect breathing only in those individuals with pulmonary disease (emphysema, COPD, etc.). Remember that blood H^+ concentration can be elevated due to increased acidity caused by anaerobic metabolism during exercise, or increased P_{CO_2}, resulting in the bicarbonate reaction. Although the peripheral chemoreceptors are sensitive to both P_{O_2} and P_{CO_2}, changes in P_{CO_2} are a stronger stimulus to change pulmonary ventilation (see Box 6-4).

The location of the peripheral chemoreceptors allows them to monitor chemical changes at two key places within the circulatory system. The carotid bodies monitor the blood supply to the head and brain, whereas the aortic bodies monitor blood that has just returned from the pulmonary circulation and is being pumped to the systemic circulation. Although both the aortic and carotid bodies impact pulmonary ventilation, the carotid bodies appear to be the more important peripheral chemoreceptors.

Other Neural Input

Other neural input also affects pulmonary ventilation. The lungs contain stretch receptors, mainly in the bronchioles, which when stimulated can terminate inspiration, limiting the end-inspiratory volume of the lungs.[5] Respiratory muscles, including the diaphragm and abdominal muscles, also contain stretch receptors and receptors sensing metabolic changes within these muscles. Similarly, skeletal muscle (muscle spindles and Golgi tendon organs; see Chapter 3) contain proprioceptors and chemoreceptors sensitive to, respectively, changes in body position and potassium (potassium concentrations in muscle increase during exercise) as well as hydrogen ion concentrations. Joints contain proprioceptors sensitive to pressure. Stimulation of any of these receptors affects pulmonary ventilation. For example, increased hydrogen ion concentration within muscle and

---

 ## Box 6-4 PRACTICAL QUESTIONS FROM STUDENTS

Why Do Swimmers Hyperventilate Before a Race?

Swimmers voluntarily hyperventilate prior to a race to remove CO_2 from their blood so they can hold their breath longer during the race. Carbon dioxide is the major stimulus for breathing. By voluntarily hyperventilating, low CO_2 concentration atmospheric air is brought into the lungs reducing the partial pressure of CO_2 in the air in the alveoli. This results in more CO_2 leaving the blood, reducing the partial pressure of CO_2 in the blood. Thus when the race starts and the swimmer holds their breath during the race it takes longer for the partial pressure of CO_2 in the blood to

increase to the point where the stimulus to breathe caused by the chemoreceptors will force the swimmer to take a breath. Voluntary hyperventilation is normally performed only by freestyle sprint swimmers. In these events whenever the swimmer turns their head and rolls their body to the side slightly to take a breath the surface area of their body exposed to the water in the direction of movement increases. This increases drag and so slows the swimmer. This is why they want to breathe as few times as possible during the race, and voluntary hyperventilation allows them to do so.

increased muscle movement both would increase pulmonary ventilation. Additionally, neural activity in the motor cortex can stimulate an increase in pulmonary ventilation. Increased pulmonary ventilation prior to the onset of exercise is normally attributed to increased motor cortex activity. Thus, many types of input affect pulmonary ventilation and gas exchange so that the needs of the body are met at rest and during exercise. Control of pulmonary ventilation during exercise is explored in the next sections.

EFFECTS OF EXCERCISE ON PULMONARY VENTILATION

During exercise, capillary gas exchange at the alveoli and muscle tissue increases to meet the greater needs for oxygen delivery and carbon dioxide removal. To increase capillary gas exchange, pulmonary ventilation increases under the control of all the factors previously discussed. To augment gas exchange at the alveoli and at active tissue, blood flow through the capillary beds of the alveoli and tissue must also increase. For blood flow to increase, factors related to the circulatory system, such as amplified cardiac output and redistribution of blood flow away from inactive tissue and into active tissue (see Chapter 5), must take place. So, although in the next sections the effect of exercise on pulmonary ventilation will be discussed, it should be understood that for increased gas exchange to take place, increased blood flow due to the acute effects of exercise on the circulatory system must also take place.

Submaximal Exercise and Pulmonary Ventilation

Although other factors are involved, during resting conditions pulmonary ventilation is primarily regulated by plasma P_{CO_2}. But during exercise, it is unclear which factors controlling pulmonary ventilation exert the greatest influence. That said, it has been shown that during submaximal exercise plasma P_{CO_2} is tightly regulated, suggesting that it is a major controlling factor of pulmonary ventilation, with other factors acting to fine-tune pulmonary ventilation to meet the needs of exercise. However, the tight control of P_{CO_2} is probably related to the effect of increased acidity (bicarbonate reaction) caused by increased plasma P_{CO_2}, as opposed to control of P_{CO_2} itself.

There appear to be three phases of pulmonary ventilation control to increase alveolar ventilation during submaximal exercise.[8] At the start of exercise, or even slightly prior to the start of exercise, pulmonary ventilation increases because of the effect of motor cortex activity on the respiratory centers. This, combined with feedback from proprioceptors in active muscles at the start of exercise, causes an abrupt increase in ventilation. This abrupt increase at the start of exercise is phase 1 of ventilatory control (Fig. 6-12). After a short plateau lasting approximately 20 seconds, pulmonary ventilation then rises almost exponentially to reach a steady-state level (exercise intensity at which the majority of metabolic needs are met by aerobic metabolism). This quick rise in pulmonary ventilation is phase 2 and is caused by the continued effect of motor cortex activity, feedback from active muscle, and feedback from peripheral chemoreceptors.[19] During phase 3, the final phase of pulmonary ventilation control, fine-tuning of pulmonary ventilation during steady-state exercise takes place due to feedback from peripheral chemoreceptors and central chemoreceptors so that pulmonary ventilation is matched to meet the demands of submaximal exercise. Increased body temperature may also have a minimal effect on pulmonary ventilation, except during extreme hyperthermia.

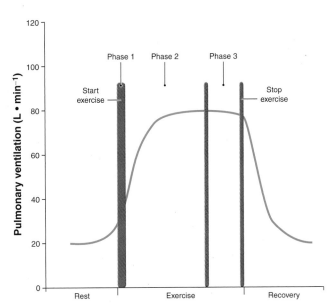

Figure 6-12. At the start of exercise, pulmonary ventilation increases to meet the needs of the body. There are three phases of changes in pulmonary ventilation from the beginning of an exercise bout to the cessation of exercise.

Upon cessation of exercise, there is a quick drop in pulmonary ventilation due to the removal of feedback from motor cortex activity and proprioceptors in active muscle. This quick drop is followed by a slower return to resting pulmonary ventilation as recovery from the metabolic stress of exercise takes place (see Chapter 2, "Post Exercise Oxygen Consumption").

Near-Maximal Exercise and Pulmonary Ventilation

As exercise intensity progresses from rest to near-maximal or maximal intensities, pulmonary ventilation goes through the three phases described above. However, during heavy exercise (beyond approximately 50%–60% of peak oxygen consumption), there is a disproportionate (you ventilate more air to get 1 L of oxygen) increase in pulmonary ventilation relative to the increase in exercise intensity. The major factor typically used to explain this disproportionate increase in pulmonary ventilation is an increase in plasma lactate and H^+ concentration (increased acidity or decreased pH) because the exercise intensity is above lactate threshold (see Chapter 2). The increased H^+ concentration stimulates the peripheral chemoreceptors to increase pulmonary ventilation. Recall that the capillary membranes of cerebral blood vessels are permeable to H^+, but not to a great extent (see "Central Chemoreceptors" above), so the central chemoreceptors respond more slowly than the peripheral chemoreceptors to changes in H^+ concentration. Increased acidity is a factor contributing to this disproportionate increase in pulmonary ventilation at high workloads.[5] There are, however, other factors that contribute to the disproportionate increase in pulmonary ventilation at near-maximal workloads. Increasing levels

of norepinephrine (a hormone associated with the fight-or-flight response and mobilization of metabolic fuels) and increased levels of potassium within the plasma probably also contribute to increased pulmonary ventilation. Likewise, an elevated body temperature may also increase pulmonary ventilation. So, although this disproportionate increase at near-maximal workloads is associated with increased acidity, other factors also affect pulmonary ventilation. The association with increased acidity and so lactate threshold has led to the use of this disproportionate increase in pulmonary ventilation as a method to noninvasively estimate lactate threshold, which is further explored in the next sections.

VENTILATION IS ASSOCIATED WITH METABOLISM

Recall that oxygen consumption has a linear relationship to workload or exercise intensity (see Chapter 5). Because of the control of pulmonary ventilation, as discussed above, you might hypothesize that pulmonary ventilation also has a linear relationship to workload. Although pulmonary ventilation is, in large part, controlled by P_{CO_2}, P_{O_2}, and H^+ concentration, all of which are related to metabolism, the relationship between its regulation and workload or oxygen consumption is not perfectly linear. In the next sections, the relationship between pulmonary ventilation, oxygen consumption, and carbon dioxide expiration are explored.

Ventilatory Equivalents

The **ventilatory equivalent of oxygen** is the ratio between pulmonary ventilation ($\dot{V}_E$) and oxygen ($\dot{V}_{O_2}$) or $\dot{V}_E/\dot{V}_{O_2}$. Similarly the **ventilatory equivalent of carbon dioxide** is the ratio of pulmonary ventilation ($\dot{V}_E$) to carbon dioxide ($\dot{V}_{CO_2}$) or $\dot{V}_E/\dot{V}_{CO_2}$. The ventilatory equivalent indicates the amount of air ventilated ($\dot{V}_E$) needed to obtain 1 L of oxygen or expire 1 L of carbon dioxide. At rest, $\dot{V}_E/\dot{V}_{O_2}$ in healthy adults is approximately 26, meaning 26 L of air is ventilated to obtain 1 L of oxygen.[5] While at rest $\dot{V}_E/\dot{V}_{CO_2}$ in healthy adults is approximately 33 meaning 33 L of air is ventilated to expire 1 L carbon dioxide.[5] Ventilatory equivalents can be used to estimate lactate threshold and indicate what factors help control pulmonary ventilation.

Ventilatory Threshold

Ventilatory threshold (VT) refers to a technique using $\dot{V}_E/\dot{V}_{O_2}$ and $\dot{V}_E/\dot{V}_{CO_2}$ to estimate lactate threshold. Whether an individual is untrained or a trained endurance athlete, the initial response to an increasing workload is a decrease of both $\dot{V}_E/\dot{V}_{O_2}$ and $\dot{V}_E/\dot{V}_{CO_2}$ (Fig. 6-13). As workload increases, $\dot{V}_E/\dot{V}_{O_2}$ also starts to increase. This increase occurs at a workload approximately 50% to 55%

Quick Review

- Increased cardiac output and redistribution of blood flow help to increase oxygen delivery and carbon dioxide removal from active tissue during exercise.
- At rest, the partial pressure of carbon dioxide within blood is tightly regulated; this regulation is probably because of changes in H^+ as opposed to partial pressure of carbon dioxide.
- Ventilation has three phases during submaximal work: phase 1, increased ventilation due to input from higher brain centers and active muscle; phase 2, increased ventilation due to continued effect of motor cortex activity, feedback from active muscle, and feedback from peripheral chemoreceptors; and phase 3, plateauing of ventilation due predominantly to input from peripheral chemoreceptors and central chemoreceptors.
- Above approximately 50% to 60% peak oxygen consumption, there is a disproportionate increase in ventilation because of increased acidity as well as other factors.

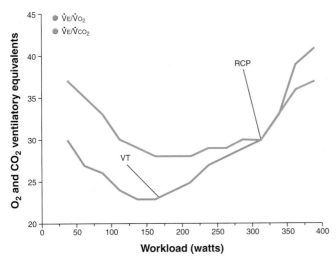

Figure 6-13. Detection of ventilatory threshold (VT) and respiratory compensation point (RCP) is shown using oxygen and carbon dioxide ventilatory equivalents. See the text for explanation of oxygen ($\dot{V}E/\dot{V}O_2$) and carbon dioxide ventilatory equivalents ($\dot{V}E/\dot{V}CO_2$). The data is for a 23-year-old triathlete with a cycling $\dot{V}O_{2peak}$ of 70.7 mL·kg·min^{-1}, maximal pulmonary ventilation of 159.4 L·min^{-1}, and maximal heart rate of 202 beats per minute. (Data courtesy of A. Lucia's laboratory, European University of Madrid, Madrid, Spain.)

of peak oxygen consumption ($\dot{V}O_{2peak}$) in untrained individuals and at higher exercise intensities in endurance trained athletes. Recall that approximately 50% to 60% of $\dot{V}O_{2peak}$ (see Chapter 2) in untrained adults is the intensity at which lactate threshold occurs, whereas in trained endurance athletes lactate threshold occurs at a higher percentage of $\dot{V}O_{2peak}$. After the initial decrease in $\dot{V}E/\dot{V}CO_2$, it remains relatively constant with increasing workload, but also eventually increases. How can this different pattern of changes in ventilatory equivalents indicate lactate threshold?

First, recall that the most important variable controlling ventilation is plasma PCO_2. This is indicated by the relatively stable $\dot{V}E/\dot{V}CO_2$ after its initial decrease with increasing workloads. This means you are ventilating the same amount of air to expire 1 L of carbon dioxide even as more carbon dioxide is produced by metabolism as the workload increases. Conversely $\dot{V}E/\dot{V}O_2$ after the initial decrease with increasing workload is stable for only a small change in workload and then increases. The stability of $\dot{V}E/\dot{V}CO_2$ over a relatively large increase in workload and the relative instability of $\dot{V}E/\dot{V}O_2$ with increasing intensity indicates plasma PCO_2 is more important than plasma PO_2 in controlling pulmonary ventilation.

VT is defined as a workload at which there is an increase in $\dot{V}E/\dot{V}O_2$ and no change in $\dot{V}E/\dot{V}CO_2$ (Fig. 6-13). The definition of VT can also include an increase in end-tidal (at the end of expiration) partial pressure of oxygen.[14] The

increase in $\dot{V}E/\dot{V}O_2$ and no change in $\dot{V}E/\dot{V}CO_2$ are related to metabolic changes that occur at, or past, the workload at which lactate threshold occurs.

Once the intensity at which lactate threshold occurs is exceeded, plasma acidity starts to increase due to a greater reliance on anaerobic energy sources, which can produce significant amounts of ATP only for short periods of time. The result is an imbalance between ATP needs and ATP production, causing increased muscle and plasma H^+ concentration (see Chapter 2). Additionally, lactic acid produced due to a reliance on anaerobic glycolysis is buffered by sodium bicarbonate, resulting in a production of carbon dioxide, which is not produced from aerobic metabolism:

$$\text{Lactic acid} + NaHCO_3 \text{ (sodium bicarbonate)} \rightleftarrows$$
$$\text{Na lactate} + H_2CO_3 \text{ (carbonic acid)} \rightleftarrows H_2O + CO_2 \quad (9)$$

The carbon dioxide produced by the buffering of lactic acid and the H^+ produced by the imbalance between ATP needs and ATP production stimulate peripheral chemoreceptors, resulting in an increase in $\dot{V}E$. However, because PCO_2 controls pulmonary ventilation to a large extent, $\dot{V}E$ stays in a constant ratio with $\dot{V}CO_2$; $\dot{V}E/\dot{V}CO_2$ is stable with increasing workloads. Conversely, because PO_2 controls pulmonary ventilation to a lesser extent, $\dot{V}E$ does not stay in a constant ratio with $\dot{V}O_2$ or $\dot{V}E/\dot{V}O_2$ with increasing exercise intensity. Although a meta-analysis indicates that VT can be used to estimate lactate threshold,[20] attempts to tightly associate the metabolic changes at lactate threshold with VT have been inconclusive. However, changes in ventilatory equivalents can be used to estimate lactate threshold.[20]

Respiratory Compensation Point

If work intensities higher than the point at which VT occurs are performed, there is a change in ventilatory equivalents. **Respiratory compensation point (RCP)** is defined as the work intensity at which both $\dot{V}E/\dot{V}O_2$ and $\dot{V}E/\dot{V}CO_2$ show an increase.[14] The definition of RCP can also include a decrease in end-tidal partial pressure of oxygen. These changes indicate an uncoupling of the control of pulmonary ventilation by plasma PCO_2 and may be due to increased acidity encountered at these higher workloads.

VT and RCP can be used to create three training zones of exercise intensity, based on heart rate,[14] in a manner similar to using lactate threshold and heart rates to estimate exercise intensity. A "light-intensity" training zone is below VT, which for trained endurance athletes would be below approximately 70% $\dot{V}O_{2peak}$. A "moderate-intensity" training zone is between VT and RCP, or between approximately 70% and 90% $\dot{V}O_{2peak}$ for trained endurance athletes. A "high-intensity" training zone is above RCP (see Box 6-5, "Use of Ventilatory Parameters to Improve Performance").

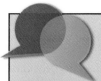

Box 6-5   AN EXPERT VIEW

Use of Ventilatory Parameters to Improve Performance

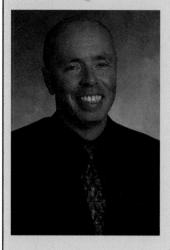

Conrad Earnest, PhD
Director Exercise Testing Core
Clinical Nutrition Unit
Pennington Biomedical Research Center
Baton Rouge, LA

Maximal oxygen consumption ($\dot{V}O_{2max}$) is determined during exercise testing and is a predictor of competition success during events relying heavily on cardiovascular ability. One might contend, however, that $\dot{V}O_{2max}$ serves only to identify the level at which an athlete might be capable of maximally performing. For example, given the relatively minimal room for $\dot{V}O_{2max}$ improvement, it is safe to say that all things being equal, an athlete with a maximal aerobic capacity of 2.5 $L \cdot min^{-1}$ is not capable of beating an individual with a $\dot{V}O_{2max}$ of 5.0 $L \cdot min^{-1}$.

Regardless of the competition level, several submaximal indices associated with exercise testing can also be used to examine an athlete's improvement and performance ability. These include assessment of lactic acid concentrations in the blood and the assessment of ventilatory threshold (VT) and respiratory compensation points (RCP). The advantage of assessing the latter indexes is that it can provide a secondary means of conforming transitions in lactate production and clearance, thus giving the practitioner even more concrete information for prescribing exercise training and assessing performance changes associated with training.[1] VT and RCP are discussed in more detail below.

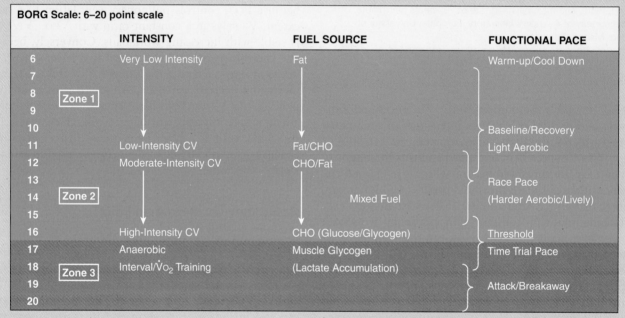

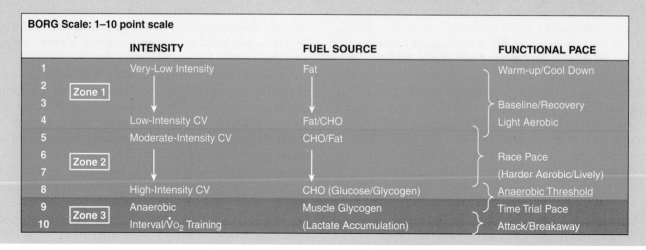

Ventilatory Threshold

Ventilatory threshold corresponds well with the concept of the lactate threshold or a rise in blood lactic acid concentration greater than 1 mmol·L^{-1} above rest. Typically, this ranges around 2 mM blood lactate in most people. Meyer et al.[1] have termed this phenomenon as the aerobic threshold. VT is obtained by using the "V-Slope Method," in which $\dot{V}O_2$ (L·min^{-1}) is plotted on the X-axis of a graph and $\dot{V}CO_2$ (L·min^{-1}) is plotted on the Y-axis. The underlying phenomenon surrounding the VT is that, at some point during an increasing exercise workload, the rise in blood lactate concentrations leads to an overproportional increase in CO_2 as related to oxygen uptake due to bicarbonate buffering of proton accumulation associated with lactate dissociation. When this occurs, there is a deflection in the line obtained from the previous graphing method. This can also be obtained by examining the first rise in the ventilatory equivalent for O_2 ($\dot{V}E/\dot{V}O_2$) without a concomitant rise in the ventilatory equivalent for CO_2 ($\dot{V}E/\dot{V}CO_2$).

Respiratory Compensation Point

The respiratory compensation point corresponds well with the concept of anaerobic threshold or the onset of blood lactic acid accumulation (OBLA). It is this point that is strongly associated with 10-km running pace and 40-km cycling time trial pace. It is also useful for delineating interval-training efforts. The underlying phenomenon is an accumulation of lactic acid equal to or greater than 4 mmol·L^{-1}, leading to the inability to buffer lactic acid via the use of the bicarbonate system. From a respiratory point of view, RCP represents the onset of exercise-induced hyperventilation due to inadequate bicarbonate buffering, thus causing an overproportional increase in ventilation ($\dot{V}E$) as related to $\dot{V}CO_2$. A synonymous term, albeit confusing, to describe this term is ventilatory threshold 2 (VT_2).

Putting It Together

The benefits of using VT and RCP as a training aid are many. When collected simultaneously, both can be used to establish basic training zones associated with heart rate, running pace, cycling power output, etc. A synopsis of these training zones is provided below.

Zone 1: The initiation of exercise through VT
  Intensity: Very low to low.
  Perceived Exertion: 6–11 on 6–20 and 1–4 on 1–10 Borg scales
  Energy Source: Fat and fat/carbohydrate
  Functional Pace: Warm-up, cool-down, baseline and recovery, light aerobic activity

Zone 2: VT through RCP
  Intensity: Moderate intensity cardiovascular through high-intensity cardiovascular
  Perceived Exertion: 12–16 on 6–20 and 5–8 on 1–10 Borg scales
  Energy Source: Carbohydrate/fat through glycolysis
  Functional Pace: Race pace

Zone 3: RCP and above
  Intensity: High-intensity cardiovascular through high-intensity cardiovascular
  Perceived Exertion: 17–20 on 6–20 and 9–10 on 1–10 Borg scales
  Energy Source: Muscle glycogen
  Functional Pace: Anaerobic threshold, interval training, attack, and breakaway pace

References

1. Meyer T, Lucia A, Earnest CP, et al. A conceptual framework for performance diagnosis and training prescription from submaximal gas exchange parameters–theory and application. Int J Sports Med. 2005;26(Suppl 1):S38–S48.
2. Lucia A, Earnest C, Arribas C. The Tour de France: a physiological review. Scand J Med Sci Sports. 2003;13(5):275–283.

Quick Review

- Ventilation is in part controlled by the partial pressure of carbon dioxide, partial pressure of oxygen, and acidity, all of which are related to metabolism. As a result, ventilation is not perfectly related to oxygen consumption.
- Because the ventilatory equivalent of carbon dioxide is a relatively stable number with increasing workloads, it indicates that partial pressure of carbon dioxide is a major factor controlling ventilation.
- Because the ventilatory equivalent of oxygen is a less stable number with increasing workloads than the ventilatory equivalent of carbon dioxide, it indicates that the partial pressure of oxygen exerts less control of ventilation than the partial pressure of carbon dioxide.
- Changes in the ventilatory equivalent of carbon dioxide and ventilatory equivalent of oxygen can be used to determine ventilatory threshold, an indirect estimate of lactate threshold.

VENTILATION LIMITS

As exercise intensity increases, so does $\dot{V}E$ because of an increase in both tidal volume and breathing frequency. At high exercise intensities, tidal volume tends to plateau so that the only way to further enhance $\dot{V}E$ is by increasing frequency. Corresponding to this, the work of ventilation is intensified, which in turn results in an increased need for oxygen by the respiratory muscles. For untrained healthy adults, the oxygen cost of ventilation is 3% to 5% of total oxygen intake ($\dot{V}O_2$) during moderate exercise, and increases to 8% to 10% of total oxygen intake at $\dot{V}O_{2peak}$.[1] As with other muscles, as exercise intensity increases, venous blood leaving the respiratory muscles shows increased oxygen desaturation, indicating an increase in a-v O_2 difference.[11]

The diaphragm is a highly oxidative muscle and therefore is fatigue resistant. Because of the diaphragm's resistance to fatigue during low- to moderate-intensity exercise in healthy adults at sea level, respiratory muscle fatigue does not appear to limit exercise performance.[7]

However, respiratory muscle fatigue does occur with some disease states, such as obstructive lung disease, and may occur at higher exercise intensities in healthy people.

Diaphragm force output in trained and untrained individuals is not decreased during exhaustive exercise at intensities less than 80% of $\dot{V}O_{2peak}$. However, during exercise at intensities greater than 80% to 85% of $\dot{V}O_{2peak}$ continued to exhaustion, diaphragm force output significantly decreases.[3,10] Fatigue of the diaphragm does not necessarily mean that the ability to ventilate the lungs is compromised, because some fatigue does not mean that the diaphragm cannot perform most of its ventilatory function. Additionally, if diaphragm fatigue is present, a greater portion of muscular work performed for ventilation may be assumed by accessory ventilatory muscles,

---

Box 6-6 DID YOU KNOW?

Diaphragm Training with Nonrespiratory Maneuvers

The diaphragm does undergo training-induced adaptations because of the need for increased pulmonary ventilation during physical activity, as well as because of the increased work of breathing with diseases such as chronic obstructive lung disease (COPD). However, the diaphragm also undergoes training-induced adaptations due to nonrespiratory maneuvers, such as physical labor and weight training exercises. During weight training exercises, such as sit-ups, bicep curls, bench press, and dead lifts, the diaphragm and abdominal musculature are recruited to help stabilize the lumbar spine area. Contraction of the abdominal musculature during weight training exercises results in an increase in intra-abdominal pressure that decreases the compressive forces on the spine and helps to stabilize the spine. The increase in intra-abdominal pressure also pushes the diaphragm into the thoracic cavity, resulting in an increase in the intrathoracic pressure. If the glottis is open due to the increase in intrathoracic pressure, air will leave the lungs. However, if the glottis is closed, a Valsalva maneuver is performed and blood pressure increases, substantially increasing the force the left ventricle must develop in order to eject blood into

the systemic circulation. This is why weight trainers are told not to perform the Valsalva maneuver or at least to minimize its effect. To decrease the intrathoracic pressure while performing a Valsalva maneuver, the diaphragm can be recruited. When active, the diaphragm flattens, resulting in an increase in intra-abdominal pressure and a decrease in intrathoracic pressure. If the diaphragm is recruited while performing a Valsalva maneuver, it decreases intrathoracic pressure, minimizing the effect of the Valsalva maneuver on blood pressure. Performing weight training exercises for 16 weeks significantly increases both the thickness of the diaphragm, indicating hypertrophy, and the maximal inspiratory pressure at the mouth, indicating an increase in force capabilities of the diaphragm.[1] Thus, the diaphragm not only adapts because of its recruitment during inspiration, but also because of recruitment during weight training exercises.

Reference

1. DePalo VA, Parker AL, Al-Bilbesi F, et al. Respiratory muscle strength training with nonrespiratory maneuvers. J Appl Physiol. 2004;96:731–734.

Box 6-7 APPLYING RESEARCH

Respiratory Muscle Training in Swimmers

It is controversial whether respiratory muscle training can increase vital capacity or total lung volume. If it is possible to increase these lung capacities, however, it would be advantageous to swimmers. An increase in vital capacity or total lung volume would increase the buoyancy of the swimmer. Passive drag while swimming (resistance to movement) is lower when lung volume is higher. This in part explains why a large total lung volume is beneficial for competitive swimmers. So, if respiratory muscle training would result in an increase in total lung capacity, it would be advantageous for the competitive swimmer.

Glossopharyngeal breathing (GPB) is the use of the glossopharyngeal muscles to assist in lung accommodation by pistoning or gulping small amounts of air (200 mL) into the lungs. This type of ventilation training is used by patients with neuromuscular disorders that affect respiratory muscles and can normalize tidal volumes within these patients.

GPB training performed for 6 weeks has been shown to increase vital capacity of healthy sedentary women by

3%.[1] GPB training performed for 5 weeks significantly increased vital capacity in female swimmers by 2%, but had no significant effect on vital capacity in male swimmers, although vital capacity did increase slightly.[2] The increase in vital capacity resulted in an increase in buoyancy of 0.17 and 0.37 kg in male and female swimmers, respectively. The authors speculated that GPB training resulting in an increase in vital capacity of swimmers would have a positive effect on the swimmers' maximal velocity through the water with filled or partially filled lungs.

References

1. Nygren-Bonnier M, Lindholm P, Markstrom A, et al. Effects of glossopharyngeal pistoning for lung insufflation on the vital capacity in healthy women. Am J Phys Med Rehabil. 2007a;86:290–294.
2. Nygren-Bonnier M, Gullstrand L, Klefbeck B, et al. Effects of glossopharyngeal pistoning for lung insufflation in elite swimmers. Med Sci Sports Exerc. 2007b;39:836–841.

and breathing frequency could also be increased to partially compensate for a decrease in tidal volume. If respiratory muscle fatigue does occur, it raises the question of whether respiratory muscles undergo training adaptations.

Research has shown that the respiratory muscles can, in fact, undergo adaptations to physical training. For example, the oxidative capacity of respiratory muscle increases due to endurance training.[16] The extra work of breathing required in those with chronic obstructive pulmonary disease (COPD), which increases airway resistance, also stimulates increased oxidative capacity of the respiratory muscles.[5] However, the concentration of glycolytic enzymes in respiratory muscles changes little with physical training. The improved oxidative capacity in the diaphragm of endurance-trained athletes allows the diaphragm to avoid indications of fatigue until

levels of $\dot{V}_E$ are reached that are higher than those of healthy, sedentary individuals. The improved oxidative capacity in the diaphragm of endurance-trained athletes allows that muscle to avoid indications of fatigue until reaching levels of $\dot{V}_E$ that are higher than those of healthy sedentary individuals.[2] Although the diaphragm is largely a respiratory muscle, it is also recruited during nonrespiratory maneuvers,[6] such as physical labor or weight training activities (see Box 6-6). In response to being recruited during nonrespiratory maneuvers, the diaphragm does hypertrophy, as indicated by an increase in diaphragm thickness and force capabilities.[6] So, it appears that respiratory muscles, like any other muscle, can undergo adaptations to physical training. One unique application of respiratory muscle training is used by swimmers and is described in Box 6-7.

CASE STUDY

Scenario

You are the coach for a Division I men's cross-country team at a university located at sea level. You are traveling to a competition at a university with a course located at 2,300 m in altitude.

Questions

How do you expect performance to be affected?

Options

Endurance events, lasting longer than 2 minutes, are highly reliant on oxygen delivery to tissue. At altitudes above sea level, partial pressure of O_2 is lower. This directly impacts the O_2 saturation of hemoglobin and oxygen transport. As P_{O_2} decreases, there is a decrease in the amount of O_2 bound to hemoglobin. Thus, the capacity to transport oxygen to exercising muscles is reduced and maximal oxygen consumption is reduced. Even with acclimatization, endurance performances will be hindered.

When exposed to low P_{O_2} at altitude, the body's response is to produce additional red blood cells to compensate for the desaturation of hemoglobin. Thus, allowing athletes sufficient time to acclimatize to the altitude may help performance. However, at altitude, training intensities will be hindered; thus, you may want your athletes to follow the model of "live high and train low." This means that athletes should live and sleep at altitude to allow enhanced red blood cell production, but to return to sea level to train to allow maintained training intensities. In addition, hypoxic masks have been used to enhance metabolic and respiratory function with training while at sea level. However, these types of training are not at your disposal. So you decide to let your athletes know this will be a difficult meet and they should just do their best.

Scenario

You are a road cycling coach and have seen advertisements for devices that are supposed to train the muscles of inspiration.

Several of your athletes have asked you if these devices work or might improve their cycling performance.

Options

You perform a literature search and find several articles related to endurance performance and use of inspiratory muscle training. These devices make it more difficult to inspire resulting in the muscles of inspiration needing to develop more force in order to perform their function. Over a period of time this results in possibly increased strength and endurance of these muscles and so less fatigue during an endurance event. This potentially results in greater pulmonary ventilation and so oxygen supply to working muscles.

Several studies do show improved performance after inspiratory muscle training in trained athletes. Mean power during 6 minutes of rowing is increased 2.7%,[1] whereas 20-, 25- and 40-km time trial performance is improved by 2.7% to 4.6%.[2,3] However, other studies also show no significant improvement in performance. It does seem that inspiratory muscle training increases strength and endurance on the inspiratory muscles. For example, training increases the inspiratory muscle pressure approximately 26% in rowers.[1] It also appears that inspiratory muscle training results in increased performance with as little as 4–6 weeks of training. With your research and the apparent lack of negative side effects, you decide to advise your athletes to try inspiratory muscle training for a short period of time.

References

1. Griffiths LA, McConnell AK. The influence of inspiratory and expiratory muscle training upon rowing performance. Eur J Appl Physiol. 2007;99:457–466.
2. Johnson MA, Sharpe GR, Brown PI. Inspiratory muscle training improves cycling time-trial performance and anaerobic work capacity but not critical power. Eur J Appl Physiol. 2007;101:761–770.
3. Rommer LM, McConnell AK, Jones DA. Effects of inspiratory muscle training on time-trial performance in train cyclists. J Sports Sci. 2002;20:547–562.

Quick Review

- In healthy individuals at submaximal workloads, respiratory muscle fatigue does not occur; however, at exercise intensities above 80% of $\dot{V}_{O_{2peak}}$, the diaphragm can show indications of some fatigue.
- The respiratory muscles, including the diaphragm, do adapt to training.

CHAPTER SUMMARY

The respiratory and circulatory systems work together to supply tissues with oxygen and to expel carbon dioxide from the body. Pulmonary ventilation and pulmonary diffusion are referred to as pulmonary respiration because these two processes occur at the alveoli in the lungs. Cellular respiration refers to the use of oxygen in aerobic metabolism and production of carbon dioxide by tissue. Partial pressure gradients between the air and blood (pulmonary respiration) and blood and tissue (cellular respiration) determine the direction and rate of the exchange of oxygen and carbon dioxide during respiration. In addition to gas exchange at the lungs, the pulmonary system also humidifies, filters, and warms air to protect the alveoli and respiratory membrane from damage. During inspiration, contraction of the inspiratory muscles, of which the diaphragm is the most important, causes a decrease in intrapulmonic pressure, resulting in air rushing into the lungs. Relaxation of the inspiratory muscles causes an increase in intrapulmonic pressure, resulting in expiration. During physical activity, expiratory muscles contract, thus aiding expiration.

During light to moderate physical activity, pulmonary ventilation is increased due to both an increase in tidal volume and frequency of breathing. At higher intensities of physical activity, tidal volume plateaus so that the only way to increase pulmonary ventilation is to increase frequency of breathing.

The majority of oxygen is transported bound to hemoglobin, whereas the majority of carbon dioxide is transported as bicarbonate. The transport of oxygen and carbon dioxide, however, is affected by increased acidity, increased temperature, and increases in partial pressure during physical activity, so that more oxygen is delivered to active tissue. This is in large part due to shifting of the oxyhemoglobin disassociation curve so that hemoglobin decreases its affinity for oxygen at working tissue.

In order to meet the body's needs, pulmonary ventilation at rest and during physical activity is controlled by the respiratory center located in the medulla and pons. The respiratory center receives input from many sources, including peripheral chemoreceptors, central chemoreceptors, higher brain centers, muscle proprioceptors, and muscle chemoreceptors. This input allows pulmonary ventilation to change to meet the needs of oxygen delivery to tissue and carbon dioxide removal. The major determinants of pulmonary ventilation are hydrogen ion concentration, oxygen partial pressure, and carbon dioxide partial pressure, which are monitored closely by chemoreceptors so that pulmonary ventilation changes to meet the metabolic needs of the body. However, as workload increases, there are several points at which there are alterations in pulmonary ventilation relative to the amount of oxygen and carbon dioxide exchanged at the lungs. These changes in pulmonary ventilation are related to performing workloads that are above lactate threshold.

Respiratory muscles can adapt to physical training, resulting in less respiratory muscle fatigue during physical activity. If it were not for the respiratory system's remarkable ability to match pulmonary ventilation with the metabolic needs of the body at rest and during physical activity and its ability to adapt to training, our ability to perform both aerobic and anaerobic exercise would be compromised.

REVIEW QUESTIONS

Fill-in-the-Blank

1. _____ are saclike structures attached to the respiratory bronchioles and are surrounded by capillaries, where gas exchange takes place.

2. If intrapulmonic pressure is _____ than atmospheric pressure, air will move into the lungs or _____ will occur; if intrapulmonic pressure is _____ than atmospheric pressure, air will move out of the lungs or _____ will occur.

3. The partial pressure of oxygen in the alveoli is _____ than the partial pressure of oxygen in the blood, which allows oxygen to diffuse into the blood. However, the partial pressure of oxygen in muscle is _____ than the partial pressure of oxygen in the blood, which allows oxygen to diffuse into the muscle.

4. When oxygen is bound to hemoglobin, _____ is formed, whereas hemoglobin not bound to oxygen is termed _____.

5. The _____ is the workload at which $\dot{V}_E$ increases disproportionately relative to $\dot{V}_{O_2}$ and changes from proportional increases in $\dot{V}_E$ relative to workload to disproportionate increases in $\dot{V}_E$ relative to workload.

Multiple Choice

1. Which of the following are muscles that aid in inspiration?

    a. intercostals, gracilis, tibialis anterior, pectoralis minor

    b. external intercostals, sartorius, brachialis, pectoralis minor

    c. trapezius, scalene muscles, sternocleidomastoid, soleus

    d. external intercostals, scalene muscles, gastrocnemius, latissimus dorsi

    e. external intercostals, scalene muscles, sternocleidomastoid, pectoralis minor

2. If the diameter of an airway is reduced by half, *resistance* to airflow will _____.

    a. increase by 16×

    b. increase by 2×

    c. decrease by 16×

    d. decrease by 2×

    e. not change

3. During inspiration, air leaving the trachea enters directly into the _____.

    a. alveoli

    b. pulmonary capillaries

    c. esophagus

    d. primary bronchus

    e. larynx

4. The majority of oxygen in the blood is transported _____, whereas the majority of carbon dioxide in the blood is transported in the form of _____.

    a. bound to myoglobin; dissolved in plasma

    b. dissolved in blood; bound to hemoglobin

    c. as bicarbonate; bound to myoglobin

    d. bound to hemoglobin; bicarbonate

    e. dissolved in blood; bicarbonate

5. Which of the following features of the oxyhemoglobin disassociation curve helps to ensure adequate oxygen delivery to tissue during exercise?

    a. the sigmoidal shape

    b. the shift in the curve to the right due to increased temperature

    c. the shift in the curve to the right due to increased acidity

    d. the shift in the curve to the right due to changing affinity of hemoglobin for 2,3-diphosphoglycerate

    e. all of the above

True/False

1. Lung tissue is capable of contracting.
2. The bottom portions of the lungs receive more ventilation at rest than the upper portions.
3. Aerobic training increases the number of alveoli.
4. All of the air inspired reaches the alveoli, where gas exchange takes place.
5. It is possible for the diaphragm to hypertrophy.

Short Answer

1. Explain how the structure of the alveoli benefit gas exchange.
2. Explain the mechanics of ventilation.
3. Why might ventilation through the mouth and nose occur during exercise as pulmonary ventilation increases?
4. Discuss how blood pressure in the pulmonary circulation differs from blood pressure in the systemic circulation.

Critical Thinking

1. Explain the role of chemoreceptors in the control of respiration.
2. Explain why the partial pressure of oxygen decreases and carbon dioxide increases from their values in the atmosphere to air within the alveoli.

KEY TERMS

alveolar ventilation: air that reaches the alveoli during pulmonary ventilation

alveoli: saclike structures surrounded by capillaries where gas exchange at the lungs takes place

anatomical dead space: air that never reaches the alveoli during pulmonary ventilation

Bohr effect: the shifting of the oxyhemoglobin disassociation curve to the right with an increase in acidity and to the left with a decrease in acidity

capillary gas exchange: the exchange of oxygen and carbon dioxide between the blood and the body's tissues

carbaminohemoglobin: hemoglobin to which carbon dioxide is bound

cellular respiration: the use of oxygen in aerobic metabolism and production of carbon dioxide

central chemoreceptors: chemoreceptors located within the medulla that stimulate changes in respiration

chemoreceptors: receptors that respond to chemical changes

chloride shift: the exchange of bicarbonate ions for chloride ions to prevent electrical imbalance within the red blood cell

Dalton's law: the law stating that the total pressure of a gas mixture is equivalent to the sum of all the pressures of all the gases that compose the mixture

deoxyhemoglobin: hemoglobin that is not bound to oxygen

diaphragm: the most important respiratory muscle, located between the thoracic and abdominal cavities

hemoglobin: an iron-containing pigment found in red blood cells that is capable of reversibly binding oxygen

Henry's law: the law stating that the amount of gas dissolved in any fluid depends on the temperature, partial pressure, and solubility of the gas

intrapleural pressure: pressure in the space or pleural cavity between the visceral and parietal membranes

intrapulmonic pressure: the air pressure within the lungs

myoglobin: an oxygen transport molecule similar to hemoglobin, except it is found within skeletal and cardiac muscle

oxyhemoglobin: hemoglobin to which oxygen is bound

partial pressure: the portion of pressure due to a particular gas in a mixture of gases

peripheral chemoreceptors: chemoreceptors located within the carotid bodies and the aortic arch that stimulate changes in respiration.

pleura: the two membranes (pulmonary and parietal) that encase the lungs

pulmonary diffusion: the movement of oxygen from air in the lungs into the blood and of carbon dioxide out of the blood to air in the lungs

pulmonary respiration: the processes of pulmonary ventilation and pulmonary diffusion, both of which occur at the lungs

pulmonary ventilation: the movement of air into and out of the lungs, commonly referred to as breathing, typically expressed as the amount of air moved per minute

residual volume: the air left in the lungs after a maximal exhalation

respiratory compensation point: exercise intensity at which both $\dot{V}E/\dot{V}O_2$ and $\dot{V}E/\dot{V}CO_2$ show an increase; respiratory compensation point occurs at an exercise intensity higher than ventilatory threshold

respiratory membrane: the membrane of the alveolar cells and the cells making up the wall of the capillary surrounding the alveoli, through which gas must pass to move between the blood and the air within the alveoli

tidal volume: the amount of air moved per breath

ventilatory equivalent of carbon dioxide: the ratio of $\dot{V}E$ to $\dot{V}CO_2$ ($\dot{V}E/\dot{V}CO_2$)

ventilatory equivalent of oxygen: the ratio of $\dot{V}E$ to $\dot{V}O_2$ ($\dot{V}E/\dot{V}O_2$)

ventilatory threshold: the use of ventilatory equivalent of oxygen ($\dot{V}E/\dot{V}O_2$) and ventilatory equivalent of carbon dioxide ($\dot{V}E/\dot{V}CO_2$) to estimate the workload at which lactate threshold occurs

REFERENCES

1. Aaron EA, Johnson BD, Seow CK, et al. Oxygen cost of exercise hyperpnea: measurement. J Appl Physiol. 1992;72:1810–1817.
2. Babcock MA, Pegelow DF, Johnson BD, et al. Aerobic fitness effects on exercise-induced low-frequency diaphragm fatigue. J Appl Physiol. 1996;81:2156–2164.
3. Babcock MA, Pegelow DF, McClaran SR, et al. Contribution of diaphragmatic power output to exercise-induced diaphragm fatigue. J Appl Physiol. 1995;78:1710–1719.
4. Cloutier MM, Thrall RS. The respiratory system. In: Levy MN, Koeppen BM, Stanton BA, eds. Berne and Levy Principles of Physiology. Saint Louis, MO, CV Mosby Company, 2005.
5. Dempsey JA, Miller JD, Romer LM. The respiratory system. In: ACSMs Advanced Exercise Physiology. Philadelphia, PA: Lippincott, Williams & Williams, 2006.
6. DePalo VA, Parker AL, Al-Bilbeisi F, et al. Respiratory muscle strength training with nonrespiratory maneuvers. J Appl Physiol. 2004;96:731–734.
7. Dodd SL, Powers SK, Thompson D, et al. Exercise performance following intense, short-term ventilatory work. Int J Sports Med. 1989;10:48–52.
8. Eldridge FL. Central integration of mechanisms in exercise hyperpnea. Med Sci Sports Exerc. 1994;26:319–327.
9. Fang TY, Zou M, Simplaceanu V, et al. Assessment of roles of surface histidyl residues in the molecular basis of the Bohr effect and of beta 143 histidine in the binding of 2,3-bisphosphoglycerate in human normal adult hemoglobin. Biochemistry. 1999;38:13423–13432.
10. Johnson BD, Babcock MA, Suman OE, et al. Exercise-induced diaphragmatic fatigue in healthy humans. J Physiol. 1993;460:385–405.
11. Legrand R, Prieur F, Marles A, et al. Respiratory muscle oxygenation kinetics: relationships with breathing pattern during exercise. Int J Sports Med. 2007;28:91–99.
12. Levitzky M. Pulmonary Physiology. New York: McGraw-Hill Companies, 1999.
13. Lijnen P, Hespel P, Van Oppens S, et al. Erythrocyte 2,3-diphosphoglycerate and serum enzyme concentrations in trained and sedentary men. Med Sci Sports Exerc. 1986;18:174–179.
14. Lucia A, Hoyos J, Santalla A, et al. Tour de France versus Vuelta a Espana: which is harder? Med Sci Sports Exerc. 2003;35:872–878.
15. Mairbaurl H, Schobersberger W, Hasibeder W, et al. Regulation of red cell 2,3-DPG and Hb-O$_2$-affinity during acute exercise. Eur J Appl Physiol Occup Physiol. 1986;55:174–180.
16. Powers SK, Coombes J, Demirel H. Exercise training-induced changes in respiratory muscles. Sports Med. 1997;24:120–131.
17. Rand PW, Norton JM, Barker N, et al. Influence of athletic training on hemoglobin-oxygen affinity. Am J Physiol. 1973;224:1334–1337.
18. Taunton JE, Taunton CA, Banister EW. Alterations in 2,3-DPG and P50 with maximal and submaximal exercise. Med Sci Sports. 1974;6:238–241.
19. Whipp BJ. Peripheral chemoreceptor control of exercise hyperpnea in humans. Med Sci Sports Exerc. 1994;26:337–347.
20. Wyatt FB. Comparison of lactate and ventilatory threshold to maximal oxygen consumption: a meta-analysis. J Strength Cond Res. 1999;13:67–71.

Suggested Readings

Aliverti A, Kayser B, Macklem PT. A human model of the pathophysiology of chronic obstructive pulmonary disease. Respirology. 2007;12(4):478–485.

Bassett DR Jr, Howley ET. Limiting factors for maximum oxygen uptake and determinants of endurance performance. Med Sci Sports Exerc. 2000;32(1):70–84.

Baughman RP, Sparkman BK, Lower EE. Six-minute walk test and health status assessment in sarcoidosis. Chest. 2007;132(1):207–213.

Florida-James G, Donaldson K, Stone V. Athens 2004: the pollution climate and athletic performance. J Sports Sci. 2004;22(10):967–980.

Harries M. ABC of sports medicine. Pulmonary limitations to performance in sport. BMJ. 1994;309(6947):113–115.

Haverkamp HC, Dempsey JA, Pegelow DF, et al. Treatment of airway inflammation improves exercise pulmonary gas exchange and performance in asthmatic subjects. J Allergy Clin Immunol. 2007;120(1):39–47.

Koppo K, Whipp BJ, Jones AM, et al. Overshoot in $\dot{V}O_2$ following the onset of moderate-intensity cycle exercise in trained cyclists. Eur J Appl Physiol. 2004;93(3):366–373.

Levitzky MG. Pulmonary Physiology (Lange Physiology), 6th ed. New York: McGraw-Hill Medical, 2003.

Macchia A, Marchioli R, Marfisi R, et al. A meta-analysis of trials of pulmonary hypertension: a clinical condition looking for drugs and research methodology. Am Heart J. 2007;153(6):1037–1047.

Miller JD, Smith CA, Hemauer SJ, et al. The effects of inspiratory intrathoracic pressure production on the cardiovascular response to submaximal exercise in health and chronic heart failure. Am J Physiol Heart Circ Physiol. 2007;292(1):H580–H592.

Romer LM, Haverkamp HC, Lovering AT, et al. Effect of exercise-induced arterial hypoxemia on quadriceps muscle fatigue in healthy humans. Am J Physiol Regul Integr Comp Physiol. 2006;290(2): R365–R375.

Romer LM, Miller JD, Haverkamp HC, et al. Inspiratory muscles do not limit maximal incremental exercise performance in healthy subjects. Respir Physiol Neurobiol. 2007;156(3):353–361.

Rossiter HB, Kowalchuk JM, Whipp BJ. A test to establish maximum O_2 uptake despite no plateau in the O_2 uptake response to ramp incremental exercise. J Appl Physiol. 2006;100(3):764–770.

Rundell KW, Jenkinson DM. Exercise-induced bronchospasm in the elite athlete. Sports Med. 2002;32(9):583–600.

Siobal MS. Pulmonary vasodilators. Respir Care. 2007;52(7):885–899.

Whipp BJ. Physiological mechanisms dissociating pulmonary CO_2 and O_2 exchange dynamics during exercise in humans. Exp Physiol. 2007;92(2):347–355.

Classic References

Filley GF, Macintosh DJ, Wright GW. Carbon monoxide uptake and pulmonary diffusing capacity in normal subjects at rest and during exercise. J Clin Invest. 1954;33(4):530–539.

Grodins FS. Analysis of factors concerned in regulation of breathing in exercise. Physiol Rev. 1950;30(2):220–239.

Hickam JB, Pryor WW, Page EB, et al. Respiratory regulation during exercise in unconditioned subjects. J Clin Invest. 1951;30(5):503–516.

Whipp BJ, Wasserman K. Alveolar-arterial gas tension differences during graded exercise. J Appl Physiol. 1969;27(3):361–365.

Whipp BJ, Wasserman K. Efficiency of muscular work. J Appl Physiol. 1969;26(5):644–648.

7

Endocrine System

After reading this chapter, you should be able to:

1. Define and describe the function of a hormone
2. Explain the organization of the endocrine system
3. Describe hormone structure and synthesis, release, transport, and degradation
4. Describe the use and side effects of anabolic drugs used by athletes
5. Explain the differences between the different hormonal feedback loops
6. Describe endocrine, autocrine, and paracrine actions and their significance in hormonal responses to exercise
7. Explain circadian rhythms and seasonal changes in hormones and how they relates to training and performance

8. Describe and distinguish peptide and steroid interactions with receptors
9. Describe the interactions of the hypothalamus and pituitary gland
10. Discuss the other forms of growth hormone and their responses to exercise
11. Describe the exercise roles, regulation, responses, interactions, and adaptations of the hormones presented in this chapter
12. Explain the impact of competition on endocrine responses

The endocrine system and the nervous system are the two major systems of communication in the body, sending out signals or messages to influence physiological responses and adaptations. The endocrine system sends a signal in the form of a **hormone**, which is a chemical substance released from a gland into the blood. A **gland** is an organized group of cells that functions as an organ to secrete chemical substances. Each hormone that is released from a gland is specifically targeted for a receptor on a specific cell. Thus, the term "targeted receptor" relates to the concept of a hormone's specific set of cellular destinations for the signal being sent from the gland. A hormone can affect many different cells but only those cells that have its receptor. The endocrine system modulates a wide range of activities in the body from cellular function to metabolism, sexual and reproductive processes, tissue growth, fluid regulation, protein synthesis and degradation, and mood states.

Increases in hormonal concentrations with exercise are important for the modulation of physiological functions as well as the repair and remodeling of body tissues. Figure 7-1 shows some of the major endocrine glands and other organs that release hormones, which also may be considered endocrine glands.

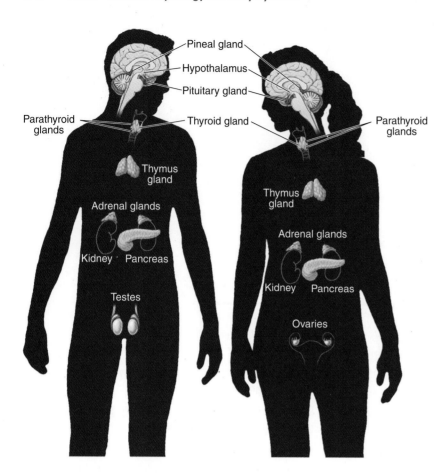

Figure 7-1. The major endocrine glands of the body. (From Cohen BJ, Taylor JJ. Memmler's The Human Body in Health and Disease. 10th ed. Baltimore, MD: Lippincott Williams & Wilkins, 2005.)

SIGNIFICANCE OF THE ENDOCRINE SYSTEM TO EXERCISE PHYSIOLOGY

Why is understanding the endocrine system so important for an exercise professional? Well, let us stop to list a few of the many different topics that involve the endocrine system and are regulated by hormones.

- Anabolic drug abuse in sports
- Insulin resistance
- Metabolic syndrome
- Menopause
- Andropause
- Diabetes

As an exercise professional, you will come across such topics every day. Understanding some of the basics about the endocrine system, how it works, and what hormones are involved in different processes will help give you the needed insights into how the body works.[66] The acute responses to exercise help the body function during activity and regulate metabolism. Recovery from exercise stress and subsequent tissue repair and remodeling is also linked with hormonal responses. Ultimately, hormones and their receptors mediate adaptations to exercise training. Adaptations are the chronic changes in physiological responses (e.g., heart rate, blood pressure); structural anatomy; or morphology (e.g., muscle fiber size, bone density).

Endocrinology is the science of intercellular and intracellular communication that was defined by Bayliss and Starling more than 100 years ago.[3,25] Exercise demands are very specific. The challenges of the physical stress associated with exercise can result in metabolic increases of 10-fold or more, and required muscular force production can reach maximal limits. The challenges of competition also span a wide spectrum of physical demands, from endurance events such as the marathon, which can be run in under 2:05:00, to power lifting, in which some can squat over 1,000 pounds. Hormones in part mediate both performance and recovery from exercise of all types.

ORGANIZATION OF THE NEUROENDOCRINE SYSTEM

In essence, the neuroendocrine system is a network of glands and substances released from these glands control physiological function at the cellular level.

Quick Review

- The endocrine system communicates messages that influence physiological responses and adaptations in the body.
- Hormonal concentrations drastically change with exercise to modulate physiological functions.

Table 7-1. The Major Hormones Secreted by Various Endocrine Glands in the Body and Their Basic Actions

Endocrine Organ	Hormone	Major Actions
Testes	Testosterone	Stimulates development and maintenance of male sex characteristics, growth, and protein anabolism
Ovaries	Estrogen	Develops female secondary sex characteristics; matures the epiphyses of the long bones
	Progesterone	Develops female sex characteristics; maintains pregnancy; develops mammary glands
Anterior pituitary	Growth hormone (GH)	Stimulates IGF-I and IGF-II synthesis; stimulates protein synthesis, growth, and intermediary metabolism
	Adrenocorticotropic hormone (ACTH)	Stimulates glucocorticoid release in adrenal cortex
	Thyroid-stimulating hormone (TSH)	Stimulates thyroid hormone synthesis and secretion
	Follicle-stimulating hormone (FSH)	Stimulates growth of follicles in ovary and seminiferous tubules in testes and sperm production
	Luteinizing hormone (LH)	Stimulates ovulation and production and secretion of sex hormones in ovaries and testes
	Prolactin (Prl)	Stimulates milk production in mammary glands
Posterior pituitary	Antidiuretic hormone (ADH)	Increases reabsorption of water by kidneys and stimulates contraction of smooth muscle
	Oxytocin	Stimulates uterine contractions and release of milk by mammary glands
Adrenal cortex	Glucocorticoids	Inhibits or retards amino acid incorporation into proteins (cortisol); stimulates conversion of proteins into carbohydrates (gluconeogenesis); maintains normal blood sugar level; conserves glucose; promotes metabolism of fat
	Mineralocorticoids (aldosterone, deoxycorticosterone, etc.)	Increases or decreases sodium–potassium metabolism; increases body water
Adrenal medulla	Epinephrine	Increases cardiac output; increases blood sugar, glycogen breakdown, and fat mobilization
	Norepinephrine (some)	Similar to epinephrine plus constriction of blood vessels
	Proenkephalins (e.g., peptide F, E)	Analgesia, enhances immune function
Thyroid	Thyroxine	Stimulates oxidative metabolism in mitochondria and cell growth
	Calcitonin	Reduces blood calcium levels; inhibits osteoclast function
Heart (cardiocytes)	Atrial natriuretic hormone	Facilitates the excretion of sodium and water; regulates blood pressure and volume homeostasis and opposes the actions of the rennin–angiotensin system
Pancreas	Insulin	Stimulates absorption of glucose and storage as glycogen
	Glucagon	Increases blood glucose levels
Parathyroids	Parathyroid hormone	Increases blood calcium; decreases blood phosphate
Skin	Vitamin D	Produces vitamin D from 7-dehydrocholesterol and sunlight
Adipose tissue	Leptin	Regulates appetite and energy expenditure

Hormones

Table 7–1 lists the major hormones secreted from the various glands, organs, tissues, and cells of the body. The most well characterized hormones are those secreted from an endocrine gland. Yet this basic function can be applied to other organs, tissues, and cells in the body. This has led to such terms as **neuroendocrine**, neuro-endocrine-immune, etc., indicating an interaction of physiological systems in the production and release of hormonal substances.

Blood Concentrations

Hormones are released into the blood from endocrine glands. The blood acts as the major transport system for hormones to their target cells. Blood samples are obtained to observe changes in hormone concentrations (i.e., the molar amount of substance) with exercise stress, or after a period of exercise training, to gain insights as to the modulation of these concentrations due to acute or chronic exercise.

Hormones can be found in the various components of blood, which is made up of **plasma** (i.e., unclotted blood versus **serum**, in which a clot has formed), packed white blood cells (leukocytes) and platelets (also called the buffy coat), and packed red blood cells (i.e., erythrocytes), as shown in Figure 7-2. Obviously, beyond hormones, many other substances are also transported in the blood, from gases such as oxygen, to fats such as cholesterol, all in this amazing transport medium which is part of the cardiovascular system.

Hormone Structure and Synthesis

There are three major types of hormones: steroids, peptides, and modified amino acid hormones, also called amines. Each has a specific chemical structure that determines how it interacts with target cell receptors. The

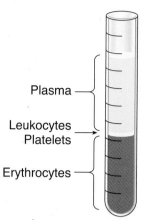

Figure 7-2. Blood components: plasma, white blood cells and platelets, and red blood cells. This makes up the major transport medium in the human body.

structures of the three major classes of hormones can be seen in Figure 7-3.

Steroid hormones are all derived from cholesterol and contain the same ring and atomic numbering system as cholesterol. It is important to understand that not all steroids have the same function. One steroid might be a medical treatment for asthma; another is a bodybuilding drug or **anabolic** (to build) steroid for building muscle (Box 7-1 and 7-2). Thus, the term "steroid" represents a large class

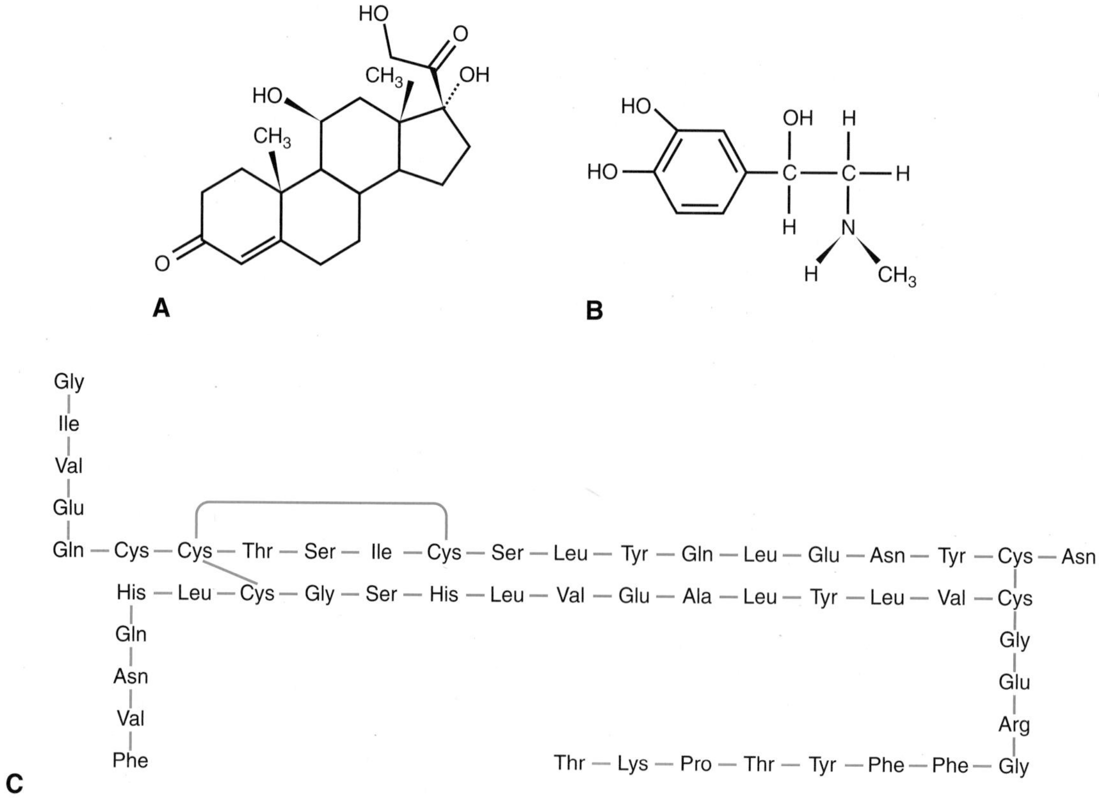

A

B

C

Figure 7-3. Structures of the major three classes of hormones. (A) Cortisol is representative of a "steroid" hormone, with its characteristic cholesterol base made of of the four membered ring structure. **(B)** Epinephrine is representative of an "amine" type hormone. **(C)** Insulin is representative of a peptide hormone made up of a sequence of amino acids.

Box 7-1 AN EXPERT VIEW

Athletes' Use of Anabolic Steroids and Human Growth Hormone

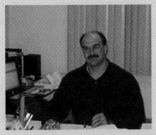

Nicholas A. Ratamess, PhD
Department of Health and Exercise Science,
The College of New Jersey
Ewing, NJ

Many athletes commonly use anabolic-androgenic steroids (AAS) and, to a lesser extent, human growth hormone (HGH) to enhance performance.[5] Although these drugs require a prescription, unfortunately they are illegally used and abused by many athletes. Historically, strength and power athletes were the predominant users of these drugs. However, use of these drugs spread as resistance training increased in popularity, and athletes from most sports have been known to experiment with them.

AASs are synthetic derivatives of *testosterone*. The androgenic effects relate to testosterone's role in the development of secondary sexual characteristics and reproductive system. However, many athletes attempt to reduce these effects by using chemically modified steroids that reduce androgenic effects, injectable steroids, or other drugs. Anabolic steroids have many ergogenic properties and increase the following: (1) muscle hypertrophy, endurance, power, and strength; (2) lipolysis; (3) cardiac tissue mass; (4) recovery ability between workouts; (5) bone mineral density; (6) glycogen storage; (7) neural transmission; (8) erythropoiesis; (9) pain tolerance; and (10) aggression. However, some potential side effects include the following[1,5]: reproductive alterations, gynecomastia, acne, hair loss, fluid retention, increased libido, increased blood pressure and LDLs, reduced HDLs, depression, mood swings, organ damage/abnormalities, connective tissue weakening, "'roid rage," higher estrogen concentrations, deepening of the voice, and cardiovascular abnormalities.

Testing for AAS is done via urine analyses, using gas and liquid chromatography-mass spectrometry and high-resolution mass spectrometry. AAS metabolites found in urine indicate a failed drug test. For detection of testosterone use, the ratio of testosterone found in urine to its metabolite epitestosterone (T:E ratio) is a common marker. Historically, a ratio of 6:1 was used, but that has been lowered to 4:1 (the average ratio is 1:1). A test showing a ratio larger than this indicates testosterone use. Athletes are known to "beat" drug tests using several techniques, including diluting urine volume, contaminating urine samples, using masking agents, gradually cycling down or discontinuing AAS use when the testing date is known, using steroids with shorter detection times, consuming epitestosterone to balance the T:E ratio, and substituting another urine sample for their own. Although undocumented, it does appear that many athletes are aware of these practices, which undoubtedly have resulted in very low numbers of AAS-using athletes testing positive.[3,4]

Human growth hormone (HGH) is released from the anterior pituitary and has several anabolic, fat-burning, and performance-enhancing functions similar to testosterone. The anabolic properties stimulate growth in bone and skeletal muscle but also affect other major organs, leading to potential side effects. Recombinant HGH has been used clinically to treat several ailments. However, athletes have been aware of HGH's anabolic potential since the late 1980s, and HGH has been used and abused by athletes ever since. HGH may enhance connective-tissue strength, which is thought to reduce injury potential.

Some clinical studies have shown that the effects of HGH alone on skeletal muscle may not be that potent. However, most athletes who use HGH (at doses far exceeding clinical recommendations) attest to benefiting greatly from it. Although HGH by itself is ergogenic, it is believed that the largest effects are seen when HGH is stacked with AAS and other anabolic drugs. The synergistic effect of the two is thought to provide greater anabolic potency than either alone.

HGH is expensive, is a protein molecule, and needs to be kept cool at all times and be injected because it would be degraded if taken orally. It is not found in urine and, therefore, cannot be detected via drug testing. Many athletes use HGH to escape detection. Various methods of determining HGH have been proposed and tested, including blood testing and measuring other secretagogue, IGF-I, and other proteins. Following such testing a new HGH doping test has been implemented by the World Anti-Doping Agency and has been used to detect HGH use in athletes.[2]

The use of HGH can lead to significant side effects, including hypoglycemia, high blood pressure, altered hormonal profiles and thyroid function, enlarged organs, kidney and liver damage, headaches, and mood swings. Visual growth of bones (*acromegaly*) also occurs. Growth in the bones in the forehead, jaw, hands, and feet are distinguishing features indicating HGH use in the athlete.

References

1. Hoffman JR, Ratamess NA. Medical issues of anabolic steroids: are they over-exaggerated? J Sports Sci Med. 2006;5:182–193.
2. Kraemer WJ, Dunn-Lewis C, Comstock BA, Thomas GA, Clark JE, Nindl BC. Growth hormone, exercise, and athletic performance: a continued evolution of complexity. Curr Sports Med Rep. 2010;9(4):242–252.
3. Parkinson AB, Evans NA. Anabolic androgenic steroids: a survey of 500 users. Med Sci Sports Exerc. 2006;38:644–651.
4. Perry PJ, Lund BC, Deninger MJ, et al. Anabolic steroid use in weightlifters and bodybuilders: an internet survey of drug utilization. Clin J Sport Med. 2005;15:326–330.
5. Ratamess NA. Coaches Guide to Performance-Enhancing Supplements. Monterey, CA: Coaches Choice Books, 2006.

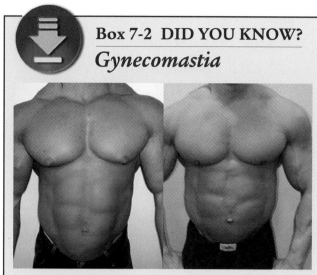

Box 7-2 DID YOU KNOW?
Gynecomastia

(Courtesy of Dr. Mordcai Blau MD, PC, Westchester New York Aesthetic Plastic Surgery, White Plains, NY.)

The development of breast tissue in men is called gynecomastia. Although the exact causes of this condition are not completely understood, it can occur in adolescent and elderly men. While very distressing, especially in young boys, it is not thought to be caused by obesity but rather an imbalance of sex hormones. Excessive amounts of estrogens (estradiol) can influence target fat cells in the chest area. With anabolic steroid abuse, the biosynthetic hormonal conversion of excess amounts of anabolic steroids (synthetic forms of the male hormone testosterone) to the estrogen compounds, estrone and estradiol, can accelerate the stimulation of breast tissue in men. This is one of the many potential negative side effects of anabolic steroid abuse among men.

of many types of hormones with different functions but with similar chemical ring structures. Steroid hormones exert their action by direct interactions with the DNA's regulatory elements. The interaction with the DNA leads to the transcription process of the activated genes signaling cells to make proteins. For example, testosterone signals an anabolic stimulus to promote protein synthesis, whereas cortisol signals a **catabolic** process for protein degradation or breakdown to preserve muscle glycogen.

Peptide hormones are made up of amino acids. They are produced in many of the endocrine glands (e.g., the anterior pituitary secretes growth hormones) and can have very complex structures and contain hundreds of amino acids (e.g., the 22-kD growth hormone contains a sequence of 191 amino acids). Peptide hormones exert their signals indirectly via secondary intracellular signaling systems.

Amine compounds make up the third type of hormones. Such organic compounds contain nitrogen and the general form of an amine, which has an alkyl group. Either one or both of the hydrogen molecules may be replaced by other groups with the compound still retaining its identity as an amine. The most commonly studied amines in exercise physiology are the catecholamines, which are derived from the amino acid tyrosine and contain catechol and amine groups. Epinephrine (also known as adrenaline) is the most

well-known of the catecholamines, as it is involved in the "fight-or-flight" response.

Hormone Release

The release of hormones occurs from specific cellular sites in the different organs and glands that produce hormones. In general, they are synthesized through a series of chemical reactions, stored, and then released from the storage site upon mechanical, neural, or hormonal signals. The stimulatory signals allow for very specific regulation and control of how much hormone is released. As noted before, an **endocrine** function is one in which the hormone is secreted directly into the blood. A **paracrine** function is one in which the hormone is released into an area to interact with other target cells nearby without any transport in the blood. Finally, **autocrine** function involves the release of a hormone from a cell (e.g., muscle cell) and the subsequent stimulation of the cell by this hormone. Thus, not all hormones are released in an endocrine fashion.

Hormone Transport, Degradation, and Half-Life

Each hormone has a specific **half-life**, or the amount of time it takes for a hormone's concentration in blood to be reduced to half of its peak value, which determines its potency to produce a signal to its intended target cell. Many hormones attach to binding proteins or other molecules or cells in the blood to lengthen their half-life. After a certain amount of time, the hormone is broken down and degraded, ending its signal to the body. Once a hormone has interacted with a receptor, it degrades and its structure and function are lost; this makes the receptor available to bind another hormone molecule and limits the stimulus duration of a hormone.

Pulsatility

Some hormones (e.g., insulin, growth hormone, luteinizing hormone) are released in bursts or pulses of a large quantity of hormone. Called "pulsatility," such a release is thought to stimulate more effective hormonal signaling. This would amplify the effect of the hormone at the target cells, making the response or adaptation greater over a given time frame. Pulsatility of hormones is potentially influenced by many different factors, including exercise intensity, drugs, nutritional intakes, and environment.[64] Exercise intensity can impact the pulsatile increase of some hormones, such as growth hormone (Fig. 7-4).

Feedback Systems

The control of hormonal secretions is affected by different feedback systems, which in part control the amount of hormone released by a gland. A number of classic feedback loops exist that demonstrate the concept of hormonal feedback loops.

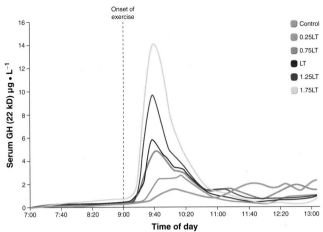

Figure 7-4. Pulsatility of a hormone in response to exercise can create a greater magnitude of response. Mean serum growth hormone (GH) concentrations during blood sampling at 10-minute intervals over 6 hours during control; 25% and 75% of difference between O$_2$ uptake ($\dot{V}$O$_2$) achieved at lactate threshold (LT) and $\dot{V}$O$_2$ at rest (0.25 LT and 0.75 LT, respectively); and 25% and 75% of difference between $\dot{V}$O$_2$ at LT and peak $\dot{V}$O$_2$ (1.25 LT and 1.75 LT, respectively) conditions. Values are means ±SE; n = 10 subjects. (Modified from Pritzlaff CJ, Wideman L, Weltman JY, et al. Impact of acute exercise intensity on pulsatile growth hormone release in men. J Appl Physiol. 1999;87(2):498–504.)

Negative Feedback

A negative feedback loop is one in which a product that is formed can feed back upon the primary structures to diminish the amount of secretion. In the case of testosterone, as shown in Figure 7-5, increased concentrations of testosterone feed back on the hypothalamus to reduce the amount of gonadotropin-releasing hormone, which reduces the amount of luteinizing hormone and follicular-stimulating hormone released from the anterior pituitary, which in turn reduces the amount of testosterone released from the testis.

Positive Feedback

A positive feedback loop accentuates the production of the hormone from the gland. Oxytocin is an example of such a mechanism (Fig. 7-6). At the end of gestation, the uterus must perform vigorous contractions for an extended period of time for the baby to be delivered. During labor, cervical and vaginal stimulation by the fetus triggers the increased release of oxytocin. This stimulates the smooth muscle of the uterus to contract more and more vigorously as labor continues, ending with the delivery of the baby. In situations in which uterine contractions are not capable of completing delivery, a physician sometimes administers oxytocin to stimulate the uterus to contract. In essence, the oxytocin helps the feed forward loop to promote the needed magnitude of smooth muscle contractions to complete the labor process.

Multiple Feedback Influences

Many different feedback loops are operational in the homeostatic control of hormones and metabolism. Another feature

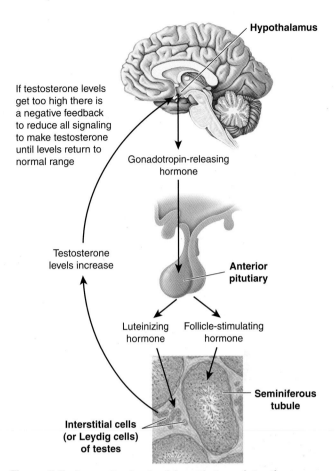

Figure 7-5. A negative feedback loop that regulates the amount of hormone released by the primary endocrine gland by feeding back on the stimulatory gland. This is one example of a negative feedback loop to control the concentration of testosterone in the blood and its signaling to target tissues. Proper modulation of a hormone signal is vital for optimal signaling to a target cell's activity.

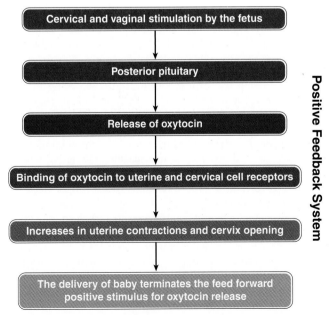

Figure 7-6. A positive feedback loop accentuates or stimulates the production of a hormone.

of the endocrine system is its redundancy in cases in which regulation is vital to survival. For example, anabolic signals are not based on only one hormonal signal but rather several hormone systems that protect one of the most important aspects for survival: repair and remodeling of tissue, most importantly skeletal muscle. Several anabolic hormones can signal protein synthesis, including testosterone, growth hormones, insulin-like growth factors, and insulin. Anabolic signals are important for exercise training adaptations (Box 7-3).

Autocrine and Paracrine Actions

As discussed above, not all hormonal secretions act via typical endocrine function, with the hormone being directly released into the blood to transport it to the target cells. Two other important functions allow hormonal signals to target cells without transport via the blood to the target tissue: autocrine and paracrine signaling.

Muscle and Autocrine Signaling

One of the most interesting autocrine secretions in exercise physiology is that of the insulin-like growth factor from muscle. When muscle fibers are activated as part of a motor unit, mechanical stimuli of force production cause the release from the muscle itself of IGF-I and a spliced genetic variant of IGF-I called mechano-growth factor (MGF). When released from the muscle fiber, these hormones then bind with IGF-I receptors on that same muscle fiber and proceed to signal protein synthesis. Thus, exercise such as a heavy set of three repetitions in the squat may not result in any hormone being released from an endocrine gland, yet autocrine release may take place at the level of the muscle fiber to stimulate protein synthesis.

Paracrine Signaling

As discussed before, paracrine actions take place when a hormone is released from a cell and its target is a cell that is nearby. Neurohormones (e.g., gonadotropin-releasing hormone) or neurotransmitters (e.g., norepinephrine) are examples of such a paracrine function. In addition, adipocytes exhibit such paracrine function by releasing leptin to alter the metabolism of neighboring fat cells. White blood cells release various cytokines and even hormones locally to affect nearby cells in a paracrine fashion.

Circadian Rhythms

Many hormones have circadian rhythms, which impact the magnitude of their response to exercise at different times of the day. Some hormones start out low in the morning and then peak later in the day and at night (e.g., growth hormone). Others start higher in the morning and decline over the day (e.g., testosterone, cortisol) (Fig. 7-7 shows the classic cortisol circadian response pattern). Circadian response patterns can be sensitive to light and dark cycles, sleep patterns, and seasonal changes. Some hormones remain relatively constant during the day and respond only to acute stressors such as exercise (e.g., IGFs, catecholamines). From a practical perspective, no study has shown any priority for a time of day in which training is optimal, unless the wake/sleep cycle impacts the "quality" of the exercise session due to feelings of tiredness or fatigue.

Box 7-3 DID YOU KNOW?

Testosterone

Testosterone is the primary anabolic hormone in men.[79] Yet, its importance in the development of strength in young men was only recently documented in a study by Kvorning et al.[48] In this study, healthy young men were randomly placed in a group that had their natural testosterone blocked by a drug (called deprivation therapy) or in a placebo group in which each subject maintained his normal testosterone function. Both groups of subjects participated in a 3-month resistance training program. The group that had their testosterone blocked demonstrated no gain in strength, whereas the placebo group did gain strength. Thus, in young men, testosterone seems to be the primary hormone mediating strength gains. Interestingly, in a study by Galvao et al.[21] examining a group of older men with prostate cancer on deprivation drug therapy, growth hormone and the prohormone dehydroepiandrosterone (DHEA) were shown to mediate strength gains with resistance training in the drug-treated group. It seems that a longer period of time with hormonal deprivation of testosterone along with resistance training causes men to switch to another anabolic system (i.e., growth hormone, IGF) and allows the prohormone to have greater potency in stimulating strength gains. This change in the primary anabolic signaling demonstrates the plasticity of the endocrine system to mediate resistance training effects under different "normal" hormonal profiles.

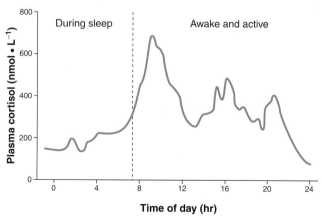

Figure 7-7. Example of a circadian pattern for the hormone cortisol.

With exercise, hormonal concentrations increase acutely. However, this exercise-induced increase is less than the increase in concentrations resulting from circadian rhythms that occur at rest. This discrepancy has fostered many coaches and trainers to think there might be an optimal time of day to train. However, no data have convincingly demonstrated this to be true, and it remains a controversial topic. It is overly simplistic to draw conclusions based upon one hormone's pattern of change. In addition, the role of epinephrine to create an arousal state must be considered.

Furthermore, even if there were an optimal time to train, it would not necessarily apply to competitions. Each sport has different duration, demands, recovery elements, frequency of competitions, and environment, making it difficult to generalize an optimal time to compete. However, in the sport of swimming, where conditions can be controlled, Kline et al.[34] demonstrated that circadian rhythm in swim performances was independent of environmental and behavioral masking effects and found that performances were significantly worse at 0200, 0500, and 0800 than at 1100, 1400, 1700, 2000, and 2300 hours. Thus, some data exist that indicate that some times of day may be more optimal than others for swimming performances that are 2 to 4 minutes in length.

Seasonal Changes in Hormones

Another controversial issue is whether hormone concentrations vary as a result of seasonal changes. This relationship is difficult to determine because other factors could affect the hormonal responses. Beyond exercise-induced training adaptations, environmental factors appear to most significantly affect hormonal response patterns. Consistent with several other cross-sectional studies, Svartberg et al.[73] studied 1,548 men living in north Norway and found that the lowest testosterone concentrations occurred in months with the highest temperatures and longest hours of daylight. If conditions are constant, limited changes occur.[68] Gravholt et al.[24] also observed no seasonal variations in insulin sensitivity in healthy men for a period of over 15 months. Plasqui et al.[63] did find seasonal variations in sleeping metabolic rates in healthy men and women, and these changes could not be explained by changes in body composition, thyroid activity, or leptin. The variations among subjects in sleeping metabolic rate were explained by fat-free mass and leptin. It was suggested by the authors that seasonal variations appear to be related to environmental conditions. It must be considered, however, that seasonal changes in physical activity levels might also explain any potential changes in hormonal response patterns.[63] Thus, seasonal variations in hormones could be affected by any or combinations of the following factors:

- Differences in environmental conditions (temperature, daylight)
- Differences in physical activity levels (training and detraining)
- Resultant behavioral responses (sleep patterns, nutritional intakes)

Receptors

Receptors are the mediators of hormonal signals to the DNA. Receptor binding is complex and differs between the different classes of hormones. For simplicity the two major types of hormone receptors are described here: peptide hormone receptors, which rely on intracellular secondary messenger systems to mediate their signals from the plasma membrane to the DNA, and steroid receptors, which are found on the DNA itself and allow more direct signal interactions.

Peptide and Receptor Interactions

Peptide hormones are made up of amino acids, and their interactions with the DNA are diverse and complex depending upon the hormone. In general, a peptide receptor can consist of an extracellular domain, an integral protein domain embedded in the plasma membrane, and an internal domain consisting of various signaling mechanisms affecting the DNA (Fig. 7-8). The so-called secondary intracellular messenger systems complete the signaling process for the specific hormone. Insulin—an important hormone in the control of glucose metabolism, metabolic syndrome, and diabetes—is one example of a peptide hormone. Examining some of the details of its interaction with a receptor might provide some insights into the receptor binding and secondary messengers systems of peptide hormones.

Quick Review

- Hormones are transported to target cells via the blood.
- Blood concentrations of a hormone give some insight to physiological function.
- The three major types of hormones are steroid, peptide, and amines, each with unique interactions with its target cell receptors.
- Positive and negative feedback systems control hormone secretions.
- Hormone release and interaction on target cells can be classified as endocrine, paracrine, or autocrine.
- Circulating hormones are influenced by circadian and seasonal factors.
- Receptors are the mediators of the hormonal signals to DNA.
- Peptide hormone receptors rely on secondary messenger systems to relay their signals to DNA.
- Steroid receptors interact directly with DNA.

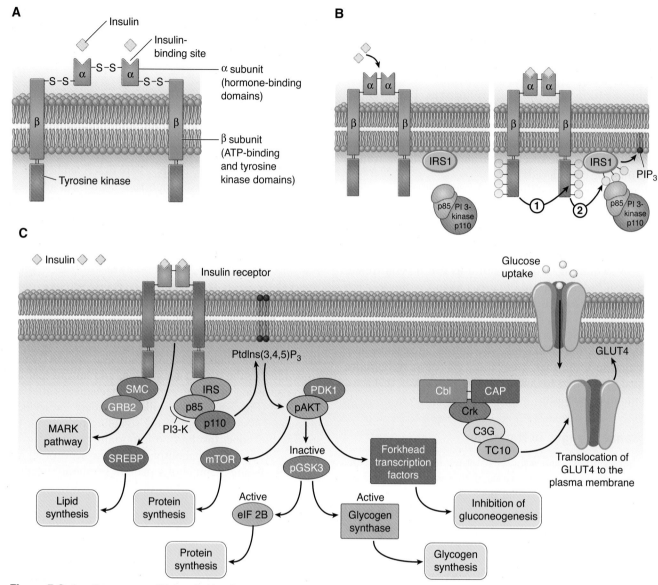

Figure 7-8. Insulin receptor. (A) A typical insulin receptor with the position of the different elements. **(B)** The interaction with the insulin receptor substrate (IRS) proteins elements and phosphorylation. **(C)** The cascade of events related to the insulin's receptors signaling systems and regulation of glucose uptake.

Steroid and Receptor Interactions

As noted before, steroid hormones interact with the regulatory elements on the DNA itself and are not reliant on secondary messenger systems. This is because steroid hormones readily diffuse across the lipid-based plasma membrane of the target cell. The receptors, located within the cell, contain specific sequences of DNA that are the targets, and these sequences are called hormone response elements (HREs). Nevertheless, receptor interaction involves a series of different interactions with cellular elements as the hormone moves from the outside of the cell to the nucleus of the cell.

Steroid receptors are different but they share similar structural and functional characteristics in that DNA binding and regulatory proteins are involved with their actions

(Fig. 7-9). Receptors for steroids such as estradiol, cortisol, testosterone, progesterone, aldosterone, thyroid hormones, and dihydroxyvitamin D3 have different variations, affinities, DNA binding sites, and regulatory proteins. The effect of steroid hormones may not be mediated by just the binding to a single protein receptor, but may be influenced by the binding of that receptor to other receptor proteins and to DNA (e.g., creating homodimers and heterodimers for receptor binding). The practical importance of such observations is that drugs designed to act as agonists or antagonists of a particular hormone receptor may have differing efficacy or effects on protein transcription. This efficacy depends on whether a receptor binds to some protein HREs as homodimers and other HREs as heterodimers.

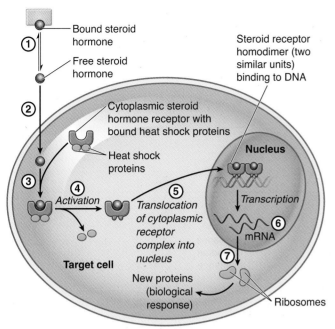

Figure 7-9. A model of steroid receptor actions related to its sequence of binding to the DNA. (1) Dissociation of steroid from binding protein, including (2) the transport of steroid into cell, the formation of binding steroid, and (3) the binding of steroid (testosterone, progesterone, estrogen) to cytoplasmic receptor with bound heat shock protein. (4) The loss of heat shock protein forms an "activated" receptor. (5) The activated cytoplasmic receptor enters the nucleus and binds DNA response elements as homodimers. (6) DNA is transcribed into messenger RNA, and mRNA leaves nucleus and is translated into protein on cytoplasmic ribosomes. (7) Finally, a newly made protein is produced (e.g., skeletal muscle proteins).

ENDOCRINE GLANDS AND EXERCISE: ROLES, REGULATION, RESPONSES, AND ADAPTATIONS

Endocrine glands, like any tissue, will adapt to exercise training. Thus, the synthesis of hormone in the gland, sensitivity of receptors, and amount of hormone released are all affected by exercise training. This adaptation is part of the specific response to an acute exercise protocol, which may be very different in its stress, and to the subsequent exercise adaptations to meet the demands of the exercise. It is important to remember that the endocrine system helps the body adapt to the demands of the stress placed on it to maintain homeostasis and needed functions in the body.

Hypothalamus and Pituitary Gland

One of the most important hormonal axes in the body is the hypothalamus-to-pituitary axis. The pituitary gland has been called the "master gland" because of its influence over so many different physiological functions in the body. There is a close relationship between these two glands in their function and coordination of a host of hormones that impact almost every tissue and system in the human body. Interestingly, the hypothalamus may be the real "master" in this process as it controls the function of the pituitary gland. Hormones secreted from the hypothalamus can either promote or inhibit hormone release from the pituitary gland.

Hypothalamus Releasing and Inhibiting Hormones

The hypothalamus influences the pituitary gland by releasing hormones that are called **releasing hormones** and **inhibiting hormones.** The hypothalamus will either promote the release of a hormone from the pituitary gland by secreting a releasing hormone or, conversely, inhibit release by secreting an inhibiting hormone. So, the true control of the pituitary and its many hormones comes from the hypothalamus.

For example, thyroid-releasing hormone is secreted from the hypothalamus, binds to peptide receptors in the anterior pituitary—a small endocrine gland located just below the brain—and stimulates the secretion of thyroid-stimulating hormone (TSH). TSH, in turn, enters the systemic circulation, binds to target receptors in the thyroid gland, and causes the release of thyroid hormones. Control of this process is mediated through negative feedback, which in turn can reverse the process by stimulating the hypothalamus to release a hormone to inhibit the release of the stimulatory hormone. In this case, thyroid-inhibitory hormone stops the production of TSH (Box 7-4).

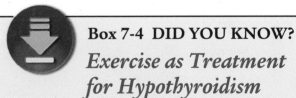

Box 7-4 DID YOU KNOW?
Exercise as Treatment for Hypothyroidism

Along with diet and medication, exercise might be an important element in dealing with hypothyroidism, in which the thyroid gland does not produce enough thyroid hormones. Without enough thyroid hormone, one can see a number of symptoms, including dry skin, hair loss, hoarseness, excessive menstruation, fatigue, lethargy, depression, intolerance to cold, constipation, and/or weight gain. Exercise can help this condition. Exercise will help to increase the sensitivity of tissue receptors to the amount of thyroid hormone produced, which allows for more effective use of the hormone secreted. With dieting, one can see a decrease in metabolic rate, especially if not done properly, and exercise can help to prevent this decline, which might be exacerbated with a hypothyroid condition. Even if taking thyroid medication (e.g., Synthroid) to replace the missing hormone synthetically, exercise is an important element for a healthy profile and more effective receptor interactions with the amount of hormone available.

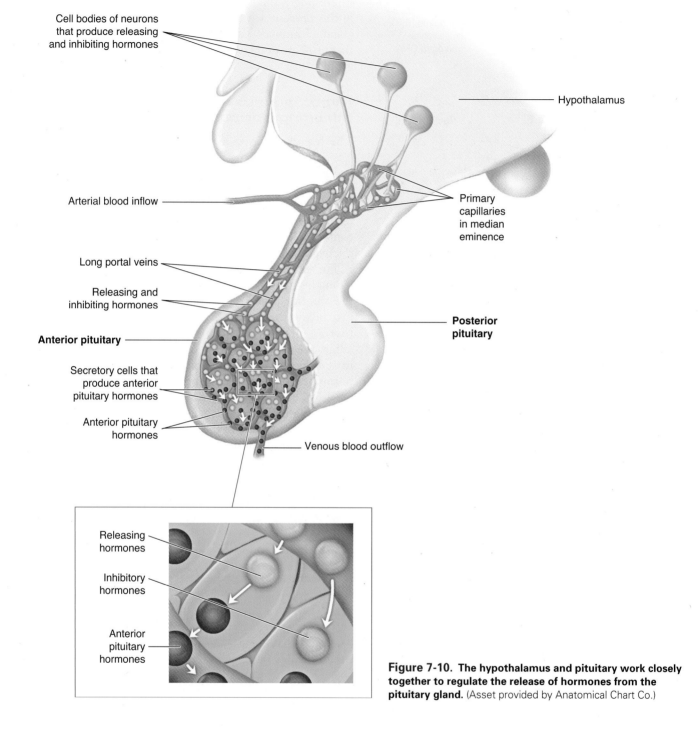

Figure 7-10. The hypothalamus and pituitary work closely together to regulate the release of hormones from the pituitary gland. (Asset provided by Anatomical Chart Co.)

Anterior Pituitary Gland

The anterior pituitary gland secretes a host of hormones that are important for physiological function and are responsive to exercise. Figure 7-10 shows the relationship between the hypothalamus and the pituitary gland.

Growth Hormone

Exercise stimulates the release of growth hormone (GH) from the anterior pituitary. GH is a 191-amino acid polypeptide hormone (Fig. 7-11). It is synthesized and secreted by cells called **somatotrophs** in the anterior pituitary. GH plays many different roles in the regulation

breakdown of triglycerides in fat cells (adipocytes) and not allowing the uptake or accumulation of lipids from the circulation (Fig. 7-12). It is easy to see why bodybuilders and other athletes might be tempted to use such a hormone as a drug. However, as you will see, its function may not be predictable and side effects (e.g., acromegaly: enlargement of flat bones in the jaw, hands, and feet, abdominal organs, nose, lips, and tongue) are negative consequences.

The 22 kD form of GH is the primary molecule produced by the DNA machinery in the pituitary somatotrophs. It is released in a pulsatile manner and is influenced by a host of factors, from exercise to sleep to stress. A hormone called growth hormone–releasing hormone is released from the hypothalamus to stimulate the synthesis and release of GH. Conversely, somatostatin—a peptide hormone secreted by

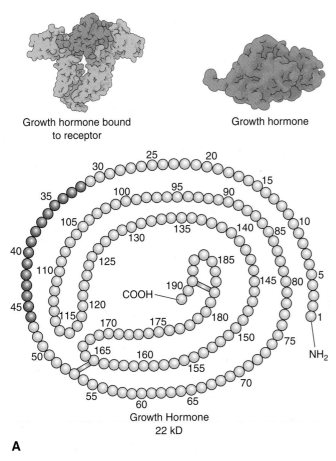

Growth hormone bound to receptor

Growth hormone

Growth Hormone 22 kD

A

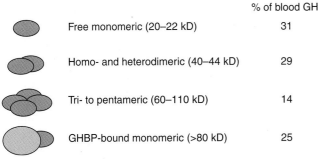

		% of blood GH
	Free monomeric (20–22 kD)	31
	Homo- and heterodimeric (40–44 kD)	29
	Tri- to pentameric (60–110 kD)	14
	GHBP-bound monomeric (>80 kD)	25

B

Figure 7-11. Growth hormone. (A) the 191-amino acid (22 kD) monomer of growth hormone is a series of amino acids that are linked with different binding mechanisms, including disulfide bonds, which help to give the molecule its ultimate shape biochemically. **(B)** Other forms of GH exist from small 5 kD, 17 kD, 20 kD to the larger aggregates of GH and binding proteins.

of numerous physiological processes, including tissue growth and metabolism. Interestingly, it has also been used as a performance-enhancing anabolic drug in sports because for many years it was not detectable in a drug test (See Box 7-1 and box reference Kraemer et al., 2010).

GH has diverse direct effects and influences on physiological functions, from stimulating protein synthesis in muscle and bone to stimulating the

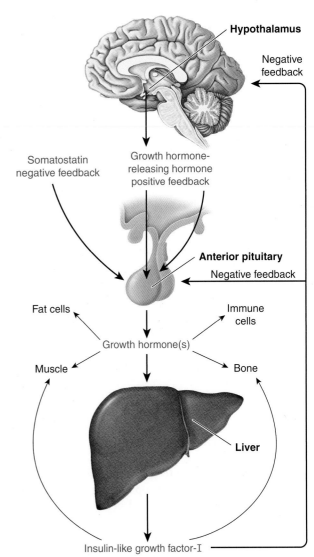

Figure 7-12. Regulatory feedback loops of growth hormone secretion and the primary targets in different tissues.

the hypothalamus—inhibits GH release. Ghrelin, a recently discovered hormone secreted from the stomach, also can stimulate GH release by binding directly to receptors on the somatotrophs. Because of GH's role in the release of IGF from the liver, high amounts of IGF in the circulation will lead to a negative feedback on the hypothalamus to release somatostatin to inhibit GH release. Over the course of a day, GH is released in a pulsatile manner, with some of the highest concentrations seen during sleep.[60] In addition, resistance exercise can affect the pattern of the GH pulsatile responses during sleep.[76] Thus, the importance of sleep to the repair and recovery process from exercise cannot be overemphasized. Also, aging can reduce the amount of GH produced over a day and the amount released with acute exercise stress.[71] This effect becomes more dramatic with each decade of aging. That is, the difference in concentrations of GH at age 20 will be much higher than concentrations at age 60. Exercise training can improve these acute responses to exercise in the aged but not to the magnitude of the response in a younger person, especially when the age span compared is greater than two decades.[40,41]

Exercise Responses and Adaptations

Exercise is a potent stimulus for GH release, and GH seems to be very sensitive to the type of exercise protocol and the mode of exercise (Figs. 7-13 and 7-14). In addition, although its levels may increase in the circulation, the true test of GH's effects is whether tissue receptors are actually available to bind with it to stimulate adaptations specific to the exercise program. For example, circulating GH might increase with walking vigorously, but the interaction with muscle to increase protein synthesis will only be with those muscle cells that were activated by the exercise and that need metabolic substrates and tissue repair during and after exercise. This underscores the importance of training specificity and the importance of exercise prescription in both resistance (Fig. 7-13) and endurance (Fig. 7-14) training protocols and programs (Box 7-5).

Proopiomelanocortin Peptides

Proopiomelanocortin (POMC) contains a host of bioactive peptides also secreted from the anterior pituitary gland (Fig. 7-15). It is also the precursor peptide for the opioid peptide "beta-endorphin." Early studies looking for these opioid peptides (the body's own morphine-like compounds) caused some to think that the POMC peptide was the source of other opioid peptides, but it is now known that two other opioid peptide families contain and biosynthesize these other opioid peptides. With stimulation of the hypothalamus to release corticotropin-releasing factor, POMC is stimulated and subsequently enzymatically cleaved into the different active peptides and to beta-endorphin, which mediates analgesia and stress responses. These other major peptides include adrenocorticotropin (ACTH) (stimulates cortisol production) and melanocyte-stimulating hormones (MSH) (stimulates melanocytes).

Exercise as a stressor stimulates release of POMC into circulation. Exercise-induced increases have been observed with both endurance exercise and resistance exercise. POMC is similar to GH in that higher values are observed with higher metabolic intensity–type exercise, during which an adequate volume of work is performed. Again, similar to GH, beta-endorphin and ACTH will increase to a greater extent with the use of a 10 RM resistance and short rest periods, potentially responding to the higher metabolic demands and the need for analgesia with such intense exercise.[37] In addition, high-intensity cycling[44] and sprint and endurance exercise[35] also result in increases in plasma concentrations of these two hormones.

Early studies indicated that beta-endorphin might be associated with positive mood states after running.[81] However, this response does not seem to be universal, as another study showed no positive changes in mood associated with beta-endorphin levels after an endurance run.[36] Another term often heard when speaking about endorphins is the feeling that runners sometimes experience, called "runner's high," or a state of euphoria while running. Exactly what this "runner's high" is remains unclear because it varies for each runner. Thus, relating "mood state" just to circulating beta-endorphin concentrations is difficult. However, in an amazing study by Boecker and colleagues[5] from Germany the link of euphoria to "opioid theory" was supported. The research team examined different regions of the brain in ten endurance runners at rest and after a 2-hr endurance run (21.5 +/− 4.7 km). Using advanced brain imaging techniques (positron emission tomography [PET] scans) and chemical labeling techniques measuring opioid ligand activity, they provided the first direct evidence supporting the theory of an opioid-mediated "runner's high" with endurance exercise.[5] We all have also heard athletes say they know when they are "in the zone," but is this a type of high, and is it related to beta-endorphin? Obviously more research is needed, but runner's high or being in the zone is not a simple phenomenon and may be related to a much larger combination of hormonal and neural contributions.

The relationship of beta-endorphin increases in humans to pain relief due to the analgesic properties of beta-endorphin is not clear. Elevations typically occur in response to stress as with the other hormones secreted from the anterior pituitary, so targeting one feature of the hormone to a symptom has been difficult to do experimentally in humans. We know from animal studies that beta-endorphin plays an analgesic role in pain relief. How the elevations of beta-endorphin in the blood with the use of various modalities used in physical therapy relate to a reduction or elimination of pain is not clear and has not been clearly documented.[4] Amazingly, pain reduction may be mediated by more local paracrine mechanisms (e.g.,

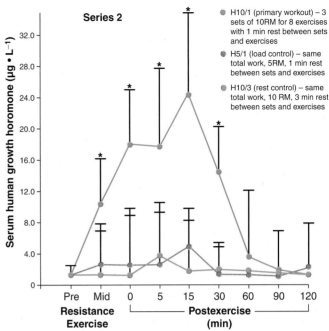

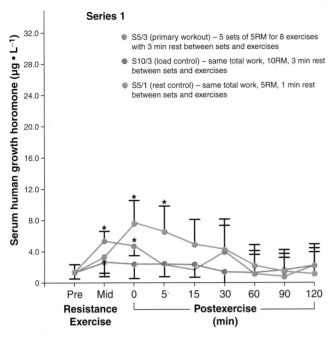

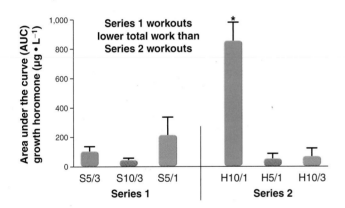

Figure 7-13. Responses of 22-kD GH to different exercise protocols using load (5 RM or 10 RM), rest period length (1 minute or 3 minutes) and volume, (series 1 lower volume and series 2 higher volume) for a resistance exercise protocol using 8 large and small muscle group exercises in men. *A significant difference from resting values. (Modified from Kraemer WJ, Marchitelli L, Gordon SE, et al. Hormonal and growth factor responses to heavy resistance exercise protocols. J Appl Physiol. 1990;69:1442–1450.) *Significant differences from pre-exercise values or in AUC data different from other workout protocols.

secretion beta-endorphin from leucocytes at the site of the pain receptor) rather than upon endocrine secretion of beta-endorphin from the anterior pituitary.[53]

Training adaptations of beta-endorphin and ACTH appear to occur with sprint interval training but not endurance training over short-term training programs.[35] This was supported in another study in which training did not affect beta-endorphin, ACTH, and cortisol concentrations consequent to a 30-minute treadmill run at 80% of the $\dot{V}o_{2max}$. Little is known about the adaptations of beta-endorphin and ATCH to resistance training.[35] However, one study revealed that 10 weeks of resistance training did not alter ACTH concentrations at rest, or its response to exercise in either 30- or 62-year-old men.[41] Cortisol did decrease in the older men, suggesting a reduction in the sensitivity of the glucocorticoid receptors with resistance training, despite a similar amount of ACTH present. Thus, training at

higher intensities may cause a greater response pattern of the POMC peptides.

Thyroid-Stimulating Hormone, Melanocyte-Stimulating Hormone, and Beta-Endorphin

Thyroid-stimulating hormone is an important signaling polypeptide from the POMC family of peptides. It stimulates the thyroid gland to secrete the hormones thyroxine (T-4) and tri-iodothyronine (T-3), which are vital for normal physiological function. Low concentrations of these hormones result in the pathological condition called "hypothyroidism," and too much production results in "hyperthyroidism." Each is characterized by abnormal metabolic function, among other negative outcomes. Thus, control of thyroid hormones is vital for normal physiological function.

Feelings of no energy, weight gain, or lethargy can many times be signs of an underactive thyroid gland (hypothyroid).

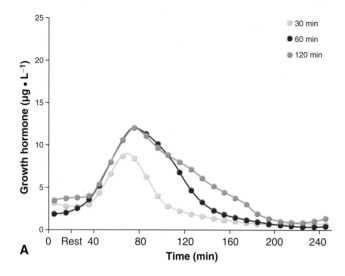

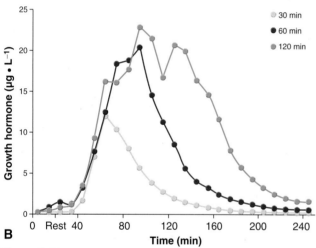

Figure 7-14. Peak responses of growth hormone in men and women during and after aerobic exercise of different durations at 70% of peak oxygen consumption. (A) Data for women and **(B)** data for men. (Modified from Wideman L, Consitt L, Patrie J, et al. The impact of sex and exercise duration on growth hormone secretion. J Appl Physiol. 2006;101:1641–1647.)

Iodide is mandatory for the production of thyroid hormones; without adequate dietary intake of iodine (e.g., iodized salt), thyroid hormones cannot be synthesized. Conversely, too much thyroid hormone can result in symptoms such as nervousness, insomnia, high heart rate, eye disease, anxiety, and Graves disease—a classic disease of the thyroid.

Thyroid hormone production is highly controlled, with TSH stimulated by thyrotropin-releasing hormone (TRH). TRH is released from the hypothalamus and stimulates the anterior pituitary gland to produce TSH. Conversely, another hormone secreted by the hypothalamus, somatostatin, inhibits the release of TSH. High concentrations of thyroid hormone also give negative feedback, letting the pituitary gland know that enough thyroid hormone is present. Both positive and negative feedback loops work to regulate the needed concentrations

of thyroid hormones in the body to meet the metabolic resting or exercise demands.

Thyroid hormones are vital for almost every chemical reaction in the body. Their presence affects in various ways many different physiological processes, including regulation of basal metabolic rate, growth and development, and metabolism of fats, proteins, and carbohydrate. In other words, thyroid hormones allow various metabolic reactions to occur by their presence or inhibits them by their absence.

Melanocyte-stimulating hormones (MSHs), which are cleaved from the POMC peptide, play a more specific physiological role. They stimulate the release of melanin by melanocytes in the hair and skin, affecting the color of these cells. MSHs exist as α-MSH (13 amino acids), β-MSH (22 amino acids), and γ-MSH (12 amino acids). Although the major biological function of MSHs is hyperpigmentation, they also stimulate aldosterone secretion from the adrenal glands. Additionally, MSHs appear to affect the blood–brain barrier for glucose, sucrose, and albumin and impact mental functions such as memory, arousal, and fear.

Beta-endorphin (31 amino acids long) is one of the body's opioid peptides, cleaved from the POMC polypeptide precursor. Thus, POMC is also considered one of the opioid peptide families. It is released from the anterior pituitary but also is found in neurons in the brain and peripheral tissues. Its levels increase in response to pain, trauma, higher exercise intensities, and various forms of stress (e.g., child birth). As noted before, when it was first discovered, some thought it was the hormone that caused "runner's high" because of its natural morphine-like qualities as an opioid peptide, but that sensation is somewhat ambiguous and highly individualized.

Exercise Roles, Responses, and Adaptations

Of the peptides derived from POMC, it is beta-endorphin, TSH, and MSH that are responsive to exercise stress, yet the most responsive is beta-endorphin, which has a similar pattern to GH and ACTH. With the important roles in metabolism for the thyroid hormones, TSH, a POMC peptide, does respond to exercise stress, even low-intensity walking.[7]

At present, the response of the different MSHs to exercise is less studied, with increases occurring with light to moderate walking. It also has possible interactions with both inflammatory processes and regulatory hormones involved in appetite and arousal in the higher brain levels. Because of its role in metabolism, exercise will increase the concentrations of TSH in the blood with light and moderate intensity.[7,78] It is not clear what adaptations occur with TSH with training. How TSH responds to long-term training is not clear. To further complicate matters, the regulation of T-3 and T-4 as measured in the blood has been shown not to be responsive to either endurance or resistance exercise.[29] A decrease from resting concentrations is observed with caloric restriction.[15]

Box 7-5 AN EXPERT VIEW

The Impact of Obesity on Growth Hormone Response During Exercise

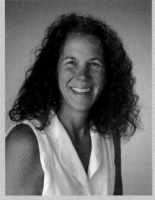

Jill A. Kanaley, PhD, FACSM
Professor
Department of Nutrition and Exercise
Physiology
University of Missouri
Columbia, MO

Growth hormone (GH) is crucial for physiological growth and development during childhood and adolescence and is also important in maintaining homeostasis of energy substrates during adulthood. Numerous factors can regulate GH release, such as diet, sleep, drugs, etc., but one of the most profound stimulators of GH release is exercise. Exercise results in a dramatic increase in GH levels in as little as 10 min,[5] and both continuous and intermittent exercise are equally effective in augmenting 24-h GH concentrations.[7] This exercise-induced GH response is related to exercise intensity in a dose–response pattern,[4] and GH levels remain elevated for a few hours postexercise. Additionally, a GH response will occur with repeated bouts of exercise (30 minutes each) without attenuation of the GH response.[2] Children also demonstrate a GH response to exercise, and an overall greater GH response to exercise is seen in late puberty than in younger children.[3]

One condition that can interfere with GH responses and have negative repercussions on health and well-being is obesity. Resting GH secretion is blunted profoundly in individuals with increased levels of body fat. More specifically, accumulation of abdominal body fat, particularly visceral fat, suppresses GH release.[6] Despite being a powerful stimulus, the exercise induced GH responses are blunted in older and obese individuals.[6] Exercise of sufficient duration and intensity will result in a small increase in GH concentrations in obese women, but this GH response is suppressed compared to that in

nonobese women.[1] Additionally, upper body obese women tend to have a lesser GH response to exercise than lower body obese women, but the impact of body fat distribution on the GH response to exercise appears to be weaker than that of obesity *per se*.[1] Furthermore, 16 weeks of aerobic training did not alter the GH response to exercise, despite the fact that aerobic exercise capacity improved significantly. Weight loss, and particularly fat loss, is crucial to see improvement in baseline and exercise GH levels in obese individuals.

Similarly, in obese children the blunted response to exercise is exacerbated with increasing severity of obesity.[3] This blunting of the GH-induced response to exercise was observed in both early- and late-pubertal children.

Thus, higher relative intensities may be necessary to stimulate adequate GH release during exercise in obese subjects, and it may take a period of time of training before substantial improvement in GH levels are seen.[6]

References

1. Kanaley JA, Weatherup-Dentes MM, Jaynes EB, et al. Obesity attenuates the growth hormone response to exercise. J Clin Endocrinol Metab. 1999;84:3156–3161.
2. Kanaley JA, Weltman JY, Veldhuis JD, et al. Human growth hormone response to repeated bouts of aerobic exercise. J Appl Physiol. 1997;79:1756–1761.
3. Oliver SR, Rosa JS, Minh TD, et al. Dose-dependent relationship between severity of pediatric obesity and blunting of the growth hormone response to exercise. J Appl Physiol. 2010;108:21–27.
4. Pritzlaff CJ, Wideman L, Weltman JY, et al. Impact of acute exercise intensity on pulsatile growth hormone release in men. J Appl Physiol. 1999;87:498–504.
5. Sauro LM, Kanaley JA. The effect of exercise duration and mode on the growth hormone responses in young women on oral contraceptives. Eur J Appl Physiol. 2003;90:69–76.
6. Weltman A, Weltman JY, Veldhuis JD, et al. Body composition, physical exercise, growth hormone and obesity. Eat Weight Disord. 2001;6:28–37.
7. Weltman A, Weltman JY, Watson Winfield DD, et al. Effects of continuous versus intermittent exercise, obesity, and gender on growth hormone secretion. J Clin Endocrinol Metab. 2008;93:4711–4720.

Beta-endorphin is the most responsive to the stress of exercise and increases in response to acute exercise (Fig. 7-16). Farrell et al.[14] had first examined the combined sequence of beta-endorphin/beta-lipotropin to controlled exercise stress. They showed the greatest increase after a 30-minute run at 60% of maximum oxygen consumption but not after the 80% and self-selected intensity runs of 30 minutes, suggesting it was not typically intensity related (Fig. 7-16). The response pattern to submaximal endurance exercise intensities still remains somewhat unclear, but it appears to be an interaction with both intensity and duration. However, increases are observed when exercising over the

anaerobic threshold or with repeat sprints.[34] Additionally, Kraemer et al.[37] showed that beta-endorphin was sensitive to the metabolic intensity of resistance exercise, similar to GH responses, with the highest values observed when using a highly metabolically demanding workout using a 10-RM resistance for eight exercises and 1-minute rest periods. Training-related changes in beta-endorphin concentrations in the blood again seem to be related to the overall stress. Specifically, combined aerobic/anaerobic sprint training results in higher concentrations of beta-endorphin, which may increase one's ability to exercise at an absolute higher intensity.[35]

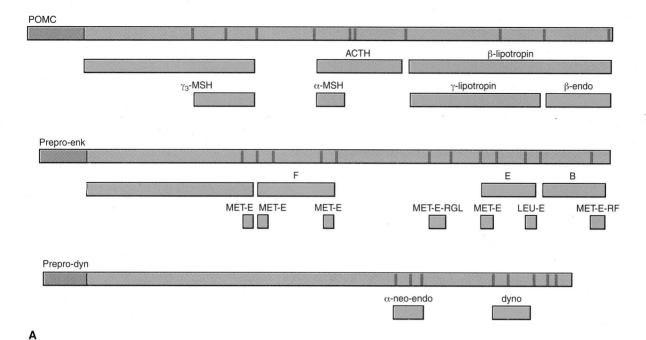

A

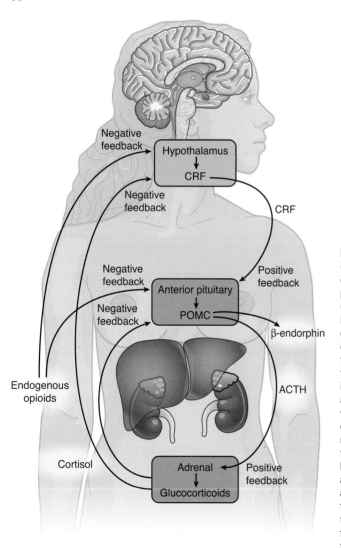

B

Figure 7-15. Opioid polypeptides and pro-opiomelanocortin (POMC) regulatory feedback control loops. (A) Three opioid families exist. Each has bioactive end products that are cleaved from the precursor by enzymes to their final sequences. Proopiomelanocotin (POMC) is the precursor for several welll known bioactive peptides including adrenocorticotropin (ACTH), which stimulates the adrenal cortex to produce cortisol, melanocyte-stimulating hormones, beta-endorphin, and beta lipotropin. The last two families discovered were the "Preproenkephlin" (Prepro-enk) a family of opoid peptides that is the precursor for bioactive peptides met- and leu-enkephalin but also important opioid fragments peptides F, E, and B found in the brain and adrenal medulla. The final family of opioid peptids discovered was "Preprodynorphin" (Prepro-dyn), which is found thoughout the central nervous system and is the precursor to bioactive peptides alpha neoendorphin and dynorphins. The physiological functions of the last two families of opioid peptides is less understood, but they potentially have been implicated in a variety of mechanisms that help mediate analgesia, immune modulation (Prepro-enk), temperature control, appetite (Prepro-dyn), and many other different functions related to the area of release. **(B)** The basic regulatory mechanisms are similar to other hypothalamic-pituitary releases, with corticotropin-releasing factor (CRF) stimulating the release of the POMC peptide, which is then cleaved via enzymatic reactions into its various bioactive peptides before release into circulation.

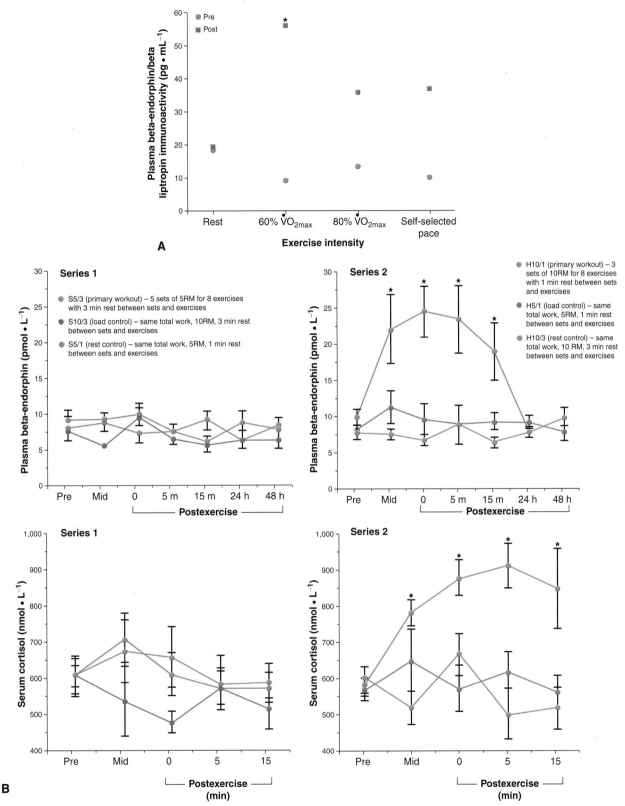

Figure 7-16. Responses of beta-endorphin to endurance exercise and resistance exercise. (A) Responses of beta-endorphin/beta-lipotropin before and after 30-minute treadmill runs at different exercise intensities. **(B)** Beta-endorphin responses to resistance exercise demonstrate that exercise with 10 RM resistances and short rest periods of 1 minute produce the highest plasma concentrations. Both examples seem to be associated with the lactate response, reflecting greater metabolic intensity stimulating higher concentrations. (Modified from Farrell PA, Gates WK, Maksud MG, Morgan WP. Increases in plasma beta-endorphin/beta-lipotropin immunoreactivity after treadmill running in humans. J Appl Physiol. 1982;52:1245–1249; and Kraemer WJ, Dziados JE, Marchitelli LJ, et al. Effects of different heavy-resistance exercise protocols on plasma beta-endorphin concentrations. J Appl Physiol. 1993;74:450–459.)

*Significant increase from pre-exercise resting concentrations.

Gonadotropins

Gonadotropins in both men and women stimulate the release of sex hormones, primarily testosterone in men and estrogen in women. Human chorionic gonadotropin (hCG) is secreted by the placenta during pregnancy. Luteinizing hormone (LH) and follicle-stimulating hormone (FSH) are the primary signal hormones to stimulate the release of the sex steroid hormones. Figure 7-17 shows a comparison of the effects of LH and FSH in men and women and their physiological targets, along with the associated feedback loops.

In women, the secretion of gonadotropin-releasing hormone (GnRH) from the hypothalamus occurs in a pulsatile manner, causing LH and FSH to be released similarly from the pituitary gland. Furthermore, the differential secretion over the month allows the menstrual cycle to vary in its estrogen concentrations to maintain the menstrual cycle. LH affects the ovarian follicle, stimulating ovulation and maintaining the corpus luteum, and FSH aids in the development of the ovarian follicle and stimulates secretion of oestradiol and progesterone. In women, FSH stimulates the production of inhibin, which also has a negative feedback on both the hypothalamus and the pituitary. The positive and negative feedback systems outlined in Figure 7-17 allow for the control of LH and FSH and the secretion of the sex steroids in women.

In men, GnRH results in the release of LH and FSH from the anterior pituitary, as with women, but it acts on a completely different target tissue, the Leydig cells, in the

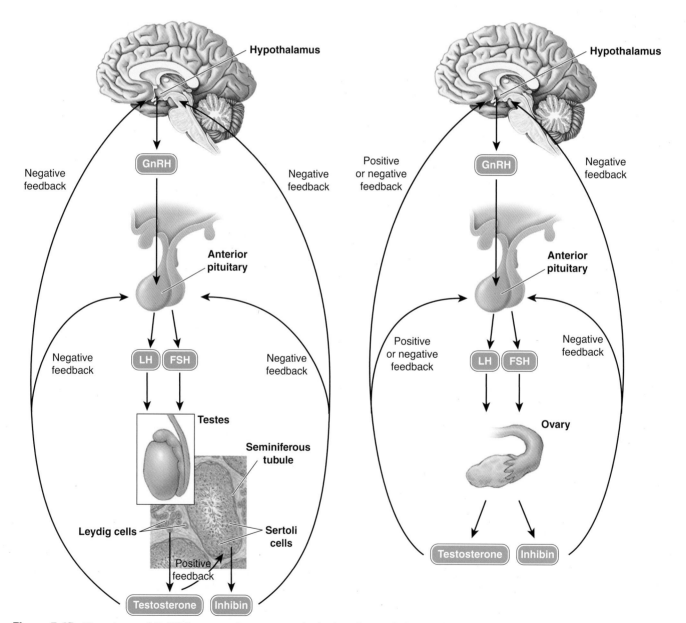

Figure 7-17. The release of GnRH in men and women results in the release of LH and FSH, which impact different tissues in men and women.

testes to produce testosterone. Interestingly, LH stimulates the theca cells of the ovaries to produce testosterone and is one source of testosterone in women (the other being the adrenal cortex). The secretion of FSH influences the Sertoli cells of the testes to help in the production of sperm and the secretion of sex-hormone binding globulin (SHBG), a major binding protein that binds to testosterone and maintains its half-life in the blood.

Androgens

Androgens, or steroid sex hormones in men and women, are the most potent regulators of sex-related physiological function. Primarily, testosterone in men and estrogens in women have important regulatory effects for each gender.

Testosterone

Testosterone is the most potent anabolic hormone in men.[79] Its role in producing the androgenic characteristics of males during pubertal development, and later in building muscle, is vital to optimal functioning. Testosterone mediates development in early infancy with the masculinization of the brain, influences the development of secondary sex characteristics of young boys, and stimulates the development of muscle and bone mass, strength, and libido in men. Blocking this hormone in young men can result in reduced

ability to build strength or muscle size.[48] Conversely, blocking LH in older men with prostate cancer, called "deprivation therapy," results in testosterone concentrations that are negligible. Thus, over about 6 months, the IGF and GH family of hormones in these men with prostate cancer seem to assume the primary anabolic function, as in women, allowing for the development of muscle size and strength with resistance training.[21] The production of testosterone is accomplished via a series of reactions. From the basic cholesterol ester, the synthesis of "prohormones" leads to the synthesis of testosterone. When too much testosterone is produced, it results in higher levels of estrogen compounds and dihydrotestosterone, which is primarily interactive with sex-linked tissue such as the prostate gland in men (Fig. 7-18).

In women, estrogens provide the basis for the menstrual cycle and impact a host of different functions related to the menstrual cycle. Testosterone concentrations are 10 to 30 times lower in women compared with men and testosterone is produced in the ovaries and in the adrenal cortex. Women rely on the GH and IGF hormonal systems more than men for anabolic actions.

Exercise Roles, Responses, and Adaptations

It is well established that both acute aerobic and resistance exercise of sufficient intensity (Fig. 7-19) will increase testosterone concentrations in the blood in both men and

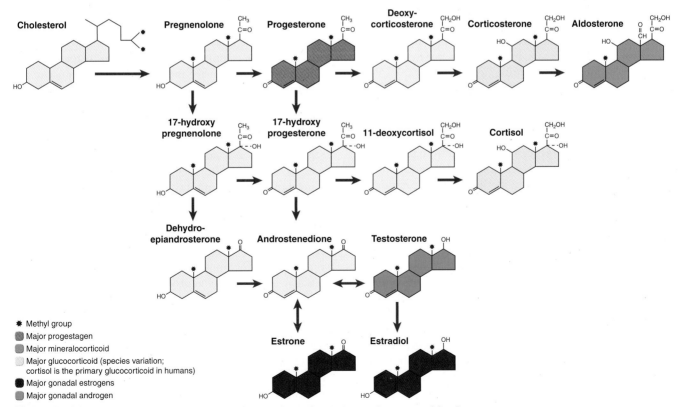

Figure 7-18. Steroidogenesis is a series of reactions from the cholesterol ester resulting in steroid hormones.

Resistance Exercise Test

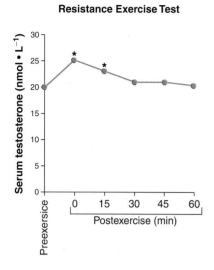

% $\dot{V}O_{2max}$ Treadmill Test

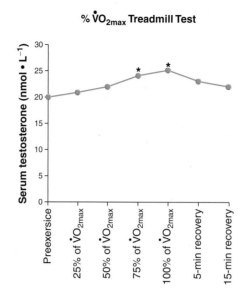

Figure 7-19. Responses of testosterone to a resistance exercise protocol consisting of 6 sets using a 10 repetition maximum (RM) and 2 minutes' rest between sets and a discontinuous graded treadmill exercise using a speed of 6–7 mph, 7-minute stages at each of the different intensities ending with a 2- to 3-minute stage at 100% $\dot{V}O_{2max}$ and 1 minute between stages for blood sampling.
*Significant increase above pre-exercise values.

women, although with dramatically lower increases in women.[31,43,45,61]

The key effects of exercise on target tissues, specifically skeletal muscle, are an increase in the amount of testosterone delivered and an increase in number of muscle fibers that become activated, which in turn will "up-regulate" a greater number of receptors. Although running and weight lifting both increase circulating concentrations of testosterone, a greater number of motor units and higher threshold motor units are typically needed to lift the heavier weights. Testosterone's signal to increase protein synthesis will therefore impact a greater number of muscle fibers, especially the type II fibers, leading to greater hypertrophy of the whole muscle when lifting heavy weights.

The effects of training on testosterone secretion are variable, depending on the fitness level of the athlete, the volume and intensity of training, and whether overtraining is present.[23,43,77] Typically, with resistance training in men, increases in resting values can be observed from pretraining values. In addition, the exercise-induced concentrations in response to the workout may be higher than pretraining levels, contributing to a greater exercise capacity.[43] In addition, testosterone responses can vary depending on the conditioning activities, as demonstrated by Moore and Fry.[59] In this study, testosterone was found to be decreased when American football players stopped weight training and did only interval sprints, agility drills, and running and blocking skill practice drills, but concentrations returned to baseline when normal weight training and conditioning were resumed. Such data indicate that caution is needed when modulating conditioning programs away from anabolic-type activities toward more catabolic- or overtraining-type protocols, as physiological function might be compromised.

Endurance training may result in no change or a decrease in resting testosterone values in both men and

women.[9,80] However, with extreme endurance training, such as that for marathons and ultraendurance events, significant reductions to hypogonadal concentrations can be observed.[16,17,39]

Because of the much lower concentration and the sources arising from the ovaries and the adrenal cortex (e.g., adrenal androgens), the training responses of testosterone in women are less clear.[79] With resistance training, small but significant increases in resting concentrations have been observed.[57] In addition, small increases in free testosterone (that which is not bound to any binding protein and thus, considered to be bioactive) have been observed in women with endurance training.[31,32] However, testosterone plays its biggest role in recovery and repair in men because of the higher molar concentrations capable of being released and secreted from the testes.[79]

Estrogens and the Menstrual Cycle

Estrogens play a major role in regulating the menstrual cycle in women. The menstrual cycle is characterized by menstruation, or monthly bleeding, which allows the woman's body to shed the lining of the uterus. Menstrual blood flows through the small opening in the cervix and passes out of the body through the vagina. Most menstrual periods last from 3 to 5 days. Menstruation prepares the woman's body for pregnancy each month and is mediated primarily by estradiol and progesterone. The average menstrual cycle is 28 days but can range anywhere from 21 to 35 days, and up to 45 days in teens.

Figure 7-20 shows the different phases of the menstrual cycle. LH stimulates the release of estradiol, and its release allows the lining of the uterus to grow and thicken. An egg (ovum) in one of the ovaries starts the maturation process. At about day 14 of 28, the egg leaves the ovary (called ovulation) and is transported via the fallopian tube to the uterus. A woman is most likely to get pregnant during the

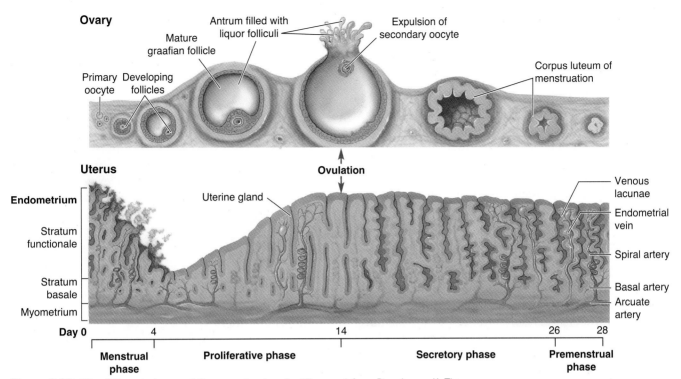

Figure 7-20. The different phases of the menstrual cycle. (*Top graph* from Premkumar K. The Massage Connection Anatomy and Physiology. Baltimore, MD: Lippincott Williams & Wilkins 2004. *Bottom image* provided by Anatomical Chart Co.)

3 days before or on the day of ovulation. If the egg is fertilized by a man's sperm and attaches to the uterine wall, pregnancy occurs. A woman will typically demonstrate shorter and more regular cycles with age, after adolescence.

Influence of Exercise on the Menstrual Cycle

The influence of exercise on the menstrual cycle has been a topic of great interest due its relationship to menstrual disturbances. The basic types of menstrual disorders are as follows:

- **Dysmenorrhea:** This disorder is characterized by painful periods with severe cramping. It is thought to be caused by the release of higher levels of prostaglandins. In younger women, it is not thought to be related to serious disease, despite the severe cramping. In older women, other pathologies, such as uterine fibroids or endometriosis, can cause the pain.
- **Amenorrhea:** This disorder is characterized by a lack of a menstrual period. There are two types of amenorrhea, primary and secondary. Primary amenorrhea is a condition in which a woman has never had a period, whereas secondary amenorrhea is the absence of menstrual period for at least 6 months, often due to pregnancy. Other causes have been related to pregnancy, breastfeeding, extreme weight loss caused by illness, eating disorders, or

stress. The role of excessive exercise, although many times blamed for this condition, might not be a primary cause; amenorrhea may be related to other factors such as nutritional insufficiency in eating disorders.
- **Menorrhagia:** This condition is characterized by prolonged menstrual bleeding and is not just heavy menstrual cycle bleeding. The very heavy bleeding lasts longer than 7 days and features large clots in the flow. It is typically caused by hormonal imbalances or uterine fibroids. Fibroids are growths in the muscular wall of the uterus and are more prevalent among women older than 35 years and those who have had multiple pregnancies.
- **Premenstrual syndrome (PMS):** This is a term given to the symptoms that may occur from 7 to 14 days before a period, which are highly variable for each woman.

The development of menstrual cycle disorders has been the topic of much study, primarily as it relates to secondary amenorrhea. Historically, extreme exercise was thought to be a major cause of menstrual disturbances. However, this does not appear to be the case. Rogol et al.[67] concluded that "a progressive exercise program of moderate distance and intensity does not adversely affect the robust reproductive system of gynecologically mature eumenorrheic women." In general, it is now believed that such disturbances may well be caused by a lack of caloric intake rather than extreme exercise alone.[84] These types of disorders appear to be related to sports that have a high level of endurance training (cross country running), demands for body image (dancing, gymnastics), weight class sports, or sports in which body size is vital to performance (diving, gymnastics, figure skating).[65] The link between secondary amenorrhea and inadequate caloric intake for activities demanding large energy expenditure underscores the importance of dietary intake matching caloric demands.[82] Recovery is linked to change in eating behavior, with increased caloric intake to meet energy demands, which may prevent or reduce menstrual disorder without any change in the exercise training program.[51]

The effect of exercise on PMS is more complex, as the symptoms and the condition itself are not universal to all women. Early data had suggested that exercise might even reduce the symptoms of PMS due to changes in hormonal balances. These changes include the concentration of estrogen, endorphin withdrawal, and decrease in progesterone concentrations during the luteal phase of the menstrual cycle. The relationship of PMS to sport and training performance has not been definitively documented because of the array of individual responses and psychological interactions. Some women believe they can perform better during this phase, with greater aggression and training intensity, whereas others feel completely shut down due to cramping and pain requiring medication. Thus, the management of PMS in athletes is highly individualized.[49]

Insulin-Like Growth Factors

Insulin-like growth factors (IGF) are a "super family" of peptides. IGF-I and IGF-II are the major forms of this hormone. Their regulation, variants produced, and signaling systems are complex and still not completely understood. They are secreted from many different cells in endocrine (i.e., liver), paracrine (e.g., fat cells) and autocrine (e.g., skeletal muscle) releases. In early research, IGFs were termed somatomedins. IGFs along with their six known binding proteins have important anabolic actions for muscle and bone. IGF-I is also a potent regulator of some of the effects of GH. The six IGF-binding proteins and an acid-labile subunit (ALS) bind to IGF-I and IGF-II. The primary functions of these binding proteins are to extend the half-life of IGFs in the circulation, transport the IGFs to the target cells, and help modulate the biological actions of the IGFs.[2] IGF-I can be broken down into three splice variants: IGF-IEa, IGF-IEb, and IGF-IEc. IGF-IEc, also called mechano-growth factor, is released from muscle as a result of the mechanical stress of exercise, with activation of motor units for muscle contraction.[22] It then acts in an autocrine manner to stimulate the muscle fiber repair and/or growth.

IGF-II is a neutral peptide with 67 amino acids and molecular weight of 7.4 kD. It is a product of a single

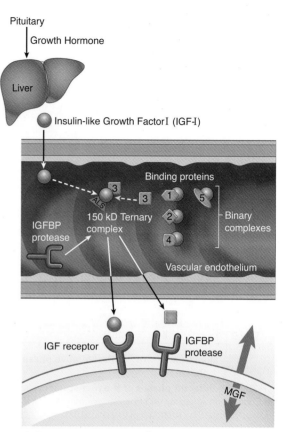

Figure 7-21. Growth hormone can stimulate IGF-I release from the liver. IGF-I circulates in the blood in association with IGF-binding proteins, creating a ternary complex made up of the IGF, IGFBP, and ALS. IGF-I penetrates the capillary and moves into the interstitial space to bind with IGF receptors, which starts the signaling process. (Courtesy of Dr Bradley C. Nindl, Military Performance Division, US Army Research Institute of Environmental Medicine, Natick, MA.)

gene and contains nine exons with four different promoter regions. It is encoded by exons 7, 8, and 9. Interestingly, unlike IGF-I, IGF-II is thought to be independent of GH control (Fig. 7-21).

Much more research remains to be done on the IGF system, as it is still poorly understood due to its complexity. IGFs are especially important in exercise physiology because of their involvement in exercise training adaptations in repair and remodeling in bone and skeletal muscle.

Signals for Protein Synthesis

A signaling system is needed to translate the hormonal message contained in IGF-I to the DNA in the nucleus of the cell. In general, exercise can stimulate IGF-I signaling mechanisms. Figure 7-22 demonstrates a common signaling pathway, in which IGF-I interacts with the receptor to stimulate the mTOR signaling pathway to increase the genetic machinery to stimulate protein synthesis. AKT blocks FOXO (FOXO proteins are a subgroup of the Forkhead family of transcription factors, and members

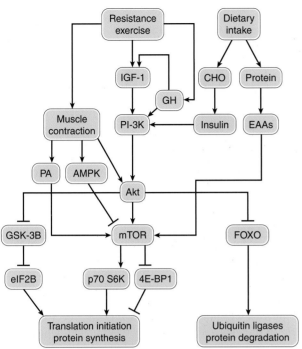

Figure 7-22. Common signaling pathway of IGF-I. The IGF-I signaling pathway results in both increased protein synthesis and decreased protein degradation. IGF-I = Insulin-like Growth Factor-I; GH = Growth Hormone; EAAs = Essential Amino Acids; CHO = carbohydrate; PI-3K = Phosphatidylinositol 3-kinase; AMPK = 5' adenosine monophosphate-activated protein kinase; Akt = a serine/threonine protein kinase family is involved in cellular survival pathways, by inhibiting apoptotic processes; mTOR = mammalian target of rapamycin; PA = phosphatidic acid; GSK-3B = Glycogen synthase kinase 3B; FOXO = FOX Proteins" are a family of transcription factors; eIF2B = eukaryotic initiation factor; P70 S6K = a serine/threonine kinase with its target S6 ribosomal protein; 4E-BP1 = Eukaryotic translation initiation factor 4E-binding protein 1.

of class 'O' share the characteristic of being regulated by the insulin/PI3K/Akt signaling pathway) to diminish any protein degradation, and adequate IGF availability is vital in the process (Box 7-6).

Exercise Responses and Adaptations

As fitness improves in an individual, the resting concentrations of IGF-I increase.[13] Acute increases with exercise stress are, again, a function of the intensity and volume of the exercise, fitness level, and carbohydrate/protein intake.[13,45,46,61,69] Note that a higher level of fitness and increased intake of carbohydrates and protein are associated with higher resting concentrations of IGF-I. Studies have shown such increases in IGF-I level with training in men and women.[13,45] The impact of exercise on circulating concentrations of IGF can be variable, but it appears that stimulation of muscle IGF concentrations are more compelling because of the mechanical signaling of muscle contraction (Box 7-7).

Adrenal Hormones

The adrenal gland has been called the "fight-or-flight" gland and is designed to assist in the response to stress. Located on top of the kidneys, its hormonal secretions influence both high-level performance and recovery from exercise stress. The adrenal gland has two functional parts, the adrenal cortex and the adrenal medulla, each with a different set of hormones that are released into the blood upon stimulation. The nervous system stimulates the adrenal medulla for a rapid response, whereas stimulatory hormones cause the release of hormones from the adrenal cortex (Fig. 7-23).

Adrenal Medulla

The stimulation and release of catecholamines from the adrenal medulla constitute an adrenergic response of the body typically reserved for the immediate response to stress, including exercise. This response affects every tissue in the body that has adrenergic receptors. It enhances the breakdown of glycogen to glucose in the liver, enhances the release of fatty acids from adipose tissue, causes vasodilation of the small arteries within muscle, increases blood pressure, and increases cardiac output.

The adrenal medulla, which is enveloped by the adrenal cortex, makes up about 10% of the adrenal mass, and secretes catecholamines (Fig. 7-23). Epinephrine (also called adrenalin) makes up about 85% of the total catecholamines within the adrenal medulla, with norepinephrine and dopamine together making up the remainder. Catecholamines are synthesized in the adrenal chromaffin granules, which are very porous, allowing movement of molecules in and out of the granule for the biosynthetic reactions (Fig. 7-24). Norepinephrine and dopamine also play roles as neurotransmitters in specific neurons in the nervous system. The hormonal release from the adrenal medulla is due to stimulation by the sympathetic nervous system (splanchnic nerve). In addition to catecholamines, one of the other opioid peptide families, proenkephalin opioid peptides, are also synthesized and released from the adrenal medulla. These opioid peptides may play important roles in recovery and immune enhancement.

Roles in Exercise Preparation and Force Production

Catecholamines (primarily epinephrine and norepinephrine) are part of the adrenergic response to stress, including exercise, and increases can be seen in the blood within seconds of a significant stressor (e.g., fright, high-intensity exercise). More interestingly, increases in epinephrine can be seen up to 24 hours, but typically 30 minutes, prior to exercise, allowing for physiological preparation for activity.[18,75] It has been shown recently that epinephrine may be important to force production. Its binding with beta-2 adrenergic receptors found in the sarcoplasmic reticulum causes more rapid release of Ca++, which leads to quicker

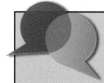

Box 7-6 AN EXPERT VIEW

Endocrine Physiology: IGF-I as a Candidate Biomarker Mediating Beneficial Aspects of Physical Activity

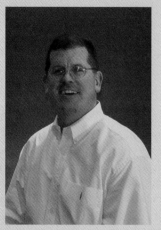

Bradley C. Nindl, PhD, FACSM

Performance Physiology Team Research Director
Military Performance Division
U.S. Army Research Institute of Environmental Medicine
Natick, MA
Adjunct Associate Professor
Department of Kinesiology
University of Connecticut
Storrs, CT
Adjunct Associate Professor
Springfield College
Springfield, MA

The endocrine system serves as a major biological communication network in which hormones act to maintain homeostasis by mediating and coordinating many of the body's physiological systems. Classic endocrine physiology literature states that a hormone is released from a gland into the systemic circulation and travels to a distant cell/organ to effect a response (i.e., endocrine action). However, major research advances in endocrine physiology over the last 15 to 20 years have also revealed that many hormones can act in other fashions as well. For example, hormones can be released from a cell to act on an adjacent cell (i.e., paracrine fashion), released from a cell to act on the same cell (i.e., autocrine fashion), or produced by a cell, never leaves the cell and acts on the same cell that produces the hormone (i.e., newly named "intocrine" fashion). In addition to the classic endocrine glands, such as the pituitary gland, the adrenal gland, the thyroid gland, the pancreas, the testes, and the ovaries, research has indicated that muscle, bone, heart, and immune cells/ tissues can also release hormones acting in these various fashions. A hormone that can act in endocrine, paracrine, autocrine, and intocrine fashions and is produced by a plethora of cell types is *insulin-like growth factor-I (IGF-I)*.

IGF-I is a small peptide hormone (7.5 kDa) that is produced primarily by the liver and is under the direct regulation of growth hormone. IGF-I has many different anabolic, metabolic, and mitogenic properties. The anabolic properties of IGF-I include its ability to facilitate muscle and bone growth. The metabolic properties of IGF-I include its ability to regulate both carbohydrate and protein metabolism. The mitogenic properties of IGF-I include its ability to act as both an initiative factor and a progression factor during cell cycle growth.

IGF-I is one of the most important and complex hormones to study and is thought to be critical in mediating many of the beneficial aspects of physical activity. The regulatory complexity of IGF-I is vast, as a family of binding proteins (BPs) serve to either stimulate or inhibit IGF-I action. Less than 2% of IGF-I circulates in a free (i.e., unbound) form. The majority (≥75%) of IGF-I circulates in a ternary form comprising IGF-I, IGFBP-3, and an acid-labile subunit (ALS). This form is quite large (150 kDa), has a long half-life (~12–15 hours), and is largely confined to the systemic circulation. Approximately 20% to 30% of IGF-I circulates in a binary form consisting of IGF-I and one of its six binding proteins. Only the free and binary forms of IGF-I are thought to be "bioavailable" and capable of escaping the circulating and trafficking toward cellular receptors. Both systemic and local proteases also serve to dissociate IGF-I from its family of binding proteins and assist IGF-I in becoming bioavailable. As IGF-I is a protein hormone, its cellular receptor is on the cell membrane and has extracellular, transmembrane, and intracellular domains. After IGF-I initiates signal transduction with its receptors, a cascade of cellular events, including multiple kinase-driven phosphorylation events, results in cellular responses.

Importantly, IGF-I has been linked to optimal health and fitness. In general, IGF-I is thought to be up-regulated with exercise, although several paradoxes exist. Activity-induced skeletal muscle adaptation is thought to be driven in part by the mitogenic and myogenic effects of IGF-I, as evidenced by positive correlations between basal levels of circulating IGF-I concentrations and indices of fitness level and lean body mass. Exercise produces changes in IGF-I, but the regulatory role of the IGF-I response to exercise has not yet been clearly defined. One reason for this is that the quantitative changes in circulating IGF-I observed in response to acute exercise interventions vary among different studies, with increases, decreases, or no changes reported. Studying circulating IGF-I remains important due to its utility as a biomarker, reflecting health and fitness status, as well as to the fact that the relationship between systemic and local IGF-I remains obscure. Furthermore, except in cancer, a low level of IGF-I usually predicts a negative health outcome. Future research efforts will need to resolve the mechanisms underlying the changes observed in circulating IGF-I and their relationship to local changes at the cell/tissue level.

Box 7-7 AN EXPERT VIEW
Growth and Development

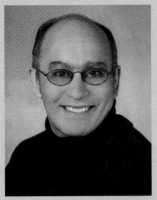

Alan D. Rogol, MD, PhD
Professor of Clinical Pediatrics
University of Virginia
President, ODR Consulting
Charlottesville, VA

Growth and adolescent development within the broad range of normal are the best signs that a child or adolescent is generally healthy. It is imperative to continue to grow as a child because "staying the same," although terrific for an adult, is really "falling behind" for a child.

Growth and sexual development occur following a genetic blueprint but are modified by hormones and the environment. The genetic plan is more than just the sum of a few genes; it represents the interplay of a great number of genes as modified by the environment—hormones and nutrition.

After birth, the most important hormonal systems for growth are the hypothalamic–pituitary–thyroid and GH/IGF-I axes. The former affects the rate of metabolism of virtually all cells. In its absence, virtually no growth occurs and the child has the signs and symptoms of hypothyroidism—slow linear growth, slow metabolism, and within the first few years of life, loss of intellectual function.

The GH/IGF-I axis is critical to achieve one's genetic potential in terms of adult height. The hypothalamus makes two hormones that affect pituitary GH release: GH-releasing hormone (GHRH) and somatostatin. The former is a signal to release GH and the latter an inhibitory signal. Intermittent, pulsatile GH release (the proper physiologic pattern) is then due to the "summation" of the GHRH and somatostatin rhythms.

GH has few effects on growth *per se*, but acts at the liver to make circulating IGF-I and in virtually every other organ to make IGF-I locally where it may act in *high concentration* in a very restricted site, such as at the ends of the bones (epiphyses) to promote linear growth. GH does have some effects on its own, for example, lipolysis—and thus its effect on the whole body—is in terms of body composition (muscle, bone, and fat tissue) as well as on the regional distribution of body fat and so is important to the risk for cardiovascular disease.

The body uses many tricks to get the most out of hormone production. GHRH and somatostatin are in relatively high concentration, but in a very limited circulation: the hypothalamic–pituitary portal system. Their half-lives are quite short for a quick "on" signal, but also a quick "off" signal is important to permit

moment-to-moment alterations in GH secretion (pulsatile). IGF-I is a potent insulin-like peptide. It would cause severe hypoglycemia if circulated in its biologically active "free" form. This potential biological activity is dampened by several large carrier proteins, permitting this potent peptide hormone to be carried around the circulation in its biologically inactive "bound" form to its sites of action. There, it might be unloaded from the binding protein to act at a "sanctuary" site where it will have its proper biological action, but will not have the whole body (systemic) effect of hypoglycemia.

At puberty, at least two things happen: the adolescent undergoes a growth spurt and begins (and completes) sexual development. The hypothalamic–pituitary gonadal axis (ovary for a female and testis for a male), however, gets an earlier start. Just after birth, especially in boys, this axis is working virtually at its adult level. Boys actually have a "mini" puberty in the first few months of life! The axis then stops working only to reawaken at the appropriate time for pubertal development. This is called the prepubertal "hiatus" and lasts 10 to 12 years. During this time, the testes and ovaries produce very small amounts of their appropriate sex hormones, estradiol for girls and testosterone for boys. These small and actually unmeasurable (by routine assays) amounts of hormones are capable of keeping the hypothalamus from secreting, again in a pulsatile fashion, gonadotropin-releasing hormone (GnRH) (luteinizing hormone [LH] for sex steroids, and follicle-stimulating hormone [FSH] for the ovum and spermatogenesis). Thus, the system is poised in the prepubertal (prereproductive) state.

Then, at puberty, the small but real secretion of testosterone and of estradiol is no longer able to inhibit the release of GnRH. Also, the testis and ovary are able to respond to the increasing levels of LH and FSH to permit the pubertal process to occur and to then operate at the adult (reproductive) state.

Another interesting phenomenon that occurs with the endocrine system is that the increasing levels of testosterone and estradiol up-regulate the hypothalamus and pituitary transiently to make more GH/IGF-I to stimulate the growth spurt so characteristic of midadolescence. After several years, these sex hormones cause the epiphyses of the long bones to fuse and linear growth ceases.

The hormones of both axes remain important to permit the attainment of the adult body composition and regional distribution of body fat, as muscle and bone continue to accrue until the middle of the third decade of life. These two hormonal axes are quite representative of the multiple endocrine organs, which use alterations in secretion, half-life in the circulation (e.g., binding proteins), action at specific receptors, and "speed" of metabolism to tune and fine tune the metabolic machinery of the body.

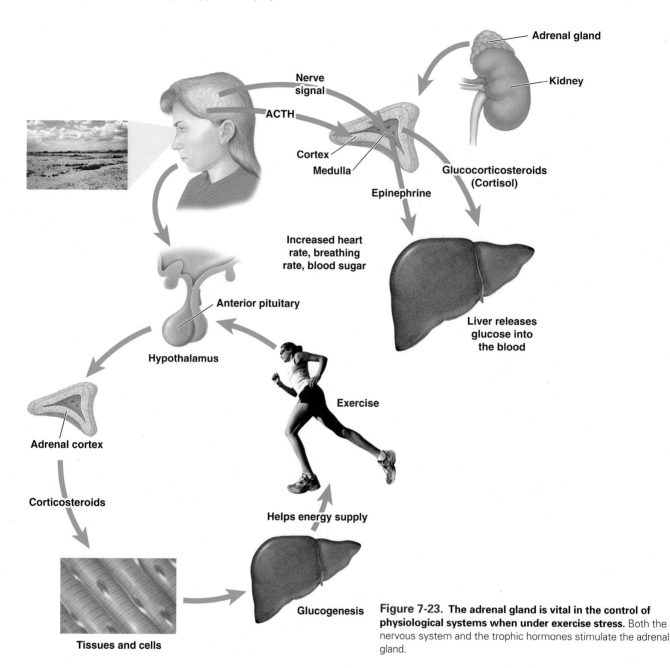

Figure 7-23. The adrenal gland is vital in the control of physiological systems when under exercise stress. Both the nervous system and the trophic hormones stimulate the adrenal gland.

interaction with troponin molecules. This quicker interaction leads to more rapid availability of troponin's active sites, which in turn leads to more rapid contraction of the sarcomere. Thus, muscle contraction is augmented by epinephrine release.

Interactions with Opioid Peptides

In 1985, it was discovered that the release of epinephrine coincides with the release of proenkephalin opioid peptides (e.g., peptide F as a marker of fragments) (Fig. 7-25).[42] Untrained men showed greater increases in levels of proenkephalin peptide F and epinephrine with higher intensity exercise. Conversely, highly trained middle distance runners had higher concentrations at rest (almost two fold higher)

and at the lower intensities, but peptide F was reduced at the higher exercise intensities, allowing significantly higher concentrations of epinephrine to be released with maximal exercise. Both groups showed increased peptide F concentrations into recovery, which also suggests a role for such opioid peptides in the recovery responses.

Recovery and Immune Interfaces

The elevations in peptide F during recovery were suggested by investigators to be due to possible interactions with immune cells. In a study by Triplett et al.,[75] it was suggested that the relationship between peptide F and the activity of B cells (which produce antibodies) indicated this fact.[75] Further study demonstrated that peptide F was found to be in the buffy coat

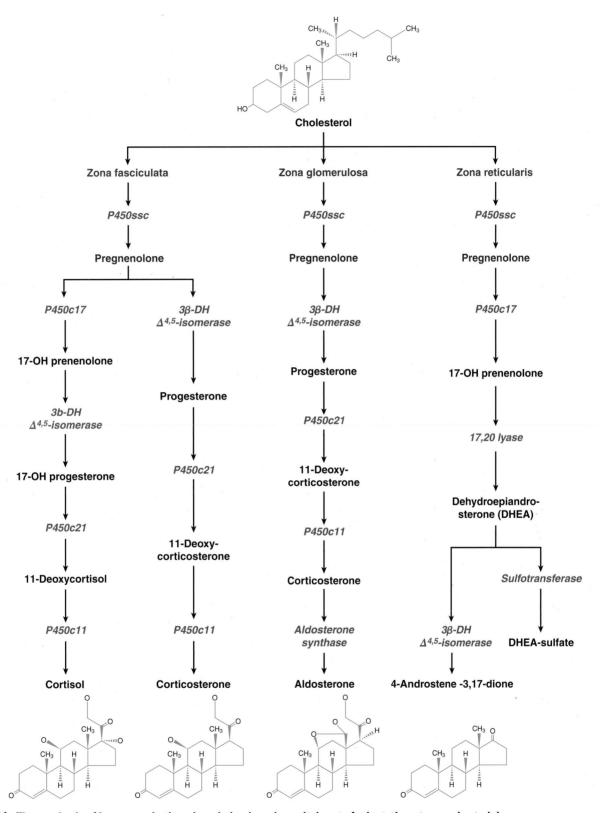

Figure 7-24. The synthesis of hormones in the adrenal gland can be a vital part of adaptations to exercise training. **(A)** Pathways of hormone synthesis in the adrenal cortex.

(continued)

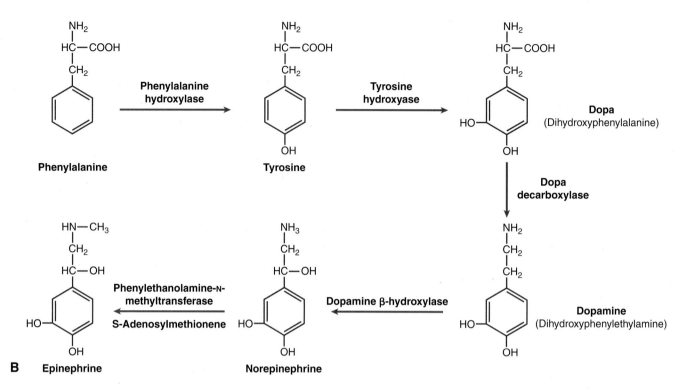

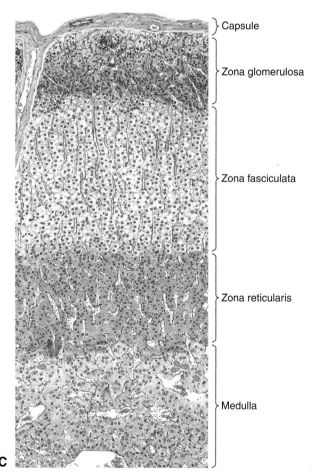

Figure 7-24. *(Continued)* The synthesis of hormones in the adrenal gland can be a vital part of adaptations to exercise training.
(B) Pathways of hormonal synthesis in the adrenal medulla.
(C) Cross-section of the adrenal medulla.

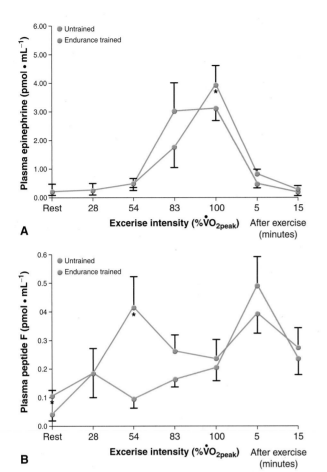

A

B

Figure 7-25. The adrenal gland synthesizes and releases more than just epinephrine, and secretion of proenkephalins influences recovery by promoting immune cell function needed for repair as well as analgesia. (A) Plasma epinephrine response to aerobic exercise. **(B)** Plasma peptide F response to aerobic exercise. The values are represented as mean and standard errors. *Significant difference between the two training groups. It is important to note that significant increases above resting values in epinephrine were seen at 83% and 100% of peak oxygen consumption for both groups, whereas for peptide F, a significant difference was seen at rest and increases above rest were observed at 54% for the trained group and 83% for the untrained group; both groups increased peptide F at and 5 and 15 after exercise (see ref. 42).

in the blood, which contains the immune cells. Thus, the adrenal gland is not only active in the response to stress but at basal levels and during recovery from stress, at which times it may well be important to immune cell activation and immune cell roles in recovery.

Exercise Roles, Responses, and Adaptations

Epinephrine and norepinephrine are typically seen to increase at approximately 50% of maximum oxygen consumption and to exponentially increase as exercise intensity reaches maximal levels. With a half-life of only about 2 minutes, epinephrine returns to resting concentrations within the first few minutes of recovery. Interestingly, if exercise stress is great enough, such as in short rest resistance training protocols, epinephrine can remain elevated 5 minutes after exercise. Dopamine levels

also increase, indicating incomplete conversion to epinephrine or a backup in the biosynthetic pathway, potentially due to acidic inactivation of reaction enzymes. Catecholamine adaptations to training show reductions in the submaximal responses, similar to heart rate responses, with greater responses to maximal exercise and reductions in proenkephalin responses at maximal exercise intensities.

Adrenal Cortex

The **adrenal cortex** produces both mineralocorticoids (aldosterone) and glucocorticoids (cortisol). Adrenal androgens are also produced in the adrenal cortex from the *zona reticularis*, and, for women, the adrenal cortex is an important synthesis site of weak androgens that can act as anabolic hormones.

Glucocorticoids

Cortisol is the primary glucocorticoid in humans secreted from the *zona fasciculata* in the adrenal cortex. As noted before, cortisol release is stimulated by the hormone ACTH, which is released from the pituitary gland. About 10% of cortisol is free, and thus bioactive, with the remainder bound to plasma proteins, primarily corticosteroid-binding globulin (also called transcortin), to extend its half-life in the blood. Cortisol interacts with glucocorticoid receptors, which are found in almost every cell in the body. Cortisol as a glucocorticoid is involved in glucose metabolism, as it stimulates several processes that together help to increase and maintain normal glucose concentrations. Such actions include gluconeogenesis, which is the synthesis of glucose from amino acids and lipids. Cortisol enhances the enzymes involved with this metabolic process. It also stimulates the release of amino acids to use in the making of glucose. Moreover, cortisol limits the uptake of glucose into muscle or adipose tissue. All of this is done to conserve glucose, which is the primary source of energy for the brain and nervous system. It preserves glycogen and glucose by providing alternate substrates to synthesize glucose (e.g., amino acids, glycerol). Cortisol also has cross-reactions with other receptors, most importantly with the androgen receptor to block protein synthesis signaling.

Cortisol is also known as the primary catabolic hormone in the body, as it attempts to protect the use of muscle glycogen or glucose by inhibiting molecular signaling for protein synthesis (e.g., inhibit mTOR system) in favor of breakdown of protein so that the resultant amino acids can be used as an energy substrate. In addition, cortisol can reduce the activity of immune cells, which use glucose as a primary energy source, again to preserve glycogen and glucose use. Thus, its bad name as a "catabolic hormone" is related to the fact that it is trying to preserve glycogen while enhancing glucose production by providing other basic substrates to synthesize it.

Cortisol plays an anti-inflammatory function by suppressing immune cell activity. Thus, it has also been used as a drug to help treat inflammatory diseases such as asthma, arthritis, or autoimmune diseases. However, because of its negative impact on protein synthesis, care must be taken clinically so as not to promote tissue breakdown. This characteristic has implications in sports medicine and is the reason why cortisone injections are not as popular as they were years ago. High glucocorticoid concentrations from a cortisone injection can reduce bone development and wound healing and negatively affect a host of other physiological functions. Excessive natural production of cortisol is called Cushing's disease.

Exercise Roles, Responses, and Adaptations. Exercise will increase cortisol concentrations with intensities from about 70% of the $\dot{V}o_{2max}$ and higher.[55] Most resistance exercise protocols will also elevate blood concentrations of cortisol, if they are of adequate volume of total work and/or intensity. Often, increases can be observed well into the recovery period, from 5 to 30 minutes. If resting concentrations are high (e.g., >450 nmol·L^{-1}), then acute exercise responses or demands really require a greater stimulus. Interestingly, although cortisol has been implicated as playing a possible role in detecting overtraining in athletes, it has not been a very predictive marker, as its elevation comes after one is already in an overtrained state.[20] Almost any severe exercise can cause an increase in cortisol for the obvious reasons of helping the body carefully use its limited stores of glycogen and reducing the magnitude of the inflammatory response due to muscle tissue damage. However, in certain circumstances, cortisol can decrease the recovery capability of the individual.

Mineralocorticoids

Aldosterone is a steroid hormone produced by the *zona glomerulosa* in the adrenal cortex. Aldosterone is one of the most important mineralocorticoids, which are a group of hormones that help to regulate water balance and electrolytes (e.g., sodium and potassium) in the blood.[52] To accomplish this, these hormones, which are produced in the adrenal cortex, influence the tubules and collecting duct in the kidney. Angiotensin II, but also ACTH and local potassium concentrations, stimulate aldosterone secretion. Aldosterone signals the kidney to retain sodium and secrete potassium, one of its more important hormonal roles. Together, these changes in electrolyte concentration cause an increase in blood pressure and blood volume, and water retention results. Aldosterone also influences acid/base balance by stimulating H$^+$ secretion by the intercalated cells in the collecting duct of the kidney, helping to regulate bicarbonate concentrations and thus acid–base balance. It also acts on the posterior pituitary gland and helps to stimulate the release of arginine vasopressin (also known as antidiuretic hormone), which causes the kidney to retain water. Interestingly, aldosterone accounts for only about 2% of the reabsorption of the sodium that would normally be found in the blood.

Exercise Roles, Responses, and Adaptations. Aldosterone plays important roles in fluid and electrolyte regulation with exercise stress. The responses to exercise are related to exercise intensity, with lower concentrations observed with lower-intensity exercise.[54] With training, one improves one's ability to perform at a higher intensity, and, accordingly, aldosterone[56] levels at maximal exercise intensities after training are higher than at maximal exercise intensities before training. With greater physiological demands and higher-intensity exercise, greater water and electrolyte regulatory demands exist, and thus intensity and volume of exercise are key signals to aldosterone release. With resistance exercise, aldosterone's response is different, as a high-intensity protocol may not impact aldosterone concentrations since no challenge is presented to the fluid and electrolyte balances. Thus, as the metabolic intensity increases due to higher volumes of total work, such as in a body-building protocol or short rest protocols, aldosterone may not increase.[30,38] The type of resistance exercise protocol used as it relates to the demands on fluid and electrolyte challenges dictate aldosterone responses.[33,58]

Pancreatic Hormones

The pancreas is located in the upper abdomen by the small intestine, deep in the body. It plays an important role in many physiological functions, from anabolic properties of the hormone insulin, to its regulation of glucose levels in the blood, to disease processes such as diabetes. It secretes pancreatic juice, which contains digestive enzymes that help neutralize stomach acids that pass from the stomach to the small intestine and that help in the process of breaking down protein, carbohydrates, and fats.

The pancreas secretes the hormones insulin, glucagon, and somatostatin. The Islets of Langerhans are specialized cells in the pancreas that secrete glucagon and insulin. Glucagon helps to increase blood glucose when it starts to drop, whereas insulin triggers cells to take up blood glucose when levels are high. The different cells types in the pancreas have different roles in the production of secretory contents, as follows:

- Beta cells secrete insulin to lower blood glucose concentrations when they are elevated; these cells make up about 60–80% of the islet cells in the adult pancreas.
- Alpha cells secrete glucagon, which causes an increase in blood glucose concentrations when they are low; these cells make up about 15% to 20% of the pancreas.
- Delta cells secrete somatostatin, which inhibits endocrine release of insulin and glucagon; these cells make up about 5% to 10% of the cells in the pancreas.
- PP cells secrete pancreatic polypeptides to inhibit the release of pancreatic juices; these cells make up about 1% of the cells in the pancreas.

The classic endocrine feedback mechanism is the interplay between insulin and glucagon, which together control blood glucose concentrations (Fig. 7-26).

Diabetes and Metabolic Syndrome

When an individual has diabetes, his or her body either does not produce insulin or has difficulty using it. Diabetes

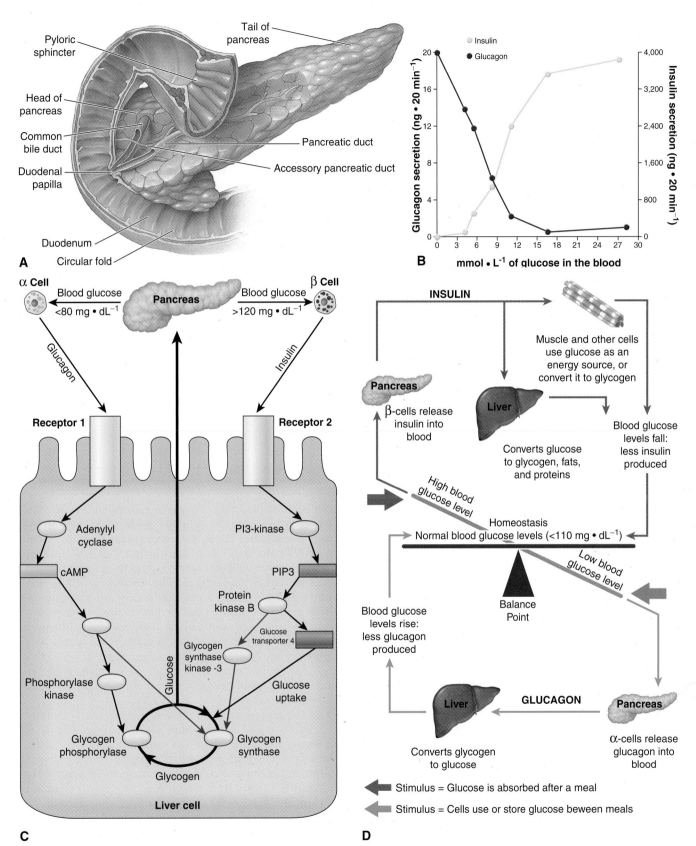

Figure 7-26. The regulation and control of glucose metabolism is one of the most important homeostatic functions in the body, and the control of glucagon and insulin synthesis and release in response to exercise assists one in meeting exercise demands. **(A)** Pancreas (asset provided by Anatomical Chart Co.). **(B)** Glucagon and insulin secretion. **(C)** Glucagon and insulin responses to blood glucose. **(D)** Glucagon and insulin actions to maintain blood glucose concentrations.

is characterized by hyperglycemia (elevated blood glucose concentrations) caused by low concentrations of insulin, or "insulin resistance," in which insulin is prevented from having its normal actions on a cell. The beta cells have problems producing enough insulin to reduce the blood glucose concentrations, which is the underlying cause of the disease. There are three types of diabetes: type 1, type 2, and gestational diabetes, the last of which typically occurs during pregnancy. Type 1 and type 2 can have serious health complications if not treated. Type 1 is usually found in children and young adults, and thus is known as juvenile diabetes. In this type, the pancreas's beta cells do not produce the needed amount of insulin. Insulin resistance characterizes type 2 diabetes, as there is a resistance to allowing insulin to impact target cells, such as muscle; thus, the cells do not respond to the hormone and its effect. Beta cells also do not function optimally in type 2 diabetes. Type 1 and type 2 diabetes are incurable but can be treated with a comprehensive program. Type 1 diabetes

must be treated with insulin injections, along with dietary and lifestyle interventions, to manage it. Type 2 diabetes can be managed with a combination of lifestyle changes, exercise and dietary treatment, and often insulin treatments.

With insulin resistance resulting in high concentrations of glucose and insulin, an individual can develop metabolic syndrome and type 2 diabetes. Metabolic syndrome is a grouping of different medical disorders that can influence one's risk for cardiovascular disease and diabetes (e.g., high blood pressure; high concentrations of certain lipids, such as triglycerides and dense LDH; high insulin concentrations; belly fat; overweight; high body fat). Exercise and diet are two of the major factors affecting metabolic syndrome (Box 7-8).

Exercise Roles, Responses, and Adaptations

One typically observes a decrease in insulin concentrations in the blood with exercise. With a decline in insulin, the

---

Box 7-8   AN EXPERT VIEW
Metabolic Syndrome

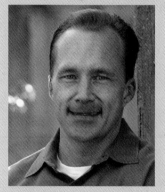

Jeff S. Volek, PhD, RD
Associate Professor
Department of Kinesiology
University of Connecticut
Storrs, CT

Metabolic syndrome (MetS; also known as insulin resistance syndrome) represents a group of markers that predispose to obesity, diabetes, and cardiovascular disease. The definition and utility of MetS have been debated, but most researchers agree that hyperinsulinemia/insulin resistance is a unifying feature. Also, impairment of the diverse downstream effects of insulin signaling provides a plausible mechanism for the features of MetS. The clinical significance of MetS is that insulin resistance and a prediabetic state indicate a hidden risk for cardiovascular risk and early mortality. The concept continues to be an important, if somewhat controversial, feature of diagnostic practice, although there is no generally agreed upon strategy for treatment. We recently suggested that the biological markers that are traditionally used to define MetS are precisely those that are improved by dietary carbohydrate restriction. These markers include obesity (high body weight, body mass index [BMI], and/or waist circumference), high glucose and insulin levels, low high-density lipoprotein cholesterol (HDL-C), and high triglyceride (TG). This finding in turn suggests that some form of reduced carbohydrate diet is a reasonable first approach to treating the syndrome.

Evidence from recent studies points to a paradigm shift in our understanding of low carbohydrate diets. Glucose

is the major stimulus for pancreatic secretion of insulin. The diverse effects of insulin point to its generally anabolic effects. These effects include stimulation of peripheral glucose uptake by recruitment of GLUT4 receptors; inhibition of glycogenolysis, gluconeogenesis, and lipolysis; and stimulation of glycogen storage and protein synthesis. The rationale of strategies based on carbohydrate restriction is that reduced dietary glucose leads to better insulin control and better regulation of this anabolic state. More specifically, the principle of carbohydrate restriction is that by keeping insulin low, metabolism is biased toward lipid oxidation rather than storage. The corollary would be that continued hyperinsulinemia may predispose to a state in which dietary fat is stored, rather than oxidized, and in which the atherogenic effects of fat, particularly saturated fats, are more readily manifested. Lipogenesis (fatty acid synthesis) is significantly inhibited on a low carbohydrate diet, and this should allow better postabsorptive management of dietary fat, reducing its adverse effects on lipoprotein metabolism and other atherogenic processes.

In the treatment of MetS and diabetes, carbohydrate restriction is the obvious and intuitive approach. It is generally acknowledged that experimentally reducing dietary carbohydrate gives better glycemic control, greater reduction in hemoglobin A1c, and more reliable reduction in medication than low fat diets, and does not require weight loss for benefit.[1] The barrier to implementing low-carbohydrate strategies in the treatment of MetS and patients with diabetes has traditionally been the concern for risk of cardiovascular disease (CVD). The major concern is that the carbohydrate removed from the diet will be replaced by dietary fat, possibly saturated fat, with a presumed increased risk of CVD. In striking contrast to this idea, recent work has demonstrated that reduction in dietary carbohydrate leads to dramatic improvement in markers of CVD, even in the absence of weight loss.

Historically, carbohydrate restriction has been viewed as a method for weight loss and has been under suspicion because of concerns about low-density lipoprotein cholesterol (LDL-C) and heart disease risk. Reduction in dietary carbohydrate has long been known to improve atherogenic dyslipidemia, that is, to increase HDL-C and to reduce plasma TG. On the other hand, total cholesterol and LDL-C are generally lowered by low-fat diets. This relationship between risk factors of LDL-C versus dyslipidemia is now complicated by the recognition that the atherogenicity of LDL-C is strongly dependent on particle size, and particle size, in turn, is strongly correlated with dietary carbohydrate. In addition, other markers, such as the apolipoproteins, may be more accurate predictors than levels of cholesterol species; the apoB/apoA-1 ratio, in particular, has been proposed as the most accurate. There is also the issue of fatty acid species, mainly saturated fat, because dietary intake of fat usually increases when carbohydrates are restricted, and this has raised concerns about potential harmful effects on lipoprotein metabolism and cardiovascular risk.

Several studies have assessed the effects of very low-carbohydrate diets on standard and emerging biomarkers of cardiac risk. The picture emerging from this recent work is that restricting carbohydrates has several advantages over low-fat diets on decreasing adiposity, improving glycemic control and insulin sensitivity, and inducing favorable TG, HDL-C, and total cholesterol/HDL-C ratio responses. In addition to these markers for MetS, low-carbohydrate diets have more favorable responses to alternative indicators of atherogenic dyslipidemia and cardiovascular risk: postprandial lipemia, apo B, apo A-1, the apo B/apo A-1 ratio, LDL particle distribution, adipokines, inflammatory markers, and postabsorptive and postprandial vascular function. We have shown in recent work that despite a threefold higher intake of dietary saturated fat, a very low-carbohydrate diet showed a consistent reduction in circulating saturated fatty acids compared with a low-fat diet. The decrease in circulating saturated fatty acids on the low-carbohydrate diet is likely due to greater oxidation of the saturated fat from both diet and endogenous lipolysis, and a reduction in *de novo* lipogenesis.

In summary, carbohydrate restriction is generally effective at improving those physiologic markers associated with metabolic syndrome: high fasting glucose and insulin, and particularly the atherogenic dyslipidemia characterized by high TG and low HDL. The effects are presumed to be attributed to better regulation of plasma glucose and insulin levels and improvement in the hyperinsulinemia/insulin resistance, which are fundamental features of MetS. The persistence of an epidemic of obesity, diabetes, and MetS suggests that alternatives to the low-fat dietary recommendations with which the epidemic is coincident should be sought. The review presented here suggests that, considered in a new light, carbohydrate restriction as a general prescription for health, independent of weight loss, is sensibly such an alternative.

Reference

1. Arora SK, McFarlane SI. The case for low carbohydrate diets in diabetes management. Nutr Metab (Lond). 2005;2:16.

---

liver also is stimulated to release glucose with breakdown of liver glycogen. Thus, maintenance of the blood glucose concentrations, one of the most tightly regulated variables in the human body, is achieved. With the acute exercise response, if one ingests carbohydrate, or carbohydrate and protein, before and after exercise, insulin can increase, showing the impact of calories and carbohydrate on blood concentrations of insulin.[46] It must also be remembered that insulin can play a potent role in protein synthesis, which is stimulated by nutrient ingestion.

With training, the target tissues become more sensitive to insulin's effect and insulin resistance is reduced. A host of molecular mechanisms have been proposed to account for these effects.[83] It has also been shown that chronic higher-intensity exercise training demonstrated more enduring benefits for insulin actions when compared with moderate- or low-intensity exercise, even in older adults.[12,50] Lower-intensity training zones demonstrated less stable training effects. Improved uptake of glucose in muscle may be related to hemodynamic adaptations, increased cellular protein content of signaling components, and the molecules needed for glucose transport and metabolism.[19] Insulin also has a dramatic influence on protein anabolism via signals modulated by carbohydrate. Strength training has been shown to improve muscle function as well as whole-body insulin sensitivity, even in individuals with type 2 diabetes.[8,62]

In a classic review on insulin's effects, Ho, Lacazar, and Goodyear[26] concluded the following:

1. Exercise and insulin both stimulate increases in glucose transport, glycogen metabolism, and protein synthesis, and help to mediate long-term increases in muscle size.
2. These effects are mediated through both common and novel signaling pathways.
3. Additive effects of exercise and insulin in the regulation of intermediary metabolism and adaptive responses have a widespread impact on both health and disease.
4. While exercise training can result in improvements in performance, chronic training can also prevent or reverse metabolic defects observed in conditions such as type 2 diabetes.

Thyroid Gland

As noted before, the thyroid gland secretes thyroid hormones (thyroxine, or T-3, and triiodothyronine, or T-4), which are vital cofactors for a great number of biochemical reactions in the body mediating physiological function. Iodine is necessary for these hormones' synthesis. To get the needed amount of iodine in the diet, iodine is available in multiple vitamins and, more commonly, is added to table salt. Thyroid hormones play a role in increasing basal metabolic rate, are important in reactions for protein synthesis, increase the effects of epinephrine at the level of the beta adrenergic receptor, and play vital roles in growth and development of human cells. T-3 plays important roles in helping to mediate changes in cardiovascular function, such as increasing cardiac output and ventilation rate. Its role in metabolism is exemplified by individuals who are "hypothyroid," that is, those whose thyroid gland does not produce enough thyroid hormones. Metabolism is dramatically slowed in such people, and undue weight gain is observed, among many other symptoms.

Exercise Roles, Responses, and Adaptations

Acute exercise-induced responses of T-3 and T-4 are many times not consistent as some experiments have observed no significant exercise-induced changes from rest,[28,72] whereas others have observed increased concentrations of thyroid hormones in the blood with aerobic exercise intensities greater than 70% of maximal oxygen consumption.[10,11] The reasons for such differences may be due to many experimental differences. Similarly, during resistance exercise, no significant changes have been observed in the blood concentrations of thyroid hormones.[29]

The many discrepancies between studies was pointed out in 1984 by Krotkiewski and colleagues,[47] who stated, "Lack of agreement in previous reports is probably due to methodological differences such as methods more or less susceptible to fatty acid interference and thyroid hormones changing differently during acute work and before and after physical training. The duration of the study may also be of importance, even 3 months possibly being too short for attaining equilibrium in thyroid homeostasis."

In addition, plasma concentration may not be representative of the uptake and use of the hormone in the biocompartments that are involved in the metabolic and biochemical reactions that thyroid hormones undergo.

Parathyroid Hormone

Parathyroid hormone (PTH), or parathormone, is secreted by the parathyroid glands, which are located on the surface of the thyroid gland. This hormone stimulates increased concentrations of calcium in the blood. Conversely, calcitonin (a hormone produced by the parafollicular cells of the thyroid gland) acts to decrease calcium concentration. PTH influences basically three target regions to increase calcium in the circulation: (1) bone, where it releases calcium from a large supply; (2) kidney, where it enhances active reabsorption of calcium; and (3) intestines, where it increases the absorption of calcium by increasing the production of vitamin D and up-regulating the key enzymes for this process. PTH is regulated by a negative feedback system in which increased calcium concentrations result in decreased production of the hormone.

Bone turnover is important in the remodeling process of bone. This process involves resorption, which is the normal destruction of bone by osteoclasts and release of calcium into the blood. PTH indirectly stimulates osteoclasts, as they have no receptors, by influencing osteoclast precursors. PTH does bind to osteoblasts, which are the cells responsible for making bone. This process is important for the repair of bones damaged from every day stress and injury. In addition, modeling of bone is a vital process, requiring exercise to maintain or increase bone mineral density.

Exercise Roles, Responses, and Adaptations

With higher-intensity exercise, increases in blood concentrations of PTH will occur.[6] This has been thought to be due to the decrease in calcium and the impact on bone turnover. It has also been observed that even moderate long-term exercise appears to increase PTH but with relatively little change in calcium concentrations, making its long-term effects on bone unclear.[1] Heavy-resistance exercise has been thought to be an effective type of exercise to strengthen bone because it also affects PTH and bone homeostasis.[70] Such interventions are important for combating bone loss from aging and osteoporosis, as well as to offset the dramatic loss of bone with spaceflight and microgravity exposure (Box 7-9).

Box 7-9　DID YOU KNOW?

Osteoporosis

Osteoporosis is a condition in which mineral density of bone is reduced, leading to an increased risk of fracture. Osteoporosis is often referred to as the "silent disease" because symptoms are not apparent until an individual actually breaks a bone. The severity of the disease becomes evident when a broken bone leads to disability, pain, and a loss of independence. About 99% of the calcium in the body is stored in the bone. Thus, the roles that parathyroid hormone and calcitonin play in maintaining circulating calcium levels influence bone remodeling, bone density, and ultimately the risk of possibly developing osteoporosis, if bone density is reduced. Parathyroid hormone increases calcium in the bloodstream by triggering the release of calcium from bone, increasing the reabsorption of calcium from the kidneys, and absorbing calcium from the intestine. On the other hand, calcitonin decreases blood calcium levels by stimulating storage in the bone and increasing excretion of calcium in the kidneys. Homeostasis of these hormones, with opposing functions in maintaining calcium in the bone and bone density, thus plays a role in the possible development of osteoporosis. To minimize the risk of developing osteoporosis, it is recommended that individuals consume a diet adequate in calcium, protein, phosphorus, vitamin D, and vitamin K, maintain a healthy body weight, and engage in weight-bearing exercise.

CASE STUDY

Scenario

You are a baseball coach at a major college and have been working with the team for 4 years. You have been impressed with two of your top players who really have potential for the majors. One day, sitting back in your chair in your office, you were reflecting on the careers of each player. Because the major league scouts were coming next week, you were getting the players' stats together, including some of their strength and conditioning data. John had made steady progress over his college career in both strength and power, but was noticeably smaller than Barton, who had in the last 2 years made a 20-pound weight gain and a corresponding upswing of his batting average and home run production. He had never tested positive for any drug during his career and was a very dedicated athlete in the weight room. With all of the controversy with anabolic drug use in the major leagues, the scouts were wondering whether this might be a problem or whether it is just normal growth. Thinking back to your studies as an undergraduate exercise science major you want to take another look at a few questions.

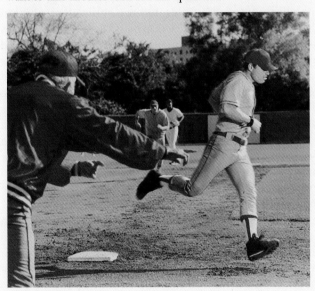

Questions

1. Is this type of growth possible for a college baseball player?
2. What might he be taking that is not detectable in drug tests?
3. Is it just solid nutrition and sound training?
4. The scouts wanted to know whether he is using some drug, as then it might be better to draft his teammate. What do you think?

Options

Upon reflection, would not such a large gain in weight also require some increase in height? You remember that increasing levels of testosterone and estradiol up-regulate the hypothalamus

and pituitary transiently to make more GH/IGF-I, which stimulates the growth spurt characteristic of mid-adolescence. But, after several years, these sex hormones cause the epiphyses of the long bones to fuse and linear growth ceases. Barton did grow several inches (cm) during the last 2 years and grew a beard. Additionally, several of the athletes have been taking the supplement creatine. These factors lead you to conclude he went through a late growth spurt, which aided his increase in body size. This, coupled with Barton's dedication in the weight room, lead you to conclude he is probably not using an illegal ergogenic aid.

Scenario

You are a high school tennis coach, and the strength and conditioning specialist at the school has asked you to pick the time you want to train your athletes for your off-season program. Your tennis practice time has been set at 3 pm to 4:30 pm each day, as the indoor tennis courts are available only at that time during the winter months in your small town in Ohio.

Questions

1. What other factors weigh into your consideration for the time of day to best train your athletes?
2. Is there an optimal time of day to train different elements, from tennis practice to strength and conditioning activities? If so, why?
3. What do you decide to choose for the time of day to train?

Options

You remember from your basic understanding of circadian patterns that many hormones have circadian rhythms, which impact the magnitude of their response to exercise at different times of the day. Some hormones start out low in the morning and peak later in the day and at night. However, you also recall that no study has shown an optimal time of day at which to train unless the wake/sleep cycle affects the quality of training. However, there is some indication that performance generally peaks in the afternoon or early evening. Your training is scheduled for the late afternoon, which is when performance may peak, and should not be affected by the wake/sleep cycle. Therefore, you decide the scheduled training time is at a good time of the day.

Scenario

As a personal trainer, you have just completed a resistance training cycle with your client. He now, for fun, wants to participate in an upcoming amateur drug-free bodybuilding contest in 3 months at the local health club in town. You have been working with him for 2 years, and his strength is very good and his muscular size from doing heavier weights is just about as good as it will get from what you can observe. However, to meet the demands for muscular definition, you know that his training program must be changed to optimize muscular definition while retaining his muscular size. Obviously, this is a drug-free contest, so you wonder whether you can create a resistance training protocol that will stimulate subcutaneous fat loss and improve his muscular definition.

Questions

1. What type of exercise protocol might that be, and how would diet interplay with this type of program?

2. What other considerations should you have in this process of trying to achieve muscular definition for such a bodybuilding contest?

Options

You remember that with intense weight training, higher concentrations of many anabolic hormones, such as growth hormone, are seen. It is these hormones, along with a higher metabolic rate, that might stimulate more fat use in metabolism compared with heavier resistances and their needed longer rest periods between sets. You decide to have your client perform a high-volume, moderate-intensity weight training program (multiple sets of approximately 10 repetitions). This exercise program, with a moderately restrictive caloric diet, will help your client achieve the muscular look they are seeking.

IMPACT OF COMPETITION ON ENDOCRINE RESPONSES

Think about the physiological arousal that occurs in athletes prior to the start of a big game or match. The endocrine glands are very much involved in this arousal phenomenon, most notably epinephrine.[27] The fight-or-flight phenomenon can have a large psychological component, especially when the athlete knows what is coming.[18] In a Davis Cup match, competitors were found to have dramatically higher epinephrine concentrations compared with practice conditions. Thus, athletes have to deal with a competitive environment that is quite different from practice. Therefore, coaches and athletes have tried to simulate the so-called "feel of the game" by exposing the athletes in training to conditions similar to those of competition. This is where experience is important, because once a dramatic fall in epinephrine occurs, getting back that "edge" is difficult.[18]

Competition can cause both anxiety and arousal due to the uncertainty involved with the outcome. Elevations in catecholamines, including epinephrine, lead to a total-body adrenergic effect that also increases other hormones, such as testosterone, shown to be related to aggressiveness in men, as well as cortisol.

Elevations in many of the hormones are important to mobilize energy substrates for the subsequent physical demands. In addition, increases in blood flow, blood pressure, and readiness for skeletal muscle contractions (e.g., increased epinephrine binding to B-2 adrenergic receptors in the sarcoplasmic reticulum to increase the output of Ca^{++}) are all part of the preparatory process prior to exercise or competition. The more intense the physical demands or the painfulness of the exercise or competition (e.g., wrestling match, 400 m intervals), the greater the preparatory adjustments that can occur anywhere from 24 hours to 15 minutes before the event or activity. Untrained individuals who are unaccustomed to exercise see epinephrine concentrations increase hours before low to moderate exercise.[75] Furthermore, Tharion et al.[74] have shown that shorter rest weight training workouts with 10 RM loads produce heightened anxiety and anger prior to the workout. All of this is part of the arousal process, which coaches, personal trainers, and scientists must acknowledge and deal with.

CHAPTER SUMMARY

The endocrine system is one of the most important systems in the body, mediating almost every physiological function. With acute exercise stress and chronic exercise training, the endocrine system sends important signaling information to the target cells. It also provides support for many metabolic functions to maintain homeostasis to meet the demands of exercise stress and recovery. Thus, understanding some of the basic aspects of the endocrine system is vital to understanding the specificity of the acute exercise stress and chronic adaptations to various types of exercise training.

Quick Review

- The endocrine system is involved in the arousal for competition.
- Elevations in catecholamines lead to a total-body adrenergic effect.
- Elevations in hormones are important for the preparatory process prior to exercise or competition.
- The more intense the physical demands, the greater the preparatory adjustments.

REVIEW QUESTIONS

Fill-in-the-Blank

1. Growth hormone is synthesized and secreted by cells called _____ in the anterior pituitary.

2. _____ is the precursor for beta-endorphin and several other bioactive peptides secreted from the anterior pituitary gland.

3. Steroid hormones are all derived from _____ and contain the same ring and atomic numbering system as _____.

4. During labor, the release of the hormone _____ is triggered by cervical and vaginal stimulation by the fetus in a positive feedback loop to stimulate the smooth muscle of the uterus to contract more and more vigorously as labor continues, ending with the delivery of the baby.

5. During exercise, the mechanical stimuli of muscle activation and force production cause the autocrine release of _____ and an isoform of IGF, called _____, from the muscle fibers.

Multiple Choice

1. Which of the following is true in explaining the magnitude of the growth hormone response to exercise?
   a. Greater response occurs when more muscle mass is recruited.
   b. Greater response occurs during eccentric than during concentric muscle actions.
   c. Greater response occurs with single-set than with multiple-set protocols.
   d. Greater acute elevations occur with lower individual strength.
   e. Greater response occurs with less amount of total work performed.

2. The endocrine system
   a. releases chemical messengers into the bloodstream for distribution throughout the body.
   b. releases hormones that alter the metabolic activities of many different tissues and organs.
   c. produces effects that can last for hours, days, or even longer.
   d. can alter gene activity of cells.
   e. All the above

3. Which of the following hormones is NOT classified as an amine?
   a. Epinephrine
   b. Melatonin
   c. Thyroxine (T-4)
   d. Norepinephrine
   e. Glucagon

4. Consuming a meal of four king-sized candy bars and a large cola would cause which hormone to be secreted at higher levels?
   a. Insulin
   b. Epinephrine
   c. Glucagon
   d. Cortisol
   e. Oxytocin

5. Which of the following factors influences the duration and intensity of messages from hormones to the DNA?
   a. Half-life of the hormone
   b. Receptor availability
   c. Degradation elements in the physiological environment
   d. Enzymes
   e. All the above

True/False

1. In a positive feedback loop, product formation can feed back upon the primary structures to diminish the amount of secretion.
2. Peptide hormone receptors rely on secondary messenger systems to mediate their signals to the DNA.
3. The thyroid gland produces a hormone that raises serum calcium levels.
4. Glucocorticoids increase circulating glucose levels.
5. Steroid hormones all exert their action by direct interactions with the DNA's regulatory element.

Short Answer

1. Describe what controls the release of anterior pituitary hormones.

Matching

1. Match the hormone type to its correct description.

Amine	• Derived from cholesterol, exerts action by direct interactions with the DNA's regulatory element
Steroid	• Composed of amino acids, exerts signals indirectly on the DNA via interactions with cellular membrane receptors and secondary molecular signaling mechanisms
Peptide	• Modifications of amino acids

2. Match the type of hormone release with its correct definition.

Paracrine	• Hormone production and secretion by glands into the bloodstream to act on target tissues
Autocrine	• Hormone secretion by a cell and acting on *adjacent cells*
Endocrine	• Hormone secretion by a cell and acting on surface receptors of the *same cell*

Critical Thinking

1. Describe hormone "pulsatility." What is the advantage of hormone "pulsatility"?

2. Describe the autocrine secretion of insulin-like growth factor in muscle.

KEY TERMS

amenorrhea: absence of a menstrual period in women

anabolic: metabolic building

androgenic: pertaining to male secondary sex characteristics

autocrine: relating to a substance secreted by and acting on surface receptors of the same cell

catabolic: pertaining to metabolic breakdown

dysmenorrhea: painful menstrual periods

endocrine: production and secretion of chemical messengers by glands that are distributed in the body by way of the bloodstream to act on target tissues

gland: a group of cells or an organized mass of cells that functions as an organ to secrete chemical substances

half-life: the amount of time it takes for a hormone's concentration in blood to be reduced to half of its peak value

hormone: a chemical substance released from a gland into the blood to interact with a cell to elicit a specific response

inhibiting hormone: a hormone that functions to block the release of another hormone

mechano-growth factor: splice variants of insulin-like growth factor 1 (IGF-1) released from the muscle due to mechanical stress

menorrhagia: prolonged menstrual bleeding

menstruation: the periodic discharging of blood, secretions, and tissue debris from the uterus that recurs in nonpregnant women at approximately monthly intervals

negative feedback: a system in which product formation decreases further formation of the product

neuroendocrine: pertaining to interaction between hormonal secretions and nerve activity

paracrine: pertaining to a substance secreted by a cell and acting on adjacent cells

plasma: the fluid portion of blood that consists of water and its dissolved constituents (proteins, electrolytes, sugars, lipids, metabolic waste products, amino acids, hormones, and vitamins)

positive feedback: a system in which product formation increases further product formation

premenstrual syndrome: symptoms that occur 7 to 14 days before a menstrual period

receptor: a cell protein that receives stimuli on the cell surface or in the cell interior that has an affinity for a specific chemical agent (as a hormone) to trigger a physiologic response

releasing hormones: hormones that function to promote the release of another hormone

serum: the fluid portion of blood remaining after clotting factors (fibrinogen, prothrombin) have been removed by clot formation

somatotrophs: cells located in the anterior pituitary gland that secrete growth hormone (GH)

REFERENCES

1. Barry DW, Kohrt WM. Acute effects of 2 hours of moderate-intensity cycling on serum parathyroid hormone and calcium. Calcif Tissue Int. 2007;80:359–365.
2. Baxter RC. Insulin-like growth factor (IGF)-binding proteins: interactions with IGFs and intrinsic bioactivities. Am J Physiol Endocrinol Metab. 2000;278:E967–E976.
3. Bayliss WM, Starling EH. The mechanism of pancreatic secretion. J Physiol. 1902;28:325–353.
4. Bender T, Nagy G, Barna I, et al. The effect of physical therapy on beta-endorphin levels. Eur J Appl Physiol. 2007;100:371–382.
5. Boecker H, Sprenger T, Spilker ME, et al. The runner's high: opioidergic mechanisms in the human brain. Cereb Cortex. 2008;18(11):2523–2531.
6. Bouassida A, Zalleg D, Zaouali Ajina M, et al. Parathyroid hormone concentrations during and after two periods of high intensity exercise with and without an intervening recovery period. Eur J Appl Physiol. 2003;88:339–344.
7. Brabant G, Schwieger S, Knoeller R, et al. Hypothalamic-pituitary-thyroid axis in moderate and intense exercise. Horm Metab Res. 2005;37:559–562.
8. Brooks N, Layne JE, Gordon PL, et al. Strength training improves muscle quality and insulin sensitivity in Hispanic older adults with type 2 diabetes. Int J Med Sci. 2007;4:19–27.
9. Bunt JC, Bahr JM, Bemben DA. Comparison of estradiol and testosterone levels during and immediately following prolonged exercise in moderately active and trained males and females. Endocr Res. 1987;13:157–172.
10. Ciloglu F, Peker I, Pehlivan A, et al. Exercise intensity and its effects on thyroid hormones. Neuro Endocrinol Lett. 2005;26:830–834.
11. Deligiannis A, Karamouzis M, Kouidi E, et al. Plasma TSH, T3, T4 and cortisol responses to swimming at varying water temperatures. Br J Sports Med. 1993;27:247–250.
12. DiPietro L, Dziura J, Yeckel CW, et al. Exercise and improved insulin sensitivity in older women: evidence of the enduring benefits of higher intensity training. J Appl Physiol. 2006;100:142–149.
13. Eliakim A, Nemet D, Cooper DM. Exercise, training and the GH-IGF-I axis. In: Kraemer WJ, Rogol AD, Committee IO, eds. The Endocrine System in Sports and Exercise. Oxford: Blackwell Publishing, 2005:165–179.
14. Farrell PA, Gates WK, Maksud MG, et al. Increases in plasma beta-endorphin/beta-lipotropin immunoreactivity after treadmill running in humans. J Appl Physiol. 1982;52:1245–1249.
15. Fontana L, Klein S, Holloszy JO, et al. Effect of long-term calorie restriction with adequate protein and micronutrients on thyroid hormones. J Clin Endocrinol Metab. 2006;91:3232–3235.
16. Fournier PE, Stalder J, Mermillod B, et al. Effects of a 110 kilometers ultra-marathon race on plasma hormone levels. Int J Sports Med. 1997;18:252–256.
17. Franca SC, Barros Neto TL, Agresta MC, et al. Divergent responses of serum testosterone and cortisol in athlete men after a marathon race. Arq Bras Endocrinol Metabol. 2006;50:1082–1087.
18. French DN, Kraemer WJ, Volek JS, et al. Anticipatory responses of catecholamines on muscle force production. J Appl Physiol. 2007;102:94–102.
19. Frosig C, Rose AJ, Treebak JT, et al. Effects of endurance exercise training on insulin signaling in human skeletal muscle: interactions at

the level of phosphatidylinositol 3-kinase, Akt, and AS160. Diabetes. 2007;56:2093–2102.

20. Fry AC, Kraemer WJ. Resistance exercise overtraining and overreaching. Neuroendocrine responses. Sports Med. 1997;23:106–129.

21. Galvao DA, Nosaka K, Taaffe DR, et al. Resistance training and reduction of treatment side effects in prostate cancer patients. Med Sci Sports Exerc. 2006;38:2045–2052.

22. Goldspink G, Yang SY, Hameed M, et al. The role of MGF and other IGF-I splice variants in muscle maintenance and hypertrophy. In: Kraemer WJ, Rogol AD, Committee IO, eds. The Endocrine System in Sports and Exercise. Oxford: Blackwell Publishing, 2005:180–193.

23. Gotshalk LA, Loebel CC, Nindl BC, et al. Hormonal responses of multiset versus single-set heavy-resistance exercise protocols. Can J Appl Physiol. 1997;22:244–255.

24. Gravholt CH, Holck P, Nyholm B, et al. No seasonal variation of insulin sensitivity and glucose effectiveness in men. Metabolism. 2000;49:32–38.

25. Henderson J. Ernest Starling and 'hormones': an historical commentary. J Endocrinol. 2005;184:5–10.

26. Ho RC, Lacazar O, Goodyear LJ. Exercise regulation of insulin action in skeletal muscle. In: Kraemer WJ, Rogol AD, Committee IO, eds. The Endocrine System in Sports and Exercise. Oxford: Blackwell Publishing, 2005:388–425.

27. Hoffman JR. Endocrinology of sport competition. In: Kraemer WJ, Rogol AD, Committee IO, eds. The Endocrine System in Sports and Exercise. Oxford: Blackwell Publishing, 2005:600–612.

28. Huanga WS, Yua MD, Leed MS, et al. Effect of treadmill exercise on circulating thyroid hormone measurements. Med Princ Pract. 2004;13:15–19.

29. Jamurtas AZ, Koutedakis Y, Paschalis V, et al. The effects of a single bout of exercise on resting energy expenditure and respiratory exchange ratio. Eur J Appl Physiol. 2004;92:393–398.

30. Jurimae T, Karelson K, Smirnova T, et al. The effect of a single-circuit weight-training session on the blood biochemistry of untrained university students. Eur J Appl Physiol Occup Physiol 1990;61:344–348.

31. Keizer H, Janssen GM, Menheere P, et al. Changes in basal plasma testosterone, cortisol, and dehydroepiandrosterone sulfate in previously untrained males and females preparing for a marathon. Int J Sports Med. 1989;10(Suppl 3):S139–S145.

32. Keizer HA, Beckers E, de Haan J, et al. Exercise-induced changes in the percentage of free testosterone and estradiol in trained and untrained women. Int J Sports Med. 1987;(8)(suppl 3):151–153.

33. Kenefick RW, Maresh CM, Armstrong LE, et al. Rehydration with fluid of varying tonicities: effects on fluid regulatory hormones and exercise performance in the heat. J Appl Physiol. 2007;102:1899–1905.

34. Kline CE, Durstine JL, Davis JM, et al. Circadian variation in swim performance. J Appl Physiol. 2007;102:641–649.

35. Kraemer RR, Blair S, Kraemer GR, et al. Effects of treadmill running on plasma beta-endorphin, corticotropin, and cortisol levels in male and female 10 K runners. Eur J Appl Physiol Occup Physiol. 1989;58:845–851.

36. Kraemer RR, Dzewaltowski DA, Blair MS, et al. Mood alteration from treadmill running and its relationship to beta-endorphin, corticotropin, and growth hormone. J Sports Med Phys Fitness. 1990;30:241–246.

37. Kraemer WJ, Dziados JE, Marchitelli LJ, et al. Effects of different heavy-resistance exercise protocols on plasma beta-endorphin concentrations. J Appl Physiol. 1993;74:450–459.

38. Kraemer WJ, Fleck SJ, Maresh CM, et al. Acute hormonal responses to a single bout of heavy resistance exercise in trained power lifters and untrained men. Can J Appl Physiol. 1999;24:524–537.

39. Kraemer WJ, Fragala MS, Watson G, et al. Hormonal responses to a 160-km race across frozen Alaska. Br J Sports Med. 2008;42:116–120, discussion 120.

40. Kraemer WJ, Hakkinen K, Newton RU, et al. Acute hormonal responses to heavy resistance exercise in younger and older men. Eur J Appl Physiol Occup Physiol. 1998;77:206–211.

41. Kraemer WJ, Hakkinen K, Newton RU, et al. Effects of heavy-resistance training on hormonal response patterns in younger vs. older men. J Appl Physiol. 1999;87:982–992.

42. Kraemer WJ, Noble B, Culver B, et al. Changes in plasma proenkephalin peptide F and catecholamine levels during graded exercise in men. Proc Natl Acad Sci USA. 1985;82:6349–6351.

43. Kraemer WJ, Patton JF, Gordon SE, et al. Compatibility of high-intensity strength and endurance training on hormonal and skeletal muscle adaptations. J Appl Physiol. 1995;78:976–989.

44. Kraemer WJ, Patton JF, Knuttgen HG, et al. Hypothalamic-pituitary-adrenal responses to short-duration high-intensity cycle exercise. J Appl Physiol. 1989;66:161–166.

45. Kraemer WJ, Ratamess NA. Hormonal responses and adaptations to resistance exercise and training. Sports Med. 2005;35:339–361.

46. Kraemer WJ, Volek JS, Bush JA, et al. Hormonal responses to consecutive days of heavy-resistance exercise with or without nutritional supplementation. J Appl Physiol. 1998;85:1544–1555.

47. Krotkiewski M, Sjostrom L, Sullivan L, et al. The effect of acute and chronic exercise on thyroid hormones in obesity. Acta Med Scand. 1984;216:269–275.

48. Kvorning T, Andersen M, Brixen K, et al. Suppression of endogenous testosterone production attenuates the response to strength training: a randomized, placebo-controlled, and blinded intervention study. Am J Physiol Endocrinol Metab. 2006;291:E1325–E1332.

49. Lambert GM. Short review: exercise and the premenstrual syndrome. J Strength Cond Res. 1988;2:16–19.

50. Lippi G, Montagnana M, Salvagno GL, et al. Glycaemic control in athletes. Int J Sports Med. 2008;29:7–10.

51. Loucks AB. Influence of energy availability on luteinizing hormone pulsatility and menstrual cyclicity. In: Kraemer WJ, Rogol AD, Committee IO, eds. The Endocrine System in Sports and Exercise. Oxford: Blackwell Publishing, 2005:232–249.

52. Luger A, Deuster PA, Debolt JE, et al. Acute exercise stimulates the renin–angiotensin–aldosterone axis: adaptive changes in runners. Horm Res. 1988;30:5–9.

53. Machelska H. Targeting of opioid-producing leukocytes for pain control. Neuropeptides. 2007;41:285–293.

54. Maresh CM, Gabaree-Boulant CL, Armstrong LE, et al. Effect of hydration status on thirst, drinking, and related hormonal responses during low-intensity exercise in the heat. J Appl Physiol. 2004;97:39–44.

55. Maresh CM, Sokmen B, Kraemer WJ, et al. Pituitary-adrenal responses to arm versus leg exercise in untrained man. Eur J Appl Physiol. 2006;97:471–477.

56. Maresh CM, Wang BC, Goetz KL. Plasma vasopressin, renin activity, and aldosterone responses to maximal exercise in active college females. Eur J Appl Physiol Occup Physiol. 1985;54:398–403.

57. Marx JO, Ratamess NA, Nindl BC, et al. Low-volume circuit versus high-volume periodized resistance training in women. Med Sci Sports Exerc. 2001;33:635–643.

58. Montain SJ, Laird JE, Latzka WA, et al. Aldosterone and vasopressin responses in the heat: hydration level and exercise intensity effects. Med Sci Sports Exerc. 1997;29:661–668.

59. Moore CA, Fry AC. Nonfunctional overreaching during off-season training for skill position players in collegiate American football. J Strength Cond Res. 2007;21:793–800.

60. Nindl BC, Hymer WC, Deaver DR, et al. Growth hormone pulsatility profile characteristics following acute heavy resistance exercise. J Appl Physiol. 2001;91:163–172.

61. Nindl BC, Kraemer WJ, Marx JO, et al. Overnight responses of the circulating IGF-I system after acute, heavy-resistance exercise. J Appl Physiol. 2001;90:1319–1326.

62. Pereira LO, Lancha AH Jr. Effect of insulin and contraction up on glucose transport in skeletal muscle. Prog Biophys Mol Biol. 2004;84:1–27.

63. Plasqui G, Kester AD, Westerterp KR. Seasonal variation in sleeping metabolic rate, thyroid activity, and leptin. Am J Physiol Endocrinol Metab. 2003;285:E338–E343.

64. Pritzlaff CJ, Wideman L, Weltman JY, et al. Impact of acute exercise intensity on pulsatile growth hormone release in men. J Appl Physiol. 1999;87:498–504.

65. Redman LM, Loucks AB. Menstrual disorders in athletes. Sports Med. 2005;35:747–755.

66. Rogol AD, Kraemer WJ. Introduction. In: Kraemer WJ, Rogol AD, Committee IO, eds. The Endocrine System in Sports and Exercise. Oxford: Blackwell Publishing, 2005:1–7.

67. Rogol AD, Weltman A, Weltman JY, et al. Durability of the reproductive axis in eumenorrheic women during 1 yr of endurance training. J Appl Physiol. 1992;72:1571–1580.

68. Ronsen O, Holm K, Staff H, et al. No effect of seasonal variation in training load on immuno-endocrine responses to acute exhaustive exercise. Scand J Med Sci Sports. 2001;11:141–148.

69. Rubin MR, Kraemer WJ, Maresh CM, et al. High-affinity growth hormone binding protein and acute heavy resistance exercise. Med Sci Sports Exerc. 2005;37:395–403.

70. Shackelford LC, LeBlanc AD, Driscoll TB, et al. Resistance exercise as a countermeasure to disuse-induced bone loss. J Appl Physiol. 2004;97:119–129.

71. Sherlock M, Toogood AA. Aging and the growth hormone/insulin like growth factor-I axis. Pituitary. 2007;10:189–203.

72. Smallridge RC, Whorton NE, Burman KD, et al. Effects of exercise and physical fitness on the pituitary–thyroid axis and on prolactin secretion in male runners. Metabolism. 1985;34:949–954.

73. Svartberg J, Jorde R, Sundsfjord J, et al. Seasonal variation of testosterone and waist to hip ratio in men: the Tromso study. J Clin Endocrinol Metab. 2003;88:3099–3104.

74. Tharion WJ, Rausch TM, Harman EA, et al. Effects of different resistance exercise protocols on mood states. J Appl Sport Sci Res. 1991;5:60–65.

75. Triplett-McBride NT, Mastro AM, McBride JM, et al. Plasma proenkephalin peptide F and human B cell responses to exercise stress in fit and unfit women. Peptides. 1998;19:731–738.

76. Tuckow AP, Rarick KR, Kraemer WJ, et al. Nocturnal growth hormone secretory dynamics are altered after resistance exercise: deconvolution analysis of 12-hour immunofunctional and immunoreactive isoforms. Am J Physiol Regul Integr Comp Physiol. 2006;291: R1749–R1755.

77. Uusitalo AL, Huttunen P, Hanin Y, et al. Hormonal responses to endurance training and overtraining in female athletes. Clin J Sport Med. 1998;8:178–186.

78. Valdemarsson S, Andersson D, Bengtsson A, et al. Gamma 2-MSH increases during graded exercise in healthy subjects: comparison with plasma catecholamines, neuropeptides, aldosterone and renin activity. Clin Physiol. 1990;10:321–327.

79. Vingren JL, Kraemer WJ, Ratamess NA, et al. Testosterone physiology in resistance exercise and training: the up-stream regulatory element. Sports Med. 2010;40(12):1037–1053.

80. Webb ML, Wallace JP, Hamill C, et al. Serum testosterone concentration during two hours of moderate intensity treadmill running in trained men and women. Endocr Res. 1984;10:27–38.

81. Wideman L, Consitt L, Patrie J, et al. The impact of sex and exercise duration on growth hormone secretion. J Appl Physiol. 2006;101:1641–1647.

82. Williams NI, DeSouza MJ. Energy balance and exercise-associated menstrual cycle disturbances: practical and clinical considerations. In: Kraemer WJ, Rogol AD, Committee IO, eds. The Endocrine System in Sports and Exercise. Oxford: Blackwell Publishing, 2005:261–278.

83. Wojtaszewski JF, Richter EA. Effects of acute exercise and training on insulin action and sensitivity: focus on molecular mechanisms in muscle. Essays Biochem. 2006;42:31–46.

84. Zanker C, Hind K. The effect of energy balance on endocrine function and bone health in youth. Med Sport Sci. 2007;51:81–101.

Suggested Reading

Kraemer WJ, Rogol AD, eds. The Endocrine System in Sports and Exercise. Malden, MA: Blackwell Publishing Inc., 2005. *The Encyclopaedia of Sports Medicine.*

Classic References

Bayliss WM, Starling EH. The mechanism of pancreatic secretion. J Physiol. 1902;28:325–353.

Selye H. Further thoughts on "stress without distress." Med Times. 1976;104(11):124–144.

Selye H. Forty years of stress research: principal remaining problems and misconceptions. Can Med Assoc J. 1976;115(1):53–56.

Selye H. Stress and distress. Compr Ther. 1975;1(8):9–13.

Selye H. Implications of stress concept. NY State J Med. 1975;75(12): 2139–2145.

Selye H. Confusion and controversy in the stress field. J Human Stress. 1975;1(2):37–44.

Selye H. The evolution of the stress concept. Am Sci. 1973;61(6): 692–699.

Selye H, The Harry G. Armstrong lecture. Stress and aerospace medicine. Aerosp Med. 1973;44(2):190–193.

Selye H, Fortier C. Adaptive reactions to stress. Res Publ Assoc Res Nerv Ment Dis. 1949;29:3–18.

Uusitalo AL, Huttunen P, Hanin Y, Uusitalo AJ, Rusko HK. Hormonal responses to endurance training and overtraining in female athletes. Clin J Sport Med. 1998;8(3):178–186.

PART III

Nutrition and Environment

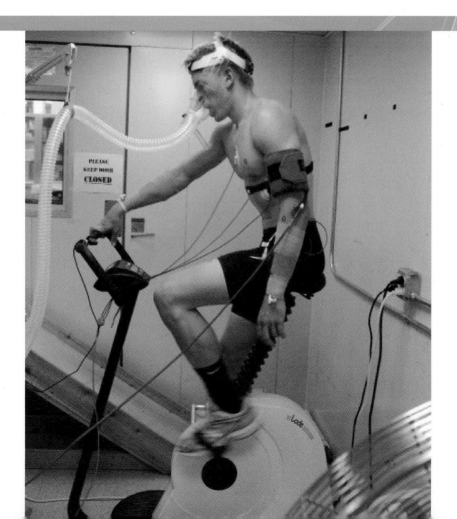

8

Nutritional Support for Exercise

After reading this chapter, you should be able to:

1. Define and distinguish the three macronutrients

2. Explain the role of the macronutrients in bodily functions and substrate metabolism

3. Identify and contrast the American Dietetic Association's nutrient recommendations for athletes

4. Explain the glycemic index of foods

5. Describe the process and objective of carbohydrate loading

6. Discuss the purpose of sports drinks

7. Discuss the composition and metabolic consequences of low-carbohydrate diets

8. Describe protein and carbohydrate supplementation strategies for both endurance and strength athletes

9. Differentiate types of triglycerides and specify roles in disease risks

10. Discuss the role of high-fat diets in sports performance

11. Understand and explain the role of vitamins and minerals in substrate metabolism

12. Explain the consequences of a mineral or vitamin deficiency

13. Describe the composition and purpose of pre- and postcompetition meals

A fitness enthusiast has trained hard for several months in preparation for the Boston Marathon. He feels like he is well conditioned for his first attempt at a marathon, and his training times for distances up to 20 miles have been quite good. On the day of the race he gets off to a good start and his times at the mile markers are what he expects all the way up to the 20th mile, at which point he feels like he has "hit the wall," and for the rest of the race his pace slows dramatically. His final time is unexpected and disappointing. Although the athlete's training program prepared him well, he overlooked an important aspect of sports performance: nutrition. The physiological occurrence that coincided with "hitting the wall" at mile 20 was a depletion of carbohydrates; the energy substrate so important to maintaining optimal performance in endurance events. He is convinced that he will not make the same mistake during his next attempt at the marathon and decides to consult with a sports nutritionist to determine what changes he can make in his diet to avoid the same carbohydrate depletion that resulted in such poor performance over the final miles of his first marathon. In his discussions with the sports nutritionist, the athlete learns much about how the carbohydrates, lipids, proteins, vitamins, and minerals we eat before, during, and after training sessions affects us not only at rest, but also during athletic performance.

In this chapter, dietary strategies on the consumption of carbohydrates, fats, proteins, vitamins, and minerals to enhance physical performance will be explored.

MACRONUTRIENTS

Carbohydrates, proteins, and lipids are needed in relatively large quantities by the human body and therefore are termed **macronutrients**. All three are organic in nature, meaning they are carbon-based substances. All three macronutrients contain carbon, hydrogen, and oxygen molecules, with protein also containing nitrogen molecules. All of the macronutrients can be used in metabolism to produce useable energy in the form of adenosine triphosphate (ATP; see Chapter 2). However, the number of kilocalories—a measure of potential energy—per gram of substrate differs among the macronutrients, with carbohydrate and protein yielding 4 kcal·g^{-1} and fat 9 kcal·g^{-1}. Thus, one reason for the need to consume relatively large amounts of the macronutrients is that they contain the energy that can be converted to ATP through aerobic and anaerobic metabolic pathways. Recall that ATP is the sole useable form of energy that can be directly used by the body to do all of its functions, including muscle contraction. In particular, carbohydrates and lipids are important to metabolism as they are responsible for the vast majority of ATP produced during metabolism. Under normal conditions, minimal amounts of protein are used for ATP production, but this can change in specific situations. For example, the use of protein for metabolism increases when one consumes a high-protein diet or when total caloric consumption does not meet the energy needs of the body (dieting or starvation). In such cases, protein comprising bodily tissue, such as skeletal muscle, is broken down and the resultant amino acids are used to synthesize ATP via aerobic metabolism.

In addition to serving as a metabolic substrate, all three macronutrients are essential for development of bodily tissue, including skeletal muscle. In this context, carbohydrates are critical for two reasons. First, they are a primary energy source during high-intensity activity, such as resistance exercise (weightlifting), which is a potent stimulant of muscle tissue growth. Second, the presence of adequate amounts of carbohydrates in the diet allows proteins that are ingested to be used for muscle growth. Skeletal muscle, like most of the body's tissues, is composed of significant amounts of protein in the form of amino acids. Thus, amino acids must be consumed to synthesize and repair skeletal muscle.

Although recommended to be consumed in limited amounts for health reasons, such as preventing cardiovascular disease, lipids are essential elements of our daily diets for many reasons. For example, lipids are needed to maintain the hormonal environment necessary for protein synthesis and reproductive function. Also, they are important components of the membranes of all cells in the body. **Adequate intake (AI)** of all three macronutrients is necessary for normal growth of the human body, maintenance of normal bodily function, and for adaptations to physical training, such as increased muscle mass due to resistance training or maintenance and repair of muscle mass due to aerobic training. In the following sections, the role of the macronutrients for potentially increasing physical performance will be explored in more detail.

Carbohydrate

Although the American Dietetic Association recommends 45% to 65% of total daily caloric intake be comprised of carbohydrates, from a practical perspective, the lower end of the range, about 45% to 50%, seems to be more prudent unless you are an endurance runner for whom the upper limits may be needed when training volume is high. High amounts of high-glycemic-index carbohydrates will interfere with needed protein and fat intakes and high-glycemic-index carbohydrates promote body fat deposition due to the role of insulin inhibiting lipolytic enzymes that break down fat.[1] The Food and Drug Administration (FDA) estimates that 130 grams per day of carbohydrate is the average minimum amount of glucose metabolized by the brain.[30] Because of this requirement, along with the fact that carbohydrates are used by so many other bodily tissues, the daily value on food labels for this macronutrient is 300 grams per day. Many high-carbohydrate foods, such as fruits and vegetables, are also relatively low in fat and high in dietary fiber. Both low-fat intake and high-fiber intake have been associated with general health benefits, such as decreased risk of some types of cancer, obesity, and cardiovascular disease. However, in terms of physical performance, perhaps the most important aspect of carbohydrate intake is meeting energy requirements for activity.

During aerobic events, such as the marathon, carbohydrate is the preferred metabolic substrate due to several factors.[13,89] The rate at which kilocalories are converted into usable ATP by the muscles is roughly twice as fast for carbohydrates as it is for lipids or proteins. This means that carbohydrate utilization allows an athlete to run, cycle, or swim at a faster sustainable pace. Another advantage of using carbohydrates as an energy substrate is that per unit of oxygen consumed by the body, approximately 6% more ATP is produced when metabolizing carbohydrates compared to lipids. So, when relying upon carbohydrate as the main energy substrate during aerobic exercise, there is a more efficient use of the oxygen consumed by the exercising muscles. In the transition from rest to activity, use of carbohydrate as a metabolic substrate increases and use of fat as a substrate decreases until at some exercise intensity,

---

🔍 *Quick Review*

- The three macronutrients are carbohydrate, lipid, and protein.
- All macronutrients are necessary for a wide array of bodily functions.
- All three macronutrients can be used as metabolic substrates, but generally minimal amounts of protein are used to produce ATP.

about 60% of $\dot{V}O_{2\,max}$ for the untrained, carbohydrate becomes the main energy substrate (see "Interactions of Substrates" in Chapter 2).

The selective use of carbohydrate as a metabolic substrate during prolonged exercise results in liver glycogen depletion as that organ attempts to maintain blood glucose levels, and to prevent glycogen depletion in the exercising muscles. For example, 1 hour of high-intensity endurance exercise decreases liver glycogen approximately 55%. However, 2 hours of strenuous activity almost completely depletes both liver and muscle glycogen. This is critical because glycogen depletion is linked to fatigue. Endurance athletes refer to the point in a race when glycogen depletion has occurred as "hitting the wall." At this point, the pace with which activity is performed must be decreased. Although the physiological mechanism(s) linking glycogen depletion to fatigue is not completely understood, several factors may be involved:

- The slower rate of energy transfer from kilocalories to ATP with lipid compared with carbohydrate, which requires that the pace of activity must decrease
- Use of blood glucose for optimal central nervous system function; this takes priority over the needs of the working muscles
- Increased reliance on type II muscle fibers as exercise intensity increases; these fibers produce more lactic acid than type I fibers

So, although it is not completely clear why glycogen depletion results in fatigue during an endurance event, it is clear that glycogen depletion is linked to fatigue.

Carbohydrate metabolism is also important during anaerobic exercise as an energy source. Only carbohydrate in the form of blood glucose or muscle glycogen can be used by glycolysis to produce ATP and lactic acid; lipids cannot be used as a substrate for anaerobic metabolism (see "Glycolysis" in Chapter 2). Research has shown that as exercise intensity increases, so does the use, and depletion, of glycogen stores. Muscle glycogen is reduced by approximately 72% during repetitive 1-minute sprint bouts of cycling at a resistance equal to 140% of that used at maximal oxygen consumption.[57] Resistance exercise, because of its anaerobic nature, is also highly dependent on glycolysis and results in glycogen depletion of the working muscles. This is especially true when performing at least a moderately high number of repetitions, and completing multiple sets with submaximal resistance.[58,79] Generally, reductions in glycogen are between approximately 30% and 40% after resistance exercise, with the reduction especially apparent in type II muscle fibers.[99] Research has clearly established that carbohydrate metabolism, and so carbohydrate ingestion, is important for performance of both aerobic and higher intensity and duration anaerobic training protocols (e.g., interval training); however, for performance of typical resistance training, which is also an anaerobic activity, it is less important. In the next sections, different dietary strategies to enhance carbohydrate availability for metabolism are discussed.

High-Carbohydrate Diets

Because of the dependence on carbohydrate as an energy substrate for performance of virtually all types of physical activity, it has been recommended that athletes consume a diet containing sufficient carbohydrate.[1] During training for most athletes, the recommended daily intake of carbohydrate should be at least 50% of total calories consumed.[1] However, carbohydrates needs may be higher for some athletes; for example, it has been recommended during high volume training carbohydrates intake may be as high as 55% to 60% of total calories consumed for bodybuilders and other strength athletes.[53] Note that this is within the range of the normally recommended 45% to 65% of the total calories consumed, and that endurance athletes' carbohydrate intake can be at the upper end of this range due to the high energy expenditure with training.[100] For all athletes, insufficient carbohydrate ingestion may result in an inability to maintain training intensity and volume, loss of muscle mass, and less-than-optimal physiological adaptations to training.[1,37,53]

Carbohydrate ingestion is correlated with muscle glycogen content. Thus, diets including sufficient carbohydrate will maintain muscle glycogen content so that fatigue can be delayed as much as possible during activity (Fig. 8-1). This is true for aerobic, anaerobic, and intermittent sports (basketball, volleyball, soccer). This is, however, perhaps most apparent for endurance activities. Studies from as early as 1939[17] and as well as later[4,34] have shown that time

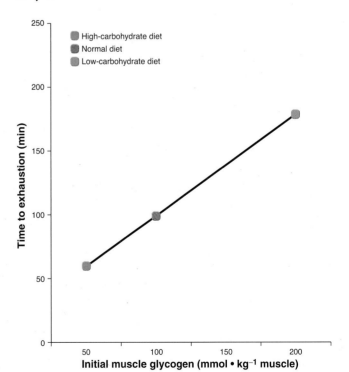

Figure 8-1. There is a correlation between carbohydrate intake, muscle glycogen content, and endurance performance. As carbohydrate ingestion increases, so does muscle glycogen content and time to exhaustion at submaximal exercise intensity. (Data from Astrand PO. Diet and athletic performance. Federation Proceedings, 1967;26:1772–1777.)

to exhaustion is increased when high-carbohydrate diets are ingested. In one study, for example, one group of subjects followed a diet in which approximately 22% of total calories were from carbohydrate and another group 52%. After 3 days of this dietary intake, time to exhaustion while cycling at 68% of peak oxygen consumption was, for both diets, approximately 65 minutes.[34] However, after a 15-minute rest time, exhaustion in a second work bout at the same workload was 9.5 and 65 minutes for the low- and high-carbohydrate-diet groups, respectively. Due to dependence on carbohydrate as a metabolic fuel in both anaerobic and aerobic activities, sufficient carbohydrate should be ingested in an athlete's diet. Although carbohydrates can be either simple, or complex in their form, the athlete should rely predominantly on complex carbohydrates in his/her regular diet. This is because complex carbohydrates take considerable time to digest, meaning that there is a slow, steady release of monosaccharides into the blood stream (all carbohydrates are converted to glucose or galactose before being released into the blood), thus avoiding a sharp insulin response. As a result, at rest, complex carbohydrates (grains, vegetables, etc.) are more likely to be stored in the body as glycogen that can be used at some later time during exercise. In contrast, simple carbohydrates (e.g., candy, soda, etc.) require very little digestion and, accordingly, glucose is released very quickly and in large amounts into the blood stream. This spike in blood glucose triggers a large insulin response and in doing so, at rest more of the glucose is converted to and stored as body fat. Clearly, the athlete and all health-conscious people should make an effort to be sure that generally the carbohydrates consumed are complex, and not simple ones. In the next section, the effects of foods resulting in quick and slow glucose release into the blood stream are explored.

Glycemic Index

The **glycemic index** is a relative measure of the increase in blood glucose concentration in the 2-hour period following ingestion of a food containing 50 grams of carbohydrate. This level is then compared with a standard carbohydrate-containing food—usually white bread or glucose—which increases blood glucose levels very quickly. The standard is assigned a glycemic index of 100. If a food raises blood glucose concentrations 45% as much as the standard, it is assigned a glycemic index of 45. High-glycemic-index foods (glycemic index = 70 or higher) offer several potential advantages compared with moderate-glycemic-index foods (glycemic index = 56–69) or low-glycemic-index foods (glycemic index = 55 or lower) because they increase blood glucose quickly. The glycemic index of some common foods is depicted in Table 8-1. If blood glucose concentrations increase quickly, the glucose can be used as a metabolic substrate quickly during exercise. Also, if blood glucose concentrations increase quickly, the blood glucose can be used to increase depleted muscle and liver

Table 8-1. Glycemic Index of Foods

Food	Glycemic Index (relative to glucose)
High-Glycemic-Index Foods (70 or greater)	
Glucose	100
Strawberry processed fruit bars	90
Puffed rice cakes	82
Jelly beans	78
Russett baked potato	78
Corn flakes	77
White bread	77
Waffles	76
Soda crackers	74
White bagel	72
Moderate-Glycemic-Index Foods (56–69)	
Special K cereal	69
Cranberry juice cocktail	68
Chocolate-flavored ice cream	68
White rice, boiled	64
Coca Cola	63
Corn chips	63
Sweet potato	61
Sweet corn	60
Pineapple, raw	59
Orange juice	57
Low-Glycemic-Index Foods (55 or lower)	
Oatmeal	54
Banana, yellow	51
Baked beans	48
Linguine noodles	46
All-bran cereal	42
Rye bread	41
Apple juice, unsweetened	40
Kidney beans	28
Reduced-fat yogurt	27
Milk, full fat	27

Data from: Foster-Powell K, Holt SHA, Brand-Miller JC. International table of glycemic index and glycemic load values: 2002. Am J Clin Nutr. 2002;76:5–56.

glycogen concentrations quickly, aiding in recovery between repeated exercise bouts.

Foods with a moderate- to high-glycemic-index rating can increase muscle glycogen more quickly than foods with a low glycemic index.[102] This effect may be of value if successive exercise bouts are close together. However, if exercise bouts or training sessions are separated by long periods of time, such as 24 hours, both high- and low-glycemic-index foods will return muscle glycogen to normal values when sufficient carbohydrate is ingested.

Surprisingly, even though high-glycemic-index foods increase blood glucose quickly and result in a more rapid replenishment of muscle glycogen following exercise, research does not confirm endurance performance benefits with ingestion of high-glycemic-index foods. For example, performance during a 64-kilometer cycling time trial did not differ between those who consumed a high-glycemic-index supplement and those who ingested a low-glycemic-index supplement during the event.

Moreover, the research conducted to date on the effect of the glycemic index of precompetition meals (30 minutes to 3 hours before activity) on endurance performance has yielded ambiguous results.[25,51,88,92,104] Overall, though, it appears that ingesting a carbohydrate mixture with a moderate glycemic index may have a more positive effect than meals with either a low or a high glycemic index. This may in part be explained by the effects of glycemic index throughout a long endurance event. For example, a high-glycemic-index food may result in more reliance on carbohydrate metabolism during the first 2 hours of activity, which results in less available carbohydrate and so more reliance on lipid metabolism after 2 hours of activity.[25] The overall result is decreased performance in long-term endurance events. Thus, for long-term endurance performance, consuming a high-glycemic-index meal prior to the event may actually result in the opposite effect desired. The best approach would be to ingest a moderate-glycemic-index carbohydrate meal before competition as it provides adequate carbohydrates to sustain endurance performance (unlike a low-glycemic-index meal) without elevating blood glucose so high as to trigger a large insulin response and the consequent "glucose crash" that occurs. The effects of glycemic index on performance requires further study, but the benefits of dietary strategies to increase muscle glycogen content resulting in increased endurance performance are well established and explored in the next section.

Carbohydrate Loading

Depletion of muscle glycogen stores happens predictably in the latter stages of an endurance activity and results in overwhelming fatigue. Because of this, dietary and training strategies were developed to increase muscle glycogen and liver glycogen stores, which have been termed **carbohydrate loading**. Carbohydrate loading resulted from

studies in the late 1960s,[2] demonstrating that several days of a low-carbohydrate diet depleted muscle glycogen and reduced endurance cycling performance compared with a moderate-carbohydrate diet.[2] With subsequent ingestion of a high-carbohydrate diet over several days, glycogen stores became supercompensated and increased cycling time to exhaustion. It is now well established that carbohydrate loading can increase muscle glycogen from normal values (approximately 90 mmol·kg⁻¹ wet weight) to values as high as approximately double (150 to 200 mmol·kg⁻¹ wet weight) the normal resting value.[13,19]

Most studies also indicate that carbohydrate loading can increase overall performance in endurance activities.[13,20,42] Although a half marathon[13] and 20.9-kilometer run[84] are too short to benefit from carbohydrate loading, performances during a 30-kilometer cross-country run, a 30-kilometer treadmill run, and a 25-kilometer treadmill run are significantly improved following carbohydrate loading. Moreover, carbohydrate loading has been found to be effective in trained as well as untrained individuals.[13,20] Typically, when endurance performance is increased, carbohydrate loading does not result in an ability to increase maximal race pace, but rather in an ability to maintain that pace for a longer period of time, resulting in a faster pace toward the end of the endurance event, such as the last 5 kilometers of a 30-kilometer run.

The original or classical method of carbohydrate loading consisted of several phases:

1. 1 day of long strenuous endurance exercise to deplete muscle glycogen stores
2. 3 days of a high-fat/protein (low-carbohydrate) diet with continued training to further deplete or maintain depletion of muscle glycogen stores
3. A high-carbohydrate diet (90% carbohydrate of total calories) with little or no training for 3 days

This classical method of carbohydrate loading has some disadvantages for the endurance athlete. For example, it requires 7 days to achieve glycogen supercompensation, which could interfere with preparation for the upcoming competitive event. Also, some athletes poorly tolerate the high-fat/protein and/or the high-carbohydrate diet portions of the carbohydrate loading strategy. To alleviate some of these practical problems and still have a glycogen supercompensation effect, modified carbohydrate loading diet and training strategies have been developed.

One such modified plan[19,83,85] has been shown to increase muscle glycogen levels to an extent similar to that of the classical method of carbohydrate loading. The modified plan (Modified Plan 1; Table 8-2) does not include the high-fat/protein or low-carbohydrate phase of the classical plan. However, this modified plan still requires several days to complete and, therefore, could interfere with training.

Another modified carbohydrate-loading strategy does not include a phase intended to bring about a severe

Table 8-2.	Types of Carbohydrate Loading		
Days Before Event	**Training Intensity**	**Training Duration**	**Carbohydrate Ingestion**
Modified Plan 1			
6	Moderate (70% $\dot{V}O_2$ peak)	90 min	Normal diet (5 g·kg^{-1} body mass)
4–5	Moderate (70% $\dot{V}O_2$ peak)	40 min	Normal diet (5 g·kg^{-1} body mass)
2–3	Moderate (70% $\dot{V}O_2$ peak)	20 min	High-carbohydrate (10 g·kg^{-1} body mass)
1	Rest	0 min	High-carbohydrate (10 g·kg^{-1} body mass)
Modified Plan 2			
6	Moderate (73% $\dot{V}O_2$ peak)	90 min	Normal diet (5 g·kg^{-1} body mass)
5	Moderate (73% $\dot{V}O_2$ peak)	40 min	Normal diet (5 g·kg^{-1} body mass)
4	Moderate (73% $\dot{V}O_2$ peak)	40 min	Normal diet (5 g·kg^{-1} body mass)
3	Moderate (73% $\dot{V}O_2$ peak)	20 min	High-carbohydrate (7.7 g·kg^{-1} body mass)
2	Moderate (73% $\dot{V}O_2$ peak)	20 min	High-carbohydrate (7.7 g·kg^{-1} body mass)
1	Rest	0 min	High-carbohydrate (7.7 g·kg^{-1} body mass)
Modified Plan 3 (Rapid Carbohydrate Loading)			
2	Cycling 130% $\dot{V}O_2$ peak	150 seconds followed by 30-second all-out sprint	Normal diet (6.67 g·kg^{-1} body mass)
1	Rest	0 min	High-carbohydrate (12.2 g·kg^{-1} lean body mass)

depletion of muscle glycogen.[84] With this strategy, training time is gradually decreased from 90 to 20 minutes over 5 days, followed by a day of rest (Modified Plan 2; Table 8-2). Additionally, during the first 3 days, a diet consisting of 50% carbohydrates is ingested, and during the last 3 days, a diet of 70% carbohydrates is ingested. This results in muscle glycogen content that is more than twice that seen under normal conditions, and about the same as that resulting from the more severe strategies of carbohydrate loading.

In addition to aerobic activity, muscle glycogen is used as a metabolic fuel during anaerobic exercise. Therefore, anaerobic activity can serve as an effective substitute for aerobic exercise in the glycogen loading protocols described above (Modified Plan 3; Table 8-2). Indeed, research has demonstrated that cycling for 150 seconds at an intensity equivalent to 130% of maximal oxygen consumption followed by a 30-second all-out cycling sprint effectively brings about the muscle glycogen depletion needed during the initial stages of glycogen loading strategies.[29] During the 24-hour period after the anaerobic cycling activity, high levels of carbohydrate are ingested and result in an approximately doubling of muscle glycogen content (109 to 198 mmol·kg^{-1} wet weight). This increase is similar to that observed when aerobic exercise is used to initially deplete muscle glycogen reserves.

Recently, it has been shown that a strategy of nothing more than rest coupled with a high intake of

carbohydrate can effectively bring about muscle glycogen supercompensation. Well-trained male endurance athletes rested for 3 days and ingested high levels of carbohydrate (10 g·kg body mass^{-1}·day^{-1}), which resulted in an approximate doubling of muscle glycogen concentration.[14] Interestingly, muscle glycogen after the first day had already approximately doubled (90 to 180 mmol·kg^{-1} wet weight) and, for the remaining 2 days, was stable, despite continued high-carbohydrate ingestion. This indicates that in trained endurance athletes, no unique carbohydrate-loading strategy is necessary and that, with adequate carbohydrate ingestion, muscle glycogen concentrations are maximized within 36 to 48 hours and possibly within 24 hours.

Although it has been well documented that carbohydrate loading can significantly improve endurance performance in events lasting more than an hour, studies have failed to find that this dietary manipulation effectively improves anaerobic performance.[37] This indicates that muscle glycogen does not limit performance in this type of activity and that other factors, such as increased acidity, limit performance in short-duration, high-power anaerobic activities. Thus, only those athletes who perform specific events, that is, endurance activities that continue for at least an hour in duration, stand to benefit from muscle glycogen loading. Athletes performing shorter duration endurance events, as well as those relying mainly on anaerobic metabolism during their sports activities, do not benefit from carbohydrate loading strategies and should simply maintain a normal diet with carbohydrates representing 45% to 50% of the total number of kilocalories consumed daily.

Carbohydrate and Electrolyte Sports Drinks

Carbohydrate and electrolyte sports drinks are meant to increase physical performance by providing an exogenous source of glucose, resulting in a sparing of muscle glycogen. In addition, they are intended to replace the valuable electrolytes lost in sweat that are necessary for proper muscle, heart, and nervous function, while at the same time replacing water lost with sweat so that dehydration can be avoided. The effectiveness of a sports drink depends on the rate at which it passes through the stomach (gastric emptying) and into the small intestine, where absorption of water, carbohydrates, and electrolytes takes place (Fig. 8-2). Sports drinks are specifically formulated in an attempt to increase the rate of carbohydrate and fluid absorption. This formulation is important because at high intensities of exercise and with dehydration, gastric emptying decreases, impairing the delivery of the sports drink to the small intestine. The carbohydrate and electrolyte content of sports drinks and the effect on carbohydrate and fluid absorption are explored in the next sections.

Carbohydrate Composition of Sports Drinks

Carbohydrate is a major component of sports drinks because it is a major substrate for metabolism (i.e., ATP production) during exercise. The type and concentration of carbohydrate are two major factors to consider when determining the proper composition of sports drinks. Both of these factors affect the **osmolality** of the sports drink, or the ratio of solutes to fluid. Since water "follows solute," a solution that has an osmolality less than bodily tissue (hypotonic) will result in water being drawn into the body's cells, while a solution with an osmolality greater than bodily tissue (hypertonic) will draw water out of the body's cells. So, tonicity is obviously an important factor when formulating a sports drink. If the sports drink's osmolality is too high, it can decrease fluid absorption, which could minimize the hydration effects of sports drinks. The osmolality of a solution depends on the number of solute molecules, and not their size. Thus, the same number of a large or complex carbohydrate (see Chapter 2) molecule creates the same osmolality as a small or simple carbohydrate molecule. However, a large carbohydrate molecule would increase the total carbohydrate content of the sports drink and, if absorbed by the small intestine, increase the total carbohydrate available for metabolism.

Different carbohydrates are absorbed by the small intestine by different mechanisms. For example, glucose is absorbed by active transport, whereas fructose is absorbed by facilitated diffusion by the cells of the small intestine. Thus, inclusion of more than one type of carbohydrate could aid in total carbohydrate absorption.[5] It must be remembered, however, that most simple carbohydrates are converted by the liver to glucose because glucose is the predominant substrate for metabolism (see Chapter 2). Most common forms of carbohydrate, such as glucose, sucrose, fructose, and glucose polymers (short chains of glucose molecules),

Gastric Factors

Volume ingested: increased stomach volume increases emptying rate

Exercise intensity: high exercise intensities decrease emptying rate

Osmolality: carbohydrate type and electrolyte content affect osmolality, increased osmolality decreases emptying rate

Hydration: dehydration slows emptying rate

Acid base: changes from a neutral pH (7.0) slow emptying rate

Small Intestine Absorption

Gastric emptying: fluid and carbohydrate must leave stomach to be absorbed

Osmolality: affected by both carbohydrate type and electrolyte content, slightly hypotonic fluid increases fluid absorption

Carbohydrate: low to moderate glucose concentration increases fluid absorption

Sodium: low to moderate sodium concentration increases fluid and glucose absorption

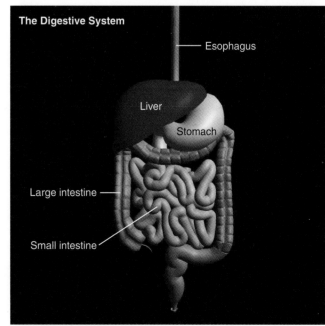

The Digestive System

Esophagus

Liver

Stomach

Large intestine

Small intestine

Figure 8-2. Several factors affect gastric emptying and carbohydrate and fluid absorption by the small intestines. Carbohydrate and electrolyte sports drinks are formulated in an attempt to increase both carbohydrate and fluid absorption by the small intestine. (LifeART image copyright (c) 2010 Lippincott Williams & Wilkins. All rights reserved.)

Box 8-1 PRACTICAL QUESTIONS FROM STUDENTS

How Do You Determine the Carbohydrate Concentration in a Sports Drink?

To determine the sports drink's carbohydrate percentage, divide the carbohydrate content in grams by the fluid volume in milliliters and multiply by 100. For example, if 60 grams of carbohydrate are contained in 1 liter (1000 milliliters) of sports drink, the carbohydrate concentration is 6%.

---

are effective in maintaining blood glucose concentration and improving endurance performance.[1,20] However, the evidence is not conclusive and is contradictory concerning the advantages or disadvantages of various carbohydrate types.

Glucose polymers, or **maltodextrins**, increase the carbohydrate content of a sports drink without an increase in osmolality and may make the sports drink taste better, which may encourage consumption. However, substitution of glucose polymers for free glucose does not affect the blood glucose response or exercise performance.[1] Likewise, use of several types of simple sugars (sucrose, fructose, glucose) in a sports drink does not significantly affect the blood glucose response or endurance exercise performance. However, a combination of glucose and fructose in equal amounts effectively increases total exogenous carbohydrate oxidation,[1] whereas fructose alone is oxidized less during exercise than glucose or glucose polymers.[60] Thus, most sports drinks contain a combination of glucose, sucrose and glucose polymers, and high-fructose corn syrup. This combination allows them to take advantage of the possible effect of several different types of carbohydrates on absorption rate, to provide better taste to encourage consumption, and to minimize the negative effect of osmolality on rates of fluid absorption into the blood.

The carbohydrate concentration in a sports drink not only affects its osmolality, but also the amount of carbohydrate available for absorption, and thus, its use as a metabolic substrate (see Box 8-1). High carbohydrate concentrations delay the gastric emptying, or absorption of fluid, but increase the total amount of carbohydrate absorbed. Additionally, if carbohydrate concentration is high enough (greater than 8% to 10%), osmolality will be high enough to cause secretion of water from the intestinal walls into the interior of the intestine (Fig. 8-3), potentially increasing dehydration.[60] High carbohydrate concentrations may also result in gastrointestinal problems.

Ingesting approximately 1 gram of carbohydrate per kilogram of body mass per hour is sufficient to improve prolonged exercise.[66] For a 55-kilogram marathon runner, this would mean ingesting approximately 0.68 liters or 680 mL·h⁻¹ of a sports drink containing 8% carbohydrate. This amount of sports drink consumption may be possible for some but not for others, as most people drink only between approximately 250 and 450 mL·h⁻¹. Ingesting some carbohydrate, even if it is not the maximal amount needed during activity, will increase performance by supplying exogenous carbohydrate, thus sparing liver and muscle glycogen stores. Beyond a certain limit, however, additional carbohydrate intake will not continue to increase the oxidation rate of exogenous carbohydrate,[1] and dilute carbohydrate solutions (1.6% carbohydrate) have been shown to be as effective in some situations as more concentrated carbohydrate solutions.[61] However, the majority of commercial sports drinks contain 6% to 8% carbohydrate. This concentration is low enough to avoid inhibiting fluid absorption but high enough to increase endurance performance, with a drink consumption rate that is tolerable by many individuals during activity.

Electrolytes in Sports Drinks

Electrolytes are formed when mineral salts, such as sodium chloride (NaCl), dissolve in water (see Chapter 9). Electrolytes are added to sports drinks for the following reasons:

- Promotion of a sustained drive to drink, which promotes voluntary fluid ingestion

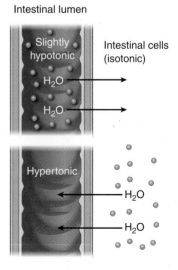

Figure 8-3. The amount of fluid absorbed by the small intestine in part depends on osmolality of the fluid. A fluid that is slightly hypotonic aids fluid absorption, whereas a fluid that is hypertonic can actually result in fluid entering the intestinal lumen.

- Maintenance of plasma volume, which helps to maintain cardiac output during exercise
- Maintenance of extracellular fluid volumes
- Reduction in the risk of hyponatremia
- Decreased urine output[1,21,66]

These factors are related. If the drive to drink is sustained (the thirst mechanism is influenced by the body's tonicity), a larger volume of the sports drink is ingested, which increases gastric emptying. If a sports drink did not contain electrolytes, ingestion of a large volume of the drink would decrease sodium concentration in the plasma, which would result in increased urine output, which would reduce plasma volume. Electrolytes in sports drinks may also help decrease the chance of decreases in sodium concentration of blood, resulting in a serious life-threatening situation (hyponatremia; see Chapter 9).

The decrease in sodium concentration of blood could occur due to ingestion of a large volume of fluid containing little or no sodium, or due to sodium loss in sweat, or some other mechanism such as diarrhea. Decreased sodium concentration of blood can occur in very long-term endurance events (3 to 4 hours), in which excessive sweating occurs. The cause of decreased sodium concentration in blood in endurance athletes is controversial, but, at least among inexperienced endurance athletes, it is more likely to result from drinking too much water rather than dehydration.[70,71]

Addition of electrolytes to a sports drink, similar to addition of carbohydrates, does increase the osmolality of the sports drink and so can affect gastric emptying. Sodium, besides helping to maintain plasma volume and extracellular fluid volume and decrease urine output, is also necessary for carbohydrate absorption by the small intestines and aids water uptake by the small intestine.[1,21,87] Glucose and sodium are cotransported across the small intestinal wall, and absorption of these molecules stimulates passive uptake of water due to osmotic action.[33,54] Sports drinks also contain potassium, the major cation in the intracellular space, at the same concentration found in plasma and sweat because it is believed that inclusion of potassium will promote rehydration. However, there is little evidence to support the inclusion of potassium in sports drinks.[1,87] Magnesium is also included in sports drinks because it is believed that decreased magnesium concentrations, which do occur with exercise, may contribute to exercise-induced cramps. This suggestion, however, has not been substantiated by science.[1] Due to the potential benefits of adding sodium to sports drinks, it is recommended that at least 20 mmol·L^{-1} (460–500 mg·L^{-1}) and not more than 50 mmol·L^{-1} (1150 mg·L^{-1}) of sodium be added.

When Are Sports Drinks Appropriate?

Carbohydrate and electrolyte sports drinks are normally associated with endurance activities or intermittent activities of a long duration, such as basketball and soccer. Studies have shown improvement in basketball skills with sports drink consumption compared with a water placebo[26] and improved performance with sports drink consumption in intermittent activities.[106] These findings indicate that adequate hydration along with carbohydrate and electrolyte consumption can improve performance in these types of activities as well.

Although guidelines for sports drink ingestion have been developed for long-duration and intermittent activities, they need to be adjusted to individuals and particular circumstances.[16,21,24] For example, an elite marathon competitor may complete a marathon in 2 hours 10 minutes in warm weather. In such a case, drinking 0.5 L·h^{-1} of fluid would not prevent the degree of dehydration that would reduce endurance performance (greater than 2% loss of body weight).[16] However, in a cool environment, drinking this same amount would be sufficient to prevent that level of dehydration. In cool weather, drinking rates of 0.5 L·h^{-1} would maintain hydration in runners with a body mass of 70 to 90 kilograms, but in smaller runners (e.g., 50 kilograms), this rate of fluid intake would result in body weight gain.[16] Guidelines recommend frequent ingestion of fluid during activity to maintain a high gastric volume, because increased gastric volume results in increased gastric emptying. However, gastric emptying rates vary among individuals, and some individuals may experience gastrointestinal distress when drinking the recommended volume of fluid.[17] Therefore, guidelines should be used to develop rehydration plans on an individual basis, and for particular activities. The plans should then be tested in simulated competitions or training, prior to use in actual competition, to ascertain whether an individual tolerates the plan without adverse symptoms.

Guidelines for carbohydrate and electrolyte sports drink consumption are presented in Box 8-2. These guidelines are applicable to events lasting longer than approximately 1 hour of continuous activity or intermittent activities of long duration. However, improved performance has been shown with carbohydrate and electrolyte drink consumption in events as short as 45 minutes.[66] The duration and environmental conditions of the event should be considered when choosing what fluid to drink during exercise (see Box 8-3). The guidelines include recommendations for fluid consumption before, during, and after training or competition. They are meant to delay dehydration and glycogen depletion during activity and result in rehydration and muscle glycogen resynthesis after activity. It may not be necessary to prevent dehydration completely during endurance activity, as athletes who win or finish near the top of endurance events are frequently dehydrated by as much as 8% to 10%.[70] This level of dehydration, however, may be more of a concern among untrained athletes, who would not tolerate this level of dehydration well. Finally, it is recommended that fluid consumption not result in body weight gain during the activity. It is also important to remember that the maintenance of plasma and extracellular fluid volumes is also important to aid in recovery. This is especially true if strenuous activity is performed in multiple training sessions per day or on successive days.

Box 8-2 APPLYING RESEARCH
Guidelines for Fluid Replacement during Long-Duration Activity

- Ingest adequate fluid during the 12 to 24 hours prior to exercise.
- Ingest 500 mL (17 oz) of fluid approximately 2 hours before exercise.
- During exercise, ingest between 600 and 1200 mL·h⁻¹ (20 to 40 oz) by drinking 150 to 300 mL (5 to 10 oz) every 15 to 20 minutes.
- After activity, drink sufficient fluid to replace water weight lost during the activity.

- Fluids should be cooler than ambient temperature (15 to 22°C, 59 to 72°F).
- Fluids should be served in containers that allow easy ingestion and minimal interruption of activity.
- Fluids may be flavored to enhance palatability and encourage drinking.

Use of carbohydrate and electrolyte sports drinks, especially high-carbohydrate sports drinks, needs to be carefully considered in individuals exercising and attempting to lose fat mass. The caloric content of the sports drink needs to be included in the daily caloric consumption in these individuals. Although less research is available concerning the use of carbohydrate and electrolyte sports drinks in anaerobic activities, such as weight training, ingestion during and after resistance training sessions does result in quicker and greater muscle glycogen resynthesis after exercise.[35,36,72] Carbohydrate supplementation before and during resistance training[36,38] does increase resistance training performance (i.e., total number of repetitions possible at a specific resistance). It has also been recommended that resistance trainers

involved in high-volume weight training programs should use carbohydrate supplementation. This supplementation, which could be in the form of a sports drink before, during, and after training sessions, can maximize muscle glycogen synthesis and improve resistance training performance.[37] The ability to recover from weight training and maintain high training volumes may ultimately result in increased protein synthesis and so greater gains in muscle mass over time.

Protein

Protein comprises approximately 22% of the mass of skeletal muscle. The majority of muscle is water, with the remainder composed of protein, glycogen, fat, vitamins, and minerals.

Box 8-3 PRACTICAL QUESTIONS FROM STUDENTS
What Fluid Should I Drink When I Go for My Daily 4-mile Run during the Hot, Muggy Days of Summer?

There are many commercial sports drinks available that contain various concentrations of carbohydrates, and electrolytes, intending to provide energy (carbohydrate) and replace the electrolytes lost by sweating. However, in the conditions described above, plain water would be the best fluid to consume during the workout. Since depletion of the body's glycogen (carbohydrate) stores is not evident in endurance activities lasting less than an hour duration, there is no need to supply the body with carbohydrates on a 4-mile run that typically will last less than an hour. Additionally, the loss of electrolytes suffered during a 4-mile run will be negligible and not result in any physiological disturbances. On the other hand, when exercising in hot, humid conditions, even for 30 to 45 minutes, the thermoregulatory challenge to the body can be considerable. Why? Because with high ambient temperatures, the temperature gradient between the body and the air is minimized so there is less potential

for the body to lose heat to its surroundings. On top of that, humid air makes the sweating mechanism inefficient because sweat can only help cool the body when it evaporates into the air. High humidity decreases the evaporative, and cooling, capacity of sweat. As a result, the body sweats even more in humid conditions in an attempt to cool the body. Accordingly, the primary concern when exercising for less than an hour in hot, humid conditions is to replace body water. This will prevent dehydration and overheating. The best, and quickest, way to replenish the body's water is to drink plain water. Anything added to water in the form of carbohydrates or electrolytes acts to slow down the uptake of water from the gastrointestinal tract into the blood stream. So, if the exercise session is less than an hour in duration, and particularly if exercising in a hot, humid environment, the best replacement fluid to drink during exercise is plain water.

Quick Review

- Carbohydrate is the major metabolic substrate for both aerobic and anaerobic activities.
- Diets containing at least 50% of total calories from carbohydrates are recommended for endurance athletes because time to exhaustion during endurance activity is increased.
- Although high-glycemic-index foods increase blood glucose concentration more quickly than low-glycemic-index foods, ingestion of high-glycemic-index foods prior to exercise does not appear to aid endurance performance.
- Carbohydrate loading can increase endurance performance by allowing a faster race pace in the latter stages of a long endurance event.
- Carbohydrate-loading strategies are effective in increasing muscle glycogen content. However, in well-trained endurance athletes, rest and sufficient carbohydrate ingestion also result in supercompensation of muscle glycogen content.
- Carbohydrate loading does not increase performance in short-duration, high-power anaerobic activities.
- Most sports drinks contain several different types of carbohydrates. Advantages to this approach include increased absorption rate, improved taste to encourage consumption, and minimizing the negative effect of increasing osmolality on water absorption.
- Electrolytes are added to sports drinks to: promote a sustained drive to drink, which promotes voluntary fluid ingestion; maintain plasma volume, which helps to maintain cardiac output during exercise; maintain extracellular fluid volumes; and reduce the risk of hyponatremia and decrease urine output.
- Carbohydrate sports drinks can be ingested before, during, and after endurance activity. They maintain hydration and supply exogenous carbohydrate for metabolism during activity, as well as aid rehydration and muscle glycogen resynthesis after activity.

Additionally, protein in the form of amino acids is needed for synthesis of virtually all bodily tissue. From a practical perspective, protein intake should tend toward the higher range of the American Dietetic Association recommendations of 10% to 35% of total caloric intake to allow for adequate protein signaling for protein synthesis, which is needed for repair and recovery of skeletal muscle and connective tissue from exercise training stress. A **recommended dietary allowance (RDA)** of a nutrient is established when there is sufficient scientific evidence indicating the average daily amount necessary to meet the needs of practically all healthy adults (98%). The RDA for protein is 0.8 g·kg^{-1} body mass·day^{-1} for healthy adults. The RDA intake can easily be accomplished on most Western diets; in fact, many individuals normally ingest substantially more protein than the RDA. The question of whether athletes require a protein intake greater than the RDA has been a subject of considerable debate. Some experts[94,95,99] believe that athletes require more protein (1.2 to 2.0 g·kg^{-1} body mass·day^{-1}), whereas others believe that the RDA is sufficient for athletes and will result in optimal training adaptations. With the demands of tissue repair and recovery with intense training and caloric expenditure, it appears prudent to increase protein intake, especially with the essential amino acids being critical for stimulating protein synthesis.

Dietary protein intake may be elevated in athletes due to increased metabolism of protein during activity and for the purpose of maintaining or increasing muscle mass during training. Although protein metabolism to obtain energy in the form of ATP normally is minimal, some amino acids are aerobically metabolized (see Chapter 2). Additionally, aerobic metabolism of amino acids may not decrease the total energy available from the aerobic metabolic pathway (Box 8-4).

Although some studies confirm increased protein metabolism during endurance activity, some of these investigations have measured protein metabolism after an overnight fast, which does not represent the dietary practices of endurance athletes.[32] Typically, endurance athletes ingest

Box 8-4 APPLYING RESEARCH

Increased Rate of Amino Acid Oxidation: Effect on Aerobic Energy during Prolonged Exercise

Prolonged exercise does increase the rate of BCCA oxidation by skeletal muscle. The Krebs cycle is an enzymatic system through which macronutrients must pass during aerobic metabolism (see Chapter 2). Increased BCCA aerobic metabolism could decrease the concentration of some Krebs cycle intermediates and so impair aerobic metabolism during prolonged exercise. During a 90-minute bout of moderate-intensity exercise, Krebs cycle intermediates increased by three times during the first initial minutes of exercise. However, after 60 and 90 minutes of exercise, Krebs cycle intermediates did not differ from resting concentrations.

Even though Krebs cycle intermediates declined initially, oxygen uptake and phosphocreatine concentration (an indicator of mitochondrial respiration) showed no significant change. This finding indicates that BCCA metabolism does not significantly affect aerobic energy production during prolonged exercise.

Further Reading

Gibala MJ, Gonzalez-Alonso J, Saltin B. Disassociation between tricarboxylic acid cycle pool size and aerobic energy provision during prolonged exercise in humans. J Appl Physiol. 2002;545:705–713.

carbohydrates before, during, and after training, which could decrease the need for protein metabolism. During 6 hours of continuous moderate-intensity aerobic exercise, total body protein turnover was not increased compared with rest.[52] However, many endurance events are contested at higher-than-moderate intensities, which could result in increased protein metabolism. Although further work is necessary to fully elucidate the protein needs of endurance athletes, currently it is recommended that the protein intake of endurance athletes should be 1.2 to 1.4 g·kg⁻¹ body mass·day⁻¹ during training,[1] which is greater than the RDA. However, due to the increased caloric needs of endurance athletes, this increased protein intake can be met with a diet containing the same protein concentration: 10% to 15% of total caloric intake (Box 8-5). The timing of protein intakes around the training session and competition may be an important practical approach to protein intake with such demands for protein and carbohydrate macronutrients.

One technique to examine protein needs is to measure the amount of protein or nitrogen ingested compared with the amount of nitrogen excreted. This technique is termed **nitrogen balance**. Recall that unlike the other macronutrients (lipids, carbohydrates), the amino acids composing proteins also include nitrogen, and thus, the consumption and use of protein can be estimated by tracking the nitrogen intake and excretion by the body. **Positive nitrogen balance** occurs when more nitrogen is ingested than excreted and indicates that nitrogen is being retained in the body and amino acids are being used to synthesize bodily tissue. **Negative nitrogen balance** occurs when more nitrogen is being excreted than ingested and indicates that amino acids are being used in

metabolism. Positive nitrogen balance indicates greater synthesis of bodily tissue than degradation, or an anabolic state of the body. On the other hand, negative nitrogen balance indicates mobilization of amino acids from bodily tissue, or a catabolic state of the body.

Nitrogen balance studies indicate that, during resistance training and in resistance-trained athletes, protein ingestion of 1.0 to 1.7 g·kg⁻¹ body mass·day⁻¹ results in a positive nitrogen balance, indicating a net increase in muscle protein synthesis.[1,6,53,95,99] This has resulted in recommendations that strength training athletes ingest approximately 1.4 g·kg⁻¹ body mass·day⁻¹ of protein or between 1.0 and 1.7 g·kg⁻¹ body mass·day⁻¹. Additionally, it has been recommended that proteins account for 25% to 35% of the total number of calories consumed by strength training athletes.

Interestingly, nitrogen balance studies have also indicated that novice strength training athletes have a protein need of approximately 1.3 to 1.5 g·kg⁻¹ body mass·day⁻¹ and that athletes who have been strength training for years require protein in the amount of 1.0 to 1.2 g·kg⁻¹ body mass·day⁻¹. Similarly for endurance training athletes, if more total calories are ingested, the percentage of total calories ingested from protein can be less and still achieve the recommended protein intake in g·kg⁻¹ body mass·day⁻¹. Not surprisingly, athletes involved in sports requiring a combination of both endurance and strength abilities also require an increased protein intake compared with the RDA.[6] Practically speaking, athletes who are building muscle (e.g., weightlifters) may need higher protein intake compared to when just maintaining muscle mass. Conversely, some endurance athletes who are performing

---

Box 8-5 APPLYING RESEARCH

Calculation of Calories from Carbohydrate, Protein, and Fat

Calculating the number of calories in a diet and the percentage of calories from each macronutrient when the amounts of carbohydrate, protein, and fat in the diet are known is relatively simple. When metabolized, there are 4 kcal per gram (17 kj·g⁻¹) of carbohydrate, 4 kcal per gram (17 kj·g⁻¹) of protein, and 9 kcal per gram (37 kj·g⁻¹) of fat. The following demonstrates how to calculate the number of calories in a diet and percentage of calories from each macronutrient:

- 90 g protein × 4 kcal·g⁻¹ = 360 kcal
- 300 g carbohydrate × 4 kcal·g⁻¹ = 1200 kcal
- 60 g fat × 9 = 540 kcal
- Total kcal = 360 kcal + 1200 kcal + 540 kcal
- Total kcal = 2100 kcal
- Percentage kcal from a macronutrient = total kcal / kcal from macronutrient
- Percentage kcal from protein = 360 kcal / 2100 kcal

- Percentage kcal from protein = 0.17 = 17%
- Percentage kcal from carbohydrate = 1200 kcal / 2100 kcal = 0.57 = 57%
- Percentage kcal from fat = 540 kcal / 2100 kcal = 0.26 = 26%

Note that if the total number of calories in the diet increases and the percentage of calories from each macronutrient is constant, the total amount of each macronutrient increases. For example, maintaining 17% of the total calories from protein and increasing total caloric consumption to 2500 kcal results in the following total grams of protein ingestion:

- Kcal from protein = 2500 kcal × 0.17
- Kcal from protein = 425 kcal from protein
- Grams of protein = 425 kcal/4 kcal·g⁻¹
- Grams of protein = 106 g

high volume training with high energy expenditure and tissue breakdown may need to maintain a higher protein intake to maintain repair processes each day. So, although more research concerning protein requirements of those undergoing intense training is needed, the evidence to date suggests that the protein requirements of athletes are much greater than the RDA, even for master athletes.

High-Protein Diets

Without adequate scientific evidence or understanding of types of higher protein diets and fears of reducing carbohydrate concentrations, clinically trained dietitians typically do not recommend high-protein diets because of their perceived association with increased risk of heart disease, some types of cancer, adult bone loss (osteoporosis), kidney disease, and difficulties with weight control.[105] However, animal protein sources tend to be rich in saturated fats, and it is difficult to separate the effects of dietary animal protein and fat. In one study attempting to do so, soy protein was substituted for animal protein, and results showed reductions in total blood cholesterol, especially in individuals whose initial total blood cholesterol levels were high.[105]

A factor that can make interpretation of the effects of a high-protein diet difficult is that there is no generally accepted definition of high-protein or low-carbohydrate diets. For example, popular weight loss diets are characterized as low-carbohydrate (Atkins), low-fat (Weight Watchers), ultralow-fat (Ornish), and moderate-protein (Zone).[100–102] Although no formal definition of very low-carbohydrate diets exists, they typically have less than 50 g·day^{-1} carbohydrate or less than 10% total calories from carbohydrate.[100,101] This generally results in ingestion of approximately 60% to 65% total calories from fat and 20% to 25% of total calories from protein. Thus, a very low-carbohydrate diet could also be characterized as high-fat and either moderate- or high-protein, as 20% to 25% total calories from protein falls within the midrange of what is typically recommended (10–35% total calories from protein).

In addition to the potentially confounding effects of saturated fats being associated with animal sources of dietary protein, proponents of high-protein diets believe that there is an adaptation period of several weeks before positive responses to these diets will occur (if at all). The presence of this adaptation period may influence the conclusions drawn from studies investigating the effects of high-protein diets. For example, 1 week after a high-protein diet (1.2 g·kg^{-1}·day^{-1}), treadmill endurance time to exhaustion at 75% of maximal oxygen consumption decreased.[75] However, endurance time to exhaustion after 6 weeks significantly increased even though subjects wore backpacks equivalent to the weight loss because of the high-protein diet. The increased time to exhaustion at 6 weeks, but not at 1 week, of ingesting the high-protein

diet was thought to be due to a lack of metabolic adaptations to the diet at 1 week.

One metabolic adaptation to high-protein diets that requires several weeks to take place is the incomplete breakdown of lipids, resulting in the formation of **ketone bodies**, which are molecules that have a C=O, or carbonyl group, between two carbons. During periods of low carbohydrate availability, such as during a high-protein diet, ketone bodies provide an alternate metabolic substrate to be used in lieu of glucose. One way to form ketone bodies is from the breakdown of acetyl CoA (see Chapter 2), as depicted in Figure 8-4. When the production of ketone bodies exceeds their use, the acid–base balance of the blood is disturbed because some ketone bodies, termed **keto acids**, contain an acid group (COOH). An increase in ketone bodies in the blood and urine is termed **ketosis** and is used in some studies as an indicator of compliance to a high-protein diet. Additionally, ketosis suppresses appetite, which is one aspect of a high-protein diet that aids weight loss. Concentrations of ketone bodies with high-protein diets, however, are not in the range of those seen with the dangerous condition of diabetic ketosis. But again, the physiological adaptations necessary for working muscles to effectively use ketone bodies to produce ATP take time, and during this interlude exercise performance may be negatively impacted by a high-protein diet. High protein diets have shown some increases in performance and

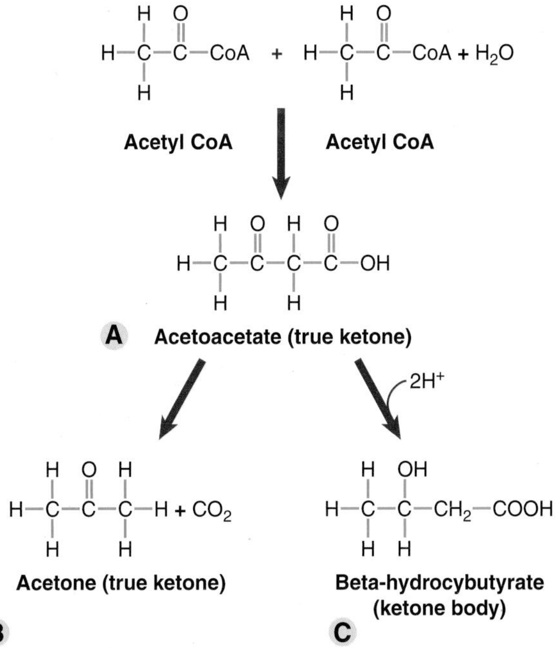

Figure 8-4. One formation method of ketone bodies.
A ketone by definition has a C=O group between two carbons. **(A)** Condensation of two acetyl CoAs results in a ketone, acetoacetate. **(B)** Acetoacetate can lose a carbon dioxide molecule, forming another ketone. **(C)** Acetoacetate can have two hydrogens added to it, forming a ketone body. Acetoacetate and acetone are true ketones, whereas beta-hydroxybutyrate is not a true ketone, but is termed a ketone body because it is formed during ketosis.

positive health benefits, such as weight loss and improved blood lipid profile. However, further research is needed to elucidate its possible benefits and future use as it relates to weight loss and combating obesity, which has continued to be epidemic despite the increase in carbohydrate and lowering of fat intakes over the past 30 years, seem to be promising.[100]

Protein Supplementation Before, During, and After Training

Protein supplementation in the form of protein bars or protein-containing sports drinks may be of value not only to individuals performing resistance training, but also to those performing endurance training. This is especially true for athletes performing high-volume and high-intensity training, because they have increased protein needs compared with sedentary individuals (see Protein section above). When endurance training increases, protein may be needed to maintain fat-free mass because amino acids are metabolized during endurance exercise. Typically, endurance athletes would not desire an increase in fat-free mass; however, loss of fat-free mass will eventually affect endurance performance. Also, high volumes of endurance training, especially running, can result in damage to muscle tissue and adequate protein intake is needed to repair damaged tissue. In contrast, resistance training is typically intended to increase fat-free mass, which requires a higher protein intake. In the next sections, the possible benefits of protein-containing supplements during both resistance and endurance training will be explored.

Resistance Training and Protein Supplementation

Ingestion and infusion of amino acids with, or without carbohydrate, stimulates protein synthesis after resistance exercise.[15,99] Protein ingestion immediately prior to,[93] or within 3 hours after exercise,[7,32,77] results in increased protein synthesis. This increased protein synthesis appears to be related not only to a greater supply of amino acids, but also to a more favorable anabolic environment due to exercise-induced changes in hormonal concentrations, such as an increase in blood insulin and growth hormone.[43,99]

Although ingestion of protein and carbohydrate either immediately prior to, or after, a resistance training session increases protein synthesis, several studies using the same supplement (6 g of essential amino acids and 35 g of sucrose) indicate that supplementation immediately prior to exercise maximizes protein synthesis.[77,93] Increased protein synthesis with supplementation prior to exercise may be related to increased blood flow during exercise, which increases amino acid availability for protein synthesis to the exercising muscle.[94,99,107] An alternative explanation is that protein synthesis is stimulated by both exercise and an increased insulin response (insulin

stimulates both carbohydrate and amino acid uptake by tissue) when a protein and carbohydrate supplement is given before exercise, and that enhanced protein synthesis continues after exercise. Yet it has also been reported that protein supplementation postexercise, particularly immediately following a resistance training session, can effectively increase muscle protein synthesis.[28] Presumably, consuming additional protein during the period in which muscles are repairing tissue damaged by intense weightlifting exercise results in gains in muscle mass. This protein repairing effect has been found to be particularly valuable during long periods (i.e., several months) of high-intensity training when performance typically suffers due to excessive and cumulative tissue damage.[78]

The research findings presented above suggest that there is a relatively large window of opportunity that extends from just before the start of resistance exercise to several hours after exercise, during which protein supplementation may increase anabolic activities within muscle tissue. But regardless of when protein supplements are ingested relative to resistance training sessions, it appears that it may take some time for increases in muscle mass to occur. In one study, it was determined that 4 weeks of resistance training, combined with protein supplementation, failed to stimulate gains in muscle mass.[55] But in another study, a 6-week resistance training program combined with protein supplementation was successful in stimulating significant increases in whole body muscle mass.[11] See Box 8-6 for more information regarding protein supplementation while resistance training.

Endurance Training and Protein Supplementation

Endurance athletes are not normally concerned with achieving an increase in fat-free mass. However, they are concerned with recovery between training sessions and after competitions, as well as possible increases in aerobic performance. Recovery includes not only maintenance of muscle glycogen levels, but also maintaining fat-free mass, and preventing muscle soreness resulting from muscle damage. It has been found that postexercise ingestion of a protein and carbohydrate supplement, as opposed to one comprised solely of carbohydrate, results in enhanced glycogen resynthesis.[45] This indicates that protein intake may influence glycogen synthesis in muscle following endurance exercise. In fact, research indicates that the ingestion of both protein and carbohydrate after exercise increases the insulinemic response compared with carbohydrate alone,[5,46,97] resulting in increased uptake of carbohydrate by muscle tissue. Because training-induced muscle damage can result not only in pain, but also in impaired performance, investigators have recently studied whether the composition of a supplement during periods of intense training can temper, or even eliminate muscle damage. Two groups of researchers have reported

Box 8-6 AN EXPERT VIEW

Supplementing to Enhance Muscle Protein Accretion Following a Resistance Exercise Training Session

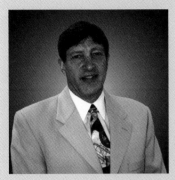

John L. Ivy, PhD, FACSM
Chairman, Kinesiology and Health Education
Teresa Lozano Long Endowed Chair
The University of Texas
Austin, TX

After resistance training exercise, the active muscle is glycogen-depleted and in a catabolic state (i.e., protein degradation exceeds protein synthesis). This state is initiated during exercise due to an increase in the catabolic hormones, such as cortisol, and a decrease in the anabolic hormones, such as insulin. The result is an increase in muscle breakdown and damage that continues after exercise unless action is taken to reverse this imbalance in protein metabolism. By consuming the appropriate types and concentrations of macronutrients, as well as timing their consumption appropriately, the resistance exercise-induced catabolic condition can be limited and the anabolic potential of the resistance exercise stimulus enhanced.

Raising the level of essential amino acids in the blood will promote protein synthesis, particularly after exercise. Insulin has also been found to promote muscle protein synthesis if sufficient amino acid levels are present. Increasing both insulin and amino acid levels simultaneously has been found to have an additive effect on protein synthesis and to reduce muscle degradation.[1]

To raise both blood amino acid and insulin levels, a supplement or meal containing protein and carbohydrate can be very effective. Importantly, the combination of protein and carbohydrate has a synergistic effect on insulin secretion. The carbohydrate or carbohydrate mixture should be readily digestible and have a high glycemic index, resulting in a high insulin response. The protein should contain all 20 amino acids and have a high concentration of the essential amino acids. Whey, a milk-based protein, has a very effective protein profile. A protein mixture should also be considered. Boirie et al.[2] found that protein synthesis increased 68% with whey supplementation and 32% with a casein supplement. The anabolic response, however, was longer lasting with casein. Therefore, it might be most beneficial to consume a combination of whey and casein when supplementing after exercise.

The timing of the protein and carbohydrate supplementation is critical. Exercise increases the muscle's anabolic potential, but with time this increased sensitivity to macronutrient activation decreases. For example, Levenhagen et al.[3] reported that protein synthesis was increased approximately threefold when supplementation occurred immediately after exercise. No increase in protein synthesis occurred when the supplement was delayed 3 hours. More recently, Cribb et al.[4] found that subjects receiving supplementation immediately before and after exercise during 10 weeks of resistance exercise training had an 86% greater increase in lean tissue mass and approximately 30% greater overall increase in strength than subjects supplemented at the beginning and end of the day.

Consumption of a carbohydrate and protein supplement immediately prior to and during exercise will reduce protein degradation and limit muscle damage. Baty et al.[5] had subjects consume a carbohydrate/protein supplement or placebo prior to and during a resistance exercise training session. Plasma cortisol and creatine kinase levels (markers of muscle damage) 24 hours after exercise were significantly lower in the subjects receiving the carbohydrate/protein supplement compared with those receiving the placebo. These results suggest that supplementation before and perhaps during exercise will reduce muscle protein degradation and limit damage.

The amount of protein and carbohydrate to consume is also of importance. If supplementing only after exercise, a carbohydrate concentration that will significantly raise plasma insulin levels and be sufficient to substantially restore muscle glycogen is recommended. This would amount to between 0.7 and 0.8 g of carbohydrate per kg body weight. The amount of protein consumed should provide approximately 6.0 g of essential amino acids. This can be accomplished with 30 to 35 g of protein. A supplement of two parts carbohydrate to one part protein, e.g., 2 g dextrose and 1 g whey, works very well. If supplementation is going to occur both before and after exercise, the amount of carbohydrate and protein in the supplementation can be equally divided.

To summarize, to promote an increase in net protein accretion following resistance exercise training, it is important to supplement immediately after exercise with both carbohydrate and protein. Supplementation prior to exercise may also be of benefit, as it appears to reduce muscle tissue damage that occurs during exercise and speed recovery. Simple carbohydrates with a high glycemic index are recommended. The protein should be a complete protein. It may also be advantageous to use several types of proteins, such as whey and casein. Supplements that contain two parts carbohydrate to one part protein are recommended for resistance training.

References

1. Miller SL, Tipton KD, Chinkes DL, et al. Independent and combined effects of amino acids and glucose after resistance exercise. Med Sci Sports Exerc. 2003;35:449–455.
2. Boirie Y, Dangin M, Gachon P, et al. Slow and fast dietary proteins differently modulate postprandial protein accretion. Proc Nat Acad Sci (U S A). 1997;94:14930–14935.
3. Levenhagen DK, Gresham JD, Carlson MG, et al. Postexercise nutrient intake timing in humans is critical to recovery of leg glucose and protein homeostasis. Am J Physiol. 2001;280:E982–E993.
4. Cribb PJ, Hayes A. Effects of supplement timing and resistance exercise on skeletal muscle hypertrophy. Med Sci Sports Exerc. 2006;38:1918–1925.
5. Baty JJ, Hwang H, Ding Z, et al. The effect of a carbohydrate and protein supplement on resistance exercise performance, hormonal response, and muscle damage. J Stren Cond Res. 2007;21:321–329.

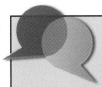

that compared to a supplement comprised solely of carbohydrate, a supplement containing a combination of protein and carbohydrate is more effective not only in stimulating muscle protein synthesis,[56] but also in reducing muscle damage and soreness.[64,80] Clearly, then, endurance athletes, like strength trained athletes, can benefit from consuming protein supplements.

Type of Amino Acid in Supplements

The amino acid composition of a protein supplement is an important consideration for the athlete. Amino acids can be classified as either essential, or those not produced by the body and accordingly must be consumed, or nonessential, or those that can be produced by the body (see Chapter 2). Further, amino acids can be categorized as those that are branched chain or those considered nonbranched chain (Table 8-3). Essential amino acids appear to be the primary stimulators of muscle protein synthesis, with little contribution from the nonessential amino acids.[7,99,107] In addition to their role as substrates for oxidation, and thus ATP production, branched-chain amino acids (BCCAs), in particular leucine, are the most important stimulators of skeletal muscle protein synthesis.[50] Thus, it may be important to include essential amino acids and BCCAs in a protein supplement, especially when a goal of supplementation is to increase or maintain fat-free mass.

Table 8-3. **Types of Amino Acids**

Essential	Nonessential
Histidine	Alanine
Isoleucine (BCCA)	Arginine
Leucine (BCCA)	Asparagine
Lysine	Aspartic acid
Methionine	Cysteine
Phenylalanine	Glutamic acid
Threonine	Glutamine
Tryptophan	Glycine
Valine (BCCA)	Proline
	Serine
	Tyrosine

BCCA, branched-chain amino acid.

Triglycerides

Triglycerides are a common member of the larger family of macronutrients known as lipids, or fats. It is triglycerides, and not free fatty acids or cholesterol, that are the most abundant member of the lipid family found circulating in the blood stream. Triglycerides are composed of a glycerol backbone to which three fatty acids are bonded (see Chapter 2). Because they represent a valuable source of potential energy, circulating triglycerides are taken up from the blood stream and stored in fat cells as well as other tissues including muscle. The enzyme **lipase** is located in fat cells and muscle fibers, and its function is to hydrolyze, or remove, the fatty acids from the glycerol backbone, resulting in "free" fatty acids. It is these free fatty acids that serve as the major substrate used in metabolism at rest, and during low-intensity exercise. There are several types of fatty acids (see Chapter 2), with a major difference between fatty acid types being whether or not the carbon atoms of the fatty acid are attached to the maximal number of hydrogen atoms possible. If so, the fatty acid is considered to be "saturated." If less than the maximal number of hydrogen atoms are bound to the carbon atoms, it is an unsaturated fatty acid. Saturated fatty acids are generally associated with greater risk of various disease states than unsaturated fatty acids. In the following sections, health risks associated with various types of fatty acids are discussed.

Degree of Fatty Acid Saturation and Disease Risk

Diets containing a high level of fat intake, whether the fat is saturated or unsaturated, can result in weight gain

---

Quick Review

- The upper range of percentages of 25% to 35% of protein intake will allow more optimal repair of muscle and connective tissue.
- Protein needs of athletes may be elevated due to the increased metabolism of protein during activity and the need to maintain or increase skeletal muscle mass.
- Recommended protein needs of endurance (1.2 to 1.4 g·kg body mass^{-1}·day^{-1}) and strength-training athletes (1.4 or greater g·kg body mass^{-1}·day^{-1}) are higher than the RDA (0.8 g·kg body mass^{-1}·day^{-1}) but may be met by the athletes' increased caloric consumption.
- There is a relatively large window of opportunity, which begins shortly before a resistance training session and ends several hours after exercise, during which supplementation may increase protein synthesis. However, long-term training studies are needed to substantiate whether supplementation increases fat-free mass.
- Supplements that contain a combination of carbohydrate and protein may aid recovery from endurance activities and maintenance of muscle mass in endurance athletes.
- Inclusion of essential and BCCAs in a protein supplement may be important because these amino acids are simulators of protein synthesis.

because fat contains a high number of kilocalories per gram (9 kcal·g^{-1}). Even moderate weight gain results in an increase in blood pressure and other cardiovascular risk factors. However, saturated fats, which are generally found in animal food sources, are of particular concern because they contribute to an increased risk of cardiovascular disease and some types of cancers.[105] Thus, because of their low content of saturated fats, it is generally recommended that lean animal protein sources, such as chicken and fish, be included in your diet.

A monounsaturated fatty acid contains one and a polyunsaturated fatty acid contains more than one double bond between carbon molecules. Good sources of monounsaturated fats are olive oil, canola oil, peanut oil, and avocados. Good sources of polyunsaturated fatty acids include nuts, seeds, and vegetable oils such as sunflower, sesame, and corn oils. Replacing saturated fats in the diet with monounsaturated and polyunsaturated fats lowers total blood cholesterol, lowers blood pressure, and decreases blood clotting factors,[86,90] reducing total cardiovascular risk.

Including high levels of saturated fats in the diet increases risk for some types of cancer, whereas including high levels of monounsaturated and polyunsaturated fats decreases risk for some types of cancer. However, it is difficult to separate the effect of saturated fatty acids, which are found in red meat, from the consumption of red meat alone. Additionally, some studies have shown a positive correlation between total caloric consumption and some types of cancer.[86] In some studies, increased total caloric consumption was in large part due to increased ingestion of saturated fatty acids and red meat, making it difficult to separate which factor or factors contributed to an increased

cancer risk. Nevertheless, saturated fat intake has been associated with increased risk of colon cancer, breast cancer, and prostate cancer.[86] Conversely, increased ingestion of monounsaturated and polyunsaturated fats generally reduces the risk of these types of cancers.

Because of the association of high-fat ingestion, in particular high-saturated-fat ingestion, with increased risk of several diseases, the FDA recommends that total fat and saturated fat intake should be limited. Total fat ingestion should not exceed 65 grams per day or 30% of total calories ingested, whereas saturated fat should not exceed 20 grams per day or 10% of total calories ingested. Fat ingestion may, however, be so low as to have negative physiological consequences. Low-fat diets and diets replacing saturated fats with polyunsaturated fats have been shown to decrease resting testosterone levels by 13% to 20%.[99] Recall that as a steroid hormone, testosterone is synthesized from a lipid precursor. Because testosterone is a potent stimulant of muscle protein synthesis, this has led some experts to recommend that strength athletes consume a moderate level of fat, with 15% to 20% of total calorie consumption, including some saturated fat.

Omega-3 and Omega-6 Fatty Acids

Omega-3 and omega-6 fatty acids are polyunsaturated fatty acids, so named because of the position of the first double bond between carbon atoms from the omega carbon of the fatty acid (Fig. 8-5). Neither of these fatty acids are produced by the human body and, accordingly, they must be consumed by eating sources that are rich in them, such as vegetable oils (e.g., sunflower, soy), fish (especially salmon

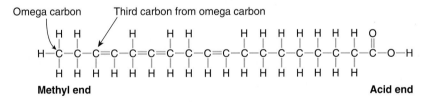

Figure 8-5. Omega-3 and omega-6 fatty acids are named due to the location of the first double bond between carbons in the fatty acid. Omega-3 and omega-6 fatty acids have the first double bond between carbons at the third and sixth carbon atom from the omega carbon, respectively. The omega carbon is the first carbon of the fatty acid starting from the methyl end of the fatty acid.

and trout). Dietary consumption of omega-3 and omega-6 fatty acids are associated with health benefits, in particular decreased cardiovascular risk and decreased risk of some types of cancer.[86,105] Improved cardiovascular health comes in the form of decreases in blood pressure, blood clots, and irregular heart beats, especially in people with those preexisting conditions.[47,65,68] Further, omega-3 fatty acids have been shown to have at least a weak association with a decrease in the risk of breast and colon cancer.[44] However, some experts consider the relationship between dietary intake of the omega acids and decreased risk of cardiovascular disease and specific forms of cancer to be minimal and not conclusive.

High-Fat Diets and Endurance Ability

The major rationale for the belief that a diet high in lipid content will positively affect endurance performance is that by a greater reliance on lipids for ATP production, there would be a glycogen sparing effect resulting in a delay of glycogen depletion and improved endurance performance.

But in reality, high-fat diets have shown positive, negative, and no effects on endurance performance measures.[39,42,75] In short-term studies, where high lipid intake persists for less than 6 days, it appears that a greater than normal fat intake (i.e., 55–85% of total daily caloric consumption) has a negative impact not only on endurance performance, but also on high-intensity exercise (greater than 95% of maximal oxygen consumption).[39] These studies show decreases in performance measures ranging from 10% to 30% compared with a high-carbohydrate diet.[62] Longer duration studies, where high lipid intake lasts for more than 7 days, have shown mixed results.[40] More specifically, while endurance performance improves during moderate-intensity exercise (less than 80% of

$\dot{V}O_{2max}$), performance during high-intensity exercise (greater than 80% of $\dot{V}O_{2max}$) has shown decreases following consumption of a high-lipid diet. One dietary strategy suggested by some would be to ingest a high-fat diet prior to competition to increase fat metabolism and then ingest a high-carbohydrate diet in the days immediately prior to an endurance competition. The objectives of this dietary strategy would be to increase fat metabolism during exercise, thus sparing muscle glycogen, as well as to increase muscle glycogen content. Presumably, both of these adaptations would increase endurance performance. Experimentation has shown that this type of dietary strategy results in a significant increase in lipid metabolism compared with a high-carbohydrate diet in well-trained cyclists during exercise at 70% of maximal oxygen consumption.[12] However, no significant difference in simulated time trial performance was noted between the diets, indicating that the dietary strategy resulted in no performance benefit.

MICRONUTRIENTS

Macronutrients are required by the body in relatively large amounts. **Micronutrients**, in contrast, are required by the body in small amounts (milligrams or micrograms per day). Vitamins and minerals are considered to be micronutrients. But just because they are found in small amounts in the body, this does not mean that they are not important for maintaining life, health, and optimal physical performance. The micronutrients most commonly associated with physical performance will be discussed in the following sections.

Vitamins

Vitamins are organic substances (i.e., they contain carbon) that facilitate enzymatic reactions. They are not necessary to cause a reaction, nor are they destroyed in metabolic reactions, but they are necessary for many enzymatic reactions to occur at their proper rates. Because of their function in essential enzymatic reactions, vitamins are referred to as "co-factors" in those reactions. Vitamin deficiencies, which can have very severe consequences, attest to the importance of vitamins. For example, a chronic lack of vitamin C, which is necessary for blood vessel integrity and bone metabolism, results in scurvy. The symptoms of scurvy include the following: bleeding of the gums; breaking of capillaries under the skin resulting in pinpoint hemorrhages; inadequate collagen synthesis resulting in further hemorrhaging; denervation of muscle, including cardiac muscle; loss of teeth; and rough skin that is brown and scaly. The symptoms of scurvy related to bone metabolism include development of osteoporosis, malformed bones, and fractures. All of these can potentially result in anemia

---

🔍 Quick Review

- Saturated fat intake is associated with increased risk of cardiovascular disease, colon cancer, breast cancer, and prostate cancer, whereas increased ingestion of monounsaturated and polyunsaturated fats reduces these disease risks.

- Omega-3 and omega-6 fatty acids are associated with health benefits such as decreased cardiovascular risk and risk for some types of cancer. However, the association with these decreased disease risks may be small, and further research is warranted before conclusions can be reached.

- Theoretically, high-fat diets should increase endurance performance by increasing fat metabolism, which would spare muscle glycogen. Although this dietary strategy does increase lipid metabolism, it does not appear to improve endurance performance.

and infections and even sudden death caused by massive internal bleeding. The variety and severity of symptoms associated with vitamin C deficiency indicate that an adequate amount of this micronutrient is important for many bodily functions and necessary for maintaining life.

Like macronutrients, some vitamins have an RDA. Other vitamins have an AI, which is the average amount of a nutrient consumed by healthy individuals and is established when there is insufficient evidence to establish an RDA. **Tolerable upper intake levels (UL)** are also established for vitamins as the amount of a nutrient that appears safe for most healthy individuals. Ingestion above the UL can result in toxic symptoms and increased health risks. Vitamins can be divided into two major subtypes: fat-soluble and water-soluble vitamins.

Fat- and Water-Soluble Vitamins

Fat-soluble vitamins can be dissolved in fat. Vitamins A, D, E, and K are the major fat-soluble vitamins. Because they are fat-soluble, these vitamins can be stored in large quantities within our body fat. Deficiencies of fat-soluble vitamins are rare because if there is inadequate dietary intake of one of these vitamins, the body can rely on its own reserves of them stored in the body's fat tissue. Although this is a positive feature of fat-soluble vitamins, the disadvantage is that it is possible for so much of these vitamins to be stored within the body that toxicity develops. Recently, vitamin D deficiencies have increased due to poor nutrition and increased appropriate use of sun blocks (which are important for skin cancer prevention but block the positive effects of the sun for vitamin D synthesis), which underscores the importance of diet and supplements to address such vitamin deficiencies.

Water-soluble vitamins can be dissolved in water and include the B vitamins and vitamin C. Niacin, folic acid, pantothenic acid, and biotin are all considered B vitamins. The majority of the B vitamins function in energy metabolism. For example, niacin is part of nicotinamide adenine dinucleotide (NAD), which functions in energy transfer from the Krebs cycle to the electron transfer chain (see Chapter 2). Vitamin C is necessary to maintain normal development of cartilage, bone, and connective tissue. Due to their water solubility, excesses of these vitamins are excreted in the urine, making it difficult to develop toxic symptoms from these vitamins. On the other hand, because there is little capacity to store the water-soluble vitamins in the body, they must be ingested on a regular basis. Fat- and water-soluble vitamin dietary sources, major functions, deficiency symptoms, and toxicity symptoms are presented in Table 8-4.

Because of the many physiological functions that vitamins participate in, mega-doses of some vitamins have been hypothesized to increase both health and physical performance. The majority of evidence, however, indicates that vitamin supplementation does not increase health or physical performance unless a person is deficient in a particular vitamin. Vitamins E and C and the B vitamins, in particular, have been thought by some to increase physical performance. The possible role of vitamins in increasing health and physical performance is examined in the following sections.

Vitamin C

Because of vitamin C's role in immune function and as an antioxidant, a person deficient in this vitamin could suffer health as well as physical performance consequences. Some endurance athletes with inadequate intake of vitamin C do, in fact, suffer from increased risk of upper respiratory tract infections, especially in the first hours after a bout of endurance activity. Daily vitamin C supplementation of 500 to 1500 mg may be of some benefit in reducing upper respiratory tract infections in these athletes, but the evidence is not conclusive.[40,73,74]

The role of vitamin C in possibly increasing physical performance is related to its role as an antioxidant. Free radicals are produced as a result of metabolism. So, exercise results in increased production of free radicals, and increased free radical production may be related to fatigue, and even contribute to exercise-induced muscle injury. Oxidative stress due to free radicals is combatted in two major ways: endogenous antioxidant capacity and non-enzymatic exogenous antioxidants, such as vitamins C and E. Exercise training can increase normal endogenous antioxidant capacity.[82] However, acute ingestion immediately prior to an exercise bout or chronic daily ingestion of vitamin C does not appear to increase either aerobic or anaerobic capabilities[63] or consistently improve exercise performance.[10,96]

Vitamin C's antioxidant properties have also been purported to reduce delayed onset muscular soreness (DOMS), or the muscle soreness that presents itself about 2 days following a training session. If supplementation does decrease DOMS, it may require high doses (3 g·day⁻¹) to do so.[48] However, at such high doses, there is also evidence that supplementation may actually promote cellular damage.[9] In general, supplementation with vitamin C does not appear warranted, since a deficiency of this micronutrient is an infrequent occurrence, and the balance of research shows that supplementation does not increase aerobic or anaerobic performance, and may even promote cellular damage.

Vitamin E

Similar to vitamin C, vitamin E is an antioxidant. Some research has indicated that exercise training may increase vitamin E stores within skeletal muscle, but this is an inconsistent finding.[45] Similarly, while some research has

Table 8-4.   **Vitamins: Summary of Functions, Deficiency Symptoms, and Food Sources**

Vitamin	Food Sources	Major Functions	Deficiency Symptoms	RDA or AI (Adult per Day)	Toxicity Symptoms or Ingestion Above UL
Fat-Soluble					
Vitamin A	Dairy products, liver, carrots, eggs, green leafy vegetables	Vision, promotes resistance to bacterial infection, skin, bone and tooth growth, antioxidant	Night blindness, drying of cornea, grey spots on eye, blindness, impaired immunity	RDA: Men: 900 µg; Women: 700 µg	Reduced bone density, liver abnormalities, birth defects
Vitamin D	Sunlight exposure causes synthesis, fortified dairy products, fortified cereals, egg yolks, fatty fish	Promotes absorption of calcium and phosphorous and bone mineralization	Rickets in children, osteomalacia in adults	AI: 5 µg	Elevated calcium in blood, calcification of soft tissues, frequent urination
Vitamin E	Leafy green vegetables, wheat germ, liver, egg yolks, nuts, polyunsaturated plant oils	Antioxidant, regulation of oxidation reactions, stabilization of cell membranes	Red blood cell hemolysis, nerve damage	RDA: 15 mg	Muscle weakness, fatigue, nausea, headache, inhibits vitamin K metabolism
Vitamin K	Bacterial synthesis in the digestive tract; leafy green vegetables, liver, milk	Synthesis of proteins, particularly blood-clotting proteins, assists bone metabolism	Hemorrhaging	AI: Men: 120 µg; Women: 90 µg	None known
Water-Soluble					
Vitamin B-1 (Thiamin)	Fortified, enriched, or whole grains and their products; pork	Coenzymes used in metabolism	Cardiac hypertrophy, cardiac failure, weakness, confusion, irritability, poor short-term memory, weight loss	RDA: Men: 1.2 mg; Women: 1.1 mg	None known
Vitamin B-2 (Riboflavin)	Dairy products, enriched or whole grains, liver	Coenzymes used in metabolism	Sensitivity to light, reddened cornea, sore throat, cracks at corners of the mouth, skin lesions	RDA: Men: 1.3 mg; Women: 1.1 mg	None known
Niacin	Milk, eggs, all protein-containing foods, whole-grain and enriched breads and cereals	Part of coenzymes used in metabolism (nicotinamide adenine dinucleotide)	Abdominal pain; vomiting; diarrhea; depression; fatigue; loss of memory; inflamed, bright red tongue	RDA: Men: 16 mg; Women: 14 mg (units are niacin equivalents: 1 mg niacin or 60 mg tryptophan)	Painful flush, hives and rash, blurred vision, liver damage, impaired glucose tolerance
Vitamin B-6	Meats, fish, poultry, legumes, noncitrus fruits, fortified cereals, soy	Coenzymes in amino acid and fatty acid metabolism, assists red blood cell production	Dermatitis, depression, confusion, convulsions, microcytic anemia	RDA: 1.3 mg	Fatigue, irritability, headaches, nerve damage, muscle weakness
Folic Acid (folate)	Fortified grains and cereals, legumes, leafy green vegetables, liver	Coenzymes for DNA synthesis	Macrocytic anemia, smooth red tongue, fatigue, headache, irritability	RDA: 400 µg	Masks vitamin B-12 deficiency symptoms

Vitamin B-12	Meats, fish, poultry, cheese, eggs, milk, fortified cereals	Coenzymes used for new cell synthesis and folate formation, maintenance of nerve cells	Anemia, poor peripheral nerve function, fatigue	RDA: 2.4 µg	None known
Pantothenic acid	Organ meats, avocados, whole grains, mushrooms	Coenzyme used in metabolism	Nausea, stomach cramps, vomiting, fatigue, irritability, insomnia, apathy, hypoglycemia, increased insulin sensitivity	AI: 5 mg	None known
Biotin	Whole grains, soybeans, organ meats, fish	Coenzyme used for energy metabolism, amino acid metabolism, fats synthesis, glycogen synthesis	Lethargy; hallucinations; depression; tingling in arms and legs; red rash around eyes, nose, and mouth	AI: 30 µg	None known
Vitamin C (ascorbic acid)	Citrus fruits, dark green vegetables, strawberries, tomatoes, potatoes, papaya, mangos	Collagen synthesis, antioxidant, amino acid metabolism, assists in iron absorption, immune function	Microcytic anemia, symptoms of scurvy, pinpoint hemorrhages, joint pain, tooth loss, poor immune function	RDA: Men: 90 mg; Women: 75 mg	Nausea, diarrhea, headache, abdominal cramps, insomnia, hot flashes, skin rashes, kidney stones

RDA, recommended dietary allowance; AI, adequate intake; UL, upper level.

shown vitamin E supplementation to result in decreased muscle and membrane damage, presumably from increased antioxidant capabilities, such decreases are not consistently shown.[96] From a performance perspective, the most important finding is that even though vitamin E supplementation may possibly decrease muscle damage, it does not significantly increase aerobic, anaerobic, or maximal strength performance.[11,64,97]

B Vitamins

The B vitamins have essential roles as coenzymes in metabolism and so could affect physical performance. Although some studies have shown effects on metabolism, such as increased carbohydrate metabolism and decreased blood lactate concentrations during activity, these have not translated into improved physical performance.[96] Supplementation with B vitamins does not increase aerobic, anaerobic, or maximal strength performance.[10,96]

Overall, the literature shows that if a deficiency exists, vitamin supplementation may aid overall health and increase physical performance. However, in the absence of a pre-existing deficiency, vitamin supplementation, even at megadoses (above the RDA, AI, or UL), does not increase physical performance. In the next sections, the potential effect of minerals on physical performance will be examined.

Minerals

Minerals are inorganic substances, meaning that they do not contain carbon-to-carbon bonds or carbon-to-hydrogen bonds. The 22 minerals found in the body account for only 4% of body mass but are involved in a myriad of chemical reactions and other bodily functions (Table 8-5). Minerals are necessary for muscle contraction, nerve transmission, protein synthesis, regulation of bodily fluid compartments, metabolism, hormone formation, and many other bodily functions. Minerals are classified as macrominerals (major) and microminerals. **Macrominerals** exist in your body in quantities of approximately 35 to 1,050 grams, depending on the mineral and body size. They include phosphorous, magnesium, sulfur, sodium, potassium, calcium, and chloride. **Microminerals** (trace) are found in your body only in quantities of less than a few grams and include iron, fluoride, iodine, zinc, selenium, copper, chromium, manganese, and molybdenum.

As with vitamins, most research indicates that mineral supplementation above recommended intakes has no effect on physical performance,[10,63,96] even though they are necessary for many physiological processes. However, deficiencies can impair overall health, aerobic performance, anaerobic performance, and maximal strength. Although most athletes, because of their increased energy intake, consume sufficient amounts of minerals, some, such as weight-class athletes and athletes involved in aesthetic sports that emphasize minimal body weight (e.g., dance, gymnastics), may be mineral-deficient.[63]

You are already familiar with why the minerals sodium, chloride, potassium, and magnesium are included in sports drinks (see "Electrolytes in Sports Drinks" above). The role of minerals in the maintenance of fluid compartment balance will be discussed in Chapter 10. In the next several sections,

Table 8-5.   Minerals: Summary of Functions, Deficiency Symptoms, and Food Sources

Mineral	Food Sources	Major Functions	Deficiency Symptoms	RDA or AI (Adult per Day)	Toxicity Symptoms or Ingestion Above UL
Macrominerals					
Calcium	Milk products, tofu, small fish with bones, legumes	Bone and teeth mineralization, muscle contraction, nerve impulse transmission, blood clotting	Osteoporosis in adults, abnormal bone growth in children	AI: 1000 mg	Risk of kidney stones, kidney dysfunction, difficulties with absorption of other minerals
Phosphorous	Meat, fish, poultry, milk	Bone and teeth mineralization, major ion of intracellular fluid, acid–base balance, phospholipids in cell membranes, part of metabolic components	Bone pain, muscle weakness	RDA: 700 mg	Calcification of nonskeletal tissue, kidney stones, kidney problems
Magnesium	Nuts, whole grain, legumes, seafood, dark green vegetables	Bone mineralization, teeth maintenance, muscle contraction, nerve impulse transmission, proper immune function	Muscle weakness, confusion, poor heart function	RDA: Men: 400 mg; Women: 310 mg	From nonfood sources: diarrhea, dehydration
Sulfur	Meat, fish, poultry, milk, nuts, eggs	Part of sulfur-containing amino acids in protein, part of insulin, part of some B vitamins (biotin, thiamin)	None known	None	Toxicity occurs only if sulfur-containing amino acids are eaten in excess; in animals, this depresses normal growth
Sodium	Table salt, soy sauce, processed foods	Major ion of extracellular fluid, maintenance of fluid compartments, nerve impulse transmission	Muscle cramps, loss of appetite, mental apathy	AI: 1500 mg	Edema, hypertension
Potassium	Meats, milk, fruits, vegetables, legumes, grains	Major ion of intracellular fluid, maintains fluid compartments, nerve impulse transmission, muscle contraction	Muscle weakness, paralysis, confusion	AI: 4700 mg	Muscle weakness, vomiting, slow heart rate apparent in kidney failure
Chloride	Table salt, soy sauce, processed foods	Major ion of extracellular fluid, maintains fluid compartments, part of stomach hydrochloric acid	Adults under normal conditions: none; convulsions in infants	AI: 2300 mg	Vomiting, linked to high blood pressure in susceptible individuals when combined with sodium
Trace Minerals					
Iron	Part of hemoglobin and myoglobin, aids immune function	Red meats, fish, poultry, shellfish, dried fruits, legumes, eggs	Anemia, low blood iron, payable red blood cells, low hemoglobin values, impaired immune function	RDA: Men: 8 mg; Women: 18 mg (19–50 yr), 8 mg (51 yr +)	Gastrointestinal distress; in children consuming iron supplements, iron overload results in nausea, vomiting, diarrhea, rapid heart rate, dizziness, shock, and confusion

Iodine	Part of thyroid hormones that regulate growth, development, and metabolic rate	Iodized salt, seafood, bread, dairy products	Underactive thyroid gland; goiter; deficiency in pregnancy causes mental and physical retardation in fetus	RDA: 150 µg	Goiter, underactive thyroid gland
Fluoride	Needed for formation of bones and teeth, makes teeth resistant to decay	Fluoridated water, tooth paste, seafood	Increased risk of tooth decay	AI: Men: 3.8 mg; Women: 3.1 mg	Pitting and discoloration of teeth
Zinc	Part of many enzymes, involved in DNA and proteins, immune reactions, taste perception, wound healing, reproduction, normal development of fetus	Red meats, shellfish, whole grains	Growth retardation, delayed sexual development, impaired immune function, hair loss, appetite and taste loss	RDA: Men: 11 mg; Women: 8 mg	Iron and copper deficiency, impaired immunity, low HDL
Selenium	Aids antioxidant system, needed for thyroid hormone regulation	Seafood, meat, whole grains, vegetables	Predisposes to heart tissue becoming fibrous, muscle pain, muscle weakness	RDA: 55 µg	Brittle and loss of hair and nails, fatigue, irritability, nervous system disorders
Copper	Needed for absorption and use of iron and formation of hemoglobin, part of enzymes	Seafood, nuts, whole grains, legumes	Anemia, low white blood cell count, bone abnormalities	RDA: 900 µg	Nervous system disorders, liver damage
Manganese	Cofactor of several enzymes, including enzymes of carbohydrate metabolism	Nuts, whole grains, tea, leafy vegetables	Rare in humans	AI: Men: 2.3 mg; Women: 1.8 mg	Nervous system disorders
Molybdenum	Cofactor for some enzymes	Legumes, cereals, organ meats	None known	RDA: 45 µg	None known

RDA, recommended dietary allowance; AI, adequate intake; UL, upper level.

the roles of the micromineral iron and the macromineral calcium will be examined.

Iron

Iron is a component of many enzymes and proteins in the human body. However, iron's roles in oxygen transport and metabolism are probably its most recognized physiological roles. Iron is a component of the cytochromes, which are part of the electron transport chain (see Chapter 2), a major enzymatic system of aerobic metabolism. It is also a component of hemoglobin and myoglobin molecules, which transport oxygen within the blood and within muscle fibers, respectively. Most of the body's iron (80%) is contained in hemoglobin and myoglobin, with the remainder being stored in the liver, spleen, and bone marrow in the form of hemosiderin and ferritin. These stores of iron are used to maintain normal hemoglobin and myoglobin levels during any period of inadequate iron ingestion. Red blood cells have a lifespan of approximately 120 days because they do not contain nuclei, which were removed as one of the last steps during their production in the bone marrow. Therefore, red blood cells are not capable of repairing the damage that occurs to them as they travel through the vascular system. Iron from red blood cells that have reached the end of their lifespan and from ingested food is transported by the iron-binding plasma glycoprotein **transferrin** to tissues needing iron, in particular to the liver, spleen, and bone marrow. This recycling of iron from red blood cells that have reached the end of their lifespan minimizes iron loss.

Heme iron, or iron found in hemoglobin and myoglobin in meat products, is the most efficiently absorbed form of iron.[4] Good sources of nonheme iron are legumes and enriched or fortified breads and cereals. The low absorption of iron from nonheme sources puts individuals, such as vegetarians, who minimize the ingestion of animal products, at risk for iron deficiency. Iron deficiency is probably the most common mineral deficiency and results in decreased oxygen transport, electron transport capabilities, protein synthesis, and neurotransmitter synthesis.[3] Athletes, particularly female ones,[22,103] may be more susceptible to iron deficiency than sedentary individuals. Due to iron's roles in aerobic metabolism and other essential bodily functions, iron deficiency can decrease physical performance.

The RDA of iron for an adult male is 8 mg·day^{-1} and for an adult female during her childbearing years is 18 mg·day^{-1}. The higher value in females is needed to replace iron loss during normal menstruation. Indeed, both before and after a woman's childbearing years, her requirements for iron intake do not differ from those of a similarly aged male. On average, adult men ingest approximately 17 mg·day^{-1} of iron, which is above the RDA, whereas adult women ingest 12 mg·day^{-1}, which is below the RDA.[105] In large part, this is due to the higher caloric intake of men compared with women. Because the average American diet contains approximately 6 mg of iron per 1000 kcal, the more calories consumed, the greater the iron ingestion.

Anemia is a medical condition in which hemoglobin concentration is lower than normal: less than 12 g·dL^{-1} and 13 g·dL^{-1} in women and men, respectively. Anemia can be caused by a large loss of blood due to hemorrhaging. However, insufficient iron intake is the most common cause of anemia in children, teenagers, and women of childbearing age.[18,76] Pregnancy may cause a moderate iron deficiency resulting in anemia due to the increased iron need of both the mother and the developing fetus. In the iron-deficient, anemic individual, low iron stores are indicated by reduced iron bound to transferrin in blood and by low levels of ferritin in the liver, spleen, and bone marrow.

In most, but not all studies, iron supplementation in individuals who are either anemic, or iron-deficient, results in increased aerobic capabilities as well as increases in hemoglobin and serum ferritin.[10,96] Iron supplementation may also benefit strength, as indicated by evidence that nonanemic but iron-deficient young women who received iron supplementation for 6 weeks demonstrated a decreased rate of fatigue during maximal voluntary isometric contractions of the knee extensors compared to their counterparts receiving a placebo.[8] Iron supplementation has been recommended for iron-deficient athletes, especially if anemia is present, and for nonanemic women with low serum iron stores, indicated by low serum ferritin levels.[10,69] Iron supplementation in nonanemic individuals may increase iron stores, without a concomitant increase in aerobic performance.[10] Supplementation, when undertaken, should not be above the UL of iron (45 mg·day^{-1}). Iron absorption is enhanced by the presence of vitamin C. So, to maximize nonheme iron absorption, one should also eat meat, fruits, or vegetables high in vitamin C.

Anemia due to iron deficiency should not be confused with sports anemia (see "Plasma Volume" in Chapter 5 and Box 5-7, "Causes of Anemia"). Sports anemia is characterized by a temporarily low hemoglobin concentration because of a training-induced increase in plasma volume during the initial stages of an aerobic training program. The total oxygen carrying capacity of the athlete with sports anemia is not decreased because there is no change in total red blood cell count. The concentration of hemoglobin in the blood is lower because the plasma volume increases with no change in the total number of red blood cells. And even though sports anemia is present, adaptations that bring about increased aerobic capabilities occur, and hemoglobin concentration returns to normal within several weeks. Whereas iron-deficient anemia does benefit from iron supplementation, iron supplementation in an athlete with sports anemia is not necessary.[105]

Calcium

The macromineral calcium is the most abundant mineral in the human body. It is necessary for muscle and heart contraction to take place, and for normal tooth development. Since 99% of the body's calcium is found within the bones, they act as a calcium store, and bones will give up some of their calcium when conditions warrant. For example, when blood calcium level decreases, bone cells (osteoclasts) break down bone, releasing calcium into the blood (stimulated by parathormone secreted from the parathyroid gland; see Chapter 7). Meanwhile, reabsorption of calcium by the kidneys and absorption of calcium by the intestines both increase, also resulting in increased calcium levels in the blood. When blood calcium levels are high, the opposite occurs (stimulated by calcitonin secreted by the thyroid gland).

Decreased bone density to the point at which there is increased risk of fractures is termed **osteoporosis**. Underweight athletes, in particular females, often show calcium ingestion lower than recommended.[63] Although this may be a factor associated with low bone mineral density in athletes or "athletic osteoporosis," there are no prospective studies concerning the effect of calcium supplementation and prevention of low bone mineral density in athletes.[63] Athletic osteoporosis is probably more related to changes in plasma hormones that affect bone metabolism than to low calcium ingestion.[63]

Peak skeletal mass normally occurs by approximately 30 years of age. After the age of 40, bone mass decreases at approximately 1% per year. By 60 years old, bone mass is reduced to a point at which the risk of fractures is increased. Women—especially older women—are typically most at risk for osteoporosis, with approximately 50% of older women suffering from osteoporosis. However, as many as one in eight men past the age of 50 years is also at risk for osteoporotic fractures. The loss in bone mass resulting in osteoporosis is due to several factors, including inadequate calcium intake, low estrogen levels in postmenopausal women, and lack of physical activity.

Calcium is most abundantly found in milk and milk products. Individuals who choose not to ingest these foods, or who are lactose-intolerant, can become calcium-deficient. If this occurs when the skeletal system is growing, bones do not reach their maximal density and mass, resulting in an increased possibility for low bone mass and density later in

> ## 🔍 *Quick Review*
>
> - The fat-soluble vitamins—A, D, E, and K—can be stored within fat tissue and released from storage if the diet is deficient in these vitamins, making it difficult to develop deficiency symptoms.
> - The water-soluble vitamins serve various roles in metabolic processes and are eliminated from the body in the urine if they are not needed, making it difficult to develop toxic symptoms of these vitamins.
> - Vitamin C is an antioxidant. However, supplementation does not appear warranted, as vitamin C deficiency is an infrequent occurrence. Most evidence indicates that supplementation does not increase aerobic or anaerobic performance and that supplementation at high doses may actually promote cellular damage.
> - Vitamin E is an antioxidant, and supplementation may possibly decrease muscle damage. However, supplementation does not significantly increase aerobic, anaerobic, or maximal strength performance.
> - The B vitamins function as coenzymes in metabolism, but supplementation does not affect aerobic, anaerobic, or maximal strength performance.
> - Macrominerals exist in your body in quantities of approximately 35 to 1,050 grams, whereas microminerals are found in your body only in quantities of less than a few grams.
> - The majority of iron within the body is found in hemoglobin and myoglobin molecules, which transport oxygen within the blood and muscle fibers, respectively.
> - Individuals with iron-deficient anemia do benefit from iron supplementation, but supplementation in nonanemic individuals does not increase physical performance.
> - Calcium deficiency can contribute to osteoporosis. Thus, recommendations to combat osteoporosis include sufficient calcium ingestion as well as exercise throughout the lifespan to minimize the loss of skeletal mass with aging.

life. If calcium ingestion is low later in life, bone mass also decreases as calcium is mobilized from the skeletal system to maintain blood calcium levels.

Decreased estrogen levels as women age are associated with increased risk of osteoporosis. Calcium supplementation with or without estrogen therapy has been shown to slow bone mineral loss in postmenopausal women.[10,67] Weight-bearing exercise during growth can increase bone mineral density, and weight-bearing exercise in young, middle-aged, and older individuals can increase bone mineral density, and minimize its loss as we age.[10,41,49,59,98] It has been demonstrated, however, that weight-bearing exercise does not affect bone mineral density equally throughout all parts of the body. This may be related to the function of bones (with bones that must bear increased stress and strain during activity increasing more in bone mineral density) as

well as to differences in the volume and intensity of activity necessary to bring about changes in bone mineral density at different places in the skeletal system. For example, resistance training in premenopausal women increases bone mineral density at the lumbar spine but not in the femoral neck,[59] even though both areas are exposed to stress and strain during weight training exercises. Recommendations to prevent osteoporosis include sufficient ingestion of calcium and exercise at a young age to maximize skeletal mass, as well as exercise throughout the lifespan to minimize the loss of skeletal mass. Ideally, calcium is ingested as part of a normal diet, but supplementation may also be used.

COMPETITION MEALS

The goal of a precompetition meal is to enhance performance in the upcoming competition. The objective of the postcompetition meal is to aid recovery so that performance in training or a successive competition (such as in a tournament setting, in which competition occurs on several successive days) is maximized. Generally, precompetition meals aim to maximize carbohydrate availability for use during metabolism in the upcoming competition. Postcompetition meals generally have as a goal replenishment of liver and muscle glycogen stores so that they are available for metabolism in an upcoming work bout. So, meals both before and after competition are comprised of easily digestible carbohydrates.

Meals Before Competition

There is convincing evidence that the composition and timing of meals before competition can influence endurance performance.[1,63] For example, endurance cyclists fed 100 grams of carbohydrate 3 hours prior to cycling to exhaustion at 70% of peak oxygen consumption cycled for 136 minutes compared with 109 minutes to those who ate no meal before competition.[81] But when carbohydrate-rich meals were consumed only 30 to 45 minutes prior to exercise at 70% to 80% of $\dot{V}O_{2max}$, performance actually decreased by up to 19%.[23,31] This diminished performance can best be explained by research revealing that eating carbohydrates too close to the start of exercise can actually result in decreased plasma glucose during the first 30 to 40 minutes of exercise.[23] These low blood glucose levels early during a prolonged event could be attributed to increased serum insulin in response to the carbohydrate-rich meal consumed shortly before exercise. Decreased free fatty acid metabolism is also noted during the initial minutes of exercise. Both of these factors increase muscle glycogen and total carbohydrate metabolism during the initial 30 to 40 minutes of exercise. This type of response to a pre-exercise meal is not the metabolic response desired, because it decreases total time to exhaustion. It should be noted, however, that not all individuals experience a decrease in blood glucose during the initial minutes of exercise when a carbohydrate meal is ingested close to the start of exercise.[1] The variability of the blood glucose response early in exercise indicates that individuals should try out any plan for meals before a major competition to ensure that the nutrient timing of the meal before competition is appropriate for them individually.

Some data suggest that ingestion of low-glycemic-index carbohydrates prior to exercise results in a slow release of glucose for metabolism, maintaining blood glucose levels longer.[63] Although such a response would seem to be beneficial for endurance performance, research has not shown that such low-glycemic-index meals before competition result in improved endurance performance.[1,63]

Appropriate meals before competition, when accompanied by nutrient intake during long-duration exercise and proper nutrition during training, have the best chance of increasing performance in any type of athletic event. The following are guidelines for meals before competition:

- The meal should not leave the athlete hungry nor with undigested food in the stomach at the start competition.
- The meal should be low in fat and fiber to increase gastric emptying and minimize gastrointestinal distress.
- The meal should contain approximately 200 to 300 grams of carbohydrate.
- A meal consumed 3 to 4 hours before exercise can be a supplement or easily digested solid food.
- If a meal is consumed within 1 hour of exercise, it should be a liquid meal to maximize gastric emptying.
- Any plan for meals before competition should be tried out before a major competition.

These general guidelines need to be customized to meet the individual needs of an athlete or sport. Meals before competition can aid performance, whereas meals after competition, the subject of the next section, may be helpful in aiding recovery so that performance in the next exercise bout is maximized, whether it is in training or in a competitive setting.

Meals After Competition

Meals after competition are an important consideration, especially when competitions consist of activity on successive days or several activity bouts on the same day, such as heats in a track meet or a tournament setting. Although here considered "postcompetition" meals, these meals could also be appropriate as posttraining meals, in some cases. For example, a triathlete performing a swimming session in the morning and a running session in the afternoon will eat after the morning session and/or prior to the afternoon session.

As discussed above (see "Resistance Training and Protein Supplementation" section), nutrient timing after activity can have an impact on the outcome. Carbohydrate ingestion starting immediately after exercise and continuing at 2-hour intervals for 6 hours results in higher muscle glycogen concentrations than when ingestion is delayed for 2 hours following the end of exercise.[1] The highest rates of glycogen synthesis occur when 0.4 grams carbohydrate·kg body mass^{-1} are ingested every 15 minutes for 4 hours after exercise.[1] However, this practice can result in greater caloric ingestion than caloric expenditure and may be most appropriate when competitive bouts are separated by only brief intervals. If the athlete has more than 24 hours between intense exercise bouts, nutrient timing is less important because carbohydrate stores will be replenished on a normal diet within this time frame.

High-glycemic-index foods result in higher muscle glycogen concentration 24 hours after exercise compared with low-glycemic-index foods.[30] However, the use of high-glycemic-index foods to increase glycogen synthesis needs to be considered within the context of the total diet and may be appropriate only during competitive—as opposed to training—settings when maximizing glycogen stores quickly is critical for performance.[1] Inclusion of protein in the meal after exercise does not hinder or aid glycogen synthesis. It may, however, provide amino acids necessary for muscle repair and promote a more anabolic hormone profile,[1] which may aid maintenance of muscle mass during long-term training.

Considering the above, the following guidelines for meals after competition seem appropriate:

- If carbohydrate stores need to be replenished quickly, 0.4 grams carbohydrate·kg body mass^{-1} should be ingested every 15 minutes for 4 hours after exercise.
- If carbohydrate stores need to be replenished less quickly, carbohydrate ingestion should start immediately after exercise and continue at 2-hour intervals for 6 hours.
- Although addition of protein to the meal after competition does not aid carbohydrate store replenishment, it does supply needed amino acids and create a more anabolic environment necessary for muscle protein repair.

Quick Review

- Meals both before and after competition typically include easily digestible carbohydrates.
- Meals before competition can increase endurance performance. However, whether the meal is composed of either high- or low-glycemic-index foods appears to have little effect on performance.
- Meals after competition do result in increased glycogen stores. Generally, carbohydrate ingestion should start immediately after exercise and continue for several hours after exercise.

CASE STUDY

Scenario

The strength and conditioning coach of a college is disappointed at the lack of muscle growth and strength gains being made by his first year shot putter on the track and field team. The other power athletes on the team are showing much more impressive gains than this young varsity athlete. This is true despite the fact that all of the team's power athletes (hammer throwers, javelin throwers, shot putters) are on the same resistance training program and are carefully supervised by the coach during weight training sessions. The coach can easily see that the young shot putter shows dedication and effort in the weight room that is at least as great as that of his teammates. The coach talks to the young man in attempting to find out what the problem might be. The athlete relates that he is sleeping well at night, he is not experiencing undue stress, nor is he suffering from injuries that might curtail his efforts in the weight room. Still perplexed as to the cause of the athlete's lack of progress, the coach asks him to keep a record of everything he eats for the next week. When the athlete turns in the dietary log, the coach realizes that the athlete is consuming a diet that is much like that of a vegetarian. It is very low in proteins, especially the complete proteins found in meat products. What is the strength and conditioning coach to do?

Options

First, the coach must instruct the athlete that it is vital to consume adequate amounts of protein in order for his muscles to respond properly to his strength training program. The coach asks the athlete whether he has made a conscious decision to become a vegetarian, or simply has unintentionally made low-protein choices in his diet. The athlete responds that he has decided to become a vegetarian, but while he avoids eating meats, he is fine with eating dairy products, such as cheese and eggs. The coach tells him that these are rich sources of the complete proteins that the body can use to build muscle tissue, and that they should comprise more of his dietary intake. The coach also explains that proteins can be found in nonanimal products, but they are considered to be incomplete proteins in that they do not contain the full complement of essential amino acids that must be obtained from dietary sources because the body cannot produce them. Because of this, it is important to eat complementary sources of vegetable proteins (different legumes, soy products) that when combined will provide the body with all the essential amino acids. The coach then sets up an appointment with the college's nutrition expert to learn what types of vegetables, nuts, and other nonanimal foods should be eaten together at a single meal to supply the athlete's body with all the essential amino acids. The coach is confident that by making these dietary adjustments, the young shot putter will be providing his body not only with the right amount, but also the right kinds of proteins that will allow his muscles to respond to his resistance training program with the same improvements in mass and strength shown by the other power athletes on the team.

Scenario

The new cross-country coach of the local high school realizes from her own training for marathons the importance of proper nutrition on performance during endurance events. In particular, she has come to appreciate the impact that carbohydrate loading has had on her performance in recent marathons. In this procedure, she couples a tapering down of her training distances with a diet in which carbohydrates account for 70% to 75% of her total caloric intake. She found that doing this several days before the marathon improved how she felt during the race, as well as her performance. In an attempt to give her cross-country runners every advantage during the upcoming state championships, she has them undergo this glycogen loading strategy several days prior to the event. On the day of the championships, however, the coach and athletes are disappointed when their times are no better, and in some cases worse, than they were during the regular competitive season.

Options

The coach finds the explanation for her team's poor performance by looking at the exercise physiology textbook used by the kinesiology department at the local state university. In it, she finds out that glycogen loading can, in fact, improve endurance performance, but is most effective for events lasting more than an hour, or with distances of at least 25 kilometers. During these types of events, it is likely that the exercising muscles will show glycogen depletion, which will force the runner to slow down his/her pace toward the end of the race. But high school cross-country events cover distances that are much shorter, perhaps only 5-kilometers long. At such distances, the cross-country runner is in no danger of glycogen depletion, assuming carbohydrates make up about 50% of her normal diet. Indeed, it is recommended by the federal government that all healthy adults consume this much carbohydrate on a daily basis. Moreover, the substandard performance of some of the cross-country runners at the state championships may have been attributed to the glycogen loading procedure they took part in. That is because for every gram of glycogen stored in the muscle, 2.6 grams of water are also stored in the muscle. So when athletes undergo glycogen loading, they often complain of feeling sluggish or bloated. Since neither the excess water nor glycogen is needed during an endurance event as short as a cross-country meet, using a glycogen loading strategy in preparation for it is unwise and may be counterproductive.

CHAPTER SUMMARY

Nutrition is important for both general health and optimal physical performance. The macronutrients carbohydrate, fat, and protein are important for a wide variety of bodily functions, not the least of which is their use as substrates for metabolism. Carbohydrate is the predominant metabolic substrate during physical activity, and diets not containing sufficient carbohydrate can result in physical performance decrements. Due to the importance of carbohydrate as a substrate, dietary and training strategies referred to as carbohydrate loading can be used to increase muscle glycogen concentration, which results in increased aerobic, but not anaerobic, performance. Carbohydrate loading regimes may not be necessary in highly trained endurance athletes because several days of rest and adequate carbohydrate ingestion from the athlete's normal diet also results in increased muscle glycogen concentrations. Carbohydrate in the form of sports drinks can be ingested before, during, and after activity. Such practices can increase performance by helping to maintain plasma volume and supplying exogenous carbohydrate as a metabolic fuel.

Protein needs of athletes are greater than the recommended dietary intake, which represents the needs of a sedentary individual. Protein needs of athletes are elevated due to the use of protein as a metabolic fuel during activity and as a source of amino acids for muscle protein synthesis. However, these needs can be met by ingestion of a normal diet due to the increased caloric consumption of most athletes. Very low-carbohydrate diets typically result in increased ingestion of fat, which is why these types of diets are associated with increased health risks, although further research is needed to elucidate their effects on health. Protein supplementation prior to, and after a resistance training session, does stimulate increased muscle protein synthesis, but the effect of such supplementation on long-term muscle mass gains requires further research. Protein and carbohydrate supplementation prior to, or after, endurance training may aid maintenance of muscle mass and recovery from exercise in endurance athletes compared with supplementation of carbohydrate alone. The effect on performance, however, is inconclusive.

Saturated fat ingestion is associated with increased health risks, whereas increased ingestion of monounsaturated, polyunsaturated, omega-3, and omega-6 fatty acids is associated with decreased risk of cardiovascular disease and several types of cancers. From a performance perspective, although high-fat diets increase lipid metabolism, they do not increase endurance performance.

Water is many times a forgotten nutrient that is important for many physiological functions, with dehydration causing decreases in both aerobic and anaerobic performance (see Chapter 9). Supplementation of either the fat-soluble or water-soluble vitamins does not increase performance unless the individual is deficient in the vitamin prior to supplementation. Supplementation with the macromineral iron is of value for increasing performance only if an individual is anemic, and supplementation with calcium is valuable in helping to combat osteoporosis.

Meals before and after competition, which typically include easily digestible carbohydrates, are an important dietary concern for athletes. Meals before competition can aid endurance performance by increasing the availability of exogenous carbohydrate for use as a substrate. Meals after competition are important for increasing glycogen stores for use in an upcoming exercise bout and for repairing damaged muscle proteins. Sound dietary practices are necessary for maintaining health and for optimal physical performance.

REVIEW QUESTIONS

Fill-in-the-Blank

1. High-glycemic-index foods (glycemic index = 70 or higher) increase blood glucose _____ compared with moderate (glycemic index = 56 to 69) or low (glycemic index = 55 or lower) glycemic index foods.

2. _____ nitrogen retention indicates anabolism, whereas _____ nitrogen balance indicates mobilization of amino acids from bodily tissue and catabolism.

3. Essential amino acids, specifically _____, appear to be the primary simulators of muscle protein synthesis, with little contribution from the nonessential amino acids.

4. When there is insufficient evidence to establish an RDA for a nutrient, an _____ is used, which is the average amount of a nutrient consumed by healthy individuals.

5. About 80% of the body's iron is contained in _____ and _____. The body's remaining iron (20%) is stored in the _____, _____, and _____ in the form of hemosiderin and ferritin.

Multiple Choice

1. Insufficient carbohydrate ingestion by an athlete may result in
   a. The ability to maintain training intensity
   b. The ability to maintain training volume
   c. The gain of muscle mass
   d. Less than optimal physiological adaptations to training
   e. Greater training adaptations

2. What is the carbohydrate percentage of a 1-liter sports drink containing 25 grams of fructose and 50 grams of glucose?

a. 7.5%

b. 2.5%

c. 25%

d. 50%

e. 5.0%

3. Which of the following is *not* a suggested guideline for a precompetition meal?

a. The meal should not leave the athlete hungry.

b. The meal should not leave undigested food in the stomach at the start competition.

c. The meal should be low in fat and fiber to increase gastric emptying and minimize gastrointestinal distress.

d. The meal should be used before a major competition even if it has not been tried out.

e. If a meal is consumed within 1 hour of exercise, it should be a liquid meal to maximize gastric emptying.

4. Which of the following strategies has been shown to be the quickest to replenish carbohydrate stores?

a. 0.4 grams carbohydrate·kg body mass^{-1} every 15 minutes for 4 hours after exercise

b. 20 grams carbohydrate every 15 minutes for 4 hours after exercise

c. 15 grams carbohydrate·kg body mass^{-1} every 0.4 minutes for 4 hours after exercise

d. 0.4 grams carbohydrate·kg body mass^{-1} every 15 minutes for 4 days after exercise

e. 4 grams carbohydrate·kg body mass^{-1} every 15 minutes for 4 hours after exercise

5. Positive nitrogen balance indicates

a. less protein ingestion than use by the body

b. equal protein ingestion and use by the body

c. more protein excretion by the body than ingestion

d. equal protein ingestion and excretion by the body

e. more protein ingestion than excretion by the body

True/False

1. Glucose is absorbed by active transport by the cells of the small intestine.

2. Inclusion of protein in the post-exercise meal does not hinder or aid glycogen synthesis, but may provide amino acids necessary for muscle repair and promote a more anabolic hormone profile.

3. It is possible for fat ingestion to be too low.

4. Minerals are organic substances (containing carbon-to-carbon bonds or carbon-to-hydrogen bonds).

5. Anemia due to iron deficiency is often confused with sports anemia, a temporarily low hemoglobin concentration due to a training-induced increase in plasma volume during the initial stages of an aerobic training program.

Short Answer

1. Explain the reason why treadmill time to exhaustion after 1 week of a high-protein or low-carbohydrate diet did not improve, whereas time to exhaustion significantly increased after 6 weeks with a high-protein or low-carbohydrate diet.

2. Why might athletes require more than the RDA for protein?

3. Describe the difference between saturated and unsaturated fatty acids.

Critical Thinking

1. Explain how protein and carbohydrate ingestion immediately prior to or within 3 hours after exercise may result in increased protein synthesis and aid recovery.

2. Why do many sports drinks contain more than one type of carbohydrate?

KEY TERMS

adequate intake (AI): average amount of a nutrient consumed by healthy individuals that is used when there is insufficient evidence to establish a recommended daily allowance

anemia: medical condition in which hemoglobin concentration is below normal

carbohydrate loading: dietary and training strategies designed to increase muscle and liver glycogen stores

fat-soluble vitamins: vitamins A, D, E, and K, which can be stored in fat tissue

glycemic index: a relative measure of the increase in blood glucose concentration in the 2-hour period following ingestion of a food containing 50 grams of carbohydrate compared with a standard carbohydrate-containing food—usually white bread or glucose—which increases blood glucose levels very quickly

keto acids: ketone bodies that contain an acid group (COOH)

ketone bodies: molecules formed from the incomplete breakdown of lipids that have a C=O between two carbons

ketosis: an increase in ketone bodies in the blood and urine

macromineral: a mineral that exists in the body in large quantities (approximately 35 to 1,050 grams, depending on the mineral and body size)

macronutrients: the nutrients carbohydrate, protein, and fat, which are needed by the body in large quantities

maltodextrins: a carbohydrate composed of glucose polymers

micromineral: a mineral found in the body in small quantities (less than a few grams)

micronutrients: nutrients, such as vitamins and minerals, that are required by the body in small amounts (milligrams or micrograms per day)

negative nitrogen balance: a nitrogen balance indicating that amino acids are being used in metabolism because more nitrogen is being excreted than ingested, indicating an overall protein loss by the body

nitrogen balance: the ratio of the amount of protein or nitrogen ingested compared with the amount of nitrogen excreted

omega-3 fatty acid: a polyunsaturated fatty acid that has the first double bond at the third bond position from the methyl group (CH_3) end of a fatty acid

omega-6 fatty acid: a polyunsaturated fatty acid that has a carbon double bond at the sixth bond position from the methyl group (CH_3) end of a fatty acid

osmolality: a measure of the ratio of solutes to liquid in a solution

osteoporosis: decreased bone density to the point where there is increased risk of fractures

positive nitrogen balance: a nitrogen balance indicating that amino acids are being used to synthesize bodily tissue because more nitrogen is ingested than excreted, indicating an overall protein synthesis condition of the body

recommended dietary allowance (RDA): dietary guideline for a nutrient established when there is sufficient scientific evidence indicating the average daily amount necessary to meet the needs of 98% of all healthy adults

transferrin: iron binding plasma glycoprotein that transports iron within the blood

water-soluble vitamins: vitamins that are soluble in water and thus may be excreted in large amounts in the urine, making it difficult for toxic symptoms to develop

REFERENCES

1. American College of Sports Medicine, American Dietetic Association, and Dietitians of Canada. Joint Position Statement: nutrition and athletic performance. American College of Sports Medicine, American Dietetic Association, and Dietitians of Canada. Med Sci Sports Exerc. 2000;32:2130–2145.
2. Alborg G, Bergstrom J, Brohult J. Human muscle glycogen content capacity for prolonged exercise after different diets. Forsvarsmedicin. 1967;3:85–99.
3. Beard J, Tobin B. Iron status and exercise. Am J Clin Nutr. 2000;72:594S–597S.
4. Bergstrom J, Hermansen L, Hultman E, et al. Diet, muscle glycogen and physical performance. Acta Physiol Scand. 1967;71:140–150.
5. Betts JA, Stevenson E, Williams C, et al. Recovery of endurance running capacity: Effect of carbohydrate–protein mixtures. Int J Sport Nutr Exerc Metab. 2005;15:590–609.
6. Boisseau N, Vermorel M, Rance M, et al. Protein requirements in male adolescent soccer players. Eur J Appl Physiol. 2007;100:27–33.
7. Borsheim E, Tipton KD, Wolf SE, et al. Essential amino acids and muscle protein recovery from resistance exercise. Am J Physiol Endocrinol Metab. 2002;283:E648–E657.
8. Brutsaert TD, Hernandez-Cordero S, Rivera J, et al. Iron supplementation improves progressive fatigue resistance during dynamic knee extensor exercise in iron-depleted, nonanemic women. Am J Clin Nutr. 2003;77:441–448.
9. Bryant RJ, Ryder J, Martino P, et al. Effects of vitamin E and C supplementation either alone or in combination on exercise-induced lipid peroxidation in trained cyclists. J Strength Cond Res. 2003;17:792–800.
10. Bucci L. Nutrition in Exercise and Sport. Boca Raton, FL: CRC Press, 1989.
11. Burke DG, Chilibeck PD, Davidson KS, et al. The effect of whey protein supplementation with and without creatine monohydrate combined with resistance training on lean tissue mass and muscle strength. Int J Sport Nutr Exerc Metab. 2001;11:349–364.
12. Burke LM, Angus DJ, Cox GR, et al. Effect of fat adaptation and carbohydrate restoration on metabolism and performance during prolonged cycling. J Appl Physiol. 2000;89:2413–2421.
13. Burke LM. Nutrition strategies for the marathon: Fuel for training and racing. Sports Med. 2007;37:344–347.
14. Bussau VA, Fairchild TJ, Rao A, et al. Carbohydrate loading in human muscle: An improved 1 day protocol. Eur J Appl Physiol. 2002;87:290–295.
15. Carroll CC, Fluckey JD, Williams RH, et al. Human soleus and vastus lateralis muscle protein metabolism with an amino acid infusion. Am J Physiol Endocrinol Metab. 2005;288:E479–E485.
16. Cheuvront SN, Montain SJ, Sawka MN. Fluid replacement and performance during the marathon. Sports Med. 2007;37:353–357.
17. Christensen E, Hansen O. Arbeitsfahigkeit und ehrnahrung. Skand Arch Physiol. 1939;81:160–175.
18. Clarkson PM, Haymes EM. Exercise and mineral status of athletes: Calcium, magnesium, phosphorus, and iron. Med Sci Sports Exerc. 1995;27:831–843.
19. Coleman E. Carbohydrate and exercise. In: Sports Nutrition: A Guide for the Professional Working with Active People. Chicago: The American Dietetic Association, 2000.
20. Convertino VA, Armstrong LE, Coyle EF, et al. American College of Sports Medicine position stand. Exercise and fluid replacement. Med Sci Sports Exerc. 1996;28:i–ix.
21. Cook JD. The effect of endurance training on iron metabolism. Semin Hematol. 1994;31:146–154.
22. Costill DL, Coyle E, Dalsky G, et al. Effects of elevated plasma FFA and insulin on muscle glycogen usage during exercise. J Appl Physiol. 1977;43:695–699.
23. Coyle EF. Fluid and fuel intake during exercise. J Sports Sci. 2004;22:39–55.
24. DeMarco HM, Sucher KP, Cisar CJ, et al. Pre-exercise carbohydrate meals: Application of glycemic index. Med Sci Sports Exerc. 1999;31:164–170.
25. Dougherty KA, Baker LB, Chow M, et al. Two percent dehydration impairs and six percent carbohydrate drink improves boys basketball skills. Med Sci Sports Exerc. 2006;38:1650–1658.
26. Earnest CP, Lancaster SL, Rasmussen CJ, et al. Low vs. high glycemic index carbohydrate gel ingestion during simulated 64-km cycling time trial performance. J Strength Cond Res. 2004;18:466–472.
27. Esmarck B, Andersen JL, Olsen S, et al. Timing of postexercise protein intake is important for muscle hypertrophy with resistance training in elderly humans. J Physiol. 2001;535:301–311.
28. Fairchild TJ, Fletcher S, Steele P, et al. Rapid carbohydrate loading after a short bout of near maximal-intensity exercise. Med Sci Sports Exerc. 2002;34:980–986.
29. Foster C, Costill DL, Fink WJ. Effects of preexercise feedings on endurance performance. Med Sci Sports. 1979;11:1–5.
30. Foster-Powell K, Holt SHA, Brand-Miller JC. International table of glycemic index and glycemic load values: 2002. Am J Clin Nutr. 2002;76:5–56.
31. Gibala MJ. Nutritional supplementation and resistance exercise: What is the evidence for enhanced skeletal muscle hypertrophy? Can J Appl Physiol. 2000;25:524–535.
32. Gisolfi CV, Summers RD, Schedl HP, et al. Effect of sodium concentration in a carbohydrate-electrolyte solution on intestinal absorption. Med Sci Sports Exerc. 1995;27:1414–1420.
33. Green HJ, Ball-Burnett M, Jones S, et al. Mechanical and metabolic responses with exercise and dietary carbohydrate manipulation. Med Sci Sports Exerc. 2007;39:139–148.

34. Haff G, Stone M, Warren B, et al. The effect of carbohydrate supplementation on multiple sessions and bouts of resistance exercise. J Strength Cond Res. 1999;13:111–117.

35. Haff GG, Koch AJ, Potteiger JA, et al. Carbohydrate supplementation attenuates muscle glycogen loss during acute bouts of resistance exercise. Int J Sport Nutr Exerc Metab. 2000;10: 326–339.

36. Haff GG, Lehmkuhl MJ, McCoy LB, et al. Carbohydrate supplementation and resistance training. J Strength Cond Res. 2003;17: 187–196.

37. Hatfield DL, Kraemer WJ, Volek JS, et al. The effects of carbohydrate loading on repetitive jump squat power performance. J Strength Cond Res. 2006;20:167–171.

38. Helge JW. Adaptation to a fat-rich diet: Effects on endurance performance in humans. Sports Med. 2000;30:347–357.

39. Hemila H. Vitamin C and common cold incidence: A review of studies with subjects under heavy physical stress. Int J Sports Med. 1996;17:379–383.

40. Hogstrom M, Nordstrom A, Alfredson H, et al. Current physical activity is related to bone mineral density in males but not in females. Int J Sports Med. 2007;28:431–436.

41. Hragraves M, Hawley J, Jeukendrup A. Pre-exercise carbohydrate and fat ingestion: Effects on metabolism and performance. J Sports Sci. 2004;22:31–38.

42. Hulmi JJ, Volek JS, Selanne H, et al. Protein ingestion prior to strength exercise affects blood hormones and metabolism. Med Sci Sports Exerc. 2005;37:1990–1997.

43. Ip C. Controversial issues of dietary fat and experimental mammary carcinogenesis. Prev Med. 1993;22:728–737.

44. Ivy JL, Goforth HW Jr, Damon BM, et al. Early postexercise muscle glycogen recovery is enhanced with a carbohydrate–protein supplement. J Appl Physiol. 2002;93:1337–1344.

45. Jackson MJ. Exercise and oxygen radical production in muscle. In: Packer CK, Hanninen PL, eds. Exercise and Oxygen Toxicity. Amsterdam: Elsevier, 1994:49–57.

46. Jentjens RL, van Loon LJ, Mann CH, et al. Addition of protein and amino acids to carbohydrates does not enhance postexercise muscle glycogen synthesis. J Appl Physiol. 2001;91:839–846.

47. Jones PJ, Lau VW. Effect of n-3 polyunsaturated fatty acids on risk reduction of sudden death. Nutr Rev. 2002;60:407–409.

48. Kaminsky M, Boal R. An effect of ascorbic acid on delayed-onset muscle soreness. Pain. 1992;50:317–321.

49. Kato T, Terashima T, Yamashita T, et al. Effect of low-repetition jump training on bone mineral density in young women. J Appl Physiol. 2006;100:839–843.

50. Kimball SR, Farrell PA, Jefferson LS. Invited review: Role of insulin in translational control of protein synthesis in skeletal muscle by amino acids or exercise. J Appl Physiol. 2002;93: 1168–1180.

51. Kirwin J, O'Gorman D, Evans W. A moderate glycemic before endurance exercise can enhance performance. J Appl Physiol. 1998;84: 53–59.

52. Koopman R, Pannemans DL, Jeukendrup AE, et al. Combined ingestion of protein and carbohydrate improves protein balance during ultra-endurance exercise. Am J Physiol Endocrinol Metab. 2004;287:E712–E720.

53. Lambert CP, Frank LL, Evans WJ. Macronutrient considerations for the sport of bodybuilding. Sports Med. 2004;34:317–327.

54. Leiper JB. Intestinal water absorption—Implications for the formulation of rehydration solutions. Int J Sports Med. 1998;19 (suppl 2):S129–S132.

55. Lemon PW, Tarnopolsky MA, MacDougall JD, et al. Protein requirements and muscle mass/strength changes during intensive training in novice bodybuilders. J Appl Physiol. 1992;73:767–775.

56. Levenhagen DK, Carr C, Carlson MG, et al. Postexercise protein intake enhances whole-body and leg protein accretion in humans. Med Sci Sports Exerc. 2002;34:828–837.

57. MacDougall JD, Ward GR, Sutton JR. Muscle glycogen repletion after high-intensity intermittent exercise. J Appl Physiol. 1977;42:129–132.

58. MacDougall JD, Ray S, Sale DG, et al. Muscle substrate utilization and lactate production. Can J Appl Physiol. 1999;24:209–215.

59. Martyn-St James M, Carroll S. Progressive high-intensity resistance training and bone mineral density changes among premenopausal women: Evidence of discordant site-specific skeletal effects. Sports Med. 2006;36:683–704.

60. Massicotte D, Peronnet F, Brisson G, et al. Oxidation of a glucose polymer during exercise: Comparison with glucose and fructose. J Appl Physiol. 1989;66:179–183.

61. Maughan RJ, Bethell LR, Leiper JB. Effects of ingested fluids on exercise capacity and on cardiovascular and metabolic responses to prolonged exercise in man. Exp Physiol. 1996;81:847–859.

62. Maughan RJ, Greenhaff PL, Leiper JB, et al. Diet composition and the performance of high-intensity exercise. J Sports Sci. 1997;15: 265–275.

63. Maughn R, Burke L, Coyle E, eds. Food, Nutrition and Sports Performance. II. The International Olympic Committee Consensus on Sports Nutrition. London: Rutledge, 2004.

64. Millard-Stafford M, Warren GL, Thomas LM, et al. Recovery from run training: Efficacy of a carbohydrate–protein beverage? Int J Sport Nutr Exerc Metab. 2005;15:610–624.

65. Morris MC, Sacks F, Rosner B. Does fish oil lower blood pressure? A meta-analysis of controlled trials. Circulation. 1993;88:523–533.

66. Murray B. The role of salt and glucose replacement drinks in the marathon. Sports Med. 2007;37:358–360.

67. Nachtigall LE, Nachtigall RH, Nachtigall RD, et al. Estrogen replacement therapy. I: A 10-year prospective study in the relationship to osteoporosis. Obstet Gynecol. 1979;53:277–281.

68. Nestel PJ. Fish oil and cardiovascular disease: Lipids and arterial function. Am J Clin Nutr. 2000;71:228S–231S.

69. Nielson P, Nachtigall D. Iron supplementation in athletes current recommendations. Sports Med. 1998;26:207–216.

70. Noakes T, Speedy D. The aetiology of exercise-associated hyponatremia is established and is not mythical. Br J Sports Med. 2007;41:111–113.

71. Noakes TD. Sports drinks: Prevention of "voluntary dehydration" and development of exercise-associated hyponatremia. Med Sci Sports Exerc. 2006;38:193; author reply 194.

72. Pascoe DD, Costill DL, Fink WJ, et al. Glycogen resynthesis in skeletal muscle following resistive exercise. Med Sci Sports Exerc. 1993;25:349–354.

73. Peters EM, Goetzsche JM, Grobbelaar B, et al. Vitamin C supplementation reduces the incidence of postrace symptoms of upper-respiratory-tract infection in ultramarathon runners. Am J Clin Nutr. 1993;57:170–174.

74. Peters EM, Anderson R, Theron AJ. Attenuation of increase in circulating cortisol and enhancement of the acute phase protein response in vitamin C-supplemented ultramarathoners. Int J Sports Med. 2001;22:120–126.

75. Phinney SD. Ketogenic diets and physical performance. Nutr Metab (Lond). 2004;1:2.

76. Rajaram S, Weaver CM, Lyle RM, et al. Effects of long-term moderate exercise on iron status in young women. Med Sci Sports Exerc. 1995;27:1105–1110.

77. Rasmussen BB, Tipton KD, Miller SL, et al. An oral essential amino acid–carbohydrate supplement enhances muscle protein anabolism after resistance exercise. J Appl Physiol. 2000;88: 386–392.

78. Ratamess NA, Kraemer WJ, Volek JS, et al. The effects of amino acid supplementation on muscular performance during resistance training overreaching. J Strength Cond Res. 2003;17:250–258.

79. Robergs RA, Pearson DR, Costill DL, et al. Muscle glycogenolysis during differing intensities of weight-resistance exercise. J Appl Physiol. 1991;70:1700–1706.

80. Saunders MJ, Kane MD, Todd MK. Effects of a carbohydrate–protein beverage on cycling endurance and muscle damage. Med Sci Sports Exerc. 2004;36:1233–1238.

81. Schabort EJ, Bosch AN, Weltan SM, et al. The effect of a preexercise meal on time to fatigue during prolonged cycling exercise. Med Sci Sports Exerc. 1999;31:464–471.

82. Sen CK. Oxidants and antioxidants in exercise. J Appl Physiol. 1995;79:675–686.

83. Sherman W. Carbohydrates, muscle glycogen, and muscle glycogen super compensation. In: Williams M, ed. Ergogenic Aids in Sports. Champagne, IL: Human Kinetics, 1983:3–26.

84. Sherman WM, Costill DL, Fink WJ, et al. Effect of exercise-diet manipulation on muscle glycogen and its subsequent utilization during performance. Int J Sports Med. 1981;2:114–118.

85. Sherman WM, Costill DL, Fink WJ, et al. Effect of a 42.2-km footrace and subsequent rest or exercise on muscle glycogen and enzymes. J Appl Physiol. 1983;55:1219–1224.

86. Shils M, Olson J, Shike M, et al. Modern Nutrition in Health and Disease. Lippincott Williams & Williams. Baltimore, MD, 1999.

87. Shirreffs SM, Armstrong LE, Cheuvront SN. Fluid and electrolyte needs for preparation and recovery from training and competition. J Sports Sci. 2004;22:57–63.

88. Sparks MJ, Selig SS, Febbraio MA. Pre-exercise carbohydrate ingestion: Effect of the glycemic index on endurance exercise performance. Med Sci Sports Exerc. 1998;30:844–849.

89. Spriet LL. Regulation of substrate use during the marathon. Sports Med. 2007;37:332–336.

90. Strak A, Madar Z. Olive oil as a functional food: Epidemiology and nutritional approaches. Nutr Rev. 2002;60:170–176.

91. Swaka M, Noakes Y. Does dehydration impaired exercise performance? Med Sci Sports Exerc. 2007;39:1209–1220.

92. Thomas DE, Brotherhood JR, Brand JC. Carbohydrate feeding before exercise: Effect of glycemic index. Int J Sports Med. 1991;12:180–186.

93. Tipton KD, Rasmussen BB, Miller SL, et al. Timing of amino acid–carbohydrate ingestion alters anabolic response of muscle to resistance exercise. Am J Physiol Endocrinol Metab. 2001;281:E197–E206.

94. Tipton KD, Wolfe RR. Protein and amino acids for athletes. J Sports Sci. 2004;22:65–79.

95. Tranopolsky M. Protein Metabolism, Strength, and Endurance Activities. In: Lamb DL, Murry R, eds. The Metabolic basis of Performance and Exercise. Carmel, IN: Cooper Publishing, 1999: 125–157.

96. Van Gammeren D. Vitamins and minerals. In: Antonio J, Kalman D, Stout J, Greenwood M. Willoughby D, Haff GG, eds. Essentials of Sports Nutrition and Supplements. Totowa, NJ: Humana Press, 2008.

97. van Loon LJ, Saris WH, Verhagen H, et al. Plasma insulin responses after ingestion of different amino acid or protein mixtures with carbohydrate. Am J Clin Nutr. 2000;72:96–105.

98. Vincente-Rodriguez G. How does exercise of the bone development during growth? Sports Med. 2006;36:561–569.

99. Volek JS. Influence of nutrition on responses to resistance training. Med Sci Sports Exerc. 2004;36:689–696.

100. Volek JS, Phinney SD, Forsythe CE, et al. Carbohydrate restriction has a more favorable impact on the metabolic syndrome than a low fat diet. Lipids. 2009;44(4):297–309.

101. Volek JS, Sharman MJ, Forsythe CE. Modification of lipoproteins by very low-carbohydrate diets. J Nutr. 2005;135:1339–1342.

102. Walton P, Rhodes EC. Glycaemic index and optimal performance. Sports Med. 1997;23:164–172.

103. Weaver CM, Rajaram S. Exercise and iron status. J Nutr. 1992;122:782–787.

104. Wee SL, Williams C, Gray S, et al. Influence of high and low glycemic index meals on endurance running capacity. Med Sci Sports Exerc. 1999;31:393–399.

105. Whitney E, Rolfes S. Understanding Nutrition 10th ed. Thompson Wadsworth, Belmont, CA, 2005.

106. Winnick JJ, Davis JM, Welsh RS, et al. Carbohydrate feedings during team sport exercise preserve physical and CNS function. Med Sci Sports Exerc. 2005;37:306–315.

107. Wolfe RR. Effects of amino acid intake on anabolic processes. Can J Appl Physiol. 2001;26(Suppl):S220–S227.

Suggested Readings

Al-Sarraj T, Saadi H, Calle MC, et al. Carbohydrate restriction, as a first-line dietary intervention, effectively reduces biomarkers of metabolic syndrome in emirati adults. J Nutr. 2009;139(9):1667–1676.

Costill DL. Carbohydrate for athletic training and performance. Bol Asoc Med P R. 1991;83(8):350–353.

Costill DL, Hargreaves M. Carbohydrate nutrition and fatigue. Sports Med. 1992;13(2):86–92.

Hatfield DL, Kraemer WJ, Volek JS, et al. The effects of carbohydrate loading on repetitive jump squat power performance. J Strength Cond Res. 2006;20(1):167–171.

Kraemer WJ, Volek JS, Bush JA, et al. Hormonal responses to consecutive days of heavy-resistance exercise with or without nutritional supplementation. J Appl Physiol. 1998;85(4):1544–1555.

Sallinen J, Pakarinen A, Fogelholm M, et al. Dietary intake, serum hormones, muscle mass and strength during strength training in 49–73-year-old men. Int J Sports Med. 2007;28(12):1070–1076.

Volek JS, Forsythe CE, Kraemer WJ. Nutritional aspects of women strength athletes. Br J Sports Med. 2006;40(9):742–748.

Volek JS, Kraemer WJ, Bush JA, et al. Testosterone and cortisol in relationship to dietary nutrients and resistance exercise. J Appl Physiol. 1997;82(1):49–54.

Volek JS, Phinney SD, Forsythe CE, et al. Carbohydrate restriction has a more favorable impact on the metabolic syndrome than a low fat diet. Lipids. 2009;44(4):297–309.

Volek JS, Sharman MJ, Love DM, et al. Body composition and hormonal responses to a carbohydrate-restricted diet. Metabolism. 2002;51(7):864–870.

Volek JS, Vanheest JL, Forsythe CE. Diet and exercise for weight loss: A review of current issues. Sports Med. 2005;35(1):1–9.

Westman EC, Feinman RD, Mavropoulos JC, et al. Low-carbohydrate nutrition and metabolism. Am J Clin Nutr. 2007;86(2):276–284.

Wood RJ, Fernandez ML, Sharman MJ, et al. Effects of a carbohydrate-restricted diet with and without supplemental soluble fiber on plasma low-density lipoprotein cholesterol and other clinical markers of cardiovascular risk. Metabolism. 2007;56(1):58–67.

Wood RJ, Volek JS, Liu Y, et al. Carbohydrate restriction alters lipoprotein metabolism by modifying VLDL, LDL, and HDL subfraction distribution and size in overweight men. J Nutr. 2006;136(2): 384–389.

Classic References

Brozek J, Keys A. Body measurements and the evaluation of human nutrition. Nutr Rev. 1956;14(10):289–291.

Costill DL, Coté R, Miller E, et al. Water and electrolyte replacement during repeated days of work in the heat. Aviat Space Environ Med. 1975;46(6):795–800.

Costill DL, Sherman WM, Fink WJ, et al. The role of dietary carbohydrates in muscle glycogen resynthesis after strenuous running. Am J Clin Nutr. 1981;34(9):1831–1836.

Keys A. Energy requirements of adults. J Am Med Assoc. 1950;142(5): 333–338.

Kirwan JP, Costill DL, Mitchell JB, et al. Carbohydrate balance in competitive runners during successive days of intense training. J Appl Physiol. 1988;65(6):2601–2606.

Neufer PD, Costill DL, Flynn MG, et al. Improvements in exercise performance: Effects of carbohydrate feedings and diet. J Appl Physiol. 1987;62(3):983–988.

Sherman WM, Costill DL, Fink WJ, et al. Effect of exercise-diet manipulation on muscle glycogen and its subsequent utilization during performance. Int J Sports Med. 1981;2(2):114–118.

Sherman WM, Plyley MJ, Sharp RL, et al. Muscle glycogen storage and its relationship with water. Int J Sports Med. 1982;3(1):22–24.

Chapter 9

Fluid and Electrolyte Challenges in Exercise

After reading this chapter, you should be able to:

1. Identify the anatomical and physiological functions of fluid and electrolytes in the body

2. Explain the effects of deficient and excessive electrolyte and fluid concentrations in the body and how to prevent such states

3. Describe optimal fluid and electrolyte consumption practices for better performance

4. Explain what electrolytes are, the functions they serve, and examples of primary processes by which electrolytes function

5. Explain how physical activity is likely to affect electrolyte function and balance

6. Explain how dehydration occurs, the systems dehydration affects, and the factors that affect the rate and extent to which dehydration occurs

7. Identify optimal strategies for assessing fluid and electrolyte balances

8. Describe hyponatremia, how it occurs, and the side effects likely to result

9. Create a hydration plan, explain why such plans are important, and identify the needed components of a complete hydration plan

In the 1982 Boston Marathon, Alberto Salazar narrowly defeated Dick Beardsley in a sprint to the finish. Almost immediately after crossing the finish line, Salazar collapsed and was brought to a medical aid station where doctors gave him 6 liters of water intravenously to replace the water he lost by sweating profusely throughout the 26.2-mile (42-kilometer) race. To maintain the pace he felt he needed to win, Salazar had avoided drinking fluids during the final 8 miles of the race. This lack of fluid intake, coupled with his extremely high rate of sweating, had left him dangerously dehydrated by the end of what came to be known as the "duel in the sun." In fact, Salazar's abnormally high sweat rate (about 3 $L \cdot h^{-1}$) had caused such severe dehydration during other distance races that he came close to dying (having had his last rites of passage read to him by a priest) on more than one occasion. These incidents underscore the health problems caused by dehydration during sports performance.

Water and electrolytes are essential for the maintenance of life. Water comprises approximately 60% of an adult's body mass, making water the most abundant substance in the human body. Electrolytes, such as sodium and chloride, are necessary for many bodily functions and create the force to hold water within cellular and extracellular compartments and to move water from one side of a cell's membrane to the other. **Dehydration**, or loss of bodily water, can decrease both aerobic and anaerobic physical performance. Likewise, decreased electrolyte content can also impair physical performance. Thus, maintenance of hydration and electrolytes within the body is necessary not just for normal bodily function but also for optimal physical performance. Aspects of maintaining hydration and electrolytes within the body are explored in this chapter.

WATER: THE OVERLOOKED NUTRIENT

Water is more important to life than any other nutrient. You need more water per day than any other nutrient and can survive only days without water. A deficiency of other nutrients, on the other hand, including carbohydrate, fat, and protein, can take weeks, months, or even years (in the case of some vitamins and minerals) before resulting in visible symptoms.

Although, as noted above, water makes up on average about 60% of body weight, body composition does affect the exact percentage of water in the body. Water constitutes approximately 75% of lean tissue weight and only 25% or less of fat weight. Thus, a greater percentage of lean tissue and lower percentage of fat tissue results in a higher proportion of water weight in the entire body. Generally, this results in a smaller percentage of water weight in

women, obese individuals, and the elderly because of their smaller percentage of lean tissue and higher percentage of fat tissue.

From a physical performance perspective, adequate water in the body is vital. Even small amounts of dehydration or loss of water weight can decrease physical performance. For example, endurance performance[9,32] and basketball skills[12] are impaired with as little as a 2% loss of body weight due to water loss. So, maintenance of normal hydration and prevention of large amounts of dehydration are important considerations for maintaining optimal physical performance (Fig. 9-1).

Importance of Water in the Body

Because water makes up such a high percentage of total body weight, it might be deduced that it serves many important functions within the body, and, in fact, it does. Water is the fluid in which life processes occur. Some functions of water within the body are quite obvious, whereas others are not. Water serves the following functions within the body:

- Forms the fluid portion of blood, which carries nutrients, waste products, oxygen, and immune cells throughout the body
- Maintains blood volume
- Participates in many metabolic reactions (see Chapter 2)
- Serves as a solvent for protein, glucose, vitamins, minerals, and many other small molecules, allowing them to participate in metabolic reactions
- Forms the fluid portion of sweat, which is necessary for maintenance of normal body temperature
- Carries heat from the internal portions of the body to the surface of the skin, which is necessary for the maintenance of normal body temperature
- Is a major constituent of lubricants in joints
- Is a major constituent of spinal fluid and the fluid within the eyes
- During pregnancy, is the major constituent of the amniotic fluid within the womb

Because water serves so many important functions within the body, it is critical to properly maintain **water balance**, which is the balance between water intake and water loss.

Water Balance

Water is taken into the body in the form of not only liquids, such as water, milk, and fruit juices, but also foods. For example, foods such as shrimp, bananas, corn, and potatoes are between 70% and 79% water. Other foods contain smaller percentages of water. For example, pizza is 40% to 49% water, whereas crackers and cereals are between 1% and 9% water. Another source of a small amount of water is that generated due to metabolic reactions, or **metabolic water** (see Chapter 2). Establishing how much

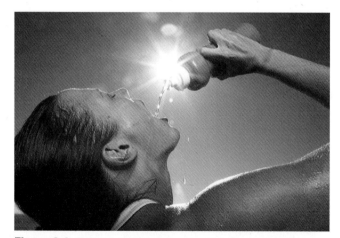

Figure 9-1. Water intake and exercise. Drinking water before, during, and after exercise is important to maintain hydration and replace lost fluids. However, caution is needed so as not to drink too much water, which can lead to hypervolemia, a serious medical condition in which there is too much fluid in the blood, which dilutes electrolytes. The longer-duration races often can cause people to overdrink. It is important to replace the fluids you lose. (See Reference 30.)

Box 9-1 DID YOU KNOW?

Recommended Water Ingestion Is Related to Metabolic Activity

Because of the relationship of water loss with physical activity, recommended water ingestion is based on energy expenditure.[23] So, an adequate intake (AI) of water can be calculated if total energy expenditure is known.

Adequate Intake for Water

For adults: 1.0 to 1.5 milliliters water per kilocalorie expended

For athletes: 1.5 milliliters water per kilocalorie expended (4.2–6.3 milliliters per kilojoule expended)

This results in the following recommended total water intake of an athlete metabolizing 3,500 kilocalories per day:

3,500 kilocalories × (1.0–1.5 mL water) = 3,500 to 5,250 mL (or 3.5–5.25 L) total daily intake from all sources (food* and fluid)

Or, convert liters to quarts:

1 L = 1.06 quarts
3.5 to 5.25 L × 1.06 quarts/L = 3.71 to 5.565 quarts

*Remember to factor a likely ~20% hydration contribution from food sources.

---

water should be ingested on a daily basis is difficult because it can vary drastically with the amount of physical activity performed, environmental temperature, and environmental humidity. However, due to the association of water loss with physical activity, experts have recommended that water ingestion should be correlated with daily energy expenditure (Box 9–1).

Water is lost from the body at the rate of approximately 2.5 liters per day. A large portion of this is lost in the form of urine to eliminate metabolic and other waste products (Table 9–1). A significant amount of water is also lost in the form of sweat; **feces**, the solid wastes excreted by the gastrointestinal tract; and what is termed **insensible water loss** (i.e., evaporation of water from the respiratory tract and the water that continuously diffuses to the surface of the skin even under nonsweating conditions). With exercise, the water loss is primarily caused by sweating to cool the body.

To maintain normal hydration, total water intake needs to match total water loss. If water intake is greater than total water loss, water loss in the form of urine increases to maintain normal hydration. Thus, to maintain a normal

hydration level, or **euhydration**, water intake must be equal to water loss (see Box 9.4 for determining hydration status). Understanding one's sweat rate will also give important practical information on how much water one needs to drink (Box 9–2). Not all individuals' sweat rates are the same, so each person must calculate his or her own sweat rate (normal sweat rates during exercise range from 0.8 to 1.4 L·min⁻¹). If water intake is not equal to water loss, **hypohydration**, or loss of body water, takes place, resulting in dehydration and possibly decreased physical performance. In the following sections, various factors related to the movement of water within the body and maintaining euhydration are explored.

ELECTROLYTES

The substances dissolved in the body's water are closely linked to maintaining hydration and controlling the movement of water within the body. Water is not distributed equally among the body's tissues. To maintain water in tissues where water is needed and control the movement

---

Table 9-1. Typical Water Loss Versus Water Ingestion

Water Loss	Milliliters	Water Ingestion	Milliliters
Urine	500–1,400	Liquids	500–1,500
Sweat	400–900 (with exercise)	Food	700–1,000
Feces	150	Metabolic water	200–300
Insensible perspiration	350		
Total per day	1,400–2,800	Total per day	1,400–2,800

Quick Review

- Water is a nutrient that is essential for many bodily functions.
- Water comprises approximately 60% of an adult's body mass.
- Dehydration (as little as 2% loss of total body mass) can decrease physical performance.
- Maintenance of euhydration depends on maintaining water balance, in which water intake is equal to water loss.
- It is important to know your sweat rate to determine how much water you need to take in during and after activity.

Box 9-2 APPLYING RESEARCH
Calculating Your Sweat Loss

- Weigh yourself in the nude before you exercise and convert pounds to ounces (1 lb = 16 oz).
- Perform a standard workout (e.g., run or cycle for 30 minutes).
- Record how much fluid you ingest in ounces.
- After the workout, weigh yourself in the nude after drying yourself of sweat.

To calculate your sweat rate, perform the following calculation:

sweat rate (oz·h⁻¹) = (pre-exercise body weight [oz] + fluid intake [oz]) – (postworkout body weight) hours you exercised

Using this calculation, you will know how much fluid you need to take in during and following exercise. Remember, environmental conditions, exercise intensity, and preexercise hydration level will impact the amount of sweat lost. Understanding your sweat rate will also help you not to overdrink.

Applying the Knowledge
Sandy weighs 125 pounds, goes out for an hour run, and drinks 12 oz of water. After the workout, she weighs in at 120 pounds. What is her sweat rate? Was her fluid intake enough to match her loss? How much water would she need to drink after her workout?

---

of water to those tissues, cells must be able to control the movement of electrolytes. What is an electrolyte? When a mineral salt such as sodium chloride (NaCl) dissolves in water, it disassociates into charged molecules termed **ions**. In the case of NaCl, a positively charged Na⁺ ion and negatively charged Cl⁻ ion result. Positively charged ions are **cations** and negatively charged ions are **anions**. Pure water does not conduct electrical current well, but if ions are dissolved in water, electricity is conducted easily. Thus, mineral salts that dissolve in water and form ions are called **electrolytes**. Because of their ability to allow electrical charges to occur, electrolytes are essential to the proper working of excitable tissues such as neurons and muscle fibers.

Cell membranes are selectively permeable, meaning that the membrane allows the movement of some molecules but not others and controls movement of these molecules. Some electrolytes, such as sodium (Na^+), calcium (Ca^{2+}), and chloride (Cl^-), are found predominantly outside of cells, whereas others, such as magnesium (Mg^{2+}) and potassium (K^+), are found predominantly inside cells.

Electrolytes are also important in the body because they create the force to hold water where needed and move water from one side of a membrane to the other. Water molecules (H_2O) have an overall electrical charge of zero. However, the oxygen of the water molecule has a slight negative charge, whereas the hydrogens have a slight positive charge. Cations and anions also have electrical charge, and both attract groups of water molecules around them. If there is a high concentration of electrolytes, protein, and other substances on one side of a cell membrane that is permeable to water, the water will move through the membrane to the side of the membrane with the higher concentration of substances until the concentration of substances is equal on both sides of the membrane (Fig. 9-2). The force created to draw water through the membrane in this situation is termed **osmotic pressure**. Cells do not control the

movement of water directly but indirectly by controlling the movements of electrolytes in and out of cells, since water follows electrolytes. A well-known mechanism by which cells control the movement of electrolytes is the sodium–potassium pump in cell membranes (see Chapter 4).

Electrolyte Balance

Electrolyte concentration must remain relatively constant within and among cells to maintain normal function of the body's tissues. Therefore, electrolyte balance within the body must be controlled. Control of **electrolyte balance** occurs primarily within the kidneys and gastrointestinal tract. If sodium content within the body is low, the kidneys conserve sodium by reabsorbing it from the urine being produced. Additionally, as the sodium is being reabsorbed, potassium is excreted. This function of the kidneys is controlled by hormonal mechanisms, such as production of aldosterone by the adrenal glands, which stimulates reabsorption of sodium back into the bloodstream (see Chapter 7). Thus, if sodium concentration within the body is low, the adrenal glands produce more **aldosterone**, resulting in a conservation of sodium.

The digestive juices within the gastrointestinal tract contain minerals. (Remember that mineral salts dissolve in water, forming electrolytes.) These minerals, as well as those within the fluid ingested, are absorbed into the bloodstream in the small intestine to match the needs of the body. If a particular mineral concentration within the body is low, more of this mineral is absorbed by the small intestine. Again, electrolyte balance, which is the amount of electrolytes lost from the body and gained by the body, is normally maintained in equilibrium by the gastrointestinal tract and kidneys. With exercise, the increase in electrolyte-containing sweat volume necessitates extra effort to ensure that equilibrium of electrolyte balance is maintained. When the body's ability to maintain equilibrium is overridden,

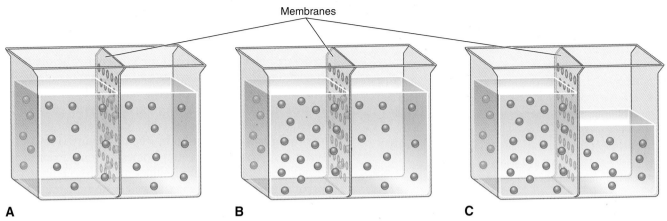

Figure 9-2. Electrolytes and osmotic pressure. (A) If a membrane permeable to water separates two volumes of water with equal concentrations of electrolytes, there is no tendency for water to move in either direction. **(B)** If more electrolytes are added to one side of the membrane, the concentration of electrolytes is now greater on one side than the other side of the membrane. **(C)** If a membrane is permeable to water, the water can move through the membrane in either direction. However, there is a tendency for the water to move toward the side of the membrane with the greater concentration of electrolytes until the concentrations of electrolytes on both sides of the membrane are equal. Osmotic pressure is the amount of pressure needed to prevent the movement of water through the membrane toward the side with the greater concentration of electrolytes.

severe injury and dysfunction are likely, with death possible in extreme cases. In most cases, supplementing the body's impressive ability to maintain electrolyte balance with precautionary dietary adjustments is sufficient to minimize the risks of electrolyte imbalances.

Sweat Electrolyte Content

Sweat is a **hypotonic** fluid, meaning it has a lower osmotic pressure than that of blood. Isotonic means having an osmotic pressure equal to that of blood, whereas **hypertonic** means having a higher osmotic pressure than that of blood. Sweat is hypotonic and so has a concentration of electrolytes less than that of blood, but it does contain some electrolytes. When sweating rates are extremely high, such as during intense activity in a hot, humid environment, up to 3 to 4 kg·h^{-1} of body weight or 3 to 4 L·h^{-1} of sweat can be lost by some individuals.[21] Acclimatization to heat may include such adaptations as higher sweat rate, earlier onset of sweating, increased resting plasma volume, and reduced electrolyte content of sweat.[20,26] Although sweat volume may increase after acclimatization, fewer electrolytes are lost per volume of sweat to help maintain electrolyte balance. The gastrointestinal tract and kidney are highly capable of reabsorbing electrolytes into the bloodstream and discouraging electrolyte imbalances from occurring.

Normally, sweating does not result in the need for ingesting additional salt (the foods we normally eat are plentiful in salt). Moreover, sweat rates are typically less than 1.5 L·h^{-1}, which results in less water and electrolyte loss than the extreme values reported for intense activity in hot, humid environments. If successive long-term exercise bouts, such as training for a triathlon or marathon, are performed in a hot environment, additional salt can be ingested in the form of lightly salted foods or fluids containing electrolytes, including various sports drinks. However, electrolyte loss by sweating can generally be compensated for by the conservation of electrolytes by the gastrointestinal tract and the kidneys. The maintenance of normal plasma mineral concentrations in athletes competing in a 20-day road race in hot and humid environments without ingestion of added mineral supplements is an example of the level of proficiency possessed by the electrolyte-saving organs and processes of the body.[13]

Urine Electrolyte Content

As described above, over time, electrolyte content of urine will vary to help ensure electrolyte balance. During exercise, there is a negative linear correlation between exercise intensity expressed as a percent of maximal oxygen consumption and sodium excretion.[21] Thus, as exercise intensity increases, sodium excretion decreases such that during maximal exercise sodium excretion is only 10% to 20% of the resting value. The decrease in sodium excretion is due to two major factors. One is that less sodium is excreted per liter of urine. The other is that urine output increases from rest (1.0 mL·min^{-1}) to light exercise (25% $\dot{V}o_{2max}$, 1.2 mL·min^{-1}) but then decreases during moderate exercise (40% $\dot{V}o_{2max}$, 0.75 mL·min^{-1}) and heavy exercise (80% $\dot{V}o_{2max}$, 0.3–0.5 mL·min^{-1}). During moderate and heavy exercise, less total urine is produced and electrolyte concentrations are lower in the urine that is produced. Consequently, the body's electrolyte stores are conserved.

Thirst Mechanism

Thirst is a conscious desire to drink and is involved in maintaining hydration and water balance. The drive to drink is controlled by several areas within the hypothalamus that sense plasma osmolality. These areas also receive input concerning cerebral spinal fluid and brain extracellular sodium concentration and extracellular fluid volume and, possibly, from peripheral receptors that sense osmolality.[21] When body water is lost, the concentration of dissolved substances within the blood and other bodily fluids increases, stimulating the thirst mechanism. This results in a drive to drink. As fluid is ingested, concentration of dissolved substances returns toward normal and the drive to drink diminishes. One of the first signs of partial dehydration is the sensation of a "dry mouth," which is a sensation that initiates drinking.[21]

When the thirst mechanism is activated or there is a drive to drink, partial dehydration has already occurred. Humans are considered slow hydrators, meaning that their thirst mechanism does not result in restoration of water balance quickly. Total volume of fluid ingestion within a 3-hour rehydration period following exercise will typically replace only 60% to 70% of the fluid lost.[21] Additionally, some of the fluid ingested after exercise will be eliminated as urine. These factors indicate that more fluid must be consumed than the thirst mechanism calls for if long-term water balance is to be maintained. Moreover, because the thirst mechanism is slow to respond and is triggered only after partial dehydration has occurred, the athlete would be wise to consume fluids before starting the exercise session.

PHYSIOLOGY OF DEHYDRATION DURING EXERCISE

Now that we understand the importance of water and electrolytes to the function of the body, we can consider the physiological effects of dehydration. First, let us review

how dehydration occurs. During exercise, dehydration most commonly results due to water lost through sweating. Sweating is the body's mechanism for dissipating the heat generated by the increased burning of energy by the body (metabolism) during exercise. The effectiveness of sweating in cooling the body depends on the relative humidity of the environment, with sweating being more effective in dryer environments since it more readily evaporates, thus removing heat from the body, when humidity is low. The water loss caused by sweating comes not only from sweat glands, but also from intracellular and extracellular compartments, including plasma, as well as from muscle tissue, skin, internal organs, and even bone, with little water coming from the brain or liver.[27] Next, we will consider how dehydration causes declines in both aerobic and anaerobic performance, explore some specific sport examples of dehydration, and learn about factors that increase susceptibility to dehydration.

Dehydration Results in Performance Decrements

Dehydration can result in decreased performance in aerobic and anaerobic activities. The levels of dehydration necessary to impact performance in aerobic and anaerobic activities are different, however. Differences in physiological responses to anaerobic and aerobic activities, along with environmental factors, help explain this difference.

Effect of Dehydration on Aerobic Capabilities

Aerobic capabilities can be compromised by dehydration. Track and field athletes dehydrated by 2% of total body mass show declines of performance in 5,000- and 10,000-meter races of approximately 5% and 3%, respectively,[2] whereas rowers show an increase of 22 seconds in the time needed to complete a 2,000-meter race.[7] These performance decreases would make the difference between winning or not winning a competition and underscore the need for athletes to maintain euhydration for optimal endurance capabilities.

Aerobic capabilities and performance depend on maintaining cardiac output so that sufficient oxygen is delivered to, and waste products are removed from, metabolically active tissue. Moreover, heat dissipation and maintaining the correct use of metabolic substrate are required for optimal aerobic capabilities. During physical activity, sweating increases at a rate that depends in part on the environment in which the activity is performed. For example, in a hot, humid environment, the sweat rates of most people during physical activity can be as great as 2 L·h^{-1}.[28,30] Also, sweat rate can vary widely in different activities but is still sufficient to induce dehydration. For instance, sweat rates are approximately 0.79 L·h^{-1} during competitive water polo but as high as 2.37 L·h^{-1} in competitive squash.[28] Thus, dehydration is not just a concern for athletes, such as marathon runners and road cyclists, who compete in what are typically thought of as aerobic activities. It is also a concern for anyone involved in a wide range of activities that depend on aerobic metabolism and aerobic capabilities for performance.

With dehydration, plasma volume decreases, resulting in a decrease in stroke volume and an increase in heart rate in an attempt to maintain cardiac output (cardiac output = heart rate × stroke volume). Dehydration also results in an increase in systemic vascular resistance due to vasoconstriction. As dehydration progresses, cardiac output and mean arterial pressure can decrease.[8,30,31] When compounded with dehydration, these factors increase cardiovascular strain, or the work the heart must perform to pump sufficient cardiac output at any particular workload, such as a certain race pace during a marathon. In short, as the level of dehydration increases, so, too, does cardiovascular strain. For example, heart rate increases 3 to 5 beats per minute for every 1% loss of body mass due to dehydration.[8]

Another factor affecting aerobic capabilities with dehydration is an increase in body temperature, or **hyperthermia**.[5,8,15,30] With dehydration, there is a decrease in skin blood flow and a decrease in sweat rate, both diminishing the ability to dissipate heat,[5,8,10] eventually resulting in hyperthermia. As a result of the intricately connected roles and functions of the cardiovascular and thermoregulatory systems of the body, hyperthermia and dehydration are likely to have compounding effects when exercising.[15,31]

Altered metabolic function is another result of dehydration, as indicated by increased reliance on carbohydrate in the form of muscle glycogen as a metabolic substrate and an increase in blood lactate levels at a particular workload when dehydrated.[5,8,30] Blood glucose concentrations may not be affected or be slightly lower when one is dehydrated.[5] These factors could result in decreased endurance performance capabilities due to fatigue resulting from glycogen depletion and increased acidity (see Chapter 2).

Still other factors can decrease endurance performance when dehydrated. Ratings of perceived exertion (RPE) increase when the same workload is performed when dehydrated.[8] Cognitive function is also disturbed with dehydration.[5,8,30] Increased perceived exertion and decreased cognitive function could decrease endurance performance by decreasing the motivation to exercise and affecting decisions during competition, such as race strategies.

All of the above factors interact to contribute to a decrease in aerobic capabilities or endurance performance when dehydrated and greater impairment of aerobic capabilities as dehydration increases (Fig. 9-3). Although individual responses exist and some people are more tolerant of dehydration than others, dehydration greater than 2%[30-32] or 3%[8] of body mass decreases aerobic power and aerobic capabilities in a temperate to hot, humid environment. However, with dehydration in a cold environment, such as might be encountered in cross-country skiing, a loss

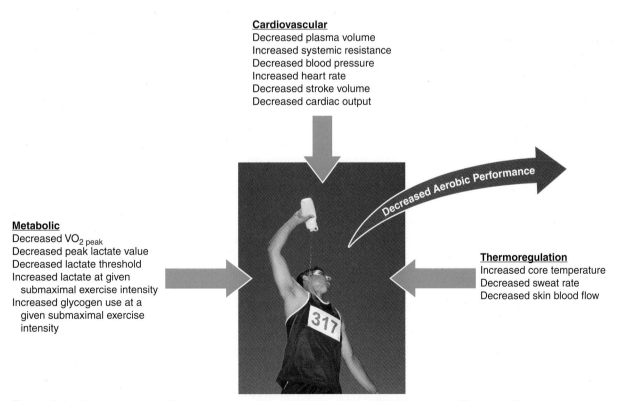

Cardiovascular
Decreased plasma volume
Increased systemic resistance
Decreased blood pressure
Increased heart rate
Decreased stroke volume
Decreased cardiac output

Decreased Aerobic Performance

Metabolic
Decreased VO$_{2\,peak}$
Decreased peak lactate value
Decreased lactate threshold
Increased lactate at given
  submaximal exercise intensity
Increased glycogen use at a
  given submaximal exercise
  intensity

Thermoregulation
Increased core temperature
Decreased sweat rate
Decreased skin blood flow

Figure 9-3. Many factors contribute to decreased aerobic performance with dehydration. Cardiovascular, thermoregulatory, and metabolic factors all contribute to decreased aerobic performance capabilities with dehydration. These factors may act independently or collectively to decrease performance.

of 3% of body mass has little impact on aerobic exercise performance.[30] These findings suggest that it is the negative impact that dehydration has on thermoregulation that is critical in modifying exercise performance.

Effect of Dehydration on Anaerobic Capabilities

Reports on the effect of dehydration on maximal strength levels and anaerobic performance capabilities are inconsistent, with some studies showing significant decreases and others showing no significant change.[5,27,29,33] There is, however, a pattern of an increased chance of a decline in performance with increased dehydration. Generally, decreases in strength are not apparent when dehydration results in less than a 5% loss of total body mass. However, dehydration resulting in a greater than 5% loss of total body mass does result in strength decrements.[8,27] Declines in muscular endurance, such as the ability to maintain grip strength, are apparent with dehydration of 3% to 4% of total body mass.[8] Anaerobic performance during maximal efforts lasting 30 seconds (Wingate cycling test) shows no significant decline following dehydration of 5% of body weight. Thus, it appears that strength and anaerobic capabilities are less affected by dehydration than are aerobic capabilities.

Several factors may explain why, compared with aerobic performance, dehydration-related decreases in strength and anaerobic capabilities are inconsistent. First, the decrease in plasma volume, and thus cardiac output, resulting from dehydration would be expected to negatively affect aerobic performance, but not strength or anaerobic performance where the delivery of oxygen to working muscle is not so crucial. Second, anaerobic capability decrements are more likely when exercise and heat exposure are used to induce dehydration as opposed to fluid restriction alone.[29] Third, dehydration-related decreases in strength performance may be more likely in upper body compared with lower body tasks.[29,33]

Although the effect of dehydration on maximal strength and anaerobic performance may be less consistently shown compared with its effect on aerobic performance, the anaerobic decrements shown in competitive athletes may be significant and could hinder performance during competition. Additionally, activities taking place in hot and humid environments warrant additional precaution when considering the compounded risks of dehydration and hyperthermia.

Sport Examples of Dehydration

Maintaining euhydration is important for optimal performance of virtually all types of physical activity. This includes not just outdoor events where high heat and humidity will affect the sweat rate, but also indoor activities and sports performed in hot arenas. To minimize the chance of dehydration in any type of environment, adequate fluid volumes must be ingested during and between training sessions leading up to the competition. The fluids consumed should contain electrolytes (sodium and potassium) to help maintain

fluid balance between the intracellular and extracellular compartments.[35] Because of obligatory urine losses, fluid consumption after a training session needs to be greater than the volume of sweat lost.[35] It is also recommended that 400 to 600 milliliters (about 17 ounces) of water be ingested 2 hours prior to the event to allow the kidneys time to regulate total body water volume prior to beginning the activity.[10] Ensuring euhydration during training, prior to competition, and during competition will help in producing the best possible performance in virtually all types of strenuous physical activity. In the following examples, hydration considerations specific to a particular sport are explored. Although these considerations are specific to the example, the concepts are also applicable to other sports and activities.

Marathon

Endurance capabilities in any event such as running a marathon (26.2 miles or 42 kilometers) are decreased by dehydration of as little as 2% of total body mass. The primary goal of fluid ingestion during the event is to prevent dehydration, with electrolyte replacement an important, but secondary concern.

Body mass and environmental conditions affect the amount of fluid ingestion needed to prevent dehydration greater than 2% of total body mass. The consideration of body mass is especially important for recreational runners, among whom body mass may vary widely. For example, during a 4-hour marathon with environmental conditions of 28°C (82.4°F) and 30% relative humidity, a 50-kilogram (110-lb) runner ingesting 0.5 liters of fluid per hour would lose body water equivalent to 0.6% of total body mass.[9] However, a 90-kilogram (198-lb) runner ingesting the same fluid volume would lose body water equivalent to 2.9% of total body mass. If the marathon were performed at environmental conditions of 14°C (57.2°F) and 70% relative humidity and fluid ingestion remained at 0.5 L·h^{-1}, the lighter runner would actually gain body mass (2.6%), whereas the heavier runner (–0.6%) would not reach a 2% of total body weight loss of fluid.

Both programmed (drinking at specific points within the race) and ad libitum drinking can be used in an attempt to maintain hydration during an event. Many marathon runners when drinking ad libitum, however, do not consume sufficient fluid volumes to prevent a water loss of greater than 2% of total body mass.[9] Both programmed and ad libitum drinking have limitations when applied to a wide range of runners' abilities, environmental conditions, and body mass, underscoring the need for an individualized hydration plan during competition, as well as training, that has been tested prior to a major event.[9]

Freestyle Wrestling

Freestyle wrestling is a weight-class sport that requires strength and power of both the upper and lower body musculature. Wrestlers typically lose 5% to 6% of total body mass to make a weight class. To lose this amount of weight, a combination of caloric and fluid restriction is used. Thus, any performance decrement may be due to either one of these factors, or a combination of them. Strength and anaerobic performance decrements have been shown in wrestlers after hypohydration of 5% to 6% of body weight;[16,18,40,41] however, an absence of effect on wrestling-specific performance measures after hypohydration has also been shown.[34,36]

Although dual meets are contested in wrestling, all significant wrestling events take place in a tournament setting, such as conference tournaments, national championships, and the Olympics. Thus, the physiological response to tournament settings is important for a wrestler's performance. After losing 6% of total body mass during 1 week prior to a simulated 2-day tournament, collegiate wrestlers (National Collegiate Athletic Association Division I) showed decreases in some, but not all tests related to wrestling ability.[18] The wrestlers showed significant decreases in grip strength and "bear hug" (hugging a padded strain gauge using a handgrip similar to a throw in wrestling) strength prior to each match compared with a baseline measure prior to the week during which weight loss took place (Fig. 9-4). Grip and bear hug strength also showed decreases as the simulated tournament progressed from match 1 to match 5. However, measures of hip and back strength, movement time, and time taken to transition from the traditional kneeling bottom position in wrestling to a standing position, were not significantly different prior to any of the five matches during the tournament compared with the baseline values. There were, however, changes in these measures after the matches compared with before the matches within the simulated tournament. Overall, during the simulated tournament, significant decreases in some but not all physiological measures were shown. These decreases were the result of a combined effect of weight loss, dehydration, and competing in the tournament; and probably do affect a wrestler's ability to maintain physical performance throughout a tournament.

Team Ball Sports: Basketball and Soccer

Dehydration can affect performance in team ball sports that are contested both indoors and outdoors. Decreased aerobic capabilities could decrease performance in the latter stages of a contest, decreased anaerobic capabilities could affect sprinting ability, and decreased strength or power could decrease jumping ability, all of which are important for performance in team ball sports.

Dehydration also decreases performance in specific skills and activities inherent in team ball sports. In basketball, players' dehydration equivalent to 2% of total body mass during a 2-hour practice session significantly decreases combined shooting percentage (3-point, 15-foot

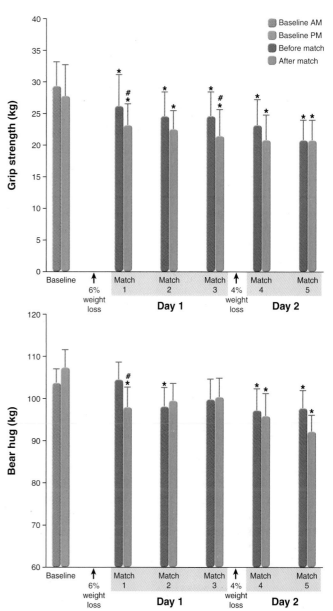

Figure 9-4. After weight loss, strength measures decrease in wrestlers throughout a simulated tournament. The simulated tournament consisted of three matches on the first day and two matches on the second day of competition. Baseline measures were obtained prior to losing 6% of total body mass during the week preceding the tournament. *Significantly different from both (morning and evening) baseline measures; #Significantly different from corresponding prematch value. (Adapted from Kraemer, et al.[18])

free-throws) by 8%, repeated sprint ability (court width suicide drill) by 2%, and lateral movement ability by 5% relative to a euhydrated state maintained with water.[12] Use of a carbohydrate electrolyte sports drink to maintain euhydration, however, significantly improved these skills relative to a euhydrated state maintained with water. Deterioration of basketball skills, such as shooting drills, shots made in a simulated game, and lateral movement ability progressively decrease as dehydration increased from 1% to 4% of total body weight.[4] Similar to deterioration of aerobic capabilities, the threshold for deterioration of basketball skills appears to be 2% body water loss of total body mass.[4] Although no significant decrease in overall shooting percentage has been shown with dehydration equal to 1.9% of total body mass, it appears that dehydration can significantly affect other basketball skills.[17]

During a soccer match, players perform repeat sprints interspaced with short rest periods. This type of performance is mimicked by the Yo-Yo Intermittent Recovery Test, which consists of 20-meter runs of ever-increasing speed interspaced with 10-second rest periods. This test has been shown to mimic the amount of high-intensity running performed in a competitive soccer match[19] and differentiates between players of varying abilities.[23] Performance of the Yo-Yo Intermittent Recovery Test by soccer players is decreased by approximately 15% after dehydration, equivalent to 1.5% to 2% of total body mass. This finding indicates that soccer performance decreases with dehydration.[14] Preventing dehydration in team ball sports helps to maintain not just general aerobic and anaerobic capabilities, but also performance in sport-specific skills.

Susceptibility to Dehydration

Various factors predispose individuals or groups to dehydration. Some of these factors are similar to factors predisposing individuals to thermoregulatory difficulties (see Chapter 10). Environmental factors such as high temperature and humidity, where sweat rates are high, increase the chance of dehydration. Environmental factors are of particular concern in long-duration events, such as a marathon, or when training or physical activity takes place on

consecutive days,[6] or more than once a day, such as the 2- or 3-a-day practice sessions that take place at the beginning of many sport seasons. Athletes in sports such as judo, boxing, wrestling, and weightlifting, who partially dehydrate themselves to make a weight class, are also susceptible to dehydration difficulties (Fig. 9-5).[8,25,37,41] Protective equipment used in some sports (e.g., American football) can interfere with heat loss and therefore increase sweat rates, placing participants at greater risk of dehydration.[6] Dark-colored clothing or equipment can result in greater heat absorption

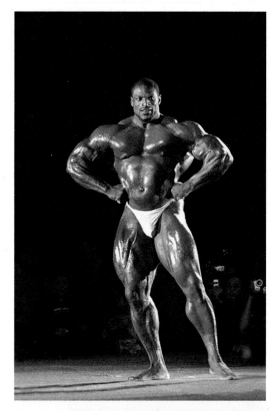

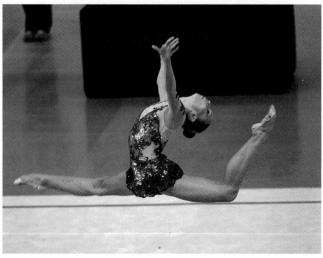

Figure 9-5. Body mass sports. Sports that use body weight classes or body image judging as a part of the competitive conditions can be susceptible to dehydration and illness with competition, in addition to a decreased performance potential.

Quick Review

- Dehydration during activity is in part due to the increase in metabolism relative to rest, resulting in sweating to dissipate heat.
- Aerobic performance decreases due to water loss are related to increased cardiovascular strain and hyperthermia.
- Physiological explanations for the decreases in anaerobic performance that accompany water loss are inconsistent and unclear.
- Dehydration can decrease performance not only in events ranging from the marathon to Olympic weightlifting, but also in events that require both aerobic and anaerobic capabilities, such as wrestling and team ball sports.
- Susceptibility to dehydration increases due to high temperature and humidity, multiple training sessions per day, participation in a weight-class sport, sports involving the subjective judging of body image, protective equipment that reduces heat loss, dark-colored uniforms, and decreased thirst sensitivity due to aging.

from the environment, resulting in increased sweat rates and possibly increasing dehydration.[6]

Illness involving a fever or diarrhea increases the probability of dehydration difficulties during activity.[6] Older individuals may be more susceptible to dehydration due to several factors.[6,30] Thirst sensitivity due to a given loss of extracellular fluid is reduced as one ages, so less fluid is ingested. Older individuals also have a decreased ability to maintain an adequate plasma volume and osmolality during exercise and are slower to restore body fluid homeostasis after water deprivation. Although, generally, older individuals are adequately hydrated, the above factors predispose them to dehydration during exercise. When one or more of the above predisposing factors to dehydration are present, it is imperative to have an adequate hydration plan.

HYDRATION ASSESSMENT METHODS

Due to the potential negative effects of dehydration on both athletic performance and health, knowing one's hydration status is important. The most common field methods of monitoring the hydration status of athletes and fitness enthusiasts involve the assessment of body weight or urine color. Although both of these methodologies have limitations, they do provide easy, noninvasive ways to monitor hydration.[25] Laboratory methods of hydration determination include urine volume, **urine specific gravity**, and **urine osmolality**. These assessment methods can also be used to monitor hydration of athletes, but do require minimal equipment and training.

Field Hydration Assessment Methods

Maintenance of body mass within plus or minus 1% of its preexercise value indicates a state of euhydration.[8,25] Body weight losses greater than 1% of pre-exercise body weight indicate increasing dehydration (Table 9-2). To accurately

Table 9-2. Hydration Status: Body Mass and Urine Color Indices

Hydration	% Body Mass Change	Urine Color
Well hydrated	± 1	1 or 2
Minimal dehydration	−1 to −3	3 or 4
Significant dehydration	−3 to −5	5 or 6
Serious dehydration	Greater than −5	Greater than 6

Adapted from Casa et al.[8]

determine preexercise body mass, at least three consecutive determinations of nude body mass should be made after urinating and ad libitum fluid and food ingestion.[28,30] However, women may require more than three determinations of body mass because menstrual cycle phase influences body water.[28,30] For example, during the luteal phase of the menstrual cycle, total body water, and thus body mass, can increase up to 2 kilograms.[28,30] Postexercise body mass should be determined in the nude after toweling off all sweat. Percent loss of body mass is calculated using this equation: pre-exercise body mass before exercise − body mass after exercise/body mass before exercise × 100. Loss of body mass during activity can also be used to calculate the amount of fluid that must be ingested to return to pre-exercise body mass (Box 9-3). Limitations of this method to determine hydration status are changes in eating habits and bowel movements, both of which affect total body weight.

Urine color can also be used to give a general indication of hydration status (Table 9-2 and, for color chart, see Casa et al.[8]). A urine light in color indicates adequate hydration, whereas a progressively darker color indicates increasing dehydration.[3] Urine color to help determine hydration status has several limitations. Ingestion of some

Box 9-3 PRACTICAL QUESTIONS FROM STUDENTS

How is the Amount of Fluid That Needs to Be Ingested After Exercise Calculated?

During physical activity, 2 kilograms of total body weight are lost. This indicates a water weight loss of 2 kilograms, excluding fluid replacement during activity. How much fluid must be ingested prior to the next bout of physical activity to maintain hydration?

$$2 \text{ kg} = 2{,}000 \text{ g} = 2{,}000 \text{ mL} = 2.0 \text{ L of fluid}$$

(in the metric system 1 g = 1 mL)

$$1 \text{ cup} = 0.24 \text{ L}$$

$$2.0 \text{ L}/0.24 \text{ L/cup} = 8.3 \text{ cups} = 2.1 \text{ qt}$$

Some of the ingested fluid between exercise bouts will be eliminated as urine, so greater than the calculated amount of fluid needs to be ingested. The fluid should be ingested in small amounts, starting immediately after exercise.

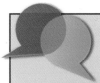

Box 9-4   AN EXPERT VIEW

Assessing Your Hydration Status

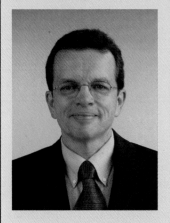

Lawrence E. Armstrong, PhD, FACSM

Professor,
Human Performance Laboratory
Department of Kinesiology
University of Connecticut
Storrs, CT

Good health, digestion, metabolism, and optimal exercise performance require that you avoid dehydration. For example, a 3% to 4% loss of body weight reduces muscular strength by approximately 2% and reduces muscular power by approximately 3%.[3] The same level of dehydration reduces high-intensity endurance performance (e.g., distance running) by approximately 10%.

Because fluid gain and loss occur continuously and because the body's network of fluid compartments (e.g., intracellular or extracellular fluid, circulating blood) is complex, no single measurement can validly represent hydration status in all situations. During periods of training or competition, when fluid compartments change continuously, one body fluid measurement is not sufficient to provide valid information about total body water or the concentration of body fluids.[1]

When you want to evaluate your hydration status during daily activities or physical training, the best approach involves comparing information from two or more hydration indices. The following paragraphs describe five simple, inexpensive techniques that you can use.

1. **Body weight difference.** Change of body weight represents an effective method of hydration assessment. It is especially appropriate for measuring dehydration that occurs over a few hours. Very simply, body weight loss equals water loss (corrected for the weight of fluid and food intake, urine and fecal losses, and sweating).

   In athletic settings, an accurate baseline body weight is required. Surprisingly, few individuals know this important number. A simple way to discover your baseline body weight is to measure it on five or six consecutive mornings, after eliminating but before eating. When three measurements lie within 0.5 lb of each other on different mornings, the average value represents your body weight accurately.

   Urine is concentrated and urine volume is low when your body is dehydrated and conserving water. When a temporary excess of body water exists, urine is dilute and plentiful. These changes of urine characteristics provide three options to evaluate your hydration status.

2. **24-hour urine volume.** Collect all urine that you produce throughout the day in a clean plastic jug. A healthy woman produces 1.13 liters (1.20 quarts) of urine per day, whereas a healthy man excretes 1.36 liters (1.44 quarts) per day. Children who are 10 to 14 years old produce proportionately less urine each day, as do adults over the age of 90.

3. **Urine specific gravity.** Place a few drops of urine on the stage of a handheld refractometer and point it toward a light source. This device measures the density (mass per volume) of a urine sample relative to the density of water. Any fluid that is denser than water has a specific gravity greater than 1.000. In dehydrated states, urine specific gravity exceeds 1.030, but when one consumes excess water, the values range from 1.001 to 1.012. Normal urine specimens range from 1.013 to 1.029 in healthy adults.

4. **Urine color.** Urine color provides a useful estimate of hydration state during everyday activities. A "pale yellow" or "straw-colored" visual reading indicates that you are within 1% of your baseline body weight (see item 1 above). Darker colors (e.g., deep yellow, tan) represent increasing levels of dehydration.[2]

5. **Thirst.** Physiological strain (i.e., significantly elevated heart rate and body temperature) increases when you lose only 1% or 2% of body weight. Similarly, when you are "a little thirsty" or "moderately thirsty," you are mildly dehydrated by 1% or 2% of body weight. However, it is important to realize that other factors may influence thirst, including the taste, volume, and contents of the fluid. Although thirst offers an estimate of the degree of your dehydration, it better serves to remind you to drink more.

The Best Approach

During daily activities, when fluid compartments are constantly fluctuating (due to meal consumption, urine loss, and sweating), a single technique will not provide valid information about dehydration. The best approach involves comparing information from two or more of the above hydration indices. When different methods agree, you can be confident of the information at that time. If the techniques do not agree, it is wise to ingest more fluid and repeat the measurements within a few hours. But remember: do not drink too much. Excessive fluid consumption can lead to illness or even death in extreme cases.

References

1. Armstrong LE. Assessing hydration status: The elusive gold standard. J Am Coll Nutr. 2007;26(5):575S–584S.
2. Armstrong LE, Herrera Soto JA, Hacker FT, et al. Urinary indices during dehydration, exercise, and rehydration. Int J Sport Nutr Exerc Metab. 1998;8:345–355.
3. Judelson DA, Maresh CM, Anderson JM, et al. Hydration and muscular performance. Does fluid balance affect strength, power and high-intensity endurance? Sports Med. (New Zealand). 2007;37:907–921.

Quick Review

- Laboratory hydration assessment methods are more accurate than field assessment methods but are not accessible or practical in many situations.
- The field hydration assessment methods of body mass loss during activity and urine color can provide valuable information concerning hydration status.
- The most common laboratory hydration assessment methods are urine osmolality and urine specific gravity.

Quick Review

- Hyponatremia is low blood sodium content, resulting in fluid movement into the brain causing swelling of the brain and disorientation, confusion, general weakness, grand mal seizures, coma, and possibly death.
- Hyponatremia may be caused by ingesting excessive volumes of low-sodium-content fluid, insufficient mobilization of sodium stores in response to a large volume of fluid ingestion, or conversion of osmotically active sodium stores in the blood to intracellular sodium, which lowers the blood sodium concentration.

supplements, such as vitamin pills, results in a darker urine color. Drinking fluids after an exercise session that caused partial dehydration results in increased urine production long before euhydration is established. When urine color is used to help determine hydration status, it is recommended that the first urine sample produced during the morning, or samples of euhydrated (rehydrated) urine after exercise, be used for assessment. Total body mass and urine color both have limitations in their accuracy in determining hydration status. However, when used in conjunction with each other, they do offer valuable information concerning hydration status.[28,30]

Laboratory Hydration Assessment Methods

Dilution methods to determine total body water via plasma osmolality measurement are the most accurate, valid, and sensitive ways to determine hydration status.[28,30] However, they are not practical for most situations. Urine volume (urination should be frequent and of normal euhydrated volume) can be used as a general indicator of hydration status but is somewhat subjective and can be confounded by fluid intake and other factors.[25,28,30] However, the more quantifiable and most-often used measures of urine specific gravity and urine osmolality are considered the best indicators of hydration status when facilities and qualified personnel are available to conduct such assessments (Box 9-4).[8,30]

HYPONATREMIA

Although failure to drink enough water or other fluids can result in dehydration, drinking too much water can also be detrimental. **Hyponatremia**, also termed "water intoxication," is a low blood sodium concentration (117–128 mmol·L^{-1}) typically resulting from drinking too much water. This condition causes an osmotic imbalance, which results in fluid movement into the brain, causing swelling of the brain. The swelling can lead to disorientation, confusion, general weakness, grand mal seizures, coma, and possibly death.[10,11,22,30] Some experts believe that the cause of the low blood sodium concentration is drinking a large volume of low-sodium-containing fluid over several hours, which can be exacerbated by sodium lost in sweat.[11] This theory

for hyponatremia is why sodium is included in rehydration drinks, such as sports drinks[10]; to minimize the possibility of hyponatremia.[22] Other experts think that hyponatremia results from insufficient mobilization of sodium stores within the body in response to drinking a large volume of fluid, or conversion of osmotically active sodium stores in the blood to intracellular sodium, which lowers the blood sodium concentration.[24] These experts believe that hyponatremia can be avoided by not ingesting excessive amounts of fluid during exercise.[24] Conversely, hyponatremia may result from excessive Na$^+$ (sodium) loss in sweat. Ultimately, low blood sodium because of an excess in water consumption is likely to have effects similar to low blood sodium resulting from profuse sweating and concomitant loss of sodium. Women may be at greater risk than men for hyponatremia when competing in marathon and ultramarathon races.[1] Several possible physiological and psychological factors could explain the greater risk in women, but the exact cause has not been explained clearly.[28,30] Whatever the exact cause of hyponatremia, its occurrence may be increased in ultraendurance athletes competing in hot weather.[39]

MAINTAINING HYDRATION

Maintaining hydration is important for the maintenance of physical performance and depends not only on hydration during activity, but also on fluid ingestion prior to and after activity so that total body water decreases do not occur as successive exercise bouts are performed. Because of the many factors that may affect hydration and fluid ingestion, individualized hydration plans are recommended to prevent body weight loss greater than 2% during activity.[30] Many factors may enter into this individualized hydration plan, such as the pressure some athletes feel to "make weight" in order to compete in a specific weight class, increased susceptibility to dehydration based on past experiences with it, and determining rehydration opportunities before, during, and after activity for fluid ingestion. Hydration guidelines have been developed and can serve as a starting point for an individualized hydration plan.

Table 9-3. Guidelines for Fluid Consumption

American College of Sports Medicine	National Athletic Trainers Association
Before exercise: 4 hours prior to event slowly drink approximately 5 to 7 mL·kg⁻¹; if no urine production or urine is dark, 2 hours prior to event drink approximately 3 to 5 L·h⁻¹	Before exercise: 2 to 3 hours prior to event drink approximately 500 to 600 mL (17–20 fl oz), 10 to 20 minutes prior to event drink 200 to 300 mL (7–10 fl oz)
During exercise: customized plans are best; a good starting point is during strenuous exercise, drink 0.4 to 0.8 L·h⁻¹	During exercise: drink 200 to 300 mL (7–10 fl oz) every 10 to 20 minutes
After exercise: time permitting, normal meals and snacks with sufficient water will restore euhydration; aggressive rehydration: drink approximately 1.5 liters of fluid for each kilogram of body weight lost	After exercise: ideally, in 2 hours, drink sufficient fluid to replace lost body weight; rapid rehydration: drink 25% to 50% more fluid than sweat lost to compensate for urine lost during rehydration

Hydration Guidelines

Hydration guidelines have been developed by professional groups concerned with maintaining a healthy hydration status during physical activity. The two sets of guidelines depicted in Table 9-3 show differences concerning how much and exactly when fluid should be ingested prior to, during, and after activity to maintain hydration. The guidelines do agree on the major tenants of maintaining hydration to enable optimal performance during activity. Developing universal guidelines is difficult because sweat rates are affected by many factors, including the following: differences in individual sweat rates even during the same type of activity, differing sweat rates that may be specific to different types of activities (running a marathon vs. playing soccer), type of clothing worn, training status, and environmental factors such as temperature, humidity, and whether wind is present.[8,30] Thus, the guidelines should be viewed as a starting point to develop individualized and customized hydration plans for a particular activity.[8,30]

Both sets of guidelines do agree that all individuals should start activity in a euhydrated state, and should attempt to maintain hydration during activity, while remembering to effectively rehydrate after activity is concluded. They also agree on other important aspects of maintaining hydration. First, fluid should be palatable and cool (10°C [50°F] to 15°C [59°F][8] or 15°C [59°F] to 21°C [69.8°F][30]) and contain electrolytes. However, for many athletes and activities, slightly salting foods will be enough to maintain proper electrolyte balance. Although the amount of fluid that should be consumed during activity is affected by the type of activity performed, and environmental conditions present, fluids should be readily available to athletes during all types of activity, and in all weather conditions.

Developing a Hydration Plan

Individualized hydration plans should be developed to maintain euhydration during training and competition. Steps that can be taken to maintain hydration involve fluid ingestion prior to, during, and after training or competition (Box 9-5). The steps presented use only body mass and urine color as indicators of hydration status because these are measures that would be available in most situations. More sensitive laboratory measures of hydration status could be incorporated into the individualized hydration

Box 9-5 PRACTICAL QUESTIONS FROM STUDENTS

What are Practical Steps to Help Maintain Euhydration?

1. Accurately determine preexercise body mass using at least three consecutive nude body masses after urinating and with ad libitum fluid and food ingestion.
2. When determining preexercise body mass, check hydration status for euhydration using urine color (Table 9-2 and Fig. 9-4).
3. If urine color does not indicate euhydration, do not use this preexercise body mass in the calculation of average preexercise body mass.
4. Use the preexercise, during exercise, and postexercise hydration guidelines (Table 9-3) to maintain hydration during training and competition.
5. Determine postactivity body mass in the nude after wiping off all sweat.

6. Calculate percent body mass loss using the following equation: preexercise body mass – postexercise body mass/preexercise body mass × 100.
7. Adjust pre-, during, and postactivity fluid ingestion to maintain a percent body mass loss in consecutive activity bouts of less than 1%.
8. Check for euhydration using body mass and urine color prior to consecutive bouts of activity.
9. Adjust fluid ingestion before, during, and after activity to maintain body mass within 1% of average body mass before exercise and urine color within the range indicating euhydration.

CASE STUDY

Scenario

You live in Minnesota and are training for a marathon to be held in Atlanta in the middle of the summer. The environment in northern Minnesota where you live and are training will generally be cooler and less humid than that in Atlanta. As one not acclimatized to a hot, humid environment, you have a higher sodium concentration (40–100 mmol·L^{-1}) in your sweat than those acclimatized to a hot, humid environment (5–30 mmol·L^{-1}). The potential greater loss of sodium in sweat in the upcoming marathon in Atlanta may place you at a greater risk for hyponatremia.

Questions

What factors put you at risk for hyponatremia?

What training adaptation could you make to prepare for the marathon?

Should you increase your intake of fluids when training or competing in an environment that is hotter and more humid than you are used to?

Options

To decrease the sodium lost in sweat, you could train in a hot, humid environment for a period of time (7–10 days) to become heat-acclimatized, which should result in a decrease of sodium lost in sweat.

You may believe that you need to ingest large volumes of fluid to compete in the marathon in Atlanta. It is noteworthy that compared to those who do not experience hyponatremia, those who do present its symptoms demonstrate only a moderate loss of body weight, which, in turn, can be attributed to drinking large volumes of hypotonic fluid during exercise. For example, athletes appearing to have hyponatremia in an iron man triathlon lost 2.5 kilograms of body mass during the event compared with a body mass loss of 2.9 kilograms in athletes who did not appear to have hyponatremia. Furthermore, one of the athletes suffering from hyponatremia drank 16 liters of fluid during the race and gained 2.5 kilograms of body mass.[38] Thus, although there is a need to ingest fluid during competition, care must be taken not to ingest too much low-sodium-content fluid because it may add to the risk of hyponatremia. These steps should minimize the chance of developing hyponatremia.

Scenario

You are the athletic trainer of a college football team. It is August and your team is getting ready to begin preseason practices, which will include two sessions per day. The hot weather of August, especially in the south where your school is located, is a concern during these strenuous preseason 2-a-days, because you can expect the players to be sweating heavily. You know that dehydration will limit the players' performance, and more seriously, threaten their health and well-being. What can you do to guard against dehydration?

Options

First, you must be aware that the thirst mechanism can be inefficient, especially during hot, humid conditions. Your players will feel the urge to drink only after they experience some degree of dehydration. Also, even when they do begin to drink, the athletes will not be able to replace fluids as quickly as they are losing them while they are sweating profusely. Further, there is a lag time between when fluids are consumed and when they actually are absorbed into the bloodstream from the gastrointestinal tract. So, it is important to have your players drink fluids before practice begins, even if they do not feel the urge to drink. Regular breaks during practice must be taken to allow for replacement fluids to be consumed, and you must be sure that all players are drinking their fluids. The fluids should be kept at a cool temperature as this will enhance palatability, and the rate at which they will be taken up into the bloodstream. Drinking water during practice should be mandatory, and not seen as a sign of weakness. After practice, players should continue to drink replacement fluids. To ensure that they are properly hydrated, you may elect to not allow the players to leave the locker room until they can demonstrate that they are normally hydrated once again. This can easily be checked by asking the players to provide urine samples. The color of the urine can be matched with a color-coded chart to determine if the players are euhydrated (the urine should be a light color). Only after this is confirmed should players be allowed to leave the practice facility.

plan if available. The steps provided here should only serve as a starting point in developing individualized hydration plans. Plans then need to be modified based on the many factors that can affect hydration and on the opportunities for fluid ingestion during exercise and sports events. The hydration plan may then need to be modified as training and the competitive season progress. For example, fluid ingestion may need to be increased before, during, and after activity as a season progresses from early spring to late summer, because heat and humidity have gradually increased as the season progressed.

Quick Review

- Because of the many factors that affect dehydration, individualized hydration plans should be developed.
- Hydration guidelines promote adequate fluid ingestion prior to, during, and after physical activity.
- Individualized hydration plans should include field tests of hydration status but can include laboratory tests of hydration status and should be used to maintain euhydration during training and competition.

CHAPTER SUMMARY

Fluid, including water, and electrolytes are necessary for many bodily functions. Water is the most abundant substance in the body, comprising 60% of an adult's body mass, and a person would not survive even several days without sufficient ingestion of water. Water balance to maintain euhydration depends on replacing water lost via sweat, feces, urine, and insensible perspiration.

Bodily fluids and cells contain electrolytes, which are substances that disassociate in water to produce charged ions. Electrolytes are necessary for many bodily functions, but are also important because cells control the movement of water by controlling the movement of electrolytes through their membranes. Moreover, the osmotic pressure created by electrolytes holds water in cells and extracellular spaces. Electrolytes are lost in sweat and urine, but electrolyte balance is maintained by increasing or decreasing, as necessary, absorption of electrolytes by the gastrointestinal tract and electrolyte content of the urine.

The thirst mechanism is activated with a loss of body water, but by the time it is activated partial dehydration has already occurred. Additionally, the human thirst mechanism does not result in fast restoration of euhydration. Thus, to restore euhydration, more fluid than indicated by the thirst mechanism must be ingested.

Loss of body water of as little as 2% of total body mass can reduce aerobic capabilities due to increased heart rate and decreased plasma volume, stroke volume, and cardiac output, all of which increase cardiovascular strain. With sufficient water loss, aerobic capabilities also decrease because of hyperthermia.

The effect of dehydration on anaerobic capabilities, such as strength, power, and sprint ability, are less consistent than the loss of aerobic capabilities. However, anaerobic abilities do decrease with body water losses equal to 3% to 5% of total body mass. Dehydration not only decreases aerobic and anaerobic performance, but also decreases performance in activities that depend on both aerobic and anaerobic metabolism, such as wrestling and team ball sports.

Although laboratory tests, such as urine osmolality and urine specific gravity, are more accurate than field tests for the determination of hydration status, they are not available in many situations. Thus, the field tests of loss of body mass during activity and urine color are used in most situations to assess hydration status.

Hyponatremia, or low blood sodium concentration, results in swelling of the brain and can occur during long-term physical activity, such as an ultramarathon. Hyponatremia can be life-threatening, and although its cause is not completely elucidated, it may be due to ingestion of high volumes of fluids that are low in sodium content during activity. Various factors, such as hot, humid environments, protective clothing or equipment that decreases heat loss, participation in a weight-class sport, and decreased functioning of the thirst mechanism due to aging, increase susceptibility to dehydration. When factors increasing susceptibility to dehydration are present, particular attention must be paid to maintaining hydration by adequate fluid ingestion.

During all activities and sports, the hydration guidelines that have been developed to encourage fluid ingestion prior to, during, and after activity should be followed to help maintain euhydration. The hydration guidelines are best applied in the context of an individualized, customized hydration plan. Although many times overlooked, water is an essential nutrient, and adequate fluid ingestion to prevent dehydration is necessary for optimal physical performance.

REVIEW QUESTIONS

Fill-in-the-Blank

1. Euhydration is possible when fluid intake is _____ to water loss.

2. Osmotic pressure caused by _____ allows water to stay where it is needed and travel throughout the body.

3. Three major factors contributing to the risk of dehydration include _____, _____, and _____.

4. When measuring hydration status, as compared with laboratory hydration assessments, _____ assessments are less accurate.

5. Hyponatremia is characterized by a loss of blood _____ to a level lower than 117 to 128 $mmol \cdot L^{-1}$.

Multiple Choice

1. Which listed electrolyte is typically found as a cation in the body?
   a. Chloride
   b. Potassium
   c. Iodide
   d. Flouride

2. Hyponatremia is characterized by deficiency in_____.
   a. nutremium
   b. potassium
   c. calcium
   d. sodium

3. Cognitive and physical performance decrements begin to occur when dehydration is at a level of:

a. >5%

b. <1%

c. 7% to 10%

d. 2%

4. When thirst occurs during physical activity,

a. the person is still euhydrated.

b. the activity should be stopped.

c. thirst is a natural component of any physical exertion; nothing needs to be done.

d. the person is in a dehydrated state already.

5. Hydration guidelines promote

a. adequate fluid ingestion before, during, and after activity.

b. the best types of hydrating fluids to consume.

c. the best sources of water.

d. the best types of activity for avoiding dehydration.

True/False

1. It is better to consume as many electrolytes as possible before a bout of physical exertion than to risk having deficiencies in electrolyte concentrations.

2. As opposed to the minerals supplied in a normally healthy diet, extra minerals should be consumed to maintain adequate hydration and electrolyte balances in athletes and exercisers.

3. Anaerobically dominant sports do not cause dehydration and do not rely on optimal hydration states for optimal performances.

4. Older athletes are at less risk of dehydration than young athletes.

5. Dehydration is affected by humidity, wind, age, clothing, and the particular activity.

Short Answer

1. What causes varying electrolyte content in urine?

2. What causes activity-related dehydration?

3. Which factors contribute to activity-related dehydration?

4. What causes hyponatremia and what are its immediate side effects?

5. How can 68% of one 180-lb man's body weight be water whereas only 59% of another 180-lb man's body weight is water?

KEY TERMS

aldosterone: a hormone secreted by the adrenal glands that is responsible for conserving bodily sodium concentrations

anion: a molecule that has a negative electrical charge

cation: a molecule that has a positive electrical charge

dehydration: loss of bodily water

electrolyte: a substance that disassociates in water, producing charged molecules

electrolyte balance: maintenance of intracellular and extracellular electrolyte concentrations for optimal bodily functioning

euhydration: referring to normal body hydration or water content of the body

feces: solid human waste excreted from the gastrointestinal tract

hyperthermia: body temperature that is above normal resting body temperature

hypertonic: a fluid having an osmotic pressure greater than that of blood

hypohydration: less than normal body hydration or water content of the body

hyponatremia: a condition characterized by blood plasma sodium levels falling below 135 $mmol \cdot L^{-1}$

hypotonic: a fluid having a lower osmotic pressure than blood

insensible water loss: unnoticed loss of water from the respiratory pathways during breathing and by evaporation from the non-sweating skin

ion: a molecule that has an electrical charge

isotonic: a fluid having an osmotic pressure equal to that of blood

metabolic water: water produced during normal metabolism

osmotic pressure: the force created by a greater concentration of osmotically active substances (electrolytes, glucose, proteins, and other substances) on one side of a membrane that draws water through the membrane toward the side with a greater concentration of substances

thirst: a conscious desire to drink fluids

urine: a fluid substance excreted to rid the body of waste products and maintain proper bodily fluid and electrolyte concentrations

urine osmolality: the quantity of substances contained within a given amount of urine fluid

urine specific gravity: density of urine compared with the density water

water balance: maintenance of normal hydration by ingesting as much water as is lost

REFERENCES

1. Almond C, Shin AY, Fortescue EB, et al. Hyponatremia among runners in the Boston Marathon. N Engl J Med. 2005;352:1550–1556.

2. Armstrong LE, Costill DL, Fink WJ. Influence of diuretic-induced dehydration on competitive running performance. Med Sci Sports Exerc. 1985;17:456–461.

3. Armstrong LE, Maresh CM, Castellani JW, et al. Urinary indices of hydration status. Int J Sport Nutr. 1994;4:265–279.

4. Baker LB, Dougherty KA, Chow M, et al. Progressive dehydration causes a progressive decline in basketball skill performance. Med Sci Sports Exerc. 2007;39:1114–1123.

5. Barr SI. Effects of dehydration on exercise performance. Can J Appl Physiol. 1999;24:164–172.

6. Binkley HM, Beckett J, Casa DJ, et al. National Athletic Trainers' Association position statement: exertional heat illnesses. J Athl Train. 2002;37:329–343.

7. Burge CM, Carey MF, Payne WR. Rowing performance, fluid balance, and metabolic function following dehydration and rehydration. Med Sci Sports Exerc. 1993;25:1358–1364.

8. Casa DJ, Armstrong LE, Hillman SK, et al. National Athletic Trainers' Association position statement: fluid replacement for athletes. J Athl Train. 2000;35:212–224.

9. Cheuvront SN, Montain SJ, Sawka MN. Fluid replacement and performance during the marathon. Sports Med. 2007;37:353–357.

10. Convertino V, Armstrong LE, Coyle EF, et al. ACSM position stand: exercise and fluid replacement. Med Sci Sports Exerc. 1996;28:i–ix.

11. Coyle EF. Fluid and fuel intake during exercise. J Sports Sci. 2004;22:39–55.

12. Dougherty KA, Baker LB, Chow M, et al. Two percent dehydration impairs and six percent carbohydrate drink improves boys basketball skills. Med Sci Sports Exerc. 2006;38:1650–1658.

13. Dressendorler R, Wade CE, Keen CL, et al. Plasma mineral levels in marathon runners during a 20-day road race. Phys Sportsmed. 1982;10:113–118.

14. Edwards AM, Mann ME, Marfell-Jones MJ, et al. Influence of moderate dehydration on soccer performance: physiological responses to 45 min of outdoor match-play and the immediate subsequent performance of sport-specific and mental concentration tests. Br J Sports Med. 2007;41:385–391.

15. Gonzalez-Alonso J, Mora-Rodriguez R, Below PR, et al. Dehydration markedly impairs cardiovascular function in hyperthermic endurance athletes during exercise. J Appl Physiol. 1997;82:1229–1236.

16. Hickner RC, Horswill CA, Welker JM, et al. Test development for the study of physical performance in wrestlers following weight loss. Int J Sports Med. 1991;12:557–562.

17. Hoffman JR, Stavsky H, Falk B. The effect of water restriction on anaerobic power and vertical jumping height in basketball players. Int J Sports Med. 1995;16:214–218.

18. Kraemer WJ, Fry AC, Rubin MR, et al. Physiological and performance responses to tournament wrestling. Med Sci Sports Exerc. 2001;33:1367–1378.

19. Krustrup P, Mohr M, Amstrup T, et al. The yo-yo intermittent recovery test: physiological response, reliability, and validity. Med Sci Sports Exerc. 2003;35:697–705.

20. Locke M. The cellular stress response to exercise: role of stress proteins. Exerc Sport Sci Rev. 1997;25:105–136.

21. Mack G. The body fluid and hemopoietic systems. In: Tipton, CM, Sawka M, Tate CA, eds. ACSM's Advanced Exercise Physiology. Phildelphia, PA: Lippincott Williams & Wilkins, 2006:501–519.

22. Maughn R, Burke LM, Coyle EF, eds. Food, Nutrition and Sports Performance II. The International Olympic Committee Consensus on Sports Nutrition. London: Routledge, 2004.

23. Mohr M, Krustrup P, Bangsbo J. Match performance of high-standard soccer players with special reference to development of fatigue. J Sports Sci. 2003;21:519–528.

24. Noakes TD. Drinking guidelines for exercise: What evidence is there that athletes should drink "as much as tolerable", "to replace the weight lost during exercise" or "ad libitum"? J Sports Sci. 2007;25:781–796.

25. Oppliger RA, Bartok C. Hydration testing of athletes. Sports Med. 2002;32:959–971.

26. Sato F, Owen M, Matthes R, et al. Functional and morphological changes in the eccrine sweat gland with heat acclimation. J Appl Physiol. 1990;69:232–236.

27. Sawka M, Montain SJ, Latzka WA. Body fluid balance during exercise-heat exposure. In: Buskirk ER, Puhl S, eds. Fluid Balance in Exercise and Sport. Boca Raton, FL: CRC Press, 1996:139–157.

28. Sawka M, Burke LM, Eicher ER, et al. Exercise and fluid replacement. Med Sci Sports Exerc. 39:377–390.

29. Sawka M, Pandolf KB. Effects of body water loss on physiological function and exercise performance. In: Gisolfi C, Lamb DR, eds. Perspectives in Exercise Science and Sports Medicine. Carmel, IN: Brown and Benchmark, 1990:1–38.

30. Sawka MN, Burke LM, Eichner ER, et al. American College of Sports Medicine position stand. Exercise and fluid replacement. Med Sci Sports Exerc. 2007;39:377–390.

31. Sawka MN, Coyle EF. Influence of body water and blood volume on thermoregulation and exercise performance in the heat. Exerc Sport Sci Rev. 1999;27:167–218.

32. Sawka MN, Noakes TD. Does dehydration impair exercise performance? Med Sci Sports Exerc. 2007;39:1209–1217.

33. Schoffstall JE, Branch JD, Leutholtz BC, et al. Effects of dehydration and rehydration on the one-repetition maximum bench press of weight-trained males. J Strength Cond Res. 2001;15:102–108.

34. Serfass R, Strull GA, Ewing JL. The effect the rapid weight loss and attempted rehydration on strength endurance of the hand gripping muscles in college wrestlers. Res Q Exerc Sport. 1984;55:46–52.

35. Shirreffs SM, Armstrong LE, Cheuvront SN. Fluid and electrolyte needs for preparation and recovery from training and competition. J Sports Sci. 2004;22:57–63.

36. Singer R, Weiss SA. Effects of weight reduction on selected anthropometric, physical, performance measures of wrestlers. Res Q. 1968;39:369–371.

37. Smith MS, Dyson R, Hale T, et al. The effects in humans of rapid loss of body mass on a boxing-related task. Eur J Appl Physiol. 2000;83:34–39.

38. Speedy DB, Faris JG, Hamlin M, et al. Hyponatremia and weight changes in an ultradistance triathlon. Clin J Sport Med. 1997;7:180–184.

39. Speedy DB, Noakes TD, Rogers IR, et al. Hyponatremia in ultradistance triathletes. Med Sci Sports Exerc. 1999;31:809–815.

40. Webster S, Rutt R, Weltman A. Physiological effects of a weight loss regimen practiced by college wrestlers. Med Sci Sports Exerc. 1990;22:229–234.

41. Wenos D, Amato HK. Weight cycling alters muscular strength and endurance, ratings of perceived exertion, and total body water in college wrestlers. Percept Motor Skills. 1998;87:975–978.

Suggested Readings

Armstrong LE. Assessing hydration status: The elusive gold standard. J Am Coll Nutr. 2007;26(5):575S–584S.

Armstrong LE, Epstein Y. Fluid–electrolyte balance during labor and exercise: Concepts and misconceptions. Int J Sport Nutr. 1999;9(1): 1–12.

Armstrong LE, Maresh CM, Castellani JW, et al. Urinary indices of hydration status. Int J Sport Nutr. 1994;4(3):265–279.

Armstrong LE. Performing in Extreme Environments. Champaign, IL: Human Kinetics Publishers, 2000.

Armstrong LE, Curtis WC, Hubbard RW, et al. Symptomatic hyponatremia during prolonged exercise in heat. Med Sci Sports Exerc. 1993;25(5):543–549.

Armstrong LE, Soto JA, Hacker FT Jr, et al. Urinary indices during dehydration, exercise, and rehydration. Int J Sport Nutr. 1998;8(4): 345–355.

Armstrong LE, Szlyk PC, De Luca JP, et al. Fluid–electrolyte losses in uniforms during prolonged exercise at 30 degrees C. Aviat Space Environ Med. 1992;63(5):351–355.

Binkley HM, Beckett J, Casa DJ, et al. National Athletic Trainers' Association position statement: exertion heat illness. J Athl Train. 2002;37:329–343.

Casa DL, Armstrong LE, Hillman SK, et al. National Athletic Trainers Association position statement: Fluid replacement for athletes. J Athl Train. 2000;35:212–224.

Corvertino VA, Armstrong LE, Coyle EF, et al. ACSM position stand: Exercise and fluid replacement. Med Sci Sports Exerc. 1996;28(10): i–ix.

Dougherty KA, Baker LB, Chow M, et al. Two percent dehydration impairs and six percent carbohydrate drink improves boys basketball skills. Med Sci Sports Exerc. 2006;38:1650–1658.

Dougherty KA, Baker LB, Chow M, et al. Progressive dehydration causes a progressive decline in basketball skill performance. Med Sci Sports Exerc. 2007;39:1114–1123.

Kraemer WJ, Fry AC, Rubin MR, et al. Physiological and performance responses to tournament wrestling. Med Sci Sports Exerc. 2001;33:1367–1378.

Oppliger RA, Bartok C. Hydration testing of athletes. Sports Med. 2002;32:959–971.

Sawka MN, Burke LM, Eicher ER, et al. Exercise and fluid replacement. Med Sci Sports Exerc. 2007;39:377–390.

Speedy DB, Noakes TD, Rogers IR, et al. Hyponatremia in ultraendurance triathletes. Med Sci Sports Exerc. 1999;31:809–821.

Classic References

Costill DL. Sweating: its composition and effects on body fluids. Ann N Y Acad Sci. 1977;301:160–174.

Costill DL, Fink WJ. Plasma volume changes following exercise and thermal dehydration. J Appl Physiol. 1974;37(4):521–525.

Dill DB, Costill DL. Calculation of percentage changes in volumes of blood, plasma, and red cells in dehydration. J Appl Physiol. 1974;37(2):247–248.

Dill DB, Hall FG, Van Beaumont W. Sweat chloride concentration: sweat rate, metabolic rate, skin temperature, and age. J Appl Physiol. 1966;21(1):99–106.

Dill DB, Horvath SM, Van Beaumont W, Gehlsen G, Burrus K. Sweat electrolytes in desert walks. J Appl Physiol. 1967;23(5):746–751.

Gisolfi CV, Summers RW, Lambert GP, et al. Effect of beverage osmolality on intestinal fluid absorption during exercise. J Appl Physiol. 1998;85(5):1941–1948.

Kenney WL, Anderson RK. Responses of older and younger women to exercise in dry and humid heat without fluid replacement. Med Sci Sports Exerc. 1988;20(2):155–160.

10

Environmental Challenges and Exercise Performance

After reading this chapter, you should be able to:

1. Explain the physiological basis and purpose of thermoregulation

2. Identify the mechanisms of heat loss

3. Describe different forms of heat illness by identifying the mechanisms by which they occur, effects on the body, and factors/mechanisms that affect and alter occurrence

4. Explain the thermoregulatory considerations of performance in the heat for both endurance and anaerobically based exertions

5. Identify and describe principle factors in the prevention of heat illness and thermoregulatory-related declines in performance capabilities

6. Describe the physiological basis of cold stress and how cold temperatures affect exertion capability

7. Identify the means of adaptation to cold environments and survival strategies when in dangerous situations

8. Explain the basis of altitude stress and identify the challenges, responses, and factors of exertion affected by high altitudes

9. Describe the nature of altitude sickness and strategies incorporating altitude training for performance

Environmental conditions are one of the major influences on the physiology of the body. Indeed, elements, such as the environment, play a major role in the body's responses and adaptations to exercise. Environmental extremes can also be a threat to survival. In athletics, they can dramatically, yet often differentially, impact performances. For example, when performed at an altitude of 2,200 m (7,218 ft), the time it takes to finish a 10-km race may be increased by 2 minutes; yet at that same altitude, performance times during a 400-m (1,312-ft) race are unaffected. In fact, world records in the 400-m race have been set while competing at altitude. Proper exercise training and progression, under the different environmental conditions, will help to offset some of the physiological stress and performance deficits. Understanding the challenges one is faced with under different environmental conditions is critical to understanding how to properly prepare the body for such physiological demands.

Three of the major environmental challenges an athlete faces are heat, cold, and altitude. Each places a specific demand on the body's physiological systems. Under each of these environmental conditions, performance can be affected. Furthermore, each of these environmental conditions can cause serious injury and even death if the body is not adequately prepared for such exposures. Exercise only increases the homeostatic demands under such environmental conditions, thereby increasing the physiological stress. Using proper training, clothing, and nutritional and acclimation/acclimatization strategies to cope with environmental challenges is vital to performance, health, and well-being.

HEAT STRESS

The challenge of heat stress, or **hyperthermia**, resides in the fact that the body must dissipate the considerable heat produced by working muscles during exercise. This stems from the fact that human beings are only about 25% to 27% efficient in converting the energy contained in food substrates into usable energy adenosine triphosphate (ATP) to supply working muscles, with the rest (~75%) being released as heat. The inability to dissipate this excess heat energy through various homeothermic mechanisms can create problems with **thermoregulation**, or the ability of the body to maintain a constant internal temperature.

Environmental conditions of elevated heat and humidity only make this a more dramatic challenge. In essence, high temperature and humidity can block heat dissipation from the body, thereby increasing the heat stress experienced by the athlete. From a normal core temperature of about 37°C (98.6°F), intense exercise in the heat can rapidly result in dangerously elevated core temperature levels of 41°C (105.8°F), leading to serious heat illness.[1] Thus, it is important to understand this environmental stressor to prevent heat illnesses and optimize performance in the heat.[1,25]

Thermoregulation

If the body is to physiologically respond to maintain its desired core temperature, it must be able to sense changes in temperature. Receptors that detect increases or decreases in temperature exist in both the periphery and the hypothalamus.[17] The peripheral receptors are located in and under the skin and in the peritoneal (abdominal) cavity. In the central nervous system, in addition to the hypothalamus, receptors are located in the brain stem and spinal cord.[8]

As it does with so many physiological functions, the hypothalamus plays a central role in integrating and regulating body temperature at 37°C (98.6°F) by controlling responses throughout the body. In other words, the hypothalamus can act like a "thermostat," sending signals to increase or decrease the temperature using different mechanisms at its command (Fig. 10-1). When body temperature increases, signals from the thermosensitive receptors as well as the temperature of the blood are detected by the hypothalamus, resulting in a host of different physiological responses, ranging from increased heart rate and cardiac output, to increased vasodilation, to accelerated rates of sweating.

The factors that determine the thermoregulatory stress that the environment imparts on the body are ambient temperature, relative humidity, and wind speed. The **relative humidity** is the percentage of water vapor held in the air. For example, a relative humidity of 30% means that air contains only 30% of the moisture it is capable of holding; a relative humidity of 90% means that only 10% more moisture can be absorbed by the surrounding air. A relative humidity of 30% with a temperature of 32.2°C (90°F) registers on the **heat stress index** as low-to-moderate risk, whereas a relative humidity of 90% at the same ambient air temperature registers as a high risk on the heat stress index. In the first case, it may be safe to hold a sport practice, but in the latter case, one should practice at another time (see Case study on page 320). Wind speed contributes to the effect of convective cooling on the body and can reduce, to a certain extent, the heat stress index.

Mechanisms of Heat Loss

The body has four basic mechanisms that can help maintain its proper core temperature and foster heat loss:

1. Convection
2. Conduction
3. Radiation
4. Evaporation

Convection

Convection is when air blowing over the surface of the skin removes the air warmed by the body and replaces it with cooler air. Think about how different it would feel going out for a run on a warm summer day with the wind blowing 1 mph versus 10 mph. This is the basis for the cooling effects of fans as well. The environment, whether artificial (fans) or natural (breeze), can effectively help the body lose heat by convection. Even during a heat wave, the risk of death can be reduced if fans are properly used (i.e., directed at the body) to promote convective cooling in the home.[7] Heat loss with convective cooling depends on the speed and temperature of the air. Obviously, replacing

Acute Regulation

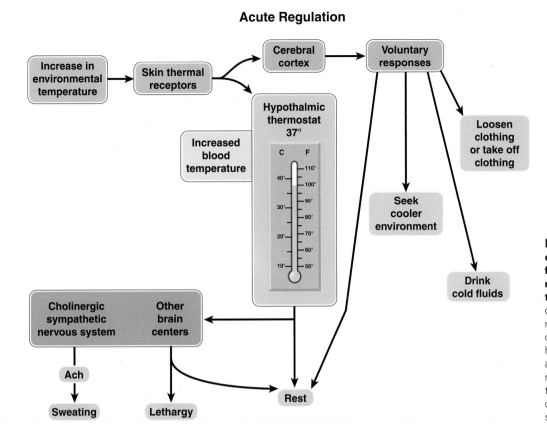

Figure 10-1. Integration of information is vital for the hypothalamus to regulate and control core temperature. Input and output mechanisms are monitored to help regulate core temperature. Input from higher blood temperature and from thermosensitive receptors will provide signals to the hypothalamus to cause skin vasodilatation and sweating.

the body's surface air layer with a warm airflow will not be as effective as with a cooler air flow. This can be easily understood by thinking about a fan blowing warm air versus a window air conditioner unit blowing cool air over your body as you stand in front of it. Interestingly, water can also have a convective heat loss element as it runs over the skin. The speed of the moving water and its temperature will impact its convective effectiveness for heat loss. Various types of water cooling suits and head covers have been experimented with for industrial, military, and space applications and have been shown to be effective.[44,53]

Conduction

Conduction occurs when there is physical contact between two surfaces and the direction of heat flow is from the warmer to the cooler object. Per the above example, a cold water flow over the skin will promote the conduction of heat from the warmer skin to the cooler water. Conversely, using a hot water whirlpool tub for a therapeutic treatment of your knee would promote the flow of heat from the water to the immersed parts of your body. Because of its conductive properties, placing a person in a cool water bath will reduce body temperature more quickly and effectively than standing in cool air even if the water and air were at the same temperature. Also, the amount of surface area in contact with the object will affect the rate of heat loss (to a cool object) or gain (from a cool object to a warm one). That is, when core temperature is high, submerging the person

in an ice water bath will have a greater cooling effect than placing ice bags on specific body parts.

Radiation

Radiation involves molecules in motion that are constantly moving and giving off heat in the form of electromagnetic waves. In a normal ambient environment of about 75°F or 23.9°C, radiation accounts for about 67% of total heat loss, whereas in a hot environment of 95°F or 35°C, only about 4% of the total amount of heat lost by the body is due to radiation. When the surrounding heat is greater than body temperature, heat can actually be gained by the body. A greater flow of radiant heat is given off if the surrounding environment is cooler. Radiant heat energy is absorbed from different sources, most obviously direct sunlight, reflected sunlight, and other sources of heat energy than the body, such as a radiator or a sauna. Thus, playing a tennis match in the Australian Open on a sunny, hot, and humid day will present a demanding set of conditions producing a high amount of heat stress. Interestingly, the radiant energy from the sun at altitude is greater than that at sea level because the sun rays are not filtered as well by the atmosphere and this results in increased light intensity resulting in more dramatic effects in shorter periods of time (e.g., sun burns).

Evaporation

Evaporation occurs when water located on the surface of the body's skin and respiratory airways transforms to

Box 10-1 DID YOU KNOW?

Sweating: Wearing a T-Shirt Versus Bare Skin

Often, when exercising in the heat, the obvious temptation is to take off a T-shirt and exercise with maximal bare skin exposure. Although at first glance this may seem to make sense, one might think again. Sweat is most valuable while it is on the surface of the body going through an evaporative cooling phenomenon to help cool the body. This cooling effect impacts the flow of blood to the skin, where it is cooled and circulated back to the core of the body to help internal cooling, as well. If the sweat drops off of the skin's surface

before it can cycle through the evaporative processes, you reduce a major cooling effect for the body. This is especially true for intense exercise or in conditions of high heat, where sweat rates are high. Wearing a white or light T-shirt or specialized shirts made of microfibers (e.g., shirts made by Under Armour and CoolMax) that allow proper retention of sweat on the skin for evaporative cooling will be more beneficial. In addition, electromagnetic UV wave exposure to the skin without sun block can also promote skin cancer.

its gaseous state (vaporization), which absorbs heat and thus cools the body. This type of evaporation occurs constantly (water continuously diffuses from the body onto the surface of the skin, and by breathing we continuously lose heat from the respiratory tract), but because we are not consciously aware of its occurrence, it is called "insensible evaporation." When there is a greater-than-usual heat load placed on the body, such as during exercise, the sweating mechanism is triggered. Sweating is a specialized form of evaporative heat loss that involves the secretion of a dilute salt solution from sweat glands found in numerous locations throughout the body. These sweat glands secrete this hypotonic solution onto the skin upon stimulation by the sympathetic nervous system. Sometimes you notice, for example, sweaty palms in a anxiety response and this should not be confused with sweating in response to thermal challenges. Thermal evaporation and body cooling occurs when a heat signal stimulates sweat glands to secrete sweat, which can be altered in its composition depending on heat acclimatization, climate, diet, and genetic factors.[39]

Because the body is warm, some surface layer sweat/water molecules have greater kinetic heat energy than other sweat/water molecules that have not absorbed as much body heat. These faster-moving molecules vaporize because they have sufficient kinetic energy for water to be converted from its liquid phase to its gaseous phase. This leaves on the skin those sweat/water molecules that have lower kinetic energy, thus causing the sweat to be at a lower temperature and resulting in evaporative cooling of the skin while allowing heat to escape. With continued exercise and heat production, this sweating cycle of molecular kinetics repeats itself over and over again, allowing the body to benefit from evaporative cooling. In the process, water is lost and the body can become seriously dehydrated, as 1 to 2 (and in extreme cases 4) L·hr^{-1} of sweat can be lost during intense exercise under hot, humid conditions. With the combination of passive and active evaporative processes, water loss can become significant, which underscores the importance of proper hydration during exercise to prevent hypohydration and dehydration (see Chapter 9).[45]

Balance of Heat Gain and Heat Loss

The challenge the body faces in heat stress or exercising in a hot environment is maintaining proper balance between heat gain and heat loss (Fig. 10-2). A very precise balance must be established if core temperature is to be maintained within acceptable limits. If this balance cannot be achieved,

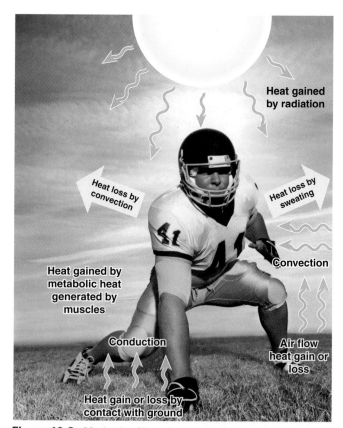

Figure 10-2. Methods of heat loss and gain. Heat produced by the body during exercise is dramatic due to the contractions of muscles and the low efficiency of the human body to use all energy. Heat is gained from conduction from contact with the ground, convection, and radiation. Heat loss is imperative to maintain normal physiological function. Heat loss is helped through convection from the peripheral vasodilation of the blood and sweating to enhance evaporative cooling.

uncontrolled hyperthermia, possibly leading to death, can occur. On one side of the scale are the factors leading to heat gain, including exercise intensity and duration, amount of muscular activation, hormonal influences, thermic effects of food, environmental conditions, hydration status, clothing, and basal metabolic rate. On the other side of the scale are the mechanisms of heat loss described earlier, in addition to extraneous cooling methods and hydration protocols. An integration of these many factors determines whether the body is capable of maintaining its core temperature within tolerable physiological limits without any resulting adverse symptoms or heat illness.

Circulatory and Metabolic Responses to Heat Stress

Circulatory responses to heat are another set of important mechanisms related to the physiological adjustments to a heat challenge. Even under resting conditions, heat increases heart rate and cardiac output and redirects circulatory flow. In essence, with this increased cardiac output, the body redistributes some of the blood flow to the periphery so that heat can be dissipated and blood cooled. Sitting or exercising in the heat results in reddened skin and flushed complexions because of the increase in peripheral blood flow. This, along with increased sweating, marks the body's attempts to dissipate heat.

Influence of Body Composition and Physical Fitness Level

Body composition can significantly influence susceptibility to heat stress. Heat production with exercise is related to an individual's body mass, and therefore, heat storage per unit of body surface area will be greater in a larger person when compared with a smaller person. For example, a National Football League (NFL) offensive linemen who is 6′6″ (1.98 m) tall and weighs 360 pounds (163.6 kg) will be at a distinct disadvantage in a hot football game in Miami in August because the amount of heat produced per unit of body surface area (where evaporation occurs) is greater than it is for a defensive back who is 6′ tall (1.83 m) and weighs 180 lbs (81.8 kg). High percentages of body fat will make matters even worse for the lineman because the insulating effect of fat will make heat loss more difficult.

One's physical fitness is also important when it comes to toleration of a hot environment. In a hot environment, redistribution of blood from the core to the peripheral tissue is needed to help dissipate heat. This means that blood that typically would be directed to the musculature during exercise is now being sent to the periphery just under the skin to allow heat to escape. If not enough heat is dissipated, hyperthermia (increase in body-core temperature) can result. Furthermore, if too much blood is sent away from the core, it would be difficult for the body to perform intense muscular activity because of

reduced blood flow. Therefore, the balance between the percentage of the cardiac output sent to the periphery to dissipate heat versus that which is needed for the core organs and musculature is very delicate. Therefore, when intense exercise is performed, this balance between the two physiological functions is at odds. Individuals who have greater maximal oxygen consumption will have greater cardiac output capabilities and, when combined with a lower body fat and favorable skin surface area to body mass ratio, will have a distinct advantage when exercising in the heat.

Heat Illness

With the onset of exercise, heat is produced and the challenge for the body is to maintain core temperature despite this greater heat load. At higher ambient temperatures, this challenge is made even more difficult because there is less of a temperature gradient between the body and its environment. Consequently, the potential for heat illness increases. Understanding and recognizing the basic forms of heat illness is vital for optimizing safety when exercising.[1,2]

Heat Cramps

Exercise-induced **heat cramps** are muscle cramps that occur when a person is exposed to heat, and often results from dehydration, a whole body sodium deficit, and neuromuscular fatigue (Fig. 10-3). Just watching various sports on television, one can see many players in soccer, American football, rugby, and lacrosse bend down, holding their thighs or calves, seemingly in pain, and athletic trainers trying to stretch the affected muscle. Typically, these cramps are brought on by intense exercise and are characterized by

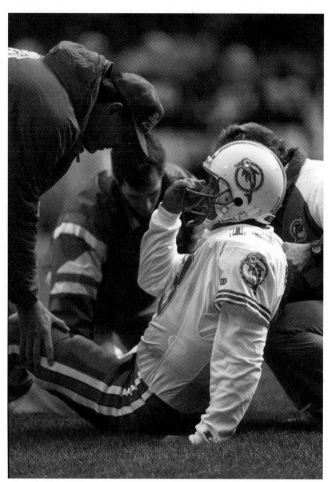

Figure 10-3. Heat cramp. Heat cramps are very common in recreational activities and sports involving intense exercise in the heat with other associated challenges from dehydration and electrolyte losses. Heat cramps are involuntary contractions of the musculature and are very painful. Heat cramps are treated by resting and cooling down, fluid and electrolyte intake, performing gentle range-of-motion stretching and gentle massage of the affected muscle group, and having a physician consult if they do not go away with in 1 hour.

very painful, involuntary muscle contractions. However, muscle cramps may even occur at rest after practices or an exercise bout. A combination of factors can contribute to heat cramps, including dehydration, electrolyte imbalances, and/or neuromuscular fatigue from multiple practices. The term "heat cramps" may be a misnomer because they often occur when core temperature is in the normal range. Interestingly, heat cramps have been found to be the most common form of heat illness in the first 3 weeks of two-a-day American football practices in hot environments.[16]

Syncope

When an athlete or any individual sits or stands for a long time in the heat, or has just completed an activity in the heat, heat **syncope**, or fainting, can occur. Dizziness or lightheadedness in the heat can be caused by too much

peripheral dilation, pooling of blood in the legs reducing venous return, dehydration, a reduction in the cardiac output, or possibly brain ischemia.[1,11] This heat illness is more common in individuals who have not been acclimated or acclimatized to a hot environment.

Heat Exhaustion

Heat exhaustion during exercise can result from a host of different factors, including heavy sweating, dehydration, sodium loss, and energy depletion. It typically occurs in hot and humid environments, making its diagnosis difficult at best for many coaches. Signs and symptoms include pallor, persistent muscular cramps, weakness, fainting, dizziness, headache, hyperventilation, nausea, diarrhea, an acute loss of drive to eat, decreased urine output, and a body-core temperature that generally ranges between 36°C (97°F) and 40°C (104°F).[1,10,18] It should be noted that heat exhaustion due to exercise is difficult to distinguish from exertional heat stroke (EHS). When in doubt, cooling treatment for heat stroke should be practiced because the potential health consequences, which include death, are more severe for heat stroke than for heat exhaustion.

Exertional Heat Stroke

Exertional heat stroke (EHS) is a genuine medical emergency, but it is often confused with heat exhaustion. If not treated quickly, heat stroke can lead to death.[10] With intense or long-duration exercise, heat production from the body or the inability to get rid of the heat can overwhelm the thermoregulatory system and heat stroke can occur. Death from EHS is a tragedy of inaction, as it can be effectively treated if proper actions are taken immediately (Fig. 10-4). With heat stroke, core temperature is typically elevated to greater than 40°C (104°F), causing cellular damage to organs and tissues, including the thermoregulatory center in the hypothalamus. Accordingly, heat loss mechanisms are typically shut down with heat stroke allowing further elevations in core temperature (death can occur at core temperatures in excess of 43°C or 109.4°F). Although many methods of measuring core temperature are available, the most accurate is rectal temperature measurement.[12] Physiological changes that occur with heat stroke include an increase in lactic acidosis, excessive potassium in the blood, acute renal failure, rhabdomyolysis (destruction of muscle tissue resulting in myoglobin and other proteins normally found in muscle appearing in blood), bleeding disorders, and other medical conditions. These changes, in combination, may result in death. Signs and symptoms of heat stroke include rapid heart rate (tachycardia), hypotension, sweating (although skin may be dry at the time of collapse), hyperventilation, altered mental state, diarrhea, seizures, and coma. Treatment must be focused on rapidly cooling the body, as the longer the delay in treatment of EHS, the greater the chance of death (Fig. 10-5).

Journal of Strength and Conditioning Research, 2006, 20(3), 462
© 2006 National Strength & Conditioning Association

SURVIVAL STRATEGY: ACUTE TREATMENT OF EXERTIONAL HEAT STROKE

DOUGLAS J. CASA,[1] JEFFREY M. ANDERSON,[1] LAWRENCE E. ARMSTRONG,[1] AND CARL M. MARESH[1]

[1]Human Performance Laboratory, Department of Kinesiology, Neag School of Education, University of Connecticut, Storrs, Connecticut 06269.

When athletes perform intense exercise in the heat, the risk of exertional heat stroke (EHS) is ever present. Although all possible efforts should be made to minimize the risk of EHS (i.e., acclimatize athletes prior to onset of twice daily practices, optimize athletes' fitness, schedule practices during the cooler times of the day, maintain good hydration, modify practice schedules based on environmental conditions, apply appropriate work-to-rest ratios, increase gradually the amount of equipment and uniform items, progressively increase the duration and intensity of practices, etc.), even the best efforts of the most proactive medical and coaching staffs cannot prevent all cases of EHS. As the twice daily practices begin in August in a wide variety of sports and across many levels of competition, the sponsoring institutions and all health care professionals need to be certain that proper precautions are in place so that if EHS occurs, tragedy is averted.

The strategy relies on the prompt assessment and rapid treatment of EHS. Assessment involves two key components: a) identification of central nervous system (CNS) dysfunction and b) rapid and accurate determination of core body temperature. Signs of CNS dysfunction include irrational behavior, altered consciousness, convulsions, coma, dizziness, irritability, emotional instability, hysteria, apathy, feeling out-of-sorts, staggering, confusion, disorientation, and delirium. A temperature greater than 105°F (40.6°C) at the time of collapse indicates possible EHS. The ability to rapidly perform both portions of the assessment is critical because an athlete may have a brief (10–15 minutes) lucid interval during which he or she may be conscious, coherent, and conversant but likely feels out-of-sorts, and a coach or athletic trainer who knows the athlete well may recognize that something is amiss. The temperature assessment must be obtained rectally. Recent research has clearly shown that when athletes perform intense exercise in the heat, axillary, oral, aural, tympanic, and temporal temperature measurements are not valid because they are influenced by hyperventilation, ingestion of oral fluids, skin temperature changes, sweat, and other mitigating factors. Therefore, these other methods do not accurately reflect core temperature. An accurate temperature becomes even more vital if the athlete has a lucid interval because critical treatment time can be lost. If the athlete with suspected EHS has a core temperature greater than 105°F and/or CNS dysfunction is evident, whole-body cooling must begin immediately.

In treating EHS, the adage "cool first, transport second" should guide immediate care if proper medical staff is on site (i.e., athletic trainer or team physician). In addition to calling an ambulance when an EHS has been identified, the medical staff should have an emergency plan in place to cool the athlete until the rectal temperature reaches 102°F (39°C; in the absence of any other emergent issues) before the athlete is transported to the nearest medical facility. Even if medical personnel are not present, we recommend cooling until the ambulance arrives because rapid cooling is the key to surviving EHS.

Although an athlete should be cooled by any means available, the best cooling rates have been found with cold-water immersion (CWI). This can be easily done in a cold tub in an athletic training facility or with a sturdy Rubbermaid tub placed near the practice facility. (A bed sheet or towel placed under the athlete's armpits and held by an assistant behind the athlete ensures that the patient does not go underwater.) The tub should be half filled with water in the shade, and three or four coolers of ice should be positioned nearby for quickly reducing the water temperature as needed. The water temperature should be kept between 45°F and 58°F (7°C to 14°C). Except for the head, as much of the body should be immersed as possible. The water should be circulated during cooling, and the athlete's rectal temperature should be monitored during cooling. Once the athlete's temperature reaches 102°F (39°C), he or she can be removed from the water. Recruit teammates or other staff to assist with lifting the EHS patient in and out of the tub. If an uninterrupted rectal temperature assessment is not possible during CWI then we recommend an initial rectal temperature assessment followed by 10 minutes of CWI and then a re-check of rectal temperature. Cooling rates with CWI will be approximately .36°F·min^{-1} (.2°C·min^{-1}) and an educated guess can be made regarding core temperature changes if an initial rectal temperature is obtained and length of cooling is recorded. Although CWI is clearly the superior cooling method, if a tub is not available, other methods may be utilized, as follows: placing cold, wet towels on the body and replacing these frequently with fresh towels; splashing cold water on the body and directing fans at the athlete; placing the athlete in a cold shower; and covering the athlete with ice.

We believe that survival is optimized (and nearly guaranteed) when accurate assessment and CWI are immediately implemented. Institutional policies and procedures may need to be modified regarding EHS to reflect these recommendations, and the details should be discussed and practiced before an incident occurs. EHS is a constant risk for athletes participating in hot environments; the risk of death from EHS need not be.

ADDITIONAL RESOURCES

BINKLEY, H.M., J. BECKETT, D.J. CASA, D. KLEINER, AND P. PLUMMER. National Athletic Trainers Association position statement: Exertional heat illnesses. *J. Athl. Train.* 37:329–343. 2002.

CASA, D.J., AND L.E. ARMSTRONG. Exertional heatstroke: A medical emergency. In: *Exertional Heat Illnesses*, L.E. Armstrong (ed.). Champaign, IL: Human Kinetics, 2003. pp. 29–56, 230–234.

CASA, D.J., L.E. ARMSTRONG, M.S. GANIO, AND S.W. YEARGIN. Exertional heat stroke in competitive athletes. *Curr. Sports Med. Rep.* 4:309–317. 2005.

Figure 10-4. Treatment of heat stroke. (Reprinted with permission from the National Strength and Conditioning Association, Colorado Springs, CO, USA. Casa DJ, Anderson JM, Armstrong LE, et al. Survival strategy: acute treatment of exertional heat stroke. J Strength Cond Res. 2006;20(3):462.)

Factors Affecting Heat Illness

Fitness level and age affect susceptibility to heat illness and responses to hot, humid conditions.[1,31] Gender, however, appears to have minimal effect.[32] Thus, gender is not a factor when evaluations are made for body size, fitness level, body fat, and acclimatization level.[31,33] This is true despite the fact that sweating is triggered at a higher core temperature in women than in men, resulting in a delayed sweat response among exercising women.

Fitness Level

Because fitness level is a modifiable risk factor, it should be carefully considered before engaging in activity in extreme environmental heat. Cardiovascular fitness, in particular, should be the primary focus of a conditioning program to enhance one's response to heat and reduce the potential for heat illnesses.[1]

Age

As one ages, cardiovascular function declines.[14,27] Training can help slow this decline, but it cannot eliminate the effects of aging. Age-related decreases in cardiac output play a major role in reducing an older person's ability to deal with heat stress. Older people cannot respond to heat with the same elevation in cardiac output that younger individuals do. Thus, the challenge to simultaneously provide enough blood to working muscles and the periphery to facilitate heat loss is greater among the aged than the young. Fortunately, like young people, older persons are capable of heat acclimatization so that their capacity to exercise under unfavorable environmental conditions can be improved.

Performance in the Heat

Getting ready to perform in the heat is a concern for many coaches and athletes, especially when they have not had the chance to acclimatize to that environmental stress. As pointed out before, cardiovascular fitness is vital to limit the negative effects of heat, yet heat stress and heat illness can occur even to the most highly conditioned athlete if precautions are not taken and warning signals not heeded.[1,10]

Quick Review

- Heat cramps, syncope, heat exhaustion, and heat stroke are conditions brought on by exposure to heat.
- Heat stroke is the most dangerous because it can be fatal, especially if it is confused with heat exhaustion and treatment is delayed.
- Core temperature measures are the only accurate diagnosis of heat stroke.
- Age and fitness level affect susceptibility to heat illness.

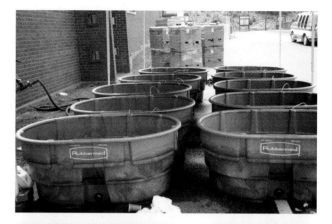

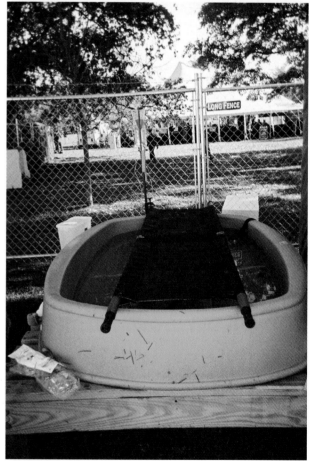

Figure 10-5. Tubs used in treatment of heat stroke. Delays because of misdiagnosis of heat stroke as heat exhaustion can be fatal. Rapid treatment of heat stroke is vital for survival. A cold water or ice bath is the most effective method and should be available at all recreational and competitive sites where heat illness is a potential problem.

Endurance Performance

Optimal performance of endurance activities in a hot environment requires prior acclimatization, proper hydration, and physical conditioning. In an interesting study by McCann and Adams,[38] endurance performance in the heat was consistently found to decrease as predicted by **wet bulb** globe temperature (**WBGT**) per the National Collegiate Athletic Association guidelines. Statistically significant linear relationships for the 3,000-m (9,843-ft) steeple chase (SC) and 10,000-m (32,808-ft) events were observed (i.e., as heat increased, times slowed), as well as when the 1,500-m (4,921-ft), 3,000-m (9,843-ft), 5,000-m (16,404-ft), and 10,000-m (32,808-ft) results were pooled. However, there were individual exceptions, and the linear relationship between WBGT and distance running performance was not seen for all running events. Most importantly, adhering to the WBGT guidelines was successful in protecting against heat illnesses during the meets.

Anaerobic Performance

Although few athletic events are wholly dependent on anaerobic metabolism, many short-duration, sprint-type activities do rely heavily on anaerobically produced ATP. But even in these all out, sprinting events, the contribution of anaerobically generated ATP gradually wanes as the event's duration increases. Limited exposure to heat during shorter anaerobic performances, say at a track meet running the 100-m (328-ft) to 800-m (2,625-ft) events, may not hamper performance at all, but in longer events such as the 1,500-m race, high ambient temperatures may, indeed, limit performance. Thus, the impact of heat exposure on any anaerobic performance is related to both the duration of that event and the length of time the athlete is exposed to the heat. Athletes who perform conditioning sessions with constant exposure to the heat and repeated high-intensity exertional outputs will suffer from the same decrements in speed with heat as will athletes performing in endurance events. In addition, susceptibility to heat illness will also be present. Thus, during competition, cooling methods, hydration, and limited exposure to heat might form the basis of successful anaerobic performances.

Strength

As with anaerobic function, the detrimental effects of heat on strength performance are a function of the length of exposure to the heat and duration of the workout. Judelson et al.[30] observed that 2% to 5% hypohydration resulting from heat exposure reduced strength, power, and muscular endurance by approximately 2%, 3%, and 10%, respectively. These findings demonstrate that a degree of hypohydration frequently experienced during exercise in high ambient temperatures significantly impairs muscle's functional capacity. This effect becomes worse with an increased number of efforts, higher training volumes, or time spent in the heat (see Box 10-2).

Prevention Strategies

To avoid declines in performance related to heat stress, athletes should use appropriate prevention strategies. These include acclimation and acclimatization over time and proper hydration before exercise.

Acclimation/Acclimatization

Artificially induced physiological adaptation to a given environment is called **acclimation**. For example, increasing the temperature of the indoor football practice facility at the University of Minnesota in December to prepare for a game in Miami would acclimate the players to heat. Conversely, practice for the same players in a naturally hot environment, such as the natural outdoor environment at the University of Mississippi, would result in **acclimatization** needed for a game in Miami. One is an artificial environment, "acclimation," and the other is a natural environment, "acclimatization."

Time Course of Adaptations

Acclimatization or acclimation to heat is a process in which different physiological systems adapt at different rates. Furthermore, it is a transient process, and so one who is acclimatized can lose acclimatization if one avoids heat for two and a half weeks to a month.[3,24] For example, a runner might be acclimatized to running in the heat and humidity of Wisconsin over the summer months, but would have to reacclimatize or reacclimate for a hot and humid 10K race environment in March in Thailand. Heat acclimatization can take up to 14 days.[3] Some of the major adjustments with heat acclimatization are discussed below.

One to five days is when early adaptations take place involving improved regulation and control of the cardiovascular system. This includes an expanded plasma volume, reduced heart rate at a specific work rate, and improvement in the autonomic nervous system to help redistribute blood flow to the capillary beds in the active musculature.

Five to eight days is when the crucial regulation of body temperature is improved, which is vital for partial protection against lethal hyperthermia. A different response occurs

Quick Review

- The ability to perform in a hot environment is a multivariable challenge involving the need for prior acclimatization, proper hydration, and physical conditioning.
- Heat hinders aerobic performance.
- The impact of hot weather on any anaerobic performance is related to the time of heat exposure, the duration of the event, and the hydration level of the athlete.
- Strength, power, and high-intensity endurance performance in the heat depend on length of exposure and hydration status.

Box 10-2   AN EXPERT VIEW
Exertional Heat Stroke

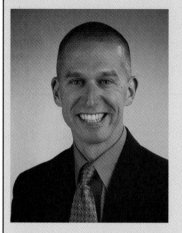

Douglas J. Casa, PhD, ATC, FACSM

Professor,
Human Performance Laboratory
Department of Kinesiology
University of Connecticut
Storrs, CT

EHS is a potentially fatal condition that is most likely to occur when athletes perform intense exercise in warm or hot conditions. Through my years of treating athletes with EHS, conducting research related to the condition, and reviewing legal documents related to cases of this condition, I have found much consistency as to causes of the condition and common errors in the recognition and treatment of it.

When EHS occurs in a practice setting, several factors are commonly present, including the following:

1. It nearly always occurs in the first 3 days of practices.
2. The athlete is often working at an intensity that is beyond his or her "normal" capacity.
3. The athlete is often wearing gear beyond just shorts and a T-shirt.
4. The athlete tends to be not very fit.
5. The practice/conditioning session was not carefully planned in terms of rest breaks, length, and hydration needs.
6. The athlete did not participate in a "phase-in" program regarding number of practices, length of practices, amount of equipment, etc. (many states have this for high school sports and the NCAA has it for football).
7. The athlete was not acclimatized or only partially acclimatized.
8. The athlete often is attempting to impress coaches, teammates, parents, or self.
9. Medical staff is often not present.
10. A faulty policy and procedures regarding EHS are in place.
11. Education of the coaches, parents, and athletes is outdated or completely absent.

When EHS occurs in a road race/triathlon scenario, it often has a few common features, including the following:

1. The athlete is trying to meet some standard (qualify for Boston, personal best) and pushes hard in the last couple miles.
2. The athlete does not plan properly for the environment, whether it be overdressing for cooler weather or not being properly acclimatized for a competition in warm weather.
3. The athlete often has an illness that causes a low-level fever before even beginning the race.
4. The athlete has pacing assistance at the end from a fresh person not doing the entire event.
5. The athlete does not have a well-rehearsed hydration strategy.

When it comes to problems related to the recognition and treatment of EHS, it often boils down to two issues. The first issue is the lack of a rapid and accurate assessment of body-core temperature and central nervous system function. The second is the delay in aggressive cooling at which the athlete is aggressively cooled. For a field setting, evaluation by rectal temperature is the only way to accurately assess body temperature. A delay in ascertaining an accurate temperature or using a mode of temperature assessment that is not valid for athletes who perform intense exercise in the heat has had fatal consequences. The process of cooling an athlete with EHS must begin as quickly as possible. Problems have arisen when cooling was delayed (due to lack of recognition or lack of proper preparation to have cooling modalities on-site) or the mode of cooling that was used had inferior cooling rates (e.g., ice bags on peripheral arteries). Cold-water immersion and rotating ice/wet towels over the entire body both provide good cooling rates and can maximize chance of survival.

See: Casa DJ, Anderson JM, Armstrong LE, et al. Survival strategy: acute treatment of exertional heat stroke. J Strength Cond Res. 2006;20(3):462.

---

depending on if the acclimatization procedure takes place in a hot, humid environment versus a hot, dry environment. Adaptations include an increased sweat rate, the onset of sweating at lower elevations in body temperature, and sweat gland adaptations (more dilute sweat), depending on the environment.

Three to nine days is when conservation of sodium chloride (NaCl) takes place during heat acclimatization. NaCl losses in the sweat and urine will decrease, which results in a better maintained extracellular fluid volume.

By 14 days, most of the changes are complete and include the following:

- Lower core temperature at the onset of sweating
- Increased heat loss via radiation and convection (skin blood flow)
- Increased plasma volume
- Decreased heart rate at a specific workload
- Decreased body-core temperature
- Decreased skin temperature
- Decreased oxygen consumption at a given workload
- Improved exercise economy

Quick Review

- Acclimatization is the process by which the human body adapts to natural changes in climate.
- Acclimation uses an artificially simulated climate to create adaptations.
- Heat acclimatization can take 14 days and lasts about 17 days.
- Sweating contributes to dehydration as the body loses water.

Hydration

Sweating contributes to the evaporative cooling of the body, which leads to heat loss. However, it also contributes to dehydration as the body loses water. Many athletes walk around in a hypohydrated state because their water intake behavior is not optimal. This makes them more susceptible to heat stress because a loss of body mass as little as 1% results in the elevation of core temperature during exercise.[46] Thus, hydration before exercise is important to optimally respond to physiological demands, especially in a hot environment. Casa et al.[11] have provided extensive guidelines for proper hydration techniques and practices that are important to eliminate or reduce the challenges of exercising in hot environments (also see Chapter 8 and Box 8-2).

COLD STRESS

At the other end of the temperature spectrum, athletes also face physiological challenges from exercise in cold environments. Downhill skiing, cross-country skiing, snowboarding, backpacking, snowmobiling, snowshoeing, and ice-skating are some of the most popular outdoor activities performed in the cold. As the external temperature falls, various physiological thermoregulatory mechanisms are engaged to maintain the body's internal temperature. Although physiological mechanisms can start the adjustment processes to help keep the body warm, appropriate clothing or shelter is typically needed to meet the challenges of cold temperatures. Clothing is vital as a shielding factor when competing or recreating in cold weather. Cold exposure to unprotected body parts or inadequately clothed body parts can have detrimental effects on performance long before cold injury is a threat (see Box 10-3).

Paradoxically, because of the production of metabolic heat with exercise and the use of too much layering of very effective protective garments, it is possible for someone to experience heat illness in the cold. Protective clothing can create a very different microclimate for the body.

Physiological Thermoregulation in the Cold

Physiological responses to the challenges of cold exposure involve many different mechanisms. The body's cold receptors monitor both the change and the rate of decrease in temperature and signal a host of different actions to occur. Cold receptors are found in fewer numbers than heat receptors and are located in the skin, abdominal viscera, and spinal cord.

The body starts its defense of body heat by making some cardiovascular adjustments, beginning with vasoconstriction of peripheral surface vessels typically used to dissipate heat. Sweating is also shut down to eliminate evaporative heat loss. The receptors send signals to the body's thermostat,

Box 10-3 PRACTICAL QUESTIONS FROM STUDENTS

How can I Acclimatize to the Cold?

For all our practices and games so far this year, my high school hockey team in Maine has used an indoor ice arena where the temperature is kept only moderately cool, i.e., 50 to 55°F (10–13°C). But in 4 weeks, we are to compete in a holiday tournament to be held at an outdoor arena at nighttime when the ambient temperature is expected to be 10 to 15°F (–12 to –9°C). Is there anything I can do to try to acclimatize my body to the cold in preparation for this upcoming outdoor hockey tournament?

It appears that unlike hot temperatures, the body undergoes few physiological adaptations as a result of exposure to cold temperatures. Still, cold ambient temperatures can negatively impact athletic performance, especially during powerful, all out sprinting efforts such as those occurring during ice hockey. The best thing to do to maintain optimal performance during cold exposure is to protect the body by wearing appropriate clothing and seeking warmer shelter when possible. So wearing thermal underwear and entering a "warming hut" between periods during the game might be the best way to deal with the cold, rather than attempting to acclimatize to it. At the same time, one should also be careful about overdressing. This may result in overheating, particularly as the game goes on and among the very active players whose intense muscular activity generates much heat that must be dissipated.

the hypothalamus, to stimulate release of thyroid-releasing hormone, which in turn stimulates the thyroid gland to release T-3 and T-4 thyroid hormones, which upregulate metabolism, resulting in heat production. In addition, integrated signals from the hypothalamus stimulate the motor cortex to activate the "shivering" of skeletal muscle to produce heat.

Moreover, the sympathetic nervous system stimulates the adrenal medulla to secrete epinephrine to increase metabolism and norepinephrine to enhance vasoconstriction of the peripheral blood vessels. Another change is the piloerection of hair (a sympathetic stimulation of hair follicles causing hair to stand), which provides insulation; however, this adaptation is more effective in animals than in humans. Ultimately, blood flow to skeletal muscle also decreases, unless voluntary behavioral responses increase muscular activity to generate heat. Other behavioral responses to cold are to curl up to preserve core heat, seek shelter or find heat sources (e.g., make a fire), eat, or put on more layers of clothing. Figure 10-6 overviews the major physiological responses to the cold. Also, one can see from the **isotherm** in Figure 10-6B how the body's temperature fluctuations are related to protecting the core organs and central nervous system, which are vital to survival.

Cold exposure can arise from a variety of situations, even when one is well clothed (Fig. 10-7). **Hypothermia** is a condition in which the body's temperature decreases to a point at which normal physiological function is impaired or not possible. Recall that the normal core temperature of humans is about 37.0°C (98.6°F).

Hypothermia has been described as consisting of three different stages during which the body's physiological systems are challenged to maintain normal core temperature. Stage 1 occurs when the body temperature drops 1 to 2°C below the normal body temperature and represents the initial challenge to body function, including a loss of the ability to perform complex motor tasks and breathing becoming rapid and shallow. Stage 2 is when the body temperature drops 2 to 4°C below normal temperature and normal neuromuscular function is affected due to the slowing of nerve conduction velocities and blood flow restrictions. Stage 3 is when the body's temperature drops below 32°C (89.6°F) and physiological systems start to dramatically shut down, such as metabolic and nervous system function, cardiac anomalies occur (e.g., tachycardia), organs fail, and, eventually, the brain dies. Thus, hypothermia is a major threat to survival.

Below a body temperature of 29.4°C (85°F), the body cools more rapidly because its natural temperature–regulating system mediated by the hypothalamus fails to effectively meet the demands of the cold environmental stress. Interestingly, there have been improbable cases in which people have survived after the body temperature had dropped to 13.9 to 15.6°C (57 to 60°F) and they had stopped breathing.

Performance Responses to the Cold

From a practical perspective, well before such potentially dramatic temperature losses, people can experience reductions in neuromuscular activity with just normal cold and damp exposure in recreational and competitive sports. Howard et al.[29] demonstrated that when men had their thighs immersed in cold water at 12°C (53.6°F) for 45 minutes, reductions in isokinetic peak torque, total work, and power were observed, indicating that neural conduction velocities of high-threshold motor units may have been slowed. In a recent study (unpublished data), the use of a warm-up activity mitigated these losses if performed immediately after the cold water immersion. Thus, performing physical activity during exposure to a cold challenge may be effective in limiting cold-induced declines in neuromuscular function.

Interestingly, precooling has been used to enhance sport performance before competition in a hot environment. This strategy was used by US marathon runners in the Athens Olympic marathon, who optimized their performances by precooling and using the first 10K as their warm-up in the hot conditions of the race. This seems to be most effective for submaximal exercise, in which the duration of the event and anaerobic enzymes are not limiting factors.[20]

Force Production

Muscle force production can be impacted by exposure of the body to cold environments. Changes in the pattern of muscle activation of the quadriceps have been observed even when those muscles were chilled with ice packs for just 3 minutes.[34] In addition, reduction in force production of the peripheral musculature appears to occur without any effect of the cooling on the body-core temperature.[13] Thus, cold exposure to the skin represents a potential threat to neuromuscular performance capability. It has been observed that when environmental temperatures are at or below 10°C (50°F) for at least 40 minutes, a significant amount of heat loss can be observed and there is a reduction in force production.[15] Interestingly, eccentric muscle actions may actually show an improvement with colder temperatures because of the added stiffness of the series component of elastic elements in the muscle.[5] Despite this, when deep cooling of a muscle occurs, force production can be reduced because of a slowing of the electrical impulses being conducted by the associated motor neurons.[50] **Nerve conduction velocity** is the rate at which neural impulses (action potentials) are conducted along the axons of motor neurons activating muscle fibers. When nerve conduction velocity is slowed, it compromises the "summation" of nerve impulses arriving at the surface of the muscle fibers and accordingly reduces force production of the muscle fibers; this is especially true with fast-twitch motor units. Prior severe cold injury can also impact nerve conduction velocities, which reflects why some people may be more sensitive to cold environments than others.[4]

Acute Regulation

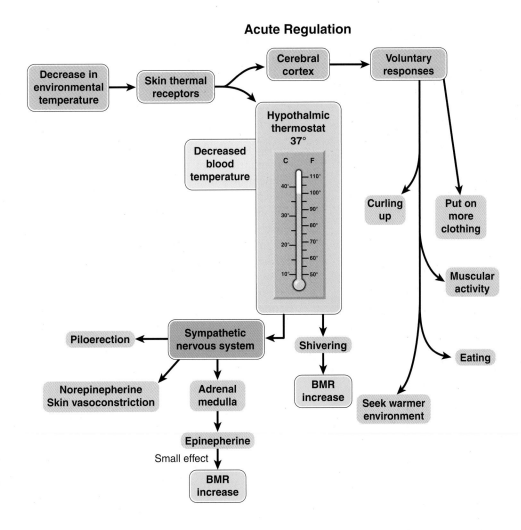

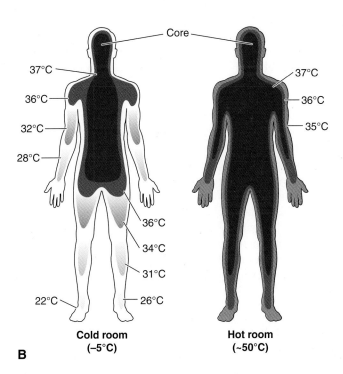

Figure 10-6. The mechanisms related to the physiological responses to cold stress. (A) A decrease in temperature is first realized by cold receptors in the body, which in turn send signals to the hypothalamus. The hypothalamus integrates and sends signals to the following: (1) the motor cortex and nervous system to increase shivering of skeletal muscle; (2) the sympathetic nervous system to cause vasoconstriction of the cutaneous vessels and stimulation of the adrenal medullas to secrete catecholamines; and (3) to the anterior pituitary to stimulate thyroid hormone and glucocorticoid release to enhance metabolic energy production. All these actions help the body to internally increase its heat production. **(B)** The layers of tissues will alter in their temperature, as shown in the mapping of body temperature depicted by a body isotherm, at different temperatures. As temperature rises, body tissues decrease in temperature from the core to the periphery, whereas under cold conditions, body temperatures increase from the periphery to the core to preserve vital organs and the central nervous system function. This is why peripheral tissues such as skin are more sensitive to cold injury.

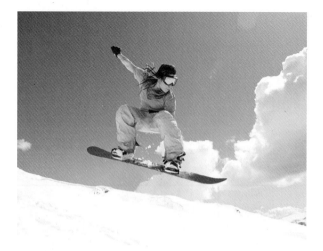

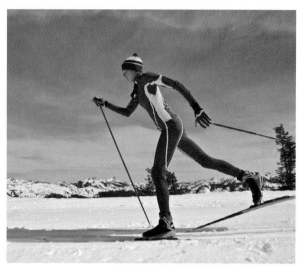

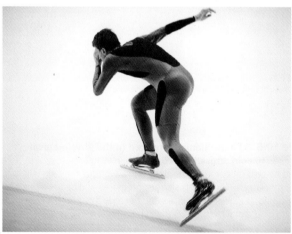

Figure 10-7. Common cold environments in sport. A variety of different environmental conditions can lead to cold exposure of different types in recreational and sport competitions. Thus, strategies to address cold exposure must be taken to support the body's own physiological mechanisms.

Acute cold water immersion (12°C or 53.6°F for 15 minutes) that mimics environmental exposures actually encountered by athletes has been shown to dramatically diminish power output, heart rate at a specific workload,

and time to peak power in highly trained cyclists.[47] Even with a very brief exposure to colder temperatures, most maximal performances are negatively altered, along with concomitant reductions in physiological function.

Cardiovascular and Endurance Performance

Unlike muscle function, submaximal and maximal oxygen consumptions are not affected by acute exposure to cold temperatures unless the body-core temperature decreases, indicating an early sign of hypothermia. Interestingly, no harmful effects in lung tissue have been documented with exercise in temperatures as low as −35°C (−31°F).

Performing endurance exercise in the cold weather has been thought to increase the potential for **exercise-induced bronchoconstriction (EIB)** (i.e., reduction in the diameter of the bronchioles in the lungs). Bronchoconstriction characterizes many asthma conditions, and EIB can be brought about by endurance exercise in people who have exercise-induced asthma. Many have thought that cold air coming into the lungs can cause a similar effect in all people. However, although running speeds and physiological parameters are affected when performing endurance exercise in the cold, only those people known to suffer from EIB experience such a bronchoconstriction effect.[49] In reality, because of clothing used by skiers and runners, the impact of typical cold weather environments on endurance performances is minimal. As temperatures increase from 5 to 25°C (41 to 77°F), marathon performances progressively slow, and thus a major threat appears to be from hyperthermia, rather than hypothermia.[21,40]

Acclimatization/Acclimation

Unlike the case with heat, acclimatization (natural exposure) or acclimation (artificial exposure) to cold typically has been related to behavioral changes, such as learning how to layer clothing or dress properly.[42] Many times, psychological adjustments can be made to view cold weather differently. In sports, some teams take pride in the ability to play in the cold, particularly on their home field. For decades, many of the warm weather teams in the National Football League hated to come to legendary Lambeau Field and play the Green Bay Packers in December (Fig. 10-8). To emphasize this psychological advantage that the cold weather did not bother them, the Packers' players would come out of the locker for pregame warm-ups with just T-shirts or much less clothing than their opponents as snow flurries swirled around the stadium. They did this to underscore the team's toughness and further "psyche out" their opponents.

Physiological adaptations to the cold, however, are less obvious than those to the heat. To determine whether such adaptations even occur, one has to consider various populations and situations in which such mechanisms may have been developed over time. Highly trained mountaineers

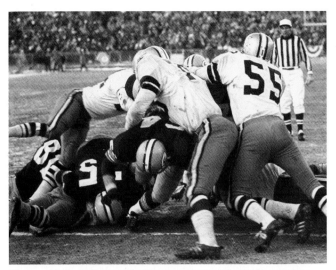

Figure 10-8. In Green Bay Wisconsin, the Green Bay Packers and Dallas Cowboys played for the National Football League (NFL) Championship in what became known as the "Ice Bowl". This was one of the most famous American football championship games ever played and that day the temperature was –26.1° C (–15° F) on Lambeau Field in 1967. The ability of this American football team to cope with the challenges of playing in the cold and winning many games contributed to the legend of Green Bay Packers and their advantage of playing at Lambeau Field known as the "Frozen Tundra" in the NFL.

have shown improved cold-induced vasodilatation responses to high altitude cold exposure compared with controls, implicating a peripheral type of acclimatization to the combination of chronic cold and high-altitude exposure.[22] This finding supports earlier work in which deep-sea fishermen demonstrated higher blood flow in the hands compared with nonacclimatized controls when exposed to cold.[23] Eskimos

Quick Review

- The body monitors cold with cold receptors.
- Vasoconstriction, shivering, reduced sweating, and stimulation of the thyroid and adrenal glands help the body regulate temperature decreases.
- Hypothermia is a condition in which the body's temperature decreases to a point at which normal physiological function is impaired or not possible.
- Exposure to dampness and cold leads to diminished nerve conduction rates and subsequent reductions in isokinetic peak torque, total work, and power.
- Precooling may be an effective technique for improving sports performance in hot climates.
- Cardiovascular and endurance performance are only impacted by cold temperatures if body-core temperature decreases.
- Acclimatization to the cold seems to have a large genetic component but can be influenced by exposure to cold in situations in which both some local physiological adaptations and psychological toleration exist.

are well suited to the study of acclimatization of humans to cold environments, as generations of these cold weather natives have had to cope with harsh weather conditions. It has been shown that Eskimos have higher basal metabolic rates (12%–46%) than non-Eskimos. Acclimatization to cold seems to have a large genetic component, but it can also be influenced by exposure to cold in situations in which both some local physiological adaptations (increased blood flow to the extremities) and psychological toleration exist.

One needs to prepare for cold weather exposure with proper clothing and shelter. Warm-up may be vital if athletes are standing around on the sideline waiting to play in a cold environment. Although exercise can help offset reductions in core temperature, exposed skin surface areas result in the cooling of the underlying musculature. This can reduce force production capabilities, which in turn might well influence sport and recreational skills, demonstrating once again that protection and warming are vital to successful performance in a cold environment (see Box 10-4).

ALTITUDE STRESS

The failed and successful attempts to scale Mount Everest have demonstrated the challenges and demands of high altitude for years. Likewise, sportscasters reporting on professional football and baseball games hosted in Denver, CO, tout the considerable effect that altitude has on the athletes at Denver's 1,609-m (5,280-ft) elevation. So, what are the demands of the different altitudes? How dramatic are the negative effects of performing at 1,609 m? Are different sport teams at an advantage or disadvantage under certain altitude conditions?

With regard to aerobic capacity, studies have shown declines in performance at altitudes as low as about 700 m (2,300 ft), becoming more obvious at roughly 1,524 m (5,000 ft). But there seems to be a threshold at about 2,200 m (7,217 ft) where the effects of altitude on performance become more pronounced. Specifically, more dramatic impairments of oxygen consumption and endurance performance begin to occur at that height (see Box 10-5). With a rise in altitude, the negative impacts on oxidative metabolism continue to increase in a curvilinear manner. Interestingly, most athletic competitions take place within the moderate altitude range, with some "high-altitude" winter sports and mountain climbing occurring at altitudes greater than 2,743 m or 9,000 ft (Fig. 10-9).

Hypoxia and Other Challenges of Altitude

The fundamental problem with increasing altitude is the associated decrease in the **barometric pressure**, which causes hypoxia. The weight of air is defined by the barometric pressure, which changes due to environmental conditions, most dramatically altitude. **Hypoxia**, or the compromised delivery of oxygen to target tissues, is a major

Box 10-4 DID YOU KNOW?
Cold Exposure: Surviving Different Cold Environmental Conditions

Whether you live in a place of constant or seasonal cold temperatures, activities in cold conditions warrant special attention. Contrary to popular belief, temperature is not the only factor to consider when determining the safety measures to take in cold environment activities. In fact, other environmental factors strongly affect the potential severity of cold exposure. When addressing the risks associated with cold temperatures, consider the effects of dry versus wet conditions, wind (or convection), and the individual in question.

Dry Conditions Versus Wet Conditions

When the environment is cold and dry, protective clothing that insulates the body is effective. Insulation works because of its ability to prevent the loss of heat that radiates from the body into the atmosphere. Because heat and air are trapped, air near the body roughly equates to body temperatures, thus preventing further heat loss, and body temperature remains stable.

Compared with cold and dry weather, cold environments with submersion or exposure to cold water can quickly become life threatening. Body heat is lost exponentially faster in water than on land because of the ability of water to rapidly absorb radiated heat from the body and to do so without quickly equating to the body's temperature (unlike air). Because water temperature does not rapidly equate to the temperature of the body, the body will continue to lose heat in a futile attempt to equate internal and external environmental temperatures, causing body temperature to quickly become fatally low.

The amount of water that must be heated to body temperature plays a large role in the rate of heat loss. For example, less bodily heat is lost to equate a water bottle to body temperature than to equate a lake to body temperature. In conditions in which relative water volume is great, swimming vigorously would likely lead to faster heat loss, without hope of equating temperatures, thus putting submersed victims at risk much more quickly.

Although submersion may be unlikely, it is important to remember the effect of water on rate of heat loss (think about how effective perspiration is because of the amount of heat water can absorb). If exposure to water is expected in cold environments, apparel isolating the skin from the external environment is integral. The worst scenario is allowing water to stand on the exposed skin, continuously cooling, and thus causing excessive heat loss.

Cold Versus Cold and Windy

Because air easily gains and loses heat to equate with the environment, increasing the rate at which air passes over the skin greatly accelerates the rate at which heat is lost. When activities take place in cold environments with wind as an additional factor, extra caution is needed because the loss of body temperature (especially skin temperature) occurs more rapidly, leading to an increased risk of injury (as shown on the wind chill chart).

If outside in cold and windy environments, wear apparel that is wind resistant. Polyester-based or waterproof material placed outside of insulating material is an optimal choice. In addition, cover all exposed body parts, especially the head, as it is one of the primary heat loss centers of the body because of the amount of superficial blood flow (or heat) it receives and can therefore easily lose and is especially prone to the dangers of wind (or convective heat loss) because of its location on the body.

Age, Body Mass, and Activity in the Cold

The status of the individual in cold environments plays a strong role in the effect of the environment on thermoregulation. Older individuals have less tolerance for cooler environments. Conversely, younger individuals have a better capacity to resist cold environment–related injuries. While younger individuals are prone to risks from warmer climates, whereas older individuals may prefer (both psychologically and physiologically) warm, but not hot, temperatures they are still prone to non-exertional heat stroke.

Additionally, quantity and composition of body mass play a strong role in thermoregulation. Some structures are capable of providing heat insulation, and some structures serve primary functions in producing heat. For example, large amounts of skeletal muscle mass create more heat, which is likely to result in a better tolerance to colder temperatures (unless wet!). Fat mass insulates vital organs and prevents loss of body-core temperature; in cold environments, this gives individuals with a higher fat mass an advantage over individuals with less fat mass.

Activity in the cold can significantly affect thermoregulatory status in potentially beneficial and harmful ways. Peripheralization of blood flow to extremities and an increased metabolic rate are likely to serve protective functions against cold injuries. Conversely, perspiration caused by vigorous activity is likely to accelerate the rate at which body heat is lost, introducing substantial risk if proper attire, drying measures, or warmer temperature relocation do not quickly take place.

---

cause of many of altitude's deleterious effects and is caused by a reduced **partial pressure** of oxygen. Because oxygen is so important for physiological function, many, including athletes and sportscasters, think it is the lack of oxygen at altitude that creates all of the problems. However, this is

not true! The percentage of oxygen (20.93%), as well as other gases (CO_2, 0.03%, and nitrogen, 79.04%), in the air is the same regardless of the altitude within earth's atmosphere. What varies is the amount of pressure exerted on the molecules of each gas. The higher the elevation, the

Box 10-5 PRACTICAL QUESTIONS FROM STUDENTS

Do Endurance Athletes from Schools and Universities Located at Altitude have an Advantage When Competing Against Athletes from Schools Located at Sea Level?

This is a good question. After living and training at altitudes over 5,000 ft (1,524 m) for several years, endurance athletes at schools such as the University of New Mexico and Colorado State University undergo physiological adaptations such as increased red blood cell volume, increased capillary density, and increased mitochondrial density of muscle fibers. These adaptations not only increase the delivery of oxygen to the working muscles, they also improve the ability of muscle fibers to produce ATP through aerobic metabolism. As a result, the athlete will be able to rely to a greater extent on aerobic metabolism to provide the necessary ATP to sustain a given pace, thus minimizing anaerobic metabolism and the fatiguing effects of increased acidity. So, yes, the physiological adaptations experienced by endurance athletes from schools located at altitude would be of benefit when they compete at sea level. This does not necessarily mean that they will win, however, since training, motivation, and natural talent all play a role in athletic performance.

lower the barometric pressure (mm Hg), and this pressure plays a major role in the ability of the body to get oxygen to the tissues. Oxygen tension, or the partial pressure of oxygen (Po_2), is calculated by multiplying the barometric pressure times the percentage of oxygen in the air (See Chapter 6). This means that the oxygen tension is reduced as altitude increases. One can then easily understand that a barometric pressure at sea level of 760 mm Hg would create a much higher partial pressure for oxygen than a barometric pressure of 596 mm Hg in Mexico City, where the 1968 Olympic Games took place (see Box 10-6).

The increasing altitude places a marked stress on the body, most directly on the ability to get oxygen to the body's tissues. Thus, the reduced barometric pressure at altitude creates a **hypobaric environment**, and this lower Po_2 reduces the effectiveness of gas transport from the pulmonary diffusion of oxygen from the lungs into the blood and then into the target tissues in the body. This reduced amount of oxygen to body tissues creates what is called a "hypoxic effect."

In addition to hypoxia, increasing altitude is associated with other environmental challenges. It is evident from the many pictures of mountain climbers reaching the summit of some of the highest peaks in the world that cold is also associated with ascent to higher altitude. By the time one reaches the peak of Mount Everest, the temperature can be as low as −44.4°C (−48°F). Cold air has a lower water vapor level than warmer air, and the gradient for water loss from the body to the environment promotes a dehydrating influence. This higher evaporative loss of moisture from the body is intensified during exercise because of the increased ventilation brought on by physical exertion (recall that water vapor is expired during breathing). These factors promoting dehydration are amplified as altitude increases. This means that one needs to monitor hydration status and fluid intake when living and exercising at altitude.

Finally, the amount of solar radiation increases as altitude increases due to a shorter distance for the sun's

Box 10-6 DID YOU KNOW?

1968 Summer Olympics

It was thought that the so-called "thin air" of Mexico City, due to its elevation of 7,349 ft (2,240 m), helped athletes shatter records in every men's and women's track and field race up to 1,500 m at the 1968 Summer Olympics. It was also thought to have played a role in U.S. long jumper Bob Beamon's incredible gold medal leap of 29 ft 2½ inches (8.9 m), beating the existing world mark by nearly 2 ft (6.1 cm). Other outstanding American performances included Al Oerter's record fourth consecutive discus title, Debbie Meyer's three individual swimming gold medals, the innovative Dick Fosbury winning the high jump with his backwards "flop," and Wyomia Tyus becoming the first woman to win back-to-back gold medals in the 100-m race.

Present day Earth topography [m]

−6,000   −4,000   −2,000   0   2,000   4,000   6,000

Figure 10-9. World map with different altitudes around the globe.

electromagnetic waves to travel and a thinning of the atmosphere. The sun emits several types of ultraviolet radiation: ultraviolet A (UVA), ultraviolet B (UVB), and ultraviolet C (UVC). UVC radiation is absorbed by the atmosphere's ozone layer. Thus, only UVA and UVB radiations reach the earth's surface, and commercially purchased sun blocks should protect against both. Although UVB exposure is beneficial in that it induces the production of vitamin D in the skin, too much of it leads to direct DNA damage and sunburn, and some forms of skin cancer.

Physiological Responses to Altitude

The first event that brought attention to altitude in sport and exercise was the 1968 Summer Olympics in Mexico City, Mexico, which is at an elevation of 2,240 m (7,349 ft). The world's athletes were going to compete at altitude for the first time in a world competition. Many scientists debated which altitude was the threshold for dramatic effects, especially in regards to maximal oxygen consumption values. Athletes, coaches, scientists, and medical professionals pondered what the impact would be and in what events. With the drop in the partial pressure of oxygen, the endurance events were of immediate concern, considering that the environment alone would add seconds if not minutes to race times. Could one acclimate to this environment, and what were the athletes to expect when arriving at the competitive venue? How long should one be at altitude before the competition to acclimatize? Was altitude sickness possible at this moderate altitude? Leading up to the Summer Olympic Games in 1968, these and many other questions haunted and challenged everyone involved.

As one ascends to even moderate altitude, many initial physiological adjustments take place in the body's attempt to maintain homeostasis. Increases in resting heart rate, blood pressure, and catecholamines all signal the stress of altitude. The body is faced with the challenge of hypoxia and the need to get oxygen to the body's tissues.

Pulmonary Ventilation

During exercise at altitude, **pulmonary ventilation** ($\dot{V}_E$) increases in response to the need for a higher arterial saturation of oxygen in the blood. Resting ventilation does not increase until one reaches about 10,000 ft or 3,048 m (Fig. 10-10). To offset the reduction in P_{O_2}, pulmonary ventilation changes in response to the stress of altitude. Under resting conditions, there is generally an increase in tidal volume, or the depth of breathing, rather than an increase in the rate of breathing. With exercise, both the volume and rate may increase to facilitate a greater availability of oxygen. But at maximal exercise, ventilation at altitude is similar to that at sea level. Evidently, there is an upper limit of pulmonary ventilation during maximal intensity exercise, regardless of whether it is performed at sea level or at altitude. At altitude, however, the body becomes more alkaline, as the increase in breathing

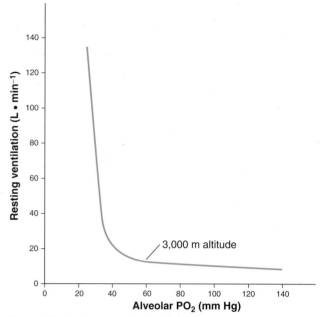

Figure 10-10. Responses of pulmonary ventilation at rest in response to alveolar Po₂ concentrations in the blood.

causes more CO_2 removal, resulting in blood pH above 7.4. With time, the kidneys help to restore homeostatic control by increasing the excretion of bicarbonate (an acid buffer), thereby allowing more acid to remain in the blood, so that it may help neutralize the alkaline substances, bringing blood back to the normal range for pH of 7.3 to 7.4. At altitude, responses in pulmonary ventilation to varying elevations may differ quite noticeably, and as a result of chronic adaptations, long-term residents of high altitude have fewer symptoms and little change in ventilation compared with those living at sea level.[19,26,41,48] The ventilatory changes and differences among individuals also appear to be driven by one's catecholamine responses to a given altitude.

Oxygen Consumption

It is well-known that maximal oxygen consumption decreases with increasing altitude and that endurance performance suffers commensurately. But an important question that has not been clearly answered pertains to the altitude at which these declines are first observed. With so many different factors, such as altitude acclimatization, training status, and test demands, a high degree of variability exists. Nonetheless, evidence generally shows that declines start at about 2,200 m (7,217 ft), with decrements estimated from 2% to 15% in maximal oxygen consumption. The high degree of variation implies that many factors contribute to the loss of aerobic power due to hypoxia.

Metabolites, Hemoglobin, and Hematocrit

Among the most notable changes with exposure to altitude is an increase in the concentrations of hemoglobin and hematocrit in the blood. Acutely, this occurs due to dehydration and a consequent decrease in blood plasma volume. However, with chronic exposure, in as little as 3 weeks the production of red blood cells by the bone marrow increases and primarily accounts for the elevations in hemoglobin and hematocrit that are part of the acclimatization process (see Box 10-7). With acute exposure to altitude, there also seems to be a greater reliance on carbohydrate metabolism, resulting in higher blood lactate concentrations. This can be explained mainly by the greater catecholamine response to altitude, more specifically, epinephrine, which promotes glycogen use. At moderate altitudes, however, acclimatized people rely more on lipid metabolism during submaximal intensity exercise than those who are not acclimatized.[36]

It is important to remember that the magnitude of the responses is proportional to the altitude one is exposed to (e.g., moderate-to-high altitude or exercising at the Olympic Training Center in Colorado Springs, CO, compared with on top of Pike's Peak, CO). Still, the basic, acute responses to altitude's hypoxia are as follows:

1. Heart rate and ventilation increase in response to the lower P_{O_2} sensed by the chemoreceptors.
2. Pulmonary diffusion is maintained.
3. Oxygen transport is reduced because of a lower saturation of hemoglobin with oxygen.
4. Ventilatory tidal volume increases at rest, and respiratory rate increases with activity and higher elevations.

Box 10-7 DID YOU KNOW?
A Comparison of Blood Doping to Altitude Training

Blood doping has been the subject of several scandals in endurance sports. In the midst of the 2007 Tour de France, professional rider Alexandre Vinokourov tested positive for a blood transfusion. Subsequent tests led to his early retirement in December 2007. His retirement occurred in the midst of a sea of controversy surrounding the 2007 race, which included multiple positive tests for blood doping and erythropoetin (EPO) use by riders such as Iban Mayo Diez.

Blood doping originally referred to the practice of injecting red blood cells into the body. Some athletes use another person's blood for this purpose. Other athletes remove their own red blood cells, wait for the body to regain natural levels, and then reinject the removed red blood cells before competition. This temporarily increases the number of red blood cells above natural values.

A newer method of doping involves EPO, a glycoprotein hormone that acts on precursors in bone marrow to stimulate red cell production. It is produced in the kidneys within the renal cortex in response to lowered oxygen levels in the blood. Some athletes inject synthetic EPO to stimulate red blood cell production. EPO use can boost the proportion of red blood cells in the blood (hematocrit levels) for 2 to 3 months.

The purpose of blood doping is to increase the number of iron-rich red blood cells (erythrocytes) in the blood. An increase in red blood cells leads to increases in the oxygen-carrying capacity of the blood, improvements in aerobic power, and increases in the ability of the aerobic respiration system to provide energy. High red blood cell levels help the blood to become more efficient at managing wastes (increasing buffering capacity), help to increase the maximum oxygen uptake ($\dot{V}_{O_{2max}}$), and improve the ability of the body to regulate temperature (thermoregulation) due to accompanying increase in total blood volume. As blood doping helps with lactic acid buffering, it may also help with anaerobic sport performance recovery.

Doping, however, does involve risks, which include increased thickness (viscosity) of the blood beyond normal levels. When viscosity is too high, circulation becomes difficult and strains the heart. This can cause a decrease in oxygen availability and $\dot{V}_{O_{2max}}$; sudden death from an inadequate heart rate, typically during sleep; antibodies against EPO, which lower production of red blood cells; blood clots, heart attacks, and paralysis; or renal failure. Doping is the suspected cause of the deaths of several otherwise healthy elite athletes over the past several years.

Blood doping also involves an inconvenient process. Blood doping that involves the removal and subsequent reinjection of red blood cells causes a temporary decrease in $\dot{V}_{O_{2max}}$ due to the anemic effect caused by removing red blood cells. If the athlete does not time the injection correctly, the athlete may still be in an anemic state or find that the red blood cells are no longer operational. The timing of the process requires a considerable amount of planning and often sophisticated equipment. Doping also has transient effects, and so it must be either scheduled around an event or performed on an ongoing basis, leading to increased health risks. Its effects on anaerobic athletes are minute, and its cost and procedures make its use practical only among the most elite endurance athletes. Blood doping of all kinds is detectable with increasingly sophisticated testing.

Although modern blood doping involves significant risks to both the athlete's health and career, if caught, blood doping arose from a fairly humble origin that offers significantly safer and more ethical training options: altitude training.

At higher altitudes, the partial pressure of oxygen is lower, making oxygen less available with each breath. During acclimatization, the body senses a reduced concentration of oxygen in the blood, prompting the release of EPO. The number of small blood vessels (capillaries) increases to help distribute the oxygen. Muscle fibers also adapt in ways that allow for improved performance, including improved oxygen extraction.

Mountain climbers go through acclimatization when they stop at camps when ascending a high mountain such as Mount Everest. These waiting periods enable climbers to avoid altitude sickness and possible death that results from ascending too quickly. It has been postulated that athletes who expose themselves to less drastic acclimatization scenarios may reap the same effects as climbers, thereby improving their performance.

When altitude training is planned, the same concerns that affect mountain climbers are taken into consideration. Simply exposing an athlete to excessively high altitudes can cause significant detriments to performance. At higher altitudes, athletes cannot reach their typical exercise intensity, leading to a decline in fitness. Excessive altitude causes the onset of altitude sickness and burdened breathing, delaying training progress. Muscle also begins to break down, particularly beyond 17,717 ft (5,400 m), and the drawbacks of training at these altitudes significantly outweigh the benefits. However, when sensible altitude levels and appropriate training techniques are used, these issues are not of concern.

Although initial research into altitude training was mixed, recent studies that included lower altitudes have shown promise. Based on this research, it is suggested that athletes live at a higher altitude (in one study, 8,202 ft or 2,500 m) while, at the same time, training at a lower altitude (4,921 ft or 1,500 m). Training at a lower altitude allows athletes to sustain a level of exertion that is not otherwise possible at higher altitudes. The detraining effect of higher altitude training is thereby avoided. This "live high and train low" style increases red blood cell mass volume by about 10%, which is comparable to the effects of direct injection of red blood cells.

Altitude training naturally increases red blood cell count to a safe and comparable level to blood doping while avoiding the complications, health concerns, and possible abnormal blood responses associated with the more drastic methods of doping. Properly performed, altitude training offers a safe and practical alternative to blood doping, which translates to improvements in performance to endurance athletes.

Suggested Readings

Associated Press. Kazakh cyclist Alexandre Vinokourov reportedly retiring after receiving doping ban. USA Today, 7 Dec. 2007.

Boyer SJ. Weight loss and changes in body composition at high altitude. J Appl Physiol. 1984;57:1580–1585.

Cazzola M. Further concerns about the medical risks of blood doping. Haematologica. 2002;87:232.

Hackett PH. High-altitude illness. N Engl J Med. 2001;345:107–114.

Holden M. Doping news update. Cycling Post, 20 Jan. 2008.

Jelkmann W. Erythropoietin: structure, control of production, and function. Physiol Rev. 1992;72:449–489.

Jones M. Blood doping—a literature review. Br J Sports Med. 1989;23: 84–88.

Levine BD, Stray-Gundersen J. "Living high-training low": effect of moderate-altitude acclimatization with low-altitude training on performance. J Appl Physiol. 1997;83:102–112.

Noakes TD. Tainted glory-doping and athletic performance. N Engl J Med. 2004;351:847–849.

Smith SL. Blood boosting. Br J Sports Med. 2004;38:99–101.

Terrados N. Effects of training at simulated altitude on performance and muscle metabolic capacity in competitive road cyclists. Eur J Appl Physiol. 1988;57:203–209.

Unal M. Gene doping in sports. Sports Med. 2004;34:357–362.

5. Increased respiration decreases blood P_{CO_2} and increases blood pH to above 7.4.

6. This increased pH results in respiratory alkalosis, which causes the oxyhemoglobin saturation curve to shift to the left and helps to keep ventilation from exceeding tolerable limits.

7. The shift of the oxyhemoglobin saturation curve to the left, which allows a greater amount of oxygen binding with hemoglobin to help compensate for the low P_{O_2}.

8. Initially, increases in heart rate compensate for a decreased stroke volume and there is a greater reliance on anaerobic glycolysis at submaximal workloads.

9. Compared to sea level, maximal exercise at altitude elicits a lower stroke volume and heart rate, resulting in decrements in cardiac output and oxygen consumption, which in turn reduces endurance performances.

Performance Responses

Not all altitudes are similar in their threat to performance. Moving even one step at the summit of Mount Everest (8,850-m or 29,035-ft) is dramatically different from running a cross-country race in Laramie, WY, at 2,195 m or 7,200 ft. Again, this is due to the dramatic differences in the P_{O_2}. In fact, most athletic competitions take place at a moderate altitude, and the challenge of such an altitude is a reality for many athletes and teams each year. Higher altitudes are typically experienced only by mountain climbers, skiers, and snowboard enthusiasts.

Short-Duration Performances

Many world or Olympic records were tied or set at the Mexico City Olympics in 1968 in sprints and jumps, as well as swimming records up to 800 m (2,625 ft). This immediately created the myth that "thin air" (a popular term referring to the lower partial pressure of oxygen in the air as altitude increases) provided an advantage in anaerobic activities, from hitting a baseball to sprinting. If a sport or activity does not rely on aerobic metabolism, the effects of altitude should be minimal. However, if one experiences sickness or is "psyched out" or "psyched up" with the thought of the competitive venue, performance might be affected. Think about it: baseball players cannot wait to bat at Coors Field in Denver and NFL kickers cannot wait to kick field goals at the Denver Broncos' stadium, INVESCO Field at Mile High, because of the perceived advantages of altitude. Conversely, players request oxygen tanks and complain of problems when performing at an altitude of 1,609 m (5,280 ft). Thus, although "thin air" might play some role, preparation, focus, and other psychological factors may contribute as well to short-term performances. Furthermore, many tracks and pools exist at elevations similar to that of Mexico City at high schools, colleges, and professional venues, and all records set at such events are not limited to these venues. Many anaerobic and power-type sports involving running, jumping, and throwing provide adequate rest between exertions, resulting in little reliance on the aerobic system. In those events, the negative effects on performance are minimized.

Long-Duration Performances

Peronnet et al.[43] showed that when competing at an altitude of about 400 m (1,312 ft), speed is dramatically reduced in running events featuring cardiovascular endurance. Thus, many coaches have come to understand that altitude is a problem for long-distance events and those dependent on aerobic metabolism. Yet many of the oxygen-carrying capabilities are improved with altitude exposure (e.g., hemoglobin increases), and this has led to altitude training concepts for endurance athletes such as "live high and train low" so that the adaptations accrued by living at high altitude can be taken advantage of during performance at sea level.[51,52] Figure 10-11 shows the theoretical effects of altitude on running performances.

> ## Quick Review
>
> - The reduced partial pressure of oxygen in the air at altitude impacts performance.
> - A decrease in the partial pressure of oxygen reduces the ability of the oxygen to get to the body's tissues.
> - Exposure to altitude results in several physiological adjustments in the attempt to maintain homeostasis.
> - During exercise at altitude, both ventilatory volume and rate may increase to facilitate greater availability of oxygen.
> - At altitude, maximal oxygen consumption, cardiac output, maximal heart rate, and stroke volume decrease.
> - Exposure to altitude causes increases in hemoglobin and hematocrit in the blood.
> - Short-duration performances are not hindered and may benefit from altitude due to the "thin air."
> - Long-duration performances, namely those dependent on aerobic metabolism, are hindered by altitude.

Getting Ready to Compete at Altitude

Beyond the "hype," competing or recreating at moderate-to-high altitude does require some preparation to minimize any negative effects. Typically, this means one needs to gain some level of acclimatization or acclimation at the altitude at which the competition or recreational outing is to take place. For moderate altitudes, typical strategies involve arriving at the site a week or so before the event or going

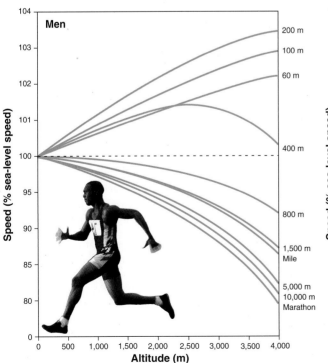
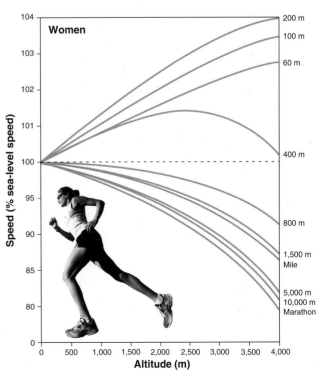

Figure 10-11. Running performances predicted at different altitudes. (Adapted with permission from the American Physiological Society.[43] In running events, as the distance of the race gets longer the negative effects of altitude on speed are observed. However, in short sprints improved performances may be observed at altitude.)

up and competing and then leaving right after the competition to minimize the exposure to altitude and not allow for any of the negative side effects of altitude to be manifested. For higher altitudes, staging from moderate elevation to allow acclimatization has been used successfully.

Altitude Sickness

Altitude sickness, which is caused by the reduction in the Po_2, is more common to higher altitudes than to lower ones and is a pathological condition that often requires medical attention. Of special concern is acute altitude sickness, also known as **acute mountain sickness (AMS)**, because it can lead to pulmonary edema (see Box 10-8). It can also progress to high-altitude cerebral edema (HACE), which is even more life-threatening and requires immediate medical attention. Treatment includes rest and removal from altitude (see Box 10-9).

Dehydration can also result in a misdiagnosis of altitude sickness, and drinking behavior is a vital factor in helping one adequately adjust to altitude. Many times, the drug acetazolamide has been effective in preventing most side effects.

Acclimatization/Acclimation

Both acclimatization (exposure to the natural environment) from living at Colorado Springs, CO, and acclimation (exposure to an artificial environment) from using a hypobaric chamber can create both short-term and long-term benefits (see Box 10-10). Short-term acclimatization/acclimation has been characterized by altitude exposure of less than 1 year. We know that even with shorter periods of 3 to 6 weeks, dramatic changes can take place and athletes can take advantage of these changes to prepare for endurance competitions. Long-term acclimatization/acclimation typically refers to people who have lived at altitude for longer than a year. However, the rate and efficiency at which acclimatization to high altitude occurs are not universal. At one end of the continuum are people who are born at moderate-to-high altitudes and live there for a lifetime. Because they have been exposed to hypoxia during their formative, growing years, these individuals undergo the proper physiological adaptations rather seamlessly. On the other end of the continuum are those who arrived during their adult years, after normal growth and development have occurred. Accordingly, their physiological systems demonstrate less plasticity, making it more difficult for adults to fully and rapidly adapt to the hypoxic and hypobaric conditions of living at altitude.

Below are changes, that can be seen with short- and long-term acclimatization/acclimation. However, it should be remembered that some variables, while gradually improving to cope with the demands of high altitude, will, nonetheless, never function as impressively as they do at sea level. For example, although the altitude-induced declines in maximum oxygen consumption and long-term endurance performance are gradually attenuated as a result acclimatization/acclimation, those variables remain lower than what they were compared to sea level. Furthermore, the changes the body experiences are highly dependent on the elevation that one has to function at, with moderate altitude much less disruptive than high altitude on body structures and functions. For example, 6 weeks of exposure to high altitude can result in a reduction in muscle size and function, whereas these effects would not be seen at moderate altitude.

Short-Term (3–6 Weeks) Effects

- Increased pulmonary ventilation compared to sea level at rest and with exercise
- Increased release of erythropoietin (EPO) from kidneys, which simulates red blood cell production above sea level values
- Increased hemoglobin concentration compared to sea level values
- Increased hematocrit compared to sea level values
- Increased plasma volume compared to initial values upon exposure to altitude, yet not equal to sea level values

Long-Term (≥3 Months) Effects

- Increased mitochondrial density compared to sea level values
- Increased capillary density compared to sea level values
- Increased pulmonary diffusing capacity compared to initial values upon exposure to altitude, yet not equal to sea level values
- Increased mitochondrial enzymes compared to sea level values
- Increased respiratory chain enzymes compared to sea level values
- Cardiac output increases at rest over initial values upon exposure to altitude, to near sea level values
- Cardiac output with maximal exercise increases over initial values upon exposure to altitude, but not to sea level values

It has been established that altitude acclimatization or acclimation allows one to perform better at altitude. However, recent controversy has questioned the advantage gained by individuals who are native to high altitude and have lived at high altitudes all their lives. Brutsaert[9] states,

"...a review of the literature suggests that indigenous HA (high altitude) natives have higher mean maximal oxygen consumption ($\dot{V}o_{2max}$) in hypoxia and smaller $\dot{V}o_{2max}$ decrement with increasing hypoxia. At present, there is insufficient information to conclude that HA natives have enhanced work economy or greater endurance capacity, although for the former a number of studies indicate that this may be the case for Tibetans."

Thus, it seems that the normal altitude acclimatization or acclimation is the basis of meeting the challenges of altitude competitions and exposure. However, even with

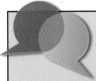

Box 10-8 AN EXPERT VIEW
Acute Mountain Sickness

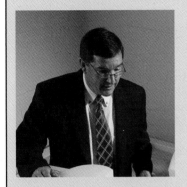

Carl M. Maresh, PhD, FACSM
Professor and Department Head
Human Performance Laboratory
Department of Kinesiology
University of Connecticut
Storrs, CT

Of the several types of altitude illnesses, AMS is the most common. AMS persists for 2 to 7 days and comprises a collection of well-recognized symptoms that can affect anyone traveling rapidly from lower to higher terrestrial elevations (especially above 2,500 m). The most recognized symptoms are headache, nausea, weakness, loss of appetite, and shortness of breath on exertion. Onset of symptoms can occur from within minutes to hours (usually 6–24 hours) after arrival, and the incidence and severity of these depend on the altitude and speed at which one travels to that altitude. Interestingly, one's susceptibility to AMS cannot be predicted from measurements obtained at low elevations, but a prior history of AMS is the best predictor of future occurrence. My interest in AMS began when I moved from Pittsburgh, PA, to Laramie, WY, as a graduate student. I was also a serious distance runner at that time with thoughts that moving from low altitude to 2,200 m would benefit my training and performance.

It was obvious that lowlanders traveling to Laramie experienced the effects of this moderate altitude as AMS. During the summer months, for example, it was very common for people traveling the interstate highway through Laramie to visit the emergency room at the community hospital with symptoms of headache, weakness, and shortness of breath. One summer, after running the Pike's Peak Marathon, I spent several days on the peak working with researchers from the altitude division at the U.S. Army Research Institute of Environmental Medicine. This project involved lowlanders who traveled overnight from Massachusetts to the top of Pike's Peak, CO (4,300 m). Symptoms of AMS occurred very rapidly in this group and remained severe during the first 48 to 72 hours. Unquestionably, headache, often accompanied with vomiting, was their most profound symptom, and virtually all subjects reported profound difficulty sleeping.

Among other experiences, these observations helped to focus my attention on one of the topics of my doctoral dissertation, the first study to compare AMS symptomatology in lowland natives (LN) and moderate altitude (2,200 m) natives (MANs) quickly taken to a higher altitude (4,300 m in a hypobaric chamber). Both groups of subjects began to report AMS symptoms 6 hours after decompression, but LNs reported far more severe headache, nausea, and vomiting. Symptoms peaked during the first 24 hours in MANs, but continued to be quite profound throughout the second day of decompression in LNs. All the MANs reported an absence of symptoms on the morning of day 3 when exercise testing was conducted, but all the LNs still experienced headaches that morning. One of the lowlanders, in particular, suffered from a headache and vomiting so severe that he was unable to perform testing. He reported a complete absence of these symptoms 2 hours after leaving the chamber.

Obviously, it is the reduction in the partial pressure of oxygen that sets into motion the ventilatory, vasoconstriction, and fluid retention mechanisms that contribute to the paradigm of AMS. If unabated, the concomitants of AMS, high-altitude pulmonary edema, and HACE can develop and are life-threatening conditions. For persons going to high altitudes, the process of staged ascent to promote altitude acclimatization and minimizing one's physical exertion are the best methods for reducing AMS susceptibility. In the absence of acclimatization, prophylaxis with acetazolamide, a carbonic anhydrase inhibitor, can be quite effective in reducing AMS symptoms, but is known to impair physical performance. The references that follow will provide more information on the topics I have presented here.

Suggested Readings

Maresh CM, Kraemer WJ, Noble BJ, et al. Exercise responses after short- and long-term residence at 2,200 meters. Aviat Space Environ Med. 1988;59:335–339.

Maresh CM, Kraemer WJ, Judelson DA, et al. The effects of high altitude and water deprivation on AVP release in man. Am J Physiol Endocrinol Metab. 2004;286:E20–E24.

Maresh CM, Noble BJ, Robertson KL, et al. Aldosterone, cortisol and electrolyte responses to hypobaric hypoxia in moderate-altitude natives. Aviat Space Environ Med. 1985;56:1078–1084.

Muza SR, Fulco CS, Cymerman A. Altitude Acclimatization Guide. USARIEM Technical Report No. TN04–05. Natick, MA: Thermal and Mountain Medicine Division, U.S. Army Research Institute of Environmental Medicine, 2004.

such physiological adaptations, endurance performances will be compromised in the hypoxic conditions of moderate or high altitude.

Live High and Train Low Theory

Given the effects of altitude discussed earlier, some have proposed the theory known as "live high and train low."

Following this approach, one lives at high altitude to gain the benefits of hypoxia, stimulating one's hematocrit and hemoglobin concentrations to aid oxygen transport, but then performs workouts at lower altitudes to stimulate cardiovascular capabilities at maximal levels and maintain quality of workouts.[1,42,51] Thus, one takes advantage of both worlds.

Box 10-9 DID YOU KNOW?
Signs and Symptoms of Altitude Sickness

General Signs and Symptoms

- Lack of appetite
- Nausea
- Vomiting
- Excessive weakness
- Dizziness
- Light-headedness
- Insomnia
- Pins and needles feeling
- Shortness of breath on exertion
- Persistent rapid pulse
- Drowsiness
- General malaise
- Peripheral edema (swelling of hands, feet, and face)

Symptoms Indicating Life-Threatening Altitude Sickness

- Pulmonary edema (fluid in the lungs)
- Persistent dry cough
- Fever
- Shortness of breath even when resting
- Cerebral edema (swelling of the brain)
- Headache that does not respond to medicine
- Motor behavior problems with walking
- Increased vomiting
- Gradual loss of consciousness

Theory to Practice

Many coaches and athletes apply this theory in a variety of ways. For example, it has been shown that intermittent exposure of 7 days to a higher altitude of 14,108 ft or 4,300 m with rest and training can improve time trial cycle exercise performance and promote physiological changes similar to those of more chronic adaptations to the same altitude.[6] It has also been seen that the natives of moderate altitudes have a physiological advantage over natives of low altitudes with respect to maximal exercise at high altitude.[36,37] This indicates that living at moderate altitude for long periods of time confers a physiological advantage to the demands of higher altitudes.[36,37]

Some teams arrive 18 to 24 hours before the competition, allowing some of the initial physiological changes in response to altitude to take place. As noted earlier, another method used by competitive athletes competing at a moderate altitude is to arrive for the competition on the same day, compete, and leave. Many American football

Box 10-10 DID YOU KNOW?
Hypoxic Tents

Hypoxic tents or rooms (A) have come into great controversy as to whether they are a legal ergogenic aid for athletes, as they change the concentration of oxygen in the air, thereby simulating altitude by creating a hypoxic environment in the air one breaths. Different from altitude, there is no change in the barometric pressure, which can only be created with the use of environmental hypobaric chambers (B).

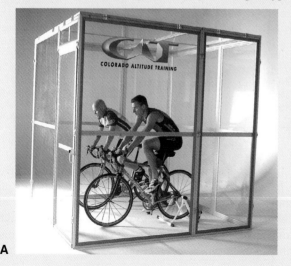

A

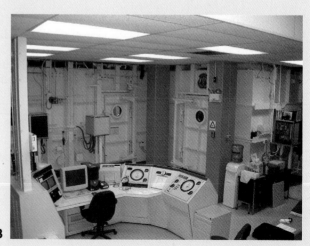

B

teams competing against the University of Wyoming practice at lower altitude and drive up on the morning of the game from a nearby lower altitude, play it, and leave to limit any impact of the moderate altitude exposure. Now, from what you have read previously, a reduced P_{O_2} should not have a very great impact on the game of American football, which focuses on anaerobic, power-type activities, but symptoms and psychology may well have an impact. Therefore, the live high and train low theory might still be part of an overall strategy for competition in American football. Even cross-country runners coming from sea level have used these above two approaches due to the inability to stay for extended time periods at moderate altitude before a competition. Its efficacy has not been clearly established, but it might be considered a practical approach to competition at moderate altitude.

Although the World Anti-Doping Agency has not banned the use of hypoxic environmental tents, controversy and concerns over their use, similar to those over blood doping, exist.[35] Still, it is not clear as to the dose that should be used to elicit the responses desired.[51] Initial data have shown that the use of such tents does not appear to have any impact on sea level performance, but more study is needed.[28]

Quick Review

- Athletes prepare for competition at altitude with strategies to gain some level of acclimatization or acclimation.
- Altitude sickness is a dangerous condition caused by reduction in P_{O_2} that can lead to HACE.
- The "live high and train low" theory allows oxidative advantages of altitude without hindering training intensity.
- Some competitive athletes do not attempt to acclimatize to altitude at all. But rather, they arrive for the competition on the same day, compete, and leave.

Practical Applications

It is vital when evaluating environmental challenges that the total picture is considered. As we have seen, one can be in a cold environment, yet suffer from heat exhaustion due to too many layers of clothing. Or, one can be at high altitude and suffer from dehydration without any heat or exercise demands. Therefore, an appreciation of the many different environmental stressors and the specific exercise to be performed is needed when workouts or strategies for competition or training are developed.

CASE STUDY

WBGT levels for modification or cancellation of workouts or athletic competition for healthy adults[a,g]

WBGT[b] °F	WBGT[b] °C	Continuous Activity and Competition	Training and Noncontinuous Activity — Nonacclimatized, Unfit, High-Risk Individuals[c]	Training and Noncontinuous Activity — Acclimatized, Fit Low-Risk Individuals[c,d]
≤50.0	≤10.0	Generally safe; Exertional heat stroke (EHS) can occur associated with individual factors	Normal activity	Normal activity
50.1–65.0	10.1–18.3		Normal activity	Normal activity
65.1–72.0	18.4–22.2	Generally safe; EHS can occur Risk of EHS and other heat illness begins to rise; high-risk individuals should be monitored or not compete	Increased risk. Increase the rest:work ratio. Monitor fluid intake.	Normal activity
72.1–78.0	22.3–25.6	Risk for all competitors is increased	Moderate risk. Increase the rest:work ratio and decrease total duration of activity.	Normal activity. Monitor fluid intake.
78.1–82.0	25.7–27.8	Risk for unfit, nonacclimatized individuals is high	Moderate-high risk. Increase the rest: work ratio, decrease intensity and total duration of activity.	Normal activity. Monitor fluid intake.
82.1–86.0	27.9–30.0	Cancel level for EHS risk	High risk.[e] Increase the rest:work ratio to 1:1, decrease intensity and total duration of activity. Limit intense exercise. Watch at-risk individuals carefully	Plan intense or prolonged exercise with discretion watch at-risk individuals carefully.
86.1–90.0	30.1–32.2		Very High-risk.[e] Cancel or stop practice and competition.	Limit intense exercise and total daily exposure to heat and humidity; watch for early signs and symptoms.
≥90.1	>32.3		Extremely high risk.[e] Cancel exercise.	Cancel exercise uncompensable heat stress[f] exists for all athletes.[g]

[a] Revised from reference (38)
[b] Wet bulb globe temperature
[c] While wearing shorts, T-shirt, socks and sneakers
[d] Acclimated to training in the heat at least 3 wk
[e] Risk of EHS and exertional heat exhaustion
[f] Internal heat production exceeds heat loss and core body temperature rises continuously, without a plateau
[g] Differences of local climate and individual heat acclimation status may allow activity at higher levels than outlined in the table, but athletes and coaches should consult with sports medicine staff and should be cautious when exceeding these limits.

Armstrong LE, et al. Position stand, American College of Sports Medicine: Exertional heat illness in training and competition. Med Sci Sports Exerc. 2007;39(3):556–572.

(continued)

The heat stress index allows one to get a handle on the risk for heat illness due to a combination of the relative humidity and air temperature. Make decisions concerning the following case studies about environmental stresses based on the information presented in this chapter.

Scenario

You are the athletic trainer for Hattiesburg High School in Hattiesburg, MS, and the football team is scheduled for an early August practice at 10:00 AM at the new stadium. You have just completed a week of one-a-day practices in shorts and helmets and are now moving into practice with full pads. You carefully checked the relative humidity and temperature and even tried to estimate the amount of change over the 90-minute practice. You measured the current conditions at 9:00 AM and found that the temperature was 29.4°C (85°F) with a relative humidity of 78%. You are getting ready to meet with the head coach and discuss the precautions needed for practice today.

Questions

- What are your recommendations going to be?
- How will you handle the coach's concerns for possible interruptions of a preplanned practice for summer training leading up to the first game?
- What else should you consider to ensure the safety of each player?

Options

Although you can expect that the players have made some physiological adaptations to the heat during the first week of practice, acclimatization will not be complete for about another week. Also, the players have not yet practiced in full gear (which impairs body heat dissipation) during the first week and so heat stress will be greater today. You should also be concerned about the ambient conditions on this day. At 9:00 AM, it is already 85°F and humidity is quite high. These conditions will limit the effectiveness of sweating to cool the body. First, you should make sure that the athletes are well hydrated before practice, consuming a sports drink containing proper a mounts of electrolytes. During practice, the players need to be monitored closely and water breaks should be taken at regular intervals. Also, you may tell the coach that practice should be limited to 60 minutes and not the 90 minutes he had planned. Explain to him that this will not only be better for performance because the desired intensity and concentration will be more readily maintained for 60 minutes, but also for the safety of his players. Finally, be sure the players consume adequate amounts of fluid after the practice session ends to promote adequate rehydration.

Scenario

You are the women's cross-country coach at East High School in Cheyenne, WY. It is August 20 and you have a scheduled run of 5 miles (8 km) at race pace for your team 3 days before the first invitational of the season. The temperature is 78°F or 25.6°C, with 39% relative humidity. The wind speed is 13 mph.

Questions

- What concerns do you have about the practice and the environmental conditions that exist?
- What other aspects of the practice should you be concerned about for your team?

Options

The ambient weather conditions are quite favorable today and will permit effective dissipation of the heat produced by the working muscles with a moderate temperature, low humidity, and a cool breeze. Overheating and dehydration are not major concerns today. However, it is only 3 days before the team's first competition, and a 5-mile run at race pace may cause muscle damage and lingering fatigue that will negatively impact performance at the invitational. It might be best not to push the athletes too hard just 3 days before the event. A more moderate pace would be in order.

Scenario

You are an athletic trainer at the University of Wisconsin in Madison, and you are getting ready to play a nonconference game against Arizona State University in Tempe, AZ, in late August. Your practices started in August, when the heat and humidity in Wisconsin are quite high. The team physician and head coach want your input on what is needed to prepare the team for the game, in which the temperature could be as high as 104°F (40°C).

Questions

- What is needed to protect the team from heat illness?
- What plans might you put in place with your sports medicine team to ensure a safe and successful performance?
- What rules govern competition in such environmental extremes?
- What other factors related to physical conditioning would you address?

Options

The best approach to this would be to mimic as closely as possible the conditions to be encountered in Tempe. This means that a very warm, but dry environment is needed. Because the ambient air in Wisconsin at this time of year can be humid and because the temperature will not match what is expected in San Diego, it would be best to have the team practice indoors in the gymnasium where the air is dry and the temperature can be elevated to match the ambient conditions of Arizona. Practicing in these conditions for 5 to 7 days before the game should allow adequate acclimation and prepare the players physiologically for the rigors of competing in a hot, dry climate. Both during practice sessions and the game itself, the training staff should be aware that such hot, dry conditions will result in much water loss via sweating (evaporation will occur at a high rate under these environmental conditions). The players, especially the linemen, should be closely monitored for signs of dehydration, and all players should be told to drink water as they come off the field. Also, large cooling fans should be placed along the benches to help cool the players during the game.

Scenario

You are the head soccer coach at the University of Virginia and travel to the Indiana University for a match. It is late in the fall, and your team will be playing a night game. Before the game, you walk out onto the field and notice that a heavy rain is starting to fall. It is now 6 PM, and the temperature has fallen from about 46°F (7.8°C) to about 39°F (3.9°C) in the past few hours. You head back into the locker room for some final pregame preparations before coming back out for warm-up and drills before the game.

Questions

- What preparations should you have taken before the trip?
- What sports medicine implications are there?
- What type of player preparation before the match might be important?
- What are some of the last-minute preparations you might make for an ever-increasing cold challenge during the game?

Options

You expected that this night game in Indiana might be played under colder conditions to which your University of Virginia players are accustomed. You made sure that you had them bring along their well-lined and insulated warm-up gear and their long-sleeved jerseys for the game. While active, the players should be warm enough, but reserves on the sideline may get cold and heaters should be stationed along the benches. Also, the goalie, who does little running during the game, may want to wear warmer clothing than he usually does. Before the game, warm-up drills should be more extensive than they would normally be in the more moderate conditions of Virginia. And at halftime of the game, it would be wise to bring the entire team into a warm locker room rather than remaining on the outdoor field.

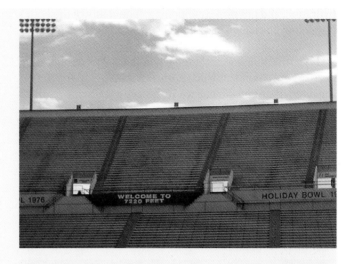

Scenario

As the head football coach of San Diego State University, you are taking your football team from San Diego to play the University of Wyoming, which is located at moderate altitude but is the highest Division-I American football stadium in the United States at 2,184 m (7,165 ft).

Questions

- What preparations would you undertake to prepare for this game in the coming week?
- Why would you select such a strategy?

Options

Although some coaches may arrive in Wyoming 18 to 24 hours before the competition to allow their athletes sufficient time for initial physiological responses to altitude to occur, it may not be necessary because football plays are short enough in duration to not tax the aerobic energy system. Because the aerobic energy system is not taxed in a football game, aerobic adaptations to altitude exposure will not likely affect performance at altitude. Thus, in football, the best strategy may be to stay and practice at low altitude until game time, drive up to the stadium in Wyoming immediately before the game, play (and win) the game, and return to lower altitude immediately afterwards. This strategy will limit any impact of the moderate altitude exposure.

CHAPTER SUMMARY

Environmental conditions such as heat, cold, and altitude affect the body's responses and ability to perform exercise. The physiological stress and performance deficits can be attenuated by training and preparation strategies.

Hyperthermia is overheating of the human body. Body size, age, fitness, temperature, humidity, and wind speed all impact the possibility of being affected by hyperthermia. Convection, conduction, radiation, and evaporation all help to dissipate excess body heat. Heat cramps, syncope, heat exhaustion, and heat stroke are conditions brought on by exposure to heat. Among them, heat stroke can be the most dangerous, as it is frequently confused for heat exhaustion, and can lead to death.

The ability to perform in a hot environment is a multivariable challenge involving the need for prior acclimatization, proper hydration, and physical conditioning. The ability of the body's physiology to change in response to environmental challenges helps it acclimatize to hot weather.

Hypothermia is a condition when the body's temperature decreases to a point at which normal physiological function is impaired or not possible. Severity ranges from Stage 1, which diminishes ability to perform motor tasks, to Stage 4, which can lead to brain death. Hypothermia can reduce athletic performance, particularly muscle force production.

High altitude leads to hypoxia as a result of the decrease in barometric pressure. High altitude particularly impacts aerobic events. Various strategies to adapt to these conditions are practiced by athletes to prepare for competition at altitude.

REVIEW QUESTIONS

Fill-in-the-Blank

1. _____ is a measure of water in the air. When it increases, it affects the body's core temperature by _____ the need for thermoregulation.

2. _____ is an environmental variable that influences core temperature. When it increases, it cools the body through _____.

3. Human beings are only about _____% efficient in using energy; the excess _____% energy is released as heat.

4. The "Live _____, train _____" strategy is practiced by some athletes to help them acclimatize to _____.

5. Acclimatization results from exposure to the _____ environment, such as from living at Colorado Springs, CO, whereas acclimation results from exposure to an _____ environment, such as using a hypobaric chamber.

Multiple Choice

1. During the first week of summer practice, your Division 1 athlete approaches you, saying that he is dizzy and nauseous and would like to sit out for a couple of plays. You notice that he is somewhat pale. What is your next step?

   a. Offer him some water, allow him to sit out for a play or two, and then check on him and see if he wants to rejoin his teammates.

   b. Take his temperature with a thermometer. If it does not seem to show heat stroke, offer him a sports beverage and tell him to resume playing as soon as he can.

   c. Immediately bring him inside and have him insert a rectal probe to check his temperature. If his temperature is elevated to heat stroke levels, place him in a cold water bath and call for medical attention.

   d. Tell him to take a cold shower, drink a sports drink, and come back to the field. When he comes back, see if he still appears sick. If so, check his temperature for heat stroke.

   e. Let him sit on the sidelines for a little while, drink some fluids, and if he has no shown signs of fainting after 1 hour, send him home.

2. It is the first day of practice, and your first day outside since last year. The first day of spring brings 98°F (36.7°C) weather with high humidity. What's your best option?

   a. Call off practice for the day.

   b. Use the day as a training day, inside the gym.

   c. Gently warm up and perform dynamic warm-ups outside to begin the process of heat acclimatization.

   d. Complete practice as usual, watching for heat illness.

3. When does cold affect exercise performance?

   a. It does not affect endurance performance unless core temperature decreases but can affect force production.

   b. It affects endurance performance but not force production.

   c. If a lot of layers are kept on in cold weather, athletes will not experience any temperature-related difficulties.

   d. The body compensates by shivering and other mechanisms, thereby negating any potential effects.

4. You are volunteering as a soccer coach for a male adult league. This is the second day of practice, and it is hot and humid outside. You decide it is safe enough to hold practice outside, although you will take the players inside partway through practice. Which group of individuals is at higher risk of heat illness from exercise in the heat?

   a. older individuals

   b. individuals with high percentage of body fat

   c. new athletes

   d. all of the above

5. Which of the following is the body's major heat loss mechanism for exercise in the heat?

   a. Convection

   b. Conduction

   c. Radiation

   d. Ventilation

   e. Evaporation

True/False

1. At acute altitude exposure, there appears to be a greater reliance on carbohydrate metabolism, resulting in higher lactate responses.

2. The percentage of oxygen in the air at altitude is reduced.
3. World and Olympic records were tied or set in the Mexico City Olympics in 1968 in sprints and jumps, as well as swimming records up to 800 m.
4. Cold receptors are fewer in number than heat receptors in the human body.
5. Limited exposure to heat for *anaerobic* performances may not hamper performance and in some cases may enhance performance due to the temperature kinetics of anaerobic enzymes.

Short Answer

1. What are some of the factors that influence regulation of body temperature?
2. What causes the reddened skin appearance common to exercise in the heat?
3. As a coach, you are holding a practice in the heat. Which aspects of performance do you expect to be hindered, which do you expect will not be affected by the heat, and what is the anticipated impact?
4. What is different about higher altitude that leads to decrements in performance?
5. What risks might one encounter when ascending a mountain?

KEY TERMS

acclimation: artificially induced adaptations to climate

acclimatization: process of adapting to a climate

acute mountain sickness: pathological condition that is caused by acute exposure to low partial pressure of oxygen at high altitudes

barometric pressure: pressure exerted by the air above you

blood doping: increasing the number of red blood cells either by transfusion or by the use of erythropoietin (EPO) to boost the production of red blood cells

bronchoconstriction: reduction in the diameter of the bronchioles in the lungs

conduction: transfer of heat between two objects in contact with each other

convection: a mechanism of cooling the body in which the air moving over the body helps the body lose heat

evaporation: a process whereby liquids absorb heat and turn into gas; when sweat evaporates from the body or humid air is released from the lungs, heat is also released from the body

exercise-induced bronchoconstriction (EIB): reduction in the diameter of the bronchioles in the lungs brought on by the onset of exercise; bronchoconstriction characterizes many asthma conditions, and EIB can be brought about by endurance exercise in people who have exercise-induced asthma

heat cramps: refer to muscle cramps that occur while in the heat, often resulting from dehydration, a whole body sodium deficit, and neuromuscular fatigue

heat exhaustion: a condition in which exposure to high temperature leads to pallor, persistent muscular cramps, weakness, fainting, dizziness, headache, hyperventilation, nausea, anorexia, diarrhea, decreased urine output, and a body-core temperature that generally ranges between 36°C (97°F) and 40°C (104°F)

heat stress index: an index combining temperature and humidity to determine the amount of physiological stress that will be experienced by the body under such conditions

heat stroke: a condition in which exposure to high temperatures leads to a rapid heart rate (tachycardia), hypotension, sweating (although skin may be dry at time of collapse), hyperventilation, altered mental state, diarrhea, seizures, and coma; the only accurate method of determining heat stroke is a rectal probe; this condition requires immediate medical attention

hyperthermia: an increase in deep internal body temperature above normal

hypobaric environment: environment epitomized by reduced pressure at altitude

hypothermia: a condition in which the body's temperature decreases to a point at which normal physiological function is impaired or not possible

hypoxia: the compromised delivery of oxygen to target tissues

isotherm: a type of contour line or surface outline connecting points of equal temperature

nerve conduction velocity: speed at which electrical impulses are conducted in a motor neuron

partial pressure: tension of a given gas (such as oxygen); calculated as a product of barometric pressure and the percentage of the given gas in the air

pulmonary ventilation: total volume of gas per minute inspired or expired

radiation: heat loss in the form of electromagnetic waves

relative humidity: the percentage of water vapor held in the air

rhabdomyolysis: destruction of muscle tissue resulting in myoglobin and other proteins normally in muscle found in the blood

syncope: fainting in response to heat exposure, often seen in those who have not been acclimatized to hot weather

thermoregulation: the process of altering physiological processes in response to stimuli to keep the body's temperature stable

wet-bulb globe temperature: a composite temperature used to estimate the effect of temperature, humidity, and solar radiation on humans

REFERENCES

1. Armstrong LE, Casa DJ, Millard-Stafford M, et al. American College of Sports Medicine position stand. Exertional heat illness during training and competition. Med Sci Sports Exerc. 2007;39:556–572.
2. Armstrong LE, Epstein Y, Greenleaf JE, et al. American College of Sports Medicine position stand. Heat and cold illnesses during distance running. Med Sci Sports Exerc. 1996;28(12):i–x.
3. Armstrong LE, Maresh CM. The induction and decay of heat acclimatization in trained athletes. Sports Med. 1991;12:302–312.
4. Arvesen A, Wilson J, Rosen L. Nerve conduction velocity in human limbs with late sequelae after local cold injury. Eur J Clin Invest. 1996;26:443–450.
5. Asmussen E, Bonde-Petersen F, Jorgensen K. Mechano-elastic properties of human muscles at different temperatures. Acta Physiol Scand. 1976;96:83–93.
6. Beidleman BA, Muza SR, Fulco CS, et al. Seven intermittent exposures to altitude improves exercise performance at 4300 m. Med Sci Sports Exerc. 2008;40:141–148.
7. Bouchama A, Dehbi M, Mohamed G, et al. Prognostic factors in heat wave related deaths: a meta-analysis. Arch Intern Med. 2007;167:2170–2176.
8. Boulant J. Hypothalamic neurons regulating body temperature. In: Fregly MJ, Blatteis CM, eds. Handbook of Physiology, Section 4: Environmental Physiology, Vol. I. Bethesda, MD: American Physiological Society, 1996:105–126.

9. Brutsaert TD. Do high-altitude natives have enhanced exercise performance at altitude? Appl Physiol Nutr Metab. 2008;33:582–592.

10. Casa DJ, Armstrong LE, Ganio MS, et al. Exertional heat stroke in competitive athletes. Curr Sports Med Rep. 2005;4:309–317.

11. Casa DJ, Armstrong LE, Hillman SK, et al. National athletic trainers' association position statement: fluid replacement for athletes. J Athl Train. 2000;35:212–224.

12. Casa DJ, Becker SM, Ganio MS, et al. Validity of devices that assess body temperature during outdoor exercise in the heat. J Athl Train. 2007;42:333–342.

13. Cheung SS, Sleivert GG. Lowering of skin temperature decreases isokinetic maximal force production independent of core temperature. Eur J Appl Physiol. 2004;91:723–728.

14. Chodzko-Zajko WJ, Proctor DN, Fiatarone Singh MA, et al. American College of Sports Medicine position stand. Exercise and physical activity for older adults. Med Sci Sports Exerc. 1998;30:992–1008.

15. Comeau MJ, Potteiger JA, Brown LE. Effects of environmental cooling on force production in the quadriceps and hamstrings. J Strength Cond Res. 2003;17:279–284.

16. Cooper ER, Ferrara MS, Broglio SP. Exertional heat illness and environmental conditions during a single football season in the southeast. J Athl Train. 2006;41:332–336.

17. Cooper KE. Some historical perspectives on thermoregulation. J Appl Physiol. 2002;92:1717–1724.

18. Degroot DW, Kenney WL. Impaired defense of core temperature in aged humans during mild cold stress. Am J Physiol Regul Integr Comp Physiol. 2007;292:R103–R108.

19. Dorrington KL, Talbot NP. Human pulmonary vascular responses to hypoxia and hypercapnia. Pflugers Arch. 2004;449:1–15.

20. Duffield R, Marino FE. Effects of pre-cooling procedures on intermittent-sprint exercise performance in warm conditions. Eur J Appl Physiol. 2007;100:727–735.

21. Ely MR, Cheuvront SN, Montain SJ. Neither cloud cover nor low solar loads are associated with fast marathon performance. Med Sci Sports Exerc. 2007;39:2029–2035.

22. Felicijan A, Golja P, Milcinski M, et al. Enhancement of cold-induced vasodilatation following acclimatization to altitude. Eur J Appl Physiol. 2008;104:201–206.

23. Frisancho AR. Human Adaptation: A Functional Interpretation. St Louis, MO: C.V. Mosby, 1979.

24. Gisolfi CV. Work-heat tolerance of distance runners. In: Milvy P, ed. The Marathon: Physiological, Medical, Epidemiological, and Psychological Studies. New York, NY: The New York Academy of Sciences, 1977:139–150.

25. Gonzalez-Alonso J, Crandall CG, Johnson JM. The cardiovascular challenge of exercising in the heat. J Physiol. 2007;586:45–53.

26. Grover RF, Reeves JT. Exercise performance of athletes at sea level and 3100 meters altitude. Schweiz Z Sportmed. 1966;14:130–148.

27. Hawkins S, Wiswell R. Rate and mechanism of maximal oxygen consumption decline with aging: implications for exercise training. Sports Med. 2003;33:877–888.

28. Hinckson EA, Hopkins WG, Edwards JS, et al. Sea-level performance in runners using altitude tents: a field study. J Sci Med Sport. 2005;8:451–457.

29. Howard RL, Kraemer WJ, Stanley DC, et al. The effects of cold immersion on muscle strength. J Strength Cond Res. 1994;8(3):129–133.

30. Judelson DA, Maresh CM, Farrell MJ, et al. Effect of hydration state on strength, power, and resistance exercise performance. Med Sci Sports Exerc. 2007;39:1817–1824.

31. Kenney WL, Munce TA. Invited review: aging and human temperature regulation. J Appl Physiol. 2003;95:2598–2603.

32. Kenney WL, Zeman MJ. Psychrometric limits and critical evaporative coefficients for unacclimated men and women. J Appl Physiol. 2002;92:2256–2263.

33. Kenney WL. A review of comparative responses of men and women to heat stress. Environ Res. 1985;37:1–11.

34. Kinugasa R, Kuchiki K, Tono T, et al. Superficial cooling inhibits force loss in damaged muscle. Int J Sports Med. 2008.

35. Lippi G, Franchini M, Guidi GC. Prohibition of artificial hypoxic environments in sports: health risks rather than ethics. Appl Physiol Nutr Metab. 2007;32:1206–1207; discussion 1208–1209.

36. Maresh CM, Kraemer WJ, Noble BJ, et al. Exercise responses after short- and long-term residence at 2,200 meters. Aviat Space Environ Med. 1988;59:335–339.

37. Maresh CM, Noble BJ, Robertson KL, et al. Maximal exercise during hypobaric hypoxia (447 Torr) in moderate-altitude natives. Med Sci Sports Exerc. 1983;15:360–365.

38. McCann DJ, Adams WC. Wet bulb globe temperature index and performance in competitive distance runners. Med Sci Sports Exerc. 1997;29:955–961.

39. Montain SJ, Cheuvront SN, Lukaski HC. Sweat mineral-element responses during 7 h of exercise-heat stress. Int J Sport Nutr Exerc Metab. 2007;17:574–582.

40. Montain SJ, Ely MR, Cheuvront SN. Marathon performance in thermally stressing conditions. Sports Med. 2007;37:320–323.

41. Noble BJ, Maresh CM. Acute exposure of college basketball players to moderate altitude: selected physiological responses. Res Q. 1979;50:668–678.

42. Patton J. The effects of acute cold exposure to exercise performance. J Strength Cond Re. 1988;2:72–78.

43. Peronnet F, Thibault G, Cousineau DL. A theoretical analysis of the effect of altitude on running performance. J Appl Physiol. 1991;70:399–404.

44. Rasch W, Cabanac M. Selective brain cooling is affected by wearing headgear during exercise. J Appl Physiol. 1993;74:1229–1233.

45. Sawka MN, Burke LM, Eichner ER, et al. American College of Sports Medicine position stand. Exercise and fluid replacement. Med Sci Sports Exerc. 2007;39:377–390.

46. Sawka MN. Physiological consequences of hypohydration: exercise performance and thermoregulation. Med Sci Sports Exerc. 1992;24:657–670.

47. Schniepp J, Campbell TS, Powell KL, et al. The effects of cold-water immersion on power output and heart rate in elite cyclists. J Strength Cond Res. 2002;16:561–566.

48. Schoene RB. Limits of respiration at high altitude. Clin Chest Med. 2005;26:405–414, vi.

49. Stensrud T, Berntsen S, Carlsen KH. Exercise capacity and exercise-induced bronchoconstriction (EIB) in a cold environment. Respir Med. 2007;101:1529–1536.

50. Swerup C. Determination of conduction velocity in A-delta and C fibres in humans from thermal thresholds. Acta Physiol Scand. 1995;153:81–82.

51. Wilber RL, Stray-Gundersen J, Levine BD. Effect of hypoxic "dose" on physiological responses and sea-level performance. Med Sci Sports Exerc. 2007;39:1590–1599.

52. Wilber RL. Application of altitude/hypoxic training by elite athletes. Med Sci Sports Exerc. 2007;39:1610–1624.

53. Williamson R, Carbo J, Luna B, et al. A thermal physiological comparison of two HAZMAT protective ensembles with and without active convective cooling. J Occup Environ Med. 1999;41:453–463.

Suggested Readings

Armstrong LE. Exertional Heat Illness. Champaign, IL: Human Kinetics, 2003.

Armstrong LE. Performing in Extreme Environments. Champaign, IL: Human Kinetics, 2000.

Armstrong LE, Epstein Y, Greenleaf JE, et al. American College of Sports Medicine position stand. Heat and cold illnesses during distance running. Med Sci Sports Exerc. 1996;28(12):i–x.

Armstrong LE, Maresh CM. Effects of training, environment, and host factors on the sweating response to exercise. Int J Sports Med. 1998;19(suppl 2):S103.

Bergh U. Human power at subnormal body temperatures. Acta Physiol Scand Suppl. 1980;478:1–39.

Fulco CS, Rock PB, Cymerman A. Improving athletic performance: is altitude residence or altitude training helpful? Aviat Space Environ Med. 2000;71:162–171.

Maresh CM, Noble BJ, Robertson KL, et al. Maximal exercise during hypobaric hypoxia (447 Torr) in moderate-altitude natives. Med Sci Sports Exerc. 1983;15:360.

Mazzeo RS. Physiological responses to exercise at altitude: an update. Sports Med. 2008;38:1–8.

Moore LG, Grover RF. Jack Reeves and his science. Respir Physiol Neurobiol. 2006;151(2/3):96–108.

Nielsen B. Heat acclimatization—mechanisms of adaptation to exercise in the heat. Int J Sports Med. 1998;19(suppl 2):S1534.

Classic References

Adams WC, Bernauer EM, Dill DB, et al. Effects of equivalent sea-level and altitude training on $\dot{V}O_{2max}$ and running performance. J Appl Physiol. 1975;39:262–266.

Dill DB, Kasch FW, Yousef MK, et al. Cardiovascular responses and temperature in relation to age. Aust J Sports Med. 1975;7:99–106.

Dill DB, Soholt LF, McLean DC, et al. Capacity of young males and females for running in desert heat. Med Sci Sports. 1977;9:137–142.

Faulkner JA, Daniels JT, Balke B. Effects of training at moderate altitude on physical performance capacity. J Appl Physiol. 1967;23(1):85–89.

Grover RF, Reeves JT. Exercise performance of athletes at sea level and 3100 meters altitude. Med Thorac. 1966;23(3):129–143.

Klausen K, Robinson S, Micahel ED, et al. Effect of high altitude on maximal working capacity. J Appl Physiol. 1966;21:1191–1194.

Training for Health and Performance

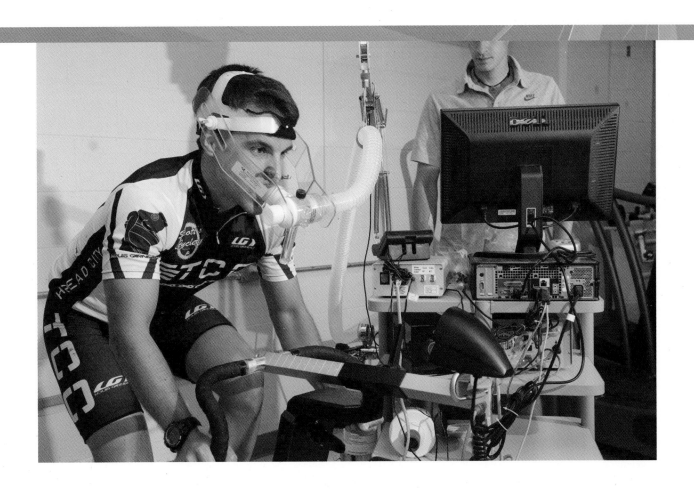

11

Understanding and Improving Body Composition

After reading this chapter, you should be able to:

1. Identify body composition and explain its specific components

2. Describe the methods and effectiveness of hydrostatic weighing, skinfolds, air-displacement plethysmography, bioelectrical impedance, and dual-energy x-ray absorptiometry (DEXA)

3. Explain essential versus nonessential body fat

4. Describe energy balance and how it can be manipulated to influence body fat percentage

5. Explain the interaction between diet, exercise, and energy balance

6. Identify the risks of severe weight loss in athletes of both sexes and normal men and women

At any given point in time, a large number of Americans are trying to change their body composition through diet and exercise. The average person attempts to decrease body fat for health-related reasons. The goal of fitness enthusiasts is typically to increase muscle mass and decrease body fat for the associated health benefits, improved body image, and increase in physical performance. Many coaches and athletes are primarily concerned with body composition because of its effect on physical performance. Although body size does affect physical performance in many sports, most measures of body size (such as height and arm length) cannot be changed. On the other hand, body mass and body composition are quite responsive to diet and exercise regimes. The goal of this chapter is to give you an understanding of how body composition is determined, the effects of diet and exercise on body composition, and the relationship between body composition and physical performance.

OVERVIEW OF BODY COMPOSITION

Body composition generally refers to the absolute amount of fat and nonfat tissue within the body as well as the ratio of fat to total body mass (TBM). **Fat mass (FM)** is the total mass (or kilograms) of all fat within the body, whereas **fat-free mass (FFM)** is the total mass of all tissues within the body excluding all fat. Some techniques of determining body composition (dual-energy x-ray absorptiometry) use the term *total lean tissue*, which is similar to the term *fat-free mass*. **Percent body fat** or **% fat** is the ratio of TBM to total FM (or FM divided by TBM). The relationships between FM, FFM, and TBM are depicted in Box 11-1, and Figure 11-1 shows the two-compartment model for body composition. In this section, we consider the current epidemic of obesity in this country and how body composition affects health and physical performance. We also cover the measures of body size and body mass index (BMI) and their relation to body composition.

Obesity, Health, and Body Composition

Despite an increased focus on a healthy diet and exercise in the U.S., obesity is now at epidemic proportions.[20] Being overweight is defined as a BMI between 25.0 and 29.9 and obesity is a BMI greater or equal to 30.0 (see Body Mass Index below). It has been estimated that ~300,000 individuals die each year from obesity-related diseases in the United States.[2] In the United States, ~65% of adults are either overweight or obese and 31% are obese,[20] despite the fact that at any given time 45% of women and 30% of men are trying to lose body mass.[58] It is also alarming that the prevalence of obesity is rapidly increasing in the United States (see Fig. 11-2). For example, in 1990, no state had an obesity prevalence rate equal to or greater than 15%, but in 2008, only one state had a prevalence less than 20%, ~60% of the states had a

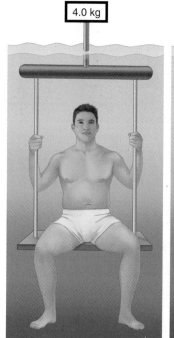
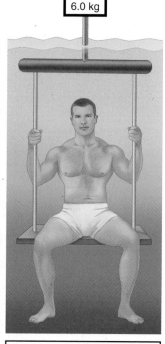

Fat mass = 23% of total body mass	Fat mass = 12% of total body mass
Fat-free mass = 77% of total body mass	Fat-free mass = 88% of total body mass

Total body mass = 90 kg
Underwater weight = 4 kg
Water displaced = 86 kg or 86 L
Body density = 1.0465 g • ml⁻¹
Siri equation %fat = 23
Fat mass = 20.7 kg
Fat-free mass = 67.4 kg

Total body mass = 90 kg
Underwater weight = 6 kg
Water displaced = 84 kg or 84 L
Body density = 1.0714 g • ml⁻¹
Siri equation %fat = 12
Fat mass = 10.8 kg
Fat-free mass = 79.2 kg

Figure 11-1. Two individuals with the same TBM can have different body compositions. Differences in % fat result in differences in underwater weight, body density, FM, and FFM.

Box 11-1 APPLYING RESEARCH
Relationships Between the Basic Measures of Body Composition

FFM, FM, and % fat are interrelated measures of body composition. All these measures of body composition are easily calculated if one or more of the measures are known. For example, if

TBM = 90 kg

% Fat = 15%

FM = TBM × % fat

FM = 90 kg × 0.15

FM = 13.5 kg

FFM = TBM − FM

FFM = 90 kg − 13.5 kg

FFM = 76.5 kg

Percent FFM (% FFM) = 100% − % fat

% FFM = 100% − 15%

% FFM = 85%

% FFM = FFM/TBM × 100

% FFM = 76.5 kg/90 kg × 100

% FFM = 0.85 × 100

% FFM = 85%

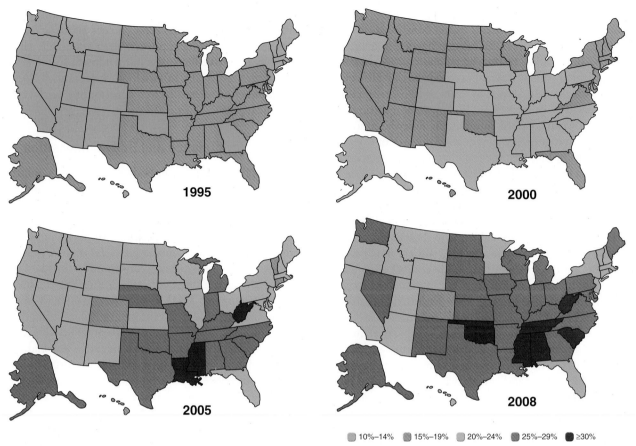

Figure 11-2. The prevalence of obesity in the United States has drastically increased from 1995 to 2005. In 1995 (*top left*), more than half the states had prevalence rates ≥15% but no state had prevalence rates ≥20%. In 2000 (*top right*), only one state had prevalence rates less than 15% (Colorado), almost half of the states had prevalence rates ≥20%, and no state had prevalence rates ≥25%. In 2005 (*bottom left*), only four states had prevalence rates <20%, about 33% of the states had prevalence rates ≥25%, and three states had prevalence he rates ≥30%. In 2008 (*bottom right*), only one state had a prevalence rate <20% (Colorado), about 60% of the states had a prevalence rate ≥25%, and six states had a prevalence rate ≥30%. (From www.cdc.gov/obesity/data/trends.html)

prevalence rate equal to or greater than 25%, and six states had a prevalence rate equal to greater than 30%. Perhaps just as alarming are the statistics from the Centers for Disease Control and Prevention for 2003–2006, which show 17% of 6- to 11-year-olds and 17.6% of 12- to 19-year-olds are obese.[12] Concerns about obesity in the general population are largely due to its association with increased mortality and risk of various diseases.[11,22,33,37,46,50] Obesity appears to be a primary factor related to hypertension, type 2 diabetes, arthritis, gout, and menstrual abnormalities. Although the strength of the association of obesity with different disease states varies, obesity has been associated with the following diseases:

1. Cardiovascular disease
2. Hypertension
3. Atherosclerosis
4. Negative effects on the blood lipid profile
5. Type 2 diabetes
6. Sleep apnea (cessation of breathing while sleeping)
7. Osteoarthritis
8. Complications in pregnancy and surgery
9. Some types of cancer (uterine, kidney, colorectal, esophageal)
10. Gallbladder disease

Fat deposition in the abdominal area, or **central obesity** (also termed *android obesity*), is more strongly associated with the majority of the above diseases than **peripheral obesity** (also termed *gynoid type obesity*), or fat deposition in the gluteal and thigh regions.[61,80] Thus, not only is obesity associated with various disease states, but the location of fat tissue in the body also affects overall health.

Causes of Obesity

Why people gain excess body fat and why the number of people doing so is increasing has no one simple answer. The basic underlying cause is people ingest more total calories than they expend. However, many interrelated factors are involved. Genetics is linked to obesity. For example, pairs of monozygotic (identical) twins eating controlled diets of 1,000 kcal·day^{-1} more than the calories needed to maintain body mass (more than resting metabolic rate [RMR]) for 100 days gained similar amounts of body mass.[6] However, the actual weight gain shown by pairs of twins ranged between 9.5 and 29.3 pounds (4.3–13.3 kg), demonstrating different pairs of twins gained substantially different amounts of weight when ingesting the same total number of calories. Although rare in humans, the inability for fat cells to produce leptin, a hormone-like substance that signals sufficient fat stores and promotes a negative energy balance, can occur. The inability to produce leptin is due to a defective ob gene, the gene that controls leptin production. Children with this disorder have minimal leptin in their blood stream, have little control over their appetite, and eat much more than other children.[47] Alterations in the control of appetite may increase the chance of obesity. For example, the insulin response to eating is correlated to a decreased appetite in normal-weight individuals.[21] In overweight or obese individuals, the insulin response to eating is not correlated to a change in appetite. This indicates that normal signals of satiety, such as the insulin response to eating, are disrupted in overweight or obese individuals, which removes the normal satiety feeling in response to eating. Physical inactivity is also a cause of obesity. The more time people spend in sedentary activities, such as watching television and playing video games, the more likely they are to be overweight.[28] Overeating for any reason is one explanation of weight gain. Overeating could be culturally biased, because of social economical factors or poor dietary habits.[52,53,74] Today, there's an abundance of high-kilocalorie, high-fat foods that are readily available, partly because of fast foods. Additionally, large portions or "super-sizing" food choices result in ingestion of more kilocalories[55] and portion sizes of virtually all foods and beverages have increased tremendously in the last several decades, especially in fast-food restaurants.[45] So, there are a number of related factors contributing to the obesity epidemic (see Box 11-2).

Physical Performance and Body Composition

As you might have guessed, body composition significantly affects physical performance. For example, an individual with a higher % fat or FM but the same FFM as another individual would have to carry more TBM in physical activities, such as running or jumping, resulting in decreased performance. Likewise, increased % fat or FM would also decrease relative peak oxygen consumption (mL·kg^{-1}·min^{-1}) because absolute oxygen consumption (L·min^{-1}) would be divided by a greater TBM. Conversely, greater FFM might be hypothesized to be an advantage in absolute strength measurements, such as one-repetition maximal bench press.

Increased body fat has shown negative correlations to performance in general physical fitness tests,[5,42] but no relationships between body composition (except for TBM) and physical performance have been shown.[65,66] In part, these inconsistent results between body composition and physical performance may be explained by the type of physical performance measured and the range of body composition (10%–15% fat or 10%–25% fat) in the populations examined. The effect of these factors on the relationship between body composition and physical performance is demonstrated by the results from several studies on athletes.

Box 11-2 AN EXPERT VIEW
The Obesity Epidemic

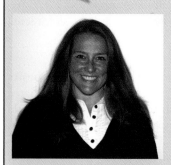

Disa L. Hatfield, PhD,
Department of Kinesiology
University of Rhode Island
Kingston, RI

The Centers for Disease Control (CDC) reports that 34% of adults aged 20 and above are obese, defined as having a BMI of 30 or more.[1] The many health risks associated with obesity include coronary heart disease, type 2 diabetes, cancers (especially endometrial, breast, and colon), hypertension, dyslipidemia, stroke, liver and gallbladder disease, sleep apnea and respiratory problems, osteoarthritis, and gynecological problems (abnormal menses and infertility).[1]

While startling, these statistics do not always cause concern in certain populations. For instance, the increased risk for disease is based upon BMI, not necessarily body fat percentage or amount of muscle mass. In fact, every player in the National Basketball Association would be considered obese by these standards, despite the fact that they are generally clearly lean and aerobically trained individuals. Further, some proponents argue that individuals who are physically active have reduced risk of disease despite their body size. For this reason, the CDC also recommends using waist circumference as a risk factor for disease since abdominal fat is closely correlated with risk.

With a 34% obesity rate, coaches and people in the health and fitness fields are going to encounter clientele who are obese. Unfortunately, the CDC and the media promote obesity as a cut and dry issue. For instance, we are bombarded with advertisements to take weight loss pills that will "melt the fat away." This gives the message that weight loss is simple and everyone should be able to decrease their weight if only they took the right medication or joined a diet or exercise program. Unfortunately, weight loss is a complex undertaking that includes balancing career and family obligations; overcoming environmental obstacles (such as living in a rural area without adequate transportation); being financially able to afford exercise equipment, gym memberships, etc.; having the knowledge to start an exercise program; and even overcoming physiological conditions, such as hormonal imbalances, that make it difficult to lose weight despite exercise and decreased caloric consumption.

Perhaps one of the largest obstacles to overcoming obesity is psychological. Discrimination against obese individuals is common in health care, the workplace, and in education, and this discrimination may impact psychological well-being.[3,4] This discrimination is often severe. A review of literature finds that 28% of grade-school teachers think that becoming obese is the worst thing that can happen to a person and that 24% of nurses are "repulsed" by individuals who are obese.[2] The invocation of such strong emotions based solely on a person's body size is alarming, and it certainly has an effect on the person these feelings are directed toward.

There are a number of ways that coaches, personal trainers, and health/fitness professionals can provide a positive and healthful way to promote weight loss in their clients who are overweight.

Educate your clients on both the risks of obesity and the benefits of physical activity. For instance, too often the focus is on weight loss, when in fact just increasing physical activity can reduce health risks for some diseases by as much as 50%.[1] You can also establish reasonable performance goals surrounding activity. Self motivation may be increased once activity goals are reached, resulting in a better mindset to reach dietary goals added later in the program.

Plan around perceived obstacles. Time, family obligations, and money are the top three barriers to actively pursuing weight loss goals. You need to be aware of each individual's barriers and be inventive in finding ways to overcome those barriers. Simply telling someone to wake up earlier for a morning walk does not work.

Help clients become autonomous in their eating habits, workout routines, and goals. Ask your clients to come up with solutions to perceived problems, instead of telling them what they should do.

Obesity is a complex and sometimes controversial issue. The most important tool for you and your obese clients is to stay informed of the social, psychological, and health consequences of obesity and to foster innovative ideas to overcoming the barriers to a healthy lifestyle.

References

1. CDC. Overweight and Obesity. Atlanta, GA: CDC. Available at: www.cdc.gov.
2. Puhl R, Brownell KD. Bias, discrimination, and obesity. Obes Res. 2001;9(12):788–805.
3. Puhl RM, Brownell KD. Psychosocial origins of obesity stigma: toward changing a powerful and pervasive bias. Obes Rev. 2003;4(4):213–227.
4. Wardle J, Cooke L. The impact of obesity on psychological well-being. Best Pract Res Clin Endocrinol Metab. 2005;19(3):421–440.

FFM of competitive power lifters shows significant correlations ($r = 0.86–0.95$) to one repetition maximum in the bench press, squat, and dead lift.[9] Collegiate American football players (% fat = 17.2 ± 5.4 [mean $\pm$ SD]) show significant but weak-to-moderate correlations between body composition and physical performance measures (Table 11-1). Similarly, collegiate soccer players (% fat = 13.9 ± 5.8) also show weak-to-moderate correlations between body composition and physical performance (Table 11-2). Note that the correlations vary from nonsignificant (FFM and vertical jump performance of soccer players, or FM and bench press ability of football players) to significant but moderate correlations (% fat and 36.5-m sprint time of football players, or total FM and 9.1-m sprint time of soccer players). Thus, the body composition measure used and the exact physical performance task attempted affect the significance of a correlation.

Table 11-1. Correlations in American Football Players between Body Composition and Physical Tasks

	9.1-m Sprint	36.5-m Sprint	Agility[a]	Vertical Jump	Bench Press
TBM	0.59*	0.64*	0.50*	−0.41*	0.40*
% Fat	0.57*	0.70*	0.52*	−0.59*	−0.03
FM	0.63*	0.74*	0.55*	−0.58*	0.10
FFM	0.35*	0.32*	0.28*	−0.10	0.56*

*Significant correlation ($P \leq 0.05$).

[a]Pro agility run.

TBM = total body mass, % fat = percent body fat, FM = fat mass, FFM = fat-free mass.

Data from Stempfle KJ, Katch FI, Petrie DE. Body composition relates poorly to performance tests in NCAA Division III football players. J Strength Cond Res. 2003;17:238–244.

Table 11-2. Correlations in Soccer Players between Body Composition and Physical Tasks

	9.1-m Sprint	36.5-m Sprint	Vertical Jump	Estimated $\dot{V}O_{2max}$[a]
TBM	0.61*	0.53*	−0.48*	−0.50
% Fat	0.69*	0.61*	−0.55*	−0.65*
Total FM	0.62*	0.60*	0.54*	−0.67*
% Lean tissue	−0.60*	−0.61*	0.55*	−0.65*
Total lean mass	0.38	0.28	0.24	−0.11

*Significant correlation ($P \leq 0.05$).

[a]$\dot{V}O_{2max}$ estimated using 20-m Yo-Yo endurance test.

TBM = total body mass, FM = fat mass, % fat = percent body fat

Data from Silvestre R, West C, Maresh CM, et al. Body composition and physical performance in men's soccer: a study of a National Collegiate Athletic Association Division I team. J Strength Cond Res. 2006;20:177–183.

Percent fat would have little effect on one repetition maximal bench press because in this physical performance task the additional body mass due to increased % fat does not need to be carried or moved during the task. However, % fat does show significant correlations to short sprint and vertical jump ability. It is important to note that for some tasks, TBM is positively correlated to physical performance, indicating that total body size may affect the performance of some tasks.

There may also be interplay between TBM and measures of body composition. For example, if two individuals have the same % fat but one has a greater TBM, the person with the greater TBM will also have a greater FFM. The person with the greater FFM would have an advantage in some physical tasks, such as the one repetition maximal bench press. Additionally, other factors (muscle fiber type, neural recruitment) not accounted for by body composition may also affect the strength of a correlation between body composition and a physical task. So, any correlation between body composition and a physical performance task depends on the measure of body composition and physical performance task examined.[59,64]

Body Size Versus Body Composition

Body size and body composition both potentially influence the ability to enjoy recreational participation in or be successful in different sports and activities (Fig. 11-3). Body composition also affects health and the risk of developing various diseases. However, body size and composition are not the same measurement. It is possible for individuals to have the same body size measure (such as TBM) and have very different body compositions (such as % fat).

Anthropometry is the measurement and study of body size. Body size typically refers to TBM and height or stature. Anthropometry, however, also includes measures of body size such as body circumferences, bone breadths, and limb

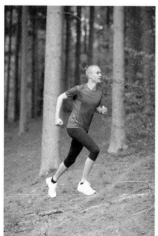 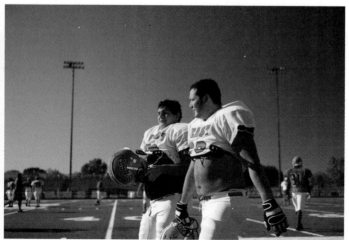 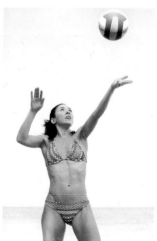

Figure 11-3. Differences in body composition and body size. Each athlete has a unique body size and composition needed for optimal performance in his or her sport.

lengths. Body size is of importance for success in some sports and activities; for example, it is advantageous for a basketball player to be tall or a shot putter to have a large TBM.

Measures of body size are significantly different between athletes of different sports and even between athletes playing at different positions within a sport. For example, in basketball, TBM, stature, and arm length are significantly greater in centers than in forwards and are greater in forwards than in guards.[1] In kayaking, 200-m time is significantly correlated to various measures of upper arm circumference, forearm circumference, and chest circumference.[69] Sweep rowers have a significantly greater TBM and stature than scull rowers,[13] and junior rowers who make the finals at the world championships are heavier and taller and generally have greater limb lengths and bone breadths than nonfinalists.[7] All the above indicate that body size does have an impact on performance in some sports and activities.

Body Mass Index

One frequently used measure of body size is **BMI**, or the ratio of body mass divided by height. BMI can be calculated using either of the following equations:

$$\text{BMI (kg/m}^2) = \frac{\text{weight (kg)}}{\text{height (m}^2)} \text{ or } \frac{\text{weight (lb)} \times 703}{\text{height (in}^2)} \quad (1)$$

If an individual is 5 feet 6 in tall (66 in, 1.45 m) and has a body mass of 136 pounds (61.8 kg), his or her BMI would be 22, which is within the normal range. An increase in BMI above a normal range indicates overweight or obesity, whereas a BMI less than the normal range identifies those who are underweight (Table 11-3). The use of the BMI as the criterion measurement for obesity in the United States has been increasing during the last several decades. According to this measure, 39% of men and 28% of women are classified as overweight (BMI = 25.0–29.9) and 31% of men and 33% of women are classified as obese (BMI ≥ 30) in the United States as of 2004.[49] This means that, using

Table 11-3. BMI Classifications

Classification	BMI (kg/m²)
Underweight	<18.5
Normal	18.5–24.9
Overweight	25.0–29.9
Obesity class I	30.0–34.9
Obesity class II	35.0–39.9
Obesity class III	>40.0

Data from Expert Panel on the Identification, Evaluation, and Treatment of Overweight and Obesity in Adults. Executive summary of the clinical guidelines on the identification, evaluation, and treatment of overweight and obesity in adults. Arch Intern Med. 1998;158:1855–1867.

BMI as an indicator, an alarming 71% of men and 62% of women are either overweight or obese.

BMI is used as a general indicator of health risks associated with obesity, severe underweight status, and % fat (Table 11-4). The accuracy with which BMI estimates % fat is between 2.5% and 4% of actual % fat. BMI does not directly account for body composition. It is quite possible for any individual or an athlete to have a BMI indicating that he or she is overweight or obese, but still have a relatively low % fat.[48] In male ($r = 0.53–0.70$) and female ($r = 0.58–0.90$) collegiate athletes from different sports, correlations between BMI and % fat are significant. However, many times, these correlations result in misclassifications of male athletes with normal % fat as either underweight or overweight, whereas female athletes who are overweight are classified as having normal % fat.[48] This is because BMI does not account for body composition. Elderly people may have a low BMI, but because of loss of muscle mass (sarcopenia) they have a high % fat. On the other hand, many individuals and athletes (because of genetics or years of training) have a higher-than-normal FFM relative to their TBM. This results in

Table 11-4. BMI Prediction of Percentage Body Fat and Health Risk

BMI (kg/m²)	Health Risk	20–39 yr	40–59 yr	60–79 yr
Men				
<18.5	Elevated	<8%	<11%	<13%
18.6–24.9	Average	8%–19%	11%–21%	13%–24%
25.0–29.9	Elevated	20%–24%	22%–27%	25%–29%
>30.0	High	>25%	>28%	>30%
Women				
<18.5	Elevated	<21%	<23%	<24%
18.6–24.9	Average	21%–32%	23%–33%	24%–35%
25.0–29.9	Elevated	33%–38%	34%–39%	36%–41%
>30.0	High	>39%	>40%	>42%

Reprinted with permission from Whaley MH, Brubaker PH, Otto RM, eds. ACSM's Guidelines for Exercise Testing and Prescription, 7th ed. Baltimore: Lippincott Williams & Wilkins; 2006:59.

Quick Review

- The basic measures of body composition are % fat, FM, and FFM.
- Obesity or high levels of % fat and FM are associated with a variety of disease states.
- Body composition is associated with physical performance; however, the body composition measure used and the physical performance task evaluated influence the correlation between body composition and performance.
- Specific body size and measures of anthropometry are related to success in certain sports.
- BMI can be used as a general indicator of being overweight or obese.
- BMI is inappropriate to determine body composition in lean, muscular athletes.

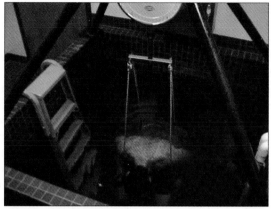

Figure 11-4. During hydrostatic weighing or densitometry, the person is completely submerged under water. As % fat increases, body volume increases, resulting in a greater displacement of water and so a decrease in underwater weight.

increased body mass, but a low % fat. High BMIs with less-than-normal % fat are prevalent in sports in which low % fat and high FFM are desirable, such as American football, body building, and Olympic weightlifting. In fact, in a study of a National Football League team, the Indianapolis Colts, players in each of the positions were considered overweight or obese according to the BMI when in fact the body fat range for players in all of the positions ranged from 6.3% to 18.5% body fat, except for the offensive linemen, who were at 25%.[35] Thus, BMI can be deceptive. In other sports, such as marathon running and road cycling, elite athletes tend to have low BMIs. Therefore, although BMI can be used as a general indicator of obesity, this measurement does have limitations when applied to certain groups of athletes.

DETERMINING BODY COMPOSITION

The major tissues within the human body are muscle, bone, nervous, adipose, and skin. Tissues are composed of various substances, including protein, adipose, carbohydrate, water, minerals, and other substances. Normally, however, the determination of body composition uses a two-component model that includes only FM and FFM (Fig. 11-1). Understanding the relationship between body density and body composition allows an understanding of the major concepts and methodologies of determining body composition.

Densitometry

Densitometry is the determination of body composition from the body's density. **Body density** is defined as TBM divided by the volume of the body:

$$\text{Body density} = \text{TBM/body volume} \qquad (2)$$

Body density can be determined by several different methodologies. The most common method is **hydrostatic weighing** (also termed *underwater weighing*), in which the

subject is totally immersed in water (Fig. 11-4). TBM can easily be determined using a scale. When submerged under water, a person is pushed toward the surface with a force equivalent to the weight of the volume of water displaced, causing underwater weight to be less than TBM. The body's tissues, as well as air in the lungs and intestinal tract, all displace water. So, the volume of water displaced must be corrected for air within the body. Volume of air in the lungs can be either measured directly or estimated. Normally, while performing hydrostatic weighing, the subject is asked to exhale as much air as possible. So, the air left in the lungs is residual lung volume. Volume of air trapped in the intestinal tract is very small and can be either ignored or estimated to be a constant (100 mL) value.[60] Although water's density can be corrected for slight changes due to temperature and its mineral content, 1 kg of water has a volume of 1 L or has a density of 1 kg·L⁻¹ or 1 g·mL⁻¹. So, body volume (after correction for air within the body) and water density are easily calculated as TBM minus underwater weight (Fig. 11-1).

Body density can then be used with an equation to determine % body fat. The most frequently used equation is the Siri equation:

$$\% \text{ Fat} = (495/\text{body density}) - 450 \qquad (3)$$

Body density varies with body composition. This variation is in large part due to FM and FFM making up different percentages of the body. Fat (or adipose tissue) has a density that is less than water and therefore floats. FFM has a density that is greater than water and therefore sinks. Because fat is less dense than FFM, if an individual has a higher % fat than another individual of the same body mass, the individual with a higher % fat will have a greater body volume and therefore a lower underwater weight (Fig. 11-1), resulting in a lower body density.

If densitometry is performed correctly, and if corrections are made for air within the body and water density, the resulting body density is quite accurate. However, densitometry does have some limitations, resulting in an error in the calculation of % fat. Many people have trouble exhaling as much air as possible or reaching residual volume, which makes them appear to have a higher % fat. Another limitation is the calculation of % fat from body density (Siri or similar equation). These equations assume the density of FM and FFM to be relatively constant in all individuals. FM density (0.9007 g·mL^{-1}) at various sites within the body is relatively consistent in all individuals.[3] On the other hand, FFM density, although relatively constant (1.099 g·mL^{-1}), does show some variability (1.072–1.114 g·mL^{-1}) amongst individuals.[73] To determine FFM density, several assumptions must be made:

1. The density of each tissue making up FFM must be known and constant.
2. The tissues comprising FFM are always in the same constant percentage of FFM.

These assumptions introduce some error into FFM density. For example, bone density is one component of FFM and typically decreases with aging and can increase with physical activity. This means that not only is bone's density changing but also that the percentage of FFM composed of bone is also changing. Despite these limitations, densitometry does estimate body composition quite accurately.

Skinfolds

Skinfolds are a method of estimating body composition that involves pinching and measuring the thickness of the skin and subcutaneous fat (Fig. 11-5) at specific anatomical sites using specialized calipers. Skinfolds are convenient and one of the most widely used methods of assessing body composition. Skinfolds predict body composition because changes in skinfold thickness relate to changes in body composition. Generally, several skinfolds at different anatomical sites are determined and used in an equation to predict body density

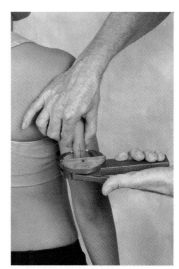

Figure 11-5. Skinfolds are determined at specific anatomical sites using a specialized caliber. Determining the triceps skinfold is shown. (Used with permission from Thompson WR, ed. ACSM's Resources for the Personal Trainer, 3e. Baltimore: Lippincott Williams & Wilkins; 2010:286.)

(Box 11-3). Body density is then used in an equation, typically the Siri equation, to predict % fat.

Determination of skinfolds when performed by an experienced technician is a relatively accurate measurement of body composition. Skinfolds, however, have several limitations. Most skinfold equations were derived using hydrostatic weighing as the correct measure of body composition. So, body composition predicted using skinfolds cannot be more accurate than hydrostatic weighing. Prediction equations have some inherent error; thus, body composition predicted using skinfolds is, in reality, less accurate than hydrostatic weighing. Although generalized skinfold equations that are applicable to a wide range of heterogeneous individuals have been developed,[29,30] many skinfold equations are population

---

Box 11-3 APPLYING RESEARCH
Generalized Skinfold Equations for Predicting Body Density in Healthy Adults

Skinfold equations typically use several skinfold measurements to determine body density. Body density is then used in an equation, such as the Siri equation, to predict % fat. Generalized equations are applicable to a wide range of heterogeneous individuals, but to obtain the most accurate prediction of body composition for a specific population, a skinfold equation developed for that specific population should be used. The equations shown are the three-site Jackson and Pollock (1978) and Jackson, Pollock, and Ward (1980) equations for men and women, respectively. These equations have a standard error of estimate of ~3.6% fat and 3.9% fat for the men and women, respectively.

Men

Skinfold sites: chest, abdomen, and thigh

Body density = $1.1125025 - (0.0013125 \times$ sum of the three skinfolds) $+ (0.0000055 \times$ sum of three skinfolds$^2) - (0.000244 \times$ age in years)

Women

Skinfold sites: thigh, suprailium, triceps

Body density = $1.089733 - (0.0009245 \times$ sum of three skinfolds) $+ (0.0000025 \times$ sum of three skinfolds$^2) - (0.0000979 \times$ age in years)

specific. Clear examples of population specificity are males versus females and individuals of different ages. Generalized equations could be used to determine body composition of any population; however, to obtain the most accurate results when determining body composition of a specific population (such as a group of athletes), equations specifically developed for that population should be used. For example, an equation developed specifically for young wrestlers (average age 11.3 years) shows no significant difference in % fat compared with the value measured by hydrostatic weighing. However, other equations show significant differences from the hydrostatic weighing value.[26]

Air-Displacement Plethysmography

Air-displacement plethysmography is a densitometry technique used to determine body composition with air displacement (instead of water displacement, as used with hydrostatic weighing) to determine body volume. The equipment consists of a closed airtight chamber (Fig. 11-6). The volume of air in the chamber when the chamber is empty is known. When a person enters the airtight chamber, he displaces his own volume in air. The volume of air remaining in the chamber is determined (with a correction for thoracic air volume). The person's body volume is the difference between the volume of air in the empty chamber minus the volume of air in the chamber when the person is in the chamber. Once body volume is known, body density and % fat can be determined using equations similar to those used for hydrostatic weighing. Air-displacement plethysmography differs from hydrostatic weighing in how body volume is determined, but has the same limitations as hydrostatic weighing in estimating FFM density in the determination of body composition.

Body composition determined by air-displacement plethysmography correlates significantly ($r = 0.96$) to that determined by hydrostatic weighing.[14,15] Similar body composition measures in groups of athletes, such as wrestlers,[15,68] have been shown between air-displacement plethysmography and hydrostatic weighing, and both measures can accurately track changes in body composition due to moderate weight loss.[77] However, air-displacement plethysmography has also been shown to significantly overestimate % fat in women collegiate athletes,[70] overestimate FM in 30-year-old women,[4] underestimate body fat in 30-year-old men,[4] and underestimate % fat in young (10- to 18-year-old) males and females compared with hydrostatic weighing.[40] Generally, air-displacement plethysmography appears to be relatively accurate in determining body composition, but differences (when compared with hydrostatic weighing) do exist in specific populations.

Bioelectrical Impedance

Determination of body composition using **bioelectrical impedance** involves placing electrodes at two or more places on the body (Fig. 11-7) and passing an undetectable electrical current between the electrodes. FFM contains more water than fat tissue; therefore, electrical conductance is greater and impedance or resistance to electrical current is lower in FFM than fat tissue. Electrical conductance is directly correlated, whereas impedance is inversely correlated, to FFM. Using these relationships, FM, FFM, and total body water are calculated.

Several types of bioelectrical impedance equipment are available, making generalizable statements concerning reliability and accuracy difficult. In healthy adults, % fat determined using bioelectrical impedance with ankle and wrist electrode placements showed significant correlations

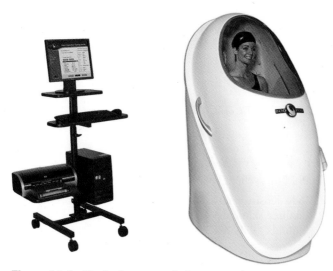

Figure 11-6. Air-displacement plethysmography uses differences in the volume of air in a sealed chamber to determine body volume. Once body volume is determined, equations similar to those used for hydrostatic weighing are used to calculate body density and other measures of body composition. (Photo courtesy of LifeMeasurment, Concord, CA.)

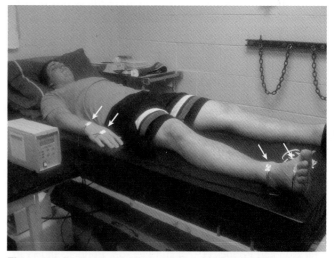

Figure 11-7. Bioelectrical impedance determines body composition by passing a weak electrical current between two electrodes at specific sites on the body. The equipment depicted uses electrode placement at the wrist and ankle (*arrows* highlight electrodes).

to % fat as measured by hydrostatic weighing ($r = 0.857$) and air-displacement plethysmography ($r = 0.859$).[4] There was also no significant difference between any of the methodologies in % fat in either men or women. In collegiate wrestlers, % fat determined using leg-to-leg bioelectrical impedance showed a significant correlation ($r = 0.80$) to % fat determined using hydrostatic weighing, but significantly underestimated % fat compared with hydrostatic weighing.[15] Additionally, leg-to-leg bioelectrical impedance significantly underestimated % fat compared with skinfolds, but not with air-displacement plethysmography. Thus, the accuracy of bioelectrical impedance in part depends on with which methodology it is compared. It must also be noted that bioelectrical impedance may be affected by hydration status, which is an important consideration for athletes, who may be partially dehydrated due to training or attempting to make a competitive weight class in part by dehydration. Additionally, some equipment has population-specific equations, making these instruments potentially more reliable.

Dual-Energy X-Ray Absorptiometry

Dual-energy x-ray absorptiometry (DEXA) uses low-energy x-ray beams and computer software to produce images of the body that can be used to determine body composition. DEXA was originally developed to determine bone density, but now it is used to determine body composition, including **regional body composition** or composition of specific areas of the body, such as the arms, legs, or trunk (Fig. 11-8). The ability to determine regional body composition is a major advantage of this methodology. For example, some research indicates that when women perform aerobic

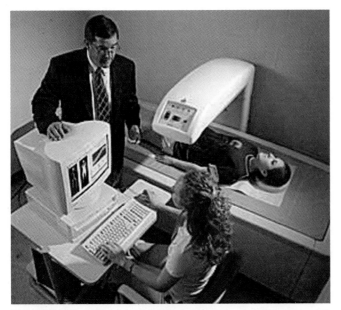

Figure 11-8. DEXA can be used to determine bone density and body composition. A major advantage of DEXA compared with other body composition methodologies is the ability to determine regional body composition and bone density.

training (cycling, running) and the same resistance training program, the increase in the upper body lean tissue mass is greater than that in the lower body lean tissue mass.[15] DEXA is highly reliable in determining body composition,[17] is sensitive to small changes in body composition,[27] and shows significant correlations ($r = 0.90$) to body composition measures determined by hydrostatic weighing.

In children, % fat determined by DEXA underestimates % fat (2.9%) determined by air-displacement plethysmography, but is not significantly different from values determined by hydrostatic weighing and shows significant correlations to measures determined by other methodologies ($r = 0.94$ to air-displacement plethysmography, $r = 0.89$ to hydrostatic weighing).[40] In adult men and women, % fat determined by DEXA is significantly correlated ($r = 0.98$) to that determined by air-displacement plethysmography, and both methodologies detected small changes in body composition due to weight loss.[77] However, changes in % fat ($r = 0.66$), FM ($r = 0.86$), and FFM ($r = 0.34$) due to weight loss showed lower correlations between the two methodologies. DEXA is now considered by many to be the most accurate, sensitive, and reliable method of determining body composition. The ability to determine regional body composition is a major advantage of this methodology. In addition, bone density is also measured in the same scan.

Other Methodologies

The aforementioned methodologies are the most frequently used methodologies to determine body composition by exercise scientists. However, several other methodologies can also be used to determine body composition. Total body water measures can be used to determine body composition because lean tissue has a higher water content than fat tissue. To determine total body water, a solution of water containing a known concentration of an isotope (^3H_2O, or ^2H_2O, or H_2O^{18}) or marker is ingested. After 4 hours, the marker is diluted equally within all water compartments of the body. A sample of body water is obtained (urine, blood, saliva), and concentration of the marker in the sample is determined. Total body water is calculated by determining the body water necessary to dilute the marker to the concentration present in the sample of body water. Body fat is then estimated using regression analyses, which depend on water content of lean and fat tissues.

Nuclear magnetic resonance imaging, also termed *magnetic resonance imaging* (MRI), uses electromagnetic waves and computer technology to produce cross sections of the body (Fig. 11-9). The electromagnetic waves are absorbed by the hydrogen molecules contained within water molecules as well as tissues. After absorption, electromagnetic waves are released at certain frequencies or resonate. The released energy is measured and can be used to produce detailed images of the body's tissues. The cross sections of the body can then be used to calculate body composition measures.

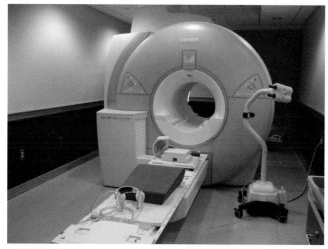

Figure 11-9. Magnetic resonance imaging (MRI). An MRI instrument can be used to assess many different anatomical structures, including bone, tendon, and muscles (photo courtesy of Department of Diagnostic Imaging and Therapeutics in Radiology at the University of Connecticut's Health Center, Farmington, CT)

Ultrasound technology transmits high-frequency sound waves through the tissues of the body (Fig. 11-10). The sound waves pass through different tissues of the body at different velocities and are reflected back to varying degrees by different tissues. The time to pass through different tissues and the amount of echo, or reflected sound waves, are used to determine thickness of various tissues. Ultrasound can be used to determine tissue thickness and volume in various regions of the body, such as the arms or legs.

The various methodologies to determine body composition all have advantages and disadvantages. For

Quick Review

- A two-component model of FM and FFM is most frequently used when determining body composition.
- The major assumptions of densitometry to determine body composition are as follows: 1) the density of each tissue making up FFM is known and constant; 2) tissues comprising FFM are always in the same constant percentage of FFM; 3) density of FM is known and constant.
- Hydrostatic weighing uses densitometry to determine body composition because it allows determination of body volume, which can be used to determine body density (TBM divided by body volume).
- Skinfold equations specific to populations are more accurate than generalized equations.
- Air-displacement plethysmography is a relatively accurate method that uses determination of body density to estimate body composition.
- Bioelectrical impedance estimates body composition on the basis of differences in resistance or conductance to electrical impulses in lean and fat tissues.
- DEXA is considered the most accurate and sensitive method of determining body composition.
- DEXA offers the ability to determine regional (arm, leg, trunk) body composition.
- Because differences in body composition measures exist, comparisons of different populations and comparisons made over time should always be made using the same methodology.

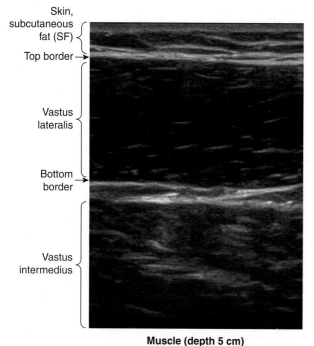

Muscle (depth 5 cm)

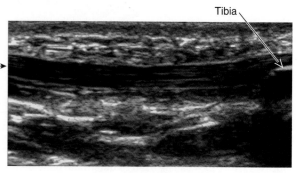

Tendon (depth 2 cm)

Figure 11-10. Ultrasound imaging. Ultrasound imaging can be used to analyze muscle and tendon thickness.

example, skinfolds are convenient and inexpensive to perform, whereas DEXA measurements are very accurate but expensive. Correlations between the various methodologies (and significant differences in body composition measures between the various methodologies) indicate that if comparisons in body composition are made, the same methodology should be used. For example, if two populations are to be compared, the same methodology should be used to determine body composition in both populations. In addition, if body composition changes over time (such as changes due to training or dieting), the same methodology should be used at all time points in the comparison.

CHANGING BODY COMPOSITION

Many people want to change their body composition and attempt to do so through dieting and exercise. Typically, people desire to decrease their FM or % fat and increase their FFM because these changes are associated with increased overall health or decreased risk of many diseases. On the other hand, an athlete desires these body composition changes because they are associated with increased physical performance in many sports and activities. Both diet and exercise are important in bringing about changes in body composition.

Body Composition of Athletes

FM serves several fundamental physiological purposes and is, in and of itself, necessary for survival. Because of sex-specific difference in fat distribution (with much greater fat in the chest and reproductive areas in women), women have a higher percentage of body fat than men of comparable health and fitness. Estimates of the body fat needed to maintain normal bodily function are in the range of 3% to 5% for men and 12% to 14% for women.[25] Although, generally, lower body fat is correlated with improved health measures, extremely low body fat is correlated with increased health risks.

Performance in certain sports and activities improves with decreases in body fat. Female athletes with the smallest percentage of body fat tend to have between 16% and 20% body fat, whereas comparable male athletes have 6% to 13% body fat. These low percentages tend to be due to the increased caloric demands of certain sports, particularly sustained endurance sports, and the need to carry body weight for sustained periods (such as the duration of a marathon or during tumbling and flipping for gymnasts).

A generally healthy body fat range for those who are not involved in competitive sport is 21% to 24% for women and 14% to 17% for men. Increased body fat in the range of 25% to 31% for women and 18% to 25% for men results in increased risk of decrements in health. Beyond 32% body fat for women and 25% for men is considered obesity.

Diet and Body Composition Changes

Ingestion of sufficient macronutrients and micronutrients is important for overall health and to maintain health while dieting to lose body mass. Macronutrients and micronutrients are also important for maintaining training volume and intensity and for bringing about training adaptations desired by athletes, such as increased FFM. Thus, maintaining a diet sufficient in macronutrients and micronutrients is important for all individuals desiring changes in body composition. Additionally, some dietary practices, such as protein and carbohydrate ingestion before and after training sessions, may help in bringing about increases in FFM. We previously discussed these issues in Chapters 8 and 9. Here, we will be focusing on the effect of diet on energy balance, common dietary mistakes, and the effects of losing large amounts of body mass.

Energy Balance

Energy balance refers to the ratio of caloric ingestion to caloric expenditure. If total caloric expenditure is greater than caloric ingestion over time, a loss in body mass will occur. If caloric expenditure is less than total caloric ingestion, a gain in body mass will occur. Total caloric expenditure includes basal metabolic rate (BMR) and caloric expenditure of physical activity. BMR and resting metabolic rate (RMR), although slightly different in definition (see Chapter 2), will be used interchangeably here. Caloric expenditure during physical activity is an important aspect of the role of exercise in causing changes in body composition.

The role of even small changes in energy balance causing changes in body composition is made apparent by the following example. If total caloric expenditure is greater than total caloric ingestion by 100 kcal·day^{-1} for an entire year, caloric expenditure will be greater than caloric ingestion by 36,500 kcal. Assuming 3,500 kcal·0.45 kg^{-1} (3,500 kcal·1 lb^{-1}), this difference in energy balance would result in a loss in FM of ~4.7 kg (10.4 lb) over the course of a year.

When caloric ingestion is restricted, RMR decreases, which affects energy balance. In sedentary populations, RMR accounts for ~60% to 75% of total caloric expenditure because most people spend the majority of the day at or close to RMR.[8,38,76] Changes in RMR can affect total caloric expenditure and thereby affect TBM or FM loss, and the change in RMR may be as large as 20% of the value before caloric restriction. Thus, the change in RMR due to caloric restriction can have a substantial effect over time. This decrease in RMR due to caloric restriction is typically viewed as a defense mechanism of the body to maintain body mass. Similarly, when caloric ingestion increases after a period of caloric restriction, RMR increases, which helps to prevent gains in body mass.

BMR is positively correlated to FFM and the mass of various tissues comprising FFM (Box 11-4). Women

Box 11-4 DID YOU KNOW?
Resting Energy Expenditure Depends on All Tissues Comprising FFM

BMR or resting energy expenditure correlates to total FFM. However, this correlation is dependent not only on skeletal muscle mass, but also on other metabolically active tissues comprising FFM. In sumo wrestlers ($r = 0.93$) and untrained college students ($r = 0.72$), the correlation between resting energy expenditure and FFM is significant.[1] The sumo wrestlers had a greater TBM (109 vs. 62 kg), FFM (78 vs. 53 kg), a greater resting energy expenditure (2,286 vs. 1,545 kcal·day^{-1}) and a greater skeletal muscle, liver, heart, and kidney mass, but not brain mass, than the college students. All these tissues are metabolically active and contribute to resting energy expenditure. When resting energy expenditure was expressed relative to FFM (resting energy expenditure, kcal·total FFM^{-1}), there was no significant difference between the sumo wrestlers and the college students (29.1 vs. 29.2 kcal·day^{-1}·kg FFM^{-1}). This indicates that not just skeletal muscle mass but all metabolic active tissues contribute to the correlation between resting energy expenditure and total FFM.

Reference

1. Midorikawa T, Masakatsu K, Beekley MD, et al. High REE in sumo wrestlers attributed to large organ-tissue mass. Med Sci Sports Exerc. 2007;39: 688–693.

and children typically have a lower FFM than their male counterparts.[39,44,51] This is one reason that both women and children have a lower BMR. However, if RMR is expressed relative to body mass or FFM, there is no difference in RMR·kg TBM^{-1} or RMR·kg FFM^{-1}.[39,44,75] This relationship is important because when dieting while performing no exercise, a substantial amount of the TBM loss can come from FFM. For example, 31% of the TBM lost came from FFM in men who lost 9.1 kg (20.0 pounds) during 12 weeks of dieting.[36] Loss of FFM can decrease RMR and so affect energy balance.

Energy balance also plays a role in the initial, relatively large weight loss that occurs when caloric ingestion is decreased drastically. On many diets, especially low-carbohydrate diets, the body's glycogen stores are depleted during the first week of dieting. This results in a relatively large weight loss because glycogen is stored with a substantial amount of water (2.6 g H_2O·g carbohydrate^{-1}). When the glycogen is used in metabolism, the water released eventually is excreted from the body, resulting in a substantial weight loss. There are dietary practices that can help ensure loss of FM while dieting and so minimize the effects of BMR on energy balance.

Dieting and Weight Loss

At any one point in time, many American adults are dieting to lose FM, indicating that attempts to lose FM and maintain the loss are not successful. Several approaches have been used, from low-fat to low-carbohydrate diets, with the latter more successful than low-fat diets in weight loss.[71,72] Whatever approach is taken, however, it is important to ensure adequate intake of all macronutrients and micronutrients when dieting. There are also other dietary guidelines that are helpful when attempting to lose FM.

Drink Sufficient Water

Water, whether ingested as part of foods (such as soup) or by itself, increases fullness and helps to reduce energy intake.[56] Water is also necessary to maintain normal hydration while eliminating normal waste products. If sufficient water is not ingested, TBM may decrease, but the decrease is due to water weight loss and not FM loss.

Make Sensible Fat Choices

Some dietary fat is necessary (see Chapter 8). However, one can make food choices to minimize total fat intake, such as drinking low-fat or skimmed milk as opposed to whole milk. The satiation effect of fat is weak, and so ingestion of a high-fat meal many times results in ingesting more total calories.[79] As with all healthy diets, when dieting to lose FM, saturated fats and trans-fats should be minimized because of their association with increased health risks.

Minimize Empty Calories

Ingested calories from foods high in caloric value but of little other nutritional value are **empty calories**. When attempting to lose FM and maintain a diet sufficient in macronutrients and micronutrients, avoid empty calories from fat, sugar, and alcohol. Alcoholic drinks, especially mixed and creamy drinks, not only add calories to the diet but also reduce the desire to maintain a dietary regime.

Do Not Reduce Calories Too Drastically

Typically, weight-loss diets provide 1,200 to 1,600 kcal·day^{-1}.[79] A prudent recommendation is to increase physical activity and reduce caloric ingestion so that a 500-kcal·day^{-1} deficit is achieved. This allows one to ingest adequate micronutrients and to minimize FFM loss due to dieting. If caloric ingestion is reduced too drastically, binge eating may result, which increases caloric ingestion, typically of empty calories.

Keep Portions Small

Portion size has increased dramatically over the years, and Americans have come to expect large portions at restaurants as well as at home. Large portions result in greater caloric ingestion. To decrease caloric ingestion, reduce your portion size while still maintaining adequate nutrient ingestion.

Using the above guidelines as well as following the dietary guidelines of macronutrient ingestion will help in achieving FM loss while minimizing FFM loss when dieting. Another aspect of FM loss is performing physical activity to increase caloric expenditure and minimize FFM loss.

Effect of Exercise on Body Composition

Physical activity can affect body composition in several ways (Box 11-5). If the caloric expenditure due to activity results in a negative energy balance (caloric ingestion less than caloric expenditure), FM will decrease over time. Physical activity can also result in an increase in FFM. Percent body fat can decrease due to physical activity because of a decrease in FM, an increase in FFM, or a combination of these two factors. As previously discussed, because of the relationship between FFM and RMR, physical activity that increases FFM will increase RMR. If an increase in RMR results in a negative energy balance, FM will decrease over time.

Any type of physical activity will increase caloric expenditure. However, estimating energy expenditure during physical activity is problematic because it depends on many factors. Body mass will affect caloric expenditure if body mass must be carried in the activity (Box 11-6). All variables related to aerobic or resistance training volume and intensity will affect total caloric expenditure. For example, in resistance training, greater energy expenditure during a training session occurs with the following: large versus small muscle mass exercises, more total sets of exercises, ten-repetition maximum sets versus five-repetition maximum sets, short (30 seconds) versus longer rest periods (2, 3, and 5 minutes), rest periods when lifting five-repetition maximum but not ten-repetition maximum resistances, and high intensity (80%–90% of one-repetition maximum) greater than moderate (60%–70% one-repetition maximum) and both high and moderate intensity greater than low intensity (20%–50% of one-repetition maximum).[54] Velocity of movement during weight training has shown mixed results, with faster velocities resulting in greater caloric expenditure than slower velocities and vice versa.[54,41] Next, we will focus on the energy expenditure of typical aerobic and weight training sessions.

Caloric Expenditure of Resistance and Aerobic Training

Comparing the caloric expenditure of resistance and aerobic training sessions is difficult because of the effects of training volume and intensity. Additionally, not just the caloric expenditure during training must be determined, but caloric expenditure immediately after the training session as estimated from excess post-oxygen consumption (see Chapter 2) must also be determined; otherwise, the total caloric expenditure will be underestimated. Studies have estimated caloric expenditure during typical training sessions.

A comparison of a weight training session, lasting 60 minutes (10 exercises, four sets of 8–12 repetitions per set) lifting 70% to 75% of one-repetition maximum, and running 60 minutes at 70% to 75% of peak oxygen consumption showed no significant difference in resting energy expenditure at 10, 24, and 48 hours after the training sessions.[31] Running resulted in a significant increase in 24-hour resting energy expenditure at 10 hours (2,150 kcal) and 48 hours (1,995 kcal) but not at 24 hours (1,914 kcal) compared with rest (1,862 kcal; see Box 11-6). However, weight training resulted in a significant increase in 24-hour resting energy expenditure at 10 hours (2,124 kcal) and 24 hours (2,081 kcal) but not at 48 hours (1,997 kcal) compared with rest (1,972 kcal). No significant difference between the two training sessions in resting energy expenditure was shown. Both training sessions elevated fat metabolism with no significant difference between training sessions for 24 hours. This finding indicates that weight and aerobic training sessions equal in length performed at the same intensity result in equivalent energy expenditure and fat metabolism, although whether running and weight training at 70% to 75% intensity is a fair comparison is debatable.

A comparison of a cycling training session and a circuit weight training session also showed no significant difference in caloric expenditure.[43] In this comparison, however, the duration of the training sessions was not equivalent. Forty-nine minutes of cycling at 70% of peak oxygen consumption resulted in 546 kcal expended during the session and a 24-hour energy expenditure of 2,787 kcal. Weight training for 70 minutes (10 exercises, three sets of 10 repetitions and a fourth set to failure using 70% of one-repetition maximum) expended 448 kcal during the session and a 24-hour energy expenditure of 2,730 kcal. Caloric expenditure while cycling was significantly greater than during weight training, but the 24-hour energy expenditures were not significantly different.

Aerobic training and weight training increase caloric expenditure during activity and increase resting energy expenditure for up to 24 or 48 hours after a training session. Weight training does increase FFM over time and so may offer the advantage of increasing BMR due to increased FFM. Typical increases in FFM due to weight training are approximately 0.66 kg·wk^{-1} (0.3 lb·wk^{-1}).[18] There may be an advantage in performing weight and aerobic training concurrently while dieting with the goal of changing body composition.[36] Men who lost 9.1 kg (20.4 lb) in 12 weeks by dieting and performing only aerobic training lost 78% of body mass from FM, whereas men losing the same

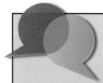

Box 11-5   AN EXPERT VIEW
Altering Body Composition with Exercise

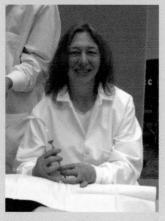

N. Travis Triplett, PhD
Professor
Department of Health, Leisure, and Exercise Science
Appalachian State University
Boone, NC

One of the more prominent health and fitness goals having the largest impact on the fitness and nutrition/nutritional supplement industries is the desire to alter one's body composition. The most common focus is to lose weight through a decrease in overall body fat, although there are many individuals who wish to increase muscle mass as well. While the experts recognize that this is best achieved through the combination of exercise and dietary modifications,[1,2] there are many companies and individuals who have focused solely on the nutritional aspects of body composition changes since individuals are often more willing to make dietary changes than to engage in a regular exercise program. However, exercise is necessary not only to achieve the desired body composition alterations but also to maintain them.[3] Different types of exercise can result in different changes in body composition and it is important to understand the basics so exercise selection can be optimized.

Aerobic exercise is excellent for promoting loss of body fat. This is because the metabolic pathways involved in providing the energy for the activity utilize fat and carbohydrate as the primary fuels. When examining the body composition of individuals who perform a lot of aerobic training, such as elite endurance athletes, it is obvious that these individuals tend to have low amounts of body fat. However they do not typically have large muscles. When examining individuals who perform a lot of resistance training, such as competitive lifters, bodybuilders, or strength/power athletes, whereas some have less body fat than others, the most common feature is a large amount of muscle mass. Resistance exercise is therefore best for promoting gains in muscle mass, although exercise selection and overall program design impact the amount of muscle increase.

Coaches and personal trainers need to emphasize to their athletes and clients that both exercise and dietary changes are necessary to alter body composition. The bottom line relates back to caloric balance: it is difficult to lose weight if more calories are consumed than expended. Likewise, it is difficult to gain weight (presumably lean weight) if the individual is not consuming enough calories. While the dietary modifications are certainly part of the overall big picture, exercise addresses the caloric expenditure side of the equation. Therefore, it is very important to:

Set realistic goals and a goal timeline for achieving desired body composition. The fitness professional must have knowledge of what the normal levels of body fat are for average and for athletic men and women,[4] and what a healthy amount of weight loss or gain consists of for a given period of time. For example, it would be unrealistic for a client or athlete to lose 20 lbs. in a month since the recommended weight loss is only 1 to 2 lb·wk^{-1}.[5] Likewise, rapid weight gain rarely results in increases in mostly lean mass. The current recommendation is the same; only 1 to 2 lb·wk^{-1} weight gain.[5]

Choose exercise modes which best address the goals. Most forms of aerobic exercise are great for promoting fat loss. The more muscles and joints that are involved in the exercise, the higher the caloric expenditure, which can mean that caloric expenditure in weight bearing exercises is often greater, but the exercise needs to fit the limitations of the client or athlete. Increasing the intensity of aerobic exercise also results in significant caloric expenditures as long as the activity can be maintained for a long enough time. If the goal is also to increase muscle mass, resistance exercise needs to be incorporated or focused upon.

Use a variety of exercise modes to optimize results. Since resistance training promotes increases in muscle mass, overall resting metabolism can increase, which will facilitate losses in body fat. This exercise variety may also help to maintain motivation for the exercise program.

Exercise should be as important as dietary changes for altering one's body composition. Once the individual begins to see results from a comprehensive program, it will be easier to maintain that success as the exercise routines and dietary changes become a lifestyle.

References

1. Heyward VH, Wagner DR. Applied Body Composition Assessment, 2nd ed. Champaign, IL: Human Kinetics, 2004.
2. Klem ML, Wing RR, McGuire MT, et al. A descriptive study of individuals successful at long-term maintenance of substantial weight loss. Am J Clin Nutr 1997;66(2):239–246.
3. Kraemer WJ, Volek JS, Clark KL, et al. Influence of exercise training on physiological and performance changes with weight loss in men. Med Sci Sports Exerc. 1999;31(9):1320–1329.
4. Reimers K. Nutritional factors in health and performance. In: Baechle T, Earle R, eds. Essentials of Strength Training and Conditioning, 3rd ed. 2008:201–233.
5. Ross R, Freeman JA, Janssen I. Exercise alone is an effective strategy for reducing obesity and related comorbidities. Exerc Sport Sci Rev. 2000;28(4):165–170.

Box 11-6 PRACTICAL QUESTIONS FROM STUDENTS

What Is the Caloric Expenditure of Walking or Running?

Caloric expenditure of walking and running increases with increasing speed and with increasing body mass because body mass must be carried in this activity. Walking or running uphill or downhill also affects caloric expenditure. An estimate of caloric expenditure while walking or running on level terrain at specific speeds can be calculated using the following equation.

Caloric expenditure (kcal) = body mass (kg) × caloric expenditure/kilogram of body mass at a specific speed × time (min)

Caloric expenditure per kilogram of body mass at a specific speed:

walking 3.5 mph = 0.077 kcal·kg^{-1}
walking 4.5 mph = 0.106 kcal·kg^{-1}
running 5 mph = 0.134 kcal·kg^{-1}
running 6 mph = 0.163 kcal·kg^{-1}

running 7.5 mph = 0.207 kcal·kg^{-1}
running 9 mph = 0.227 kcal·kg^{-1}
running 10 mph = 0.251 kcal·kg^{-1}
running 11 mph = 0.288 kcal·kg^{-1}
1 kg = 2.2 lb

If an individual had a TBM of 70 kg (154 lb) and ran 30 minutes at a speed of 6 mph (10-min miles), her estimated caloric expenditure would be as follows:

Caloric expenditure (kcal) = 70 kg × 0.163 kcal·kg^{-1} × 30 minutes
Caloric expenditure (kcal) = 342.3 kcal

Caloric expenditure data obtained from Ainsworth BE, Haskell WL, Leon AS, et al. Compendium of physical activities: classification of energy cost of human physical activities. Med Sci Sports Exerc. 1993;25:71–80.

amount of body mass by dieting and performing aerobic and resistance training lost 97% of the mass from FM. Thus, the combination of dieting and aerobic and resistance training resulted in a greater loss of FM and smaller loss of FFM.

Spot Reduction

Spot reduction refers to the localized loss of subcutaneous fat in a body part or muscle group, more so than in other places on the body, as a result of exercising that particular body part or muscle group. For example, if spot reduction occurred when doing sit-ups, it would result in more fat reduction in the abdominal area than in other parts of the body. Most evidence concerning spot reduction, however, does not support its occurrence due to the performance of resistance exercise in either men or women.[34] There is, however, greater metabolism of fat in muscle adjacent to exercising muscle compared with muscle adjacent to resting muscle because of aerobic exercise lasting 30 and 120 minutes.[62] This indicates that spot reduction may occur. However, the majority of evidence indicates spot reduction does not occur.

Appetite and Exercise

During long-term, high-volume, or high-intensity physical training, energy intake needs to increase or TBM and eventually FFM would decrease, resulting in decreased physical performance. This would seem to indicate that appetite increases with physical training, but this is not entirely true. The immediate effect of physical activity

in most people is a decrease in appetite after exercise.[79] Physical activity and control of appetite involve many factors. The hypothalamus is the area of the brain that primarily controls appetite and **satiety**, the feeling of satisfaction that occurs after a meal and inhibits further eating. Elevated blood catecholamine concentrations and elevated body temperature after exercise may decrease appetite. Hot and cold environmental temperatures affect body temperature and could decrease and increase appetite, respectively. The hormone ghrelin, primarily secreted by the stomach in response to eating, stimulates appetite and promotes energy storage.[67] Leptin, a protein produced by fat cells when fat storage is sufficient, acts like a hormone that suppresses appetite.[63] Insulin and blood glucose response to eating also affect appetite.[21] Although physiological control of appetite is not completely clear, it appears that in most individuals the response to physical activity is a decrease in appetite immediately after exercise, but an overall increase in appetite to offset the increased caloric expenditure due to physical activity.

Losing Body Mass Wisely

Most people, including athletes, who want to lose weight do not want the loss to come from FFM but from FM and want to be able to maintain the loss once it is achieved. Achieving both these goals normally means the loss in FM must take place slowly over a relatively long period of time. To maximize FM loss and minimize FFM loss, a combination of diet and exercise should be used to create the needed caloric deficit. Not all people will respond with the same body mass loss because of the same diet and exercise regime. Previously, people who did not lose body mass on a diet and exercise regime were thought to be not following the prescribed regime or were "noncompliers." It is now clear that because of individual differences, such as differences in metabolic rate and caloric expenditure during exercise, some will comply with the same diet and exercise regime but may not lose as much TBM as others. Thus, there are low responders and high responders to the same weight loss program. Knowing this will help low responders to not become discouraged and to continue with the weight loss program.

To maximize FM loss, the average person should lose about 1 to 2 lb·wk^{-1} (0.45–0.90 kg·wk^{-1}). Although this seems slow, if this rate were continued for 1 year, one would lose 52 to 104 lb (23.6–47.3 kg)! Losing body mass at this rate helps to ensure loss of FM and not FFM. Remember that loss of FFM will decrease BMR, which will make FM loss more difficult and will decrease physical performance in many sports and activities. Exercise and not just diet should be used to lose FM because exercise minimizes FFM loss and may increase fat oxidation.[24] Assuming there are 3,500 kcal·lb^{-1} fat (7,700 kcal·kg^{-1} fat), to achieve a body mass loss of 1 to 2 lb·wk^{-1} (0.45–0.91 kg·wk^{-1}) a daily caloric deficit of 500 to 1,000 kcal needs to be achieved.

Energy expenditure in physical activity of 150 to 400 kcal·day^{-1} is recommended and should be coupled with a diet to achieve a total caloric deficit of 500 to 1,000 kcal·day^{-1}.[78] The lower end of this range should be the goal of previously sedentary individuals. The upper end of this range is the goal of more physically fit individuals and the goal of sedentary individuals as their fitness levels improve. To maintain a body mass loss, a caloric expenditure in physical activity of more than 2,000 kcal·wk^{-1} is recommended.[78] One characteristic of people who are successful in maintaining weight loss is that they are vigorous exercisers. This shows that the need for exercise cannot be underestimated in bringing about losses of FM, maintaining FFM, and the maintenance of TBM loss once it is achieved.

For many people, dietary habits are at least in part responsible for gains in FM. Generally, a weight loss diet should supply between 1,200 and 1,600 kcal·day^{-1}.[79] Caloric ingestion in this range helps to ensure that the diet is sufficient in macronutrients and micronutrients. Using both exercise and diet, it is possible to achieve a caloric deficit in the range of 500 to 1,000 kcal·day^{-1}, which, over time, does result in substantial TBM loss primarily from FM. One question many have is what should I weigh if I currently have a certain % fat and desire to lose body mass to reach a lower % fat. This question is answered in Box 11-7, but it must be remembered that this calculation assumes no loss in FFM, which is difficult to achieve on any diet and exercise weight loss program.

Mean % Fat

Because of its effect on physical performance and association with various health risks, % fat is of interest to both athletes and people concerned with general health and fitness. Athletes generally have lower-than-average % fat (Table 11-5) compared with the mean values of ~15% and 25% for healthy young adult males and females, respectively. However, % fat must be kept in perspective. Minimal % fat values of 5% for adult males and 12% to 14% for adult females are probably close estimates of the lower limits of body fat needed to maintain normal physiological and metabolic function.[25] Other factors that must be considered concerning % fat include, as discussed earlier, the fact that different techniques to determine body composition do potentially result in different % fat values and the fact that, due to individual differences, not all athletes will achieve optimum physical performance when at the % fat of elite athletes. Body composition can also vary substantially among athletes at different positions within the same sport. For example,

---

Box 11-7 PRACTICAL QUESTIONS FROM STUDENTS

What Would I Weigh at a Lower % Fat?

The calculation to answer this question is relatively simple. However, the calculation does assume that FFM will not change. On any dietary and exercise program, to lose TBM, some loss in FFM will take place. So, the assumption that FFM will not change does introduce error into this calculation.

New body mass (kg) = present FFM/desired % FFM at new body mass
Present TBM = 88 kg

Present FFM = 74.8 kg
Present % fat = 15
Desired % fat = 10
Desired % FFM at new body mass = 100% − desired % fat (100% − 10% = 90% = 0.90)
New body mass (kg) = 74.8 kg/0.90 = 83.1 kg
Body mass loss (kg) = 88 kg − 83.1 kg = 4.9 kg

So, 4.9 kg (10.8 lb) must be lost to achieve the desired 10% fat.

Table 11-5. Mean % Fat of Athletes

Sport	% Fat	
	Men	Women
Basketball	13	15
Bodybuilding	5	9
Cycling (road)	9	15
Football (American)	12	–
Gymnastics	8	14
Judo	11	16
Rowing	11	14
Skiing		
Alpine	10	18
Nordic	8	14
Swimming	9	16
Track and field		
Distance running	8	12
Sprinting	8	13
Shot put	16	25
Volleyball	12	18

Selected data from Callister R, Callister RJ, Fleck SJ, et al. Physiological and performance responses to overtraining in elite judo athletes. Med Sci Sports Exerc. 1990;22:816–824; De Gary A. Genetic and Anthropological Studies of Olympic Athletes. New York: Academic Press, 1974; Fleck SJ. Body composition of elite American athletes. American J Sports Med. 1983;11:398–403; Fleck SJ, Kraemer WJ. Designing Resistance Training Programs, 3rd ed. Champaign, IL: Human Kinetics, 2004.

Quick Review

- Diet-only strategies to lose FM may cause a substantial amount of FFM loss, which decreases BMR.
- When dieting to lose FM, healthy dietary practices should be followed and caloric ingestion normally should be maintained at 1,200 to 1,600 kcal·day^{-1} to ensure adequate ingestion of macro- and micronutrients.
- Exercise can help with body mass loss due to increased caloric expenditure while exercising and increased BMR.
- Aerobic or weight training aids loss of FM while dieting.
- The greatest loss of FM and smallest loss of FFM may occur when both aerobic exercise and resistance exercise are performed.
- Exercise reduces appetite immediately after activity but overall increases appetite to offset the increased caloric expenditure due to exercise.
- To successfully lose FM and minimize FFM loss, a combination of diet and exercise should be used to achieve a caloric deficit of 500 to 1,000 kcal·day^{-1}.

Division I American football running backs and offensive linemen have % fats of 8.8% and 19.2%, respectively. Thus, % fat should be viewed as an estimate and as only one factor in a multitude of factors affecting health and physical performance.

SEVERE WEIGHT LOSS

Severe body mass loss, as occurs on a "crash" diet or in athletes attempting to make a weight class, does have negative physiological consequences. Weight class athletes, such as wrestlers and boxers, many times lose weight rapidly to compete in the lowest weight class possible to gain an advantage over their competitors. Losing body mass rapidly has performance as well as health consequences in both males and females.

Dehydration

Rapid weight loss due to fasting or severe caloric restriction brings about a quick decrease in body mass, but this decrease is largely due to dehydration. As discussed earlier, glycogen within the body is stored with a substantial amount of water (2.6 g H_2O·g carbohydrate^{-1}). When the glycogen is used in metabolism, the water is released and eventually excreted from the body. This results in a significant body mass loss, but the loss is primarily due to loss of body water. Of special concern to athletes, if glycogen stores are reduced, they are not available for either aerobic or anaerobic metabolism in an upcoming competition.

Athletes using techniques such as water restriction, sitting in a steam room, and exercising in rubberized suits to make a weight class have demonstrated decreases in performance. Dehydration of 3% to 4% of TBM significantly decreases aerobic capabilities (see Chapter 9). Although decreases in anaerobic and strength capabilities occur with this same level of dehydration, they are not as consistently shown with rapid dehydration (see Chapter 9). Thus, the magnitude of decreased performance due to rapid dehydration depends in part on what sport an athlete is competing.

Female Athlete Triad

The **female athlete triad** refers to a syndrome consisting of three interrelated conditions that affect female athletes and active women, including menstrual cycle irregularities, osteoporosis, and eating disorders (see Chapter 15). All these factors relate to aspects of body composition and diet. Menstrual cycle irregularities in athletes are correlated to low % fat, but dietary restriction of calories may be the real culprit for menstrual cycle irregularities.[10,32] Menstrual cycle irregularities can result in decreased estrogen levels.[32,57] Estrogen increases osteoblast (bone cells) proliferation and inhibits bone resorption. Thus, decreased estrogen levels result in a decrease in bone mineral density. Moreover, eating disorders are strongly related to menstrual cycle irregularities. Thus, the three factors are interrelated.

There are two major types of eating disorders. **Anorexia nervosa** is an eating disorder characterized by determined dieting, often accompanied by compulsive exercise, resulting in sustained low body mass. **Bulimia nervosa** is characterized by binge eating followed by some type of compensatory behavior, most typically purging. Both types of eating disorders are viewed as psychiatric disorders and are most prevalent in women (~0.7%–2.0% of the population), but men also are affected by eating disorders.[57,16] Some groups of athletes may be more susceptible than others to eating disorders[10,23]; these include the following:

- Weight class sports: martial arts, wrestling, and rowing
- Subjectively scored sports: dance, figure skating, gymnastics, and diving
- Endurance sports in which a low body weight is an advantage: distance running, cycling, and cross-country skiing
- Sports in which body contour–revealing clothing is worn: volleyball, swimming, diving, and running

Quick Review

- Severe weight loss can result in dehydration, loss of FFM, and decreased aerobic and anaerobic performance.
- Eating disorders are more prevalent in women than in men and in athletes participating in sports that involve weight classes or are subjectively scored.
- The female athlete triad factors (eating disorders, menstrual cycle irregularities, and bone mineral density loss) are all interrelated and can result in decreased physical performance.

Perfectionism may play a role in eating disorders in the general population and in athletes, but being an athlete for some people may also be a protective factor from developing an eating disorder.[23] It seems that, depending in part on the sport, anywhere from 1% to 62% of female athletes may be affected by an eating disorder.[10] Coaches and athletes need to be aware that eating disorders and the female athlete triad can result in decreased performance and an increased chance of injury. To minimize the chance of injury and prevent decreases in performance, any athlete displaying signs of an eating disorder or the female athlete triad should be referred to a healthcare professional for treatment.

CASE STUDY

Scenario

A college cross-country skier comes in for a yearly DEXA body composition analysis. One year ago, Stephanie had a body fat percentage of 16% and weighted 125 pounds (56.8 kg). You complete Stephanie's profile in the laboratory and are surprised after examining her DEXA results because she is now at a body mass of 100 pounds (45.5 kg), has a 9.5% body fat percentage, and her bone mineral density is now lower when compared to that last year. She says the coach thought she was too fat and some weight loss would help her performance. You ask her what she is eating. She says she eats pretty well but has cut down on her calories.

Questions

1. To what do these warning signs point?
2. What is your next step?

Options

You notice the dramatic weight loss, hear that she is cutting calories, and note that she has a dramatically lower bone density this year. You also note that an authority figure has stated she needs to lose weight. After thinking about it, you realize that you are in over your head and this could be a serious medical or eating disorder. You refer her to the team physician with your observations because you understand that anorexia nervosa or bulimia nervosa are serious medical conditions requiring intervention by a physician team with psychiatric specialties.

Scenario

A muscular male athlete comes to you and says his BMI, which is 26, indicates he is overweight. What do you do?

Options

You first explain that BMI only takes into account the weight and height of an individual. BMI does not account for differences in body composition, such as FFM and FM. You go on to explain that BMI indicates for many athletes that they are overweight or even obese due to their large FFM, which increases their TBM relative to their height. This results in a high BMI. To put the athlete's doubts completely to rest, you perform a body composition analysis using hydrostatic weighing. The results show that the athlete has 10% fat, which is below the average adult male value of 15%. You advise the athlete not to be concerned about his BMI because his body composition indicates he is not overweight and in fact he is quite lean.

CHAPTER SUMMARY

Body composition is related to health and physical performance, with most individuals desiring a decrease in % fat and an increase in FFM. Both these factors are responsive to diet and exercise and so can be changed over time. On the other hand, anthropometric measures, such as height and arm and leg length, although related to performance in various sports, cannot be changed except through normal growth. When attempting to alter body composition, a combination of diet and aerobic and weight training should be used to slowly change body composition so that FFM loss is minimized and FM loss is maximized. Severe fast weight loss should normally be avoided because it results in dehydration, FFM loss, and decreased physical performance. Several techniques to determine body composition have been shown to be sensitive and reliable, but the results from different techniques can vary, and so when tracking body composition changes, the same technique should always be used. In the next chapter, we turn our attention to the development of endurance and strength training programs and their effects on health and performance rather than body composition.

REVIEW QUESTIONS

Fill-in-the-Blank

1. The three components of the female athletic triad are: _____, _____, and _____.

2. _____ and _____ use the volume of the body to estimate % fat.

3. _____ is purported by experts to be the most accurate method of measuring body fat percentage.

4. The ideal total caloric deficit per day for weight loss is between _____ and _____.

5. _____, or the minimal level of energy needed by the body to stay alive, can decrease if caloric intake is _____ significantly.

Multiple Choice

1. Obesity could be in part due to
   a. genetics of a person
   b. having a positive caloric balance
   c. increased portion sizes
   d. physical inactivity
   e. all of the above

2. You are performing a field study on body composition in wrestlers before the national tournament to see what their body composition profiles are after a season of wrestling. Under these conditions, what method of body composition would you use?
   a. DEXA
   b. Underwater weighing
   c. Skinfold calipers
   d. Any bioelectrical impedance device
   e. Air-displacement plethysmography

3. The average % fat of adult males and females are approximately
   a. 15% and 25%, respectively.
   b. 5% and 10% to 15%, respectively.
   c. 20% for both sexes.
   d. 8% and 18%, respectively.
   e. none of the above

4. A college football player says his mother says he is fat based on his BMI as determined by a local insurance document. What do you tell him?
   a. Talk to him about the weaknesses of BMI and body composition
   b. Evaluate his body composition with a valid technique before any decisions are made
   c. Tell him to get on a diet to make his mother happy
   d. Help to develop a new and better weight training program for the athlete
   e. a and b

5. Which of the following equations can be used to calculate FFM?
   a. TBM × % FFM
   b. FFM × % fat
   c. % FFM × % fat
   d. TBM × % fat
   e. TBM × FM

True/False

1. Strength training is counterproductive for decreasing body fat percentage.
2. Eating disorders happen primarily in people who are undisciplined.
3. Three percent dehydration can result in decrements in physical performance.
4. Appetite can be decreased by factors such as heat and exercise.

5. The suggested minimal caloric ranges were established, in part, to ensure that adequate macro- and micronutrients are consumed each day.
6. Dieting alone to achieve fat loss may result in losses of and decreases in lean tissue.

Short Answer

1. Describe briefly the problems with the traditional weight loss strategy of crash dieting. What can be done to counteract the problems?
2. What type of exercise protocol would you prescribe to someone who told you she wanted to lose fat around the waist?
3. Athletes in which sports might be most susceptible to an eating disorder?
4. What are the two components of body composition, and of what are they composed?
5. Why is the prevalence of obesity in the U.S. of concern?

Critical Thinking Questions

1. What are the assumptions of skinfold measurements to determine body composition?
2. What precautions should be taken when losing body mass to ensure the majority of weight loss comes from FM?

KEY TERMS

air-displacement plethysmography: a densitometry technique to determine body composition using air displacement to determine body volume

anorexia nervosa: an eating disorder characterized by a refusal to maintain a minimal normal body mass, which is often accompanied by compulsive exercise resulting in sustained low body mass

anthropometry: the measurement and study of body size, such as stature, body mass, and leg length

bioelectrical impedance: estimation of body composition involving placing electrodes at two or more places on the body and passing an undetectable electrical current between the electrodes

body density: total body mass divided by the volume of the body

body mass index (BMI): the ratio of body mass divided by height squared

bulimia nervosa: an eating disorder characterized by binge eating, followed by a compensatory behavior, such as purging

central obesity (android obesity): fat deposition in the abdominal area

densitometry: determination of body composition from the body's density

dual-energy x-ray absorptiometry (DEXA): use of low-energy x-ray beams and computer software to produce images of the body that can be used to determine body composition

empty calories: calories from foods high in caloric value but of little other nutritional value

energy balance: ratio of caloric ingestion versus caloric expenditure

fat-free mass: the total mass of all tissues within the body excluding all fat

fat mass: the total mass of fat within the body

female athlete triad: a syndrome consisting of three interrelated conditions that affect female athletes and active women, including menstrual irregularities, osteoporosis, and eating disorders

hydrostatic weighing: a technique of determining body density by complete submersion in water

percent body fat (% fat): the ratio of total body mass to total fat mass

peripheral obesity (gynoid-type obesity): fat deposition in the gluteal and thigh regions

regional body composition: tissue composition of specific areas of the body, such as the arms, legs, or trunk

satiety: the feeling of satisfaction that occurs after a meal that inhibits further eating

skinfolds: a method of estimating body composition by measuring the thickness of the skin and subcutaneous fat at specific anatomical sites using a specialized caliber

spot reduction: the false concept that body fat will be lost predominantly from an area of the body by performing exercise using that area of the body

REFERENCES

1. Ackland TR, Schreiner AB, Kerr DA. Absolute size and proportionality characteristics of World Championship female basketball players. J Sports Sci. 1997;15:485–490.
2. Allison DB, Fontaine KR, Manson JE, et al. Annual deaths attributable to obesity in the United States. J Am Med Assoc. 1999;282:1530–1538.
3. Astrand PO. Diet and athletic performance. Fed Proc. 1967;26:1772–1777.
4. Biaggi RR, Vollman MW, Nies MA, et al. Comparison of air-displacement plethysmography with hydrostatic weighing and bioelectrical impedance analysis for the assessment of body composition in healthy adults. Am J Clin Nutr. 1999;69:898–903.
5. Boileau RA, Lohman TG. The measurement of human physique and its effect on physical performance. Orthop Clin North Am. 1977;8:563–581.
6. Bouchard C, Tremblay A, Despres JP, et al. The response to long-term overfeeding in identical twins. N Engl J Med. 1990;322:1477–1482.
7. Bourgois J, Claessens AL, Vrjens J, et al. Anthropometric characteristics of elite male junior rowers. Br J Sports Med. 2000;34:213–217.
8. Bray GA. Effect of caloric restriction on energy expenditure in obese patients. Lancet. 1969;2:397–400.
9. Brechue WF, Takashi A. The role of FFM accumulation and skeletal muscle architecture and powerlifting performance. Eur J Appl Physiol. 2002;86:237–336.
10. Burnett M. Female athlete triad. Clin Sports Med. 2005;21:623–636.
11. Calle EE, Rodriguez C, Walker-Thurmond K, et al. Overweight, obesity, and mortality from cancer in a prospectively studied cohort of U.S. adults. N Engl J Med. 2003;348:1625–1638.
12. CDC. Overweight and Obesity. Atlanta, GA: CDC, 2010. Available at: www.cdc.gov/obesity.
13. Classens AL, Bourgois J, Vrijens J. The relevance of kinanthropometry to rowing performance: the Hazewinkel anthropometric project. Acta Kinesiologiae Univesitatis Tartuensis. 2001;6:15S–21S.
14. Dempster P, Aitkens S. A new air displacement method for the determination of human body composition. Med Sci Sports Exerc. 1995;27:1692–1697.
15. Dixon CB, Deitrick RW, Pierce JR, et al. Evaluation on the BOD POD and leg-to-leg bioelectrical impedance analysis for estimating percent body fat in National Collegiate Athletic Association Division III collegiate wrestlers. J Strength Cond Res. 2005;19:85–91.
16. Fairburn CG, Harrison PJ. Eating disorders. Lancet. 2003;361:407–416.

17. Figueroa-Colan R, Mayo MS, Treuth MS, et al. Reproducibility of dual-energy X-ray absorptiometry in prepubertal girls. Obes Res. 1998;6:262–267.
18. Fleck SJ, Kraemer WJ. Designing Resistance Training Programs, 3rd ed. Champaign, IL: Human Kinetics, 2004.
19. Fleck SJ, Mattie C, Martensen HC III. Effect of resistance and aerobic training on regional body composition in previously recreationally trained middle-aged women. Appl Physiol Nutr Metab. 2006;31:261–270.
20. Flegal KM, Carroll MD, Ogden CL, et al. Prevalence and trends in obesity among U.S. adults, 1999–2000. J Am Med Assoc. 2002;288:1723–1727.
21. Flint A, Gregersen NT, Gluud LL, et al. Associations between postprandial insulin and blood glucose responses, appetite sensations and energy intake in normal weight and overweight individuals: a meta-analysis of test meal studies. Br J Nutr. 2007;98:17–25.
22. Fontain KR, Redden DT, Wang C, et al. Years of life lost due to obesity. J Am Med Assoc. 2003;289:187–193.
23. Fosberg LJ. The relationship between perfectionism, eating disorders and athletes: a review. Minerva Pediatr. 2006;58:525–536.
24. Fulton JE, McGuire MT, Casoersen CJ, et al. Interventions for weight loss and weight gain prevention among youth current issues. Sports Med. 2001;31:153–165.
25. Heyward VH, Wagner DR. Applied Body Composition Assessment, 2nd ed. Champaign, IL: Human Kinetics, 2004.
26. Housh TJ, Johnson GO, Housh DJ, et al. Estimation of body density in young wrestlers. J Strength Cond Res. 2000;14:477–482.
27. Houtkooper LB, Going SB, Sproul J, et al. Comparison of methods for assessing body composition changes over 1 year in postmenopausal women. Am J Clin Nutr. 2000;72:401–406.
28. Hu F. Television watching and other sedentary behaviors in relation to risk of obesity and type 2 diabetes mellitus in women. J Am Med Assoc. 2003;289:1785–1791.
29. Jackson A, Pollock ML. Generalized equations for predicting body density of men. Br J Nutr. 1978;40:497–504.
30. Jackson AS, Pollock ML, Ward A. Generalized equations for predicting body density of women. Med Sci Sports Exerc. 1980;12:175–182.
31. Jamurtas AZ, Koutedakis Y, Paschalis V, et al. The effects of a single bout of exercise on resting energy expenditure and respiratory exchange ratio. Eur J Appl Physiol. 2004;92:393–398.
32. Jayasinghe Y, Grover SR, Zacharin M. Current concepts in bone and reproductive health in adolescents with anorexia nervosa. Br J Obstet Gynaecol. 2008;115:304–315.
33. Kannel WB, Cupples LA, Ramaswami R, et al. Regional obesity and risk of cardiovascular disease: the Framingham study. J Clin Epidemiol. 1991;44:183–190.
34. Kostek MA, Pescatello LS, Seip RL, et al. Subcutaneous fat alterations resulting from an upper-body resistance training program. Med Sci Sports Exerc. 2007;39:1177–85.
35. Kraemer WJ, Torine JC, Silvestre R, et al. Body size and composition of National Football League players. J Strength Cond Res. 2005;19:485–489.
36. Kraemer WJ, Volek JS, Clark KL, et al. Influence of exercise training on physiological and performance changes with weight loss in men. Med Sci Sports Exerc. 1999;31:1320–1329.
37. Krauss RM, Winston M, Fletcher BJ, et al. Obesity: impact on cardiovascular disease. Circulation. 1998;980:1472–1476.
38. Leibel RL, Rosenbaum M, Hirsch J. Changes in energy expenditure resulting from altered body weight. N Engl J Med. 1995;332:673–674.
39. Lemmer JT, Ivey FM, Ryan AS, et al. Effect of strength training on resting metabolic rate and physical activity: age and gender comparisons. Med Sci Sports Exerc. 2001;33:532–541.
40. Lockner DW, Heyward VH, Baumgartner RN, et al. Comparison of air-displacement plethysmography, hydrodensitometry, and dual X-ray absorptiometry for assessing body composition of children 10 to 18 years of age. Ann NY Acad Sci. 2000;904:72–78.
41. Mazzetti S, Douglas M, Yocum A, et al. Effect of explosive versus slow contractions and exercise intensity on energy expenditure. Med Sci Sports Exerc. 2007;39:1291–1301.
42. McLeod WD, Hunter SC, Etchison B. Performance measurement and body fat in the high school athlete. Am J Sports Med. 1983;11:390–397.
43. Melanson EL, Sharp TA, Seagle HM, et al. Resistance and aerobic exercise have similar effects on 24-h nutrient oxidation. Med Sci Sports Exerc. 2002;34:1793–1800.
44. Midorikawa T, Masakatsu K, Beekley MD, et al. High REE in sumo wrestlers attributed to large organ-tissue mass. Med Sci Sports Exerc. 2007;39:688–693.
45. Nielsen S, Popkin BM. Patterns and trends in food portion sizes, 1977–1998. J Am Med Assoc. 2003;289:450–453.
46. NIH. Clinical Guidelines on the Identification, Evaluation, and Treatment of Overweight and Obesity in Adults: The Evidence Report. Bethesda, MD: National Institutes of Health, 1998: 51S–209S.
47. O'Rahilly S, Farooqi IS, Yeo GS, et al. Minireview: human obesity—lessons from monogenic disorders. Endocrinology. 2003;144: 3757–3764.
48. Ode JJ, Pivarnik JM, Reeves MJ, et al. Body mass index as a predictor of percent fat in college athletes and nonathletes. Med Sci Sports Exerc. 2007;39:403–409.
49. Ogden CL CM, Curtin LR, McDowell MA, et al. Prevalence of overweight and obesity in the United States, 1999–2004. J Am Med Assoc. 2006;295(13):1549–1555.
50. Pi-Sunyer FX. The obesity epidemic: pathophysiology and consequences of obesity. Obes Res. 2002;10:97S–104S.
51. Poehlman ET, Toth PA, Ades PA, et al. Gender differences in resting metabolic rate and noradrenaline kinetics in older individuals. Eur J Clin Invest. 1997;27:23–28.
52. Puhl R, Brownell KD. Bias, discrimination, and obesity. Obes Res. 2001;9:788–805.
53. Puhl RM, Brownell KD. Psychosocial origins of obesity stigma: toward changing a powerful and pervasive bias. Obes Rev. 2003;4: 213–227.
54. Ratamess NA, Falvo MJ, Mangine GT, et al. The effect of rest period length on metabolic responses to the bench press exercise. Eur J Appl Physiol. 2007;100:1–17.
55. Rolls B, Morris EL, Roe LS. Portion size of food affects energy intake in normal-weight and overweight men and women. Am J Clin Nutr. 2002;76:1207–1213.
56. Rolls BJ, Bell A, Thorwart ML. Water incorporated into a food but not served with a food decreases energy intake in lean women. Am J Clin Nutr. 1999;70 448–455.
57. Rome ES. Eating disorders. Obstet Gynecol Clin. 2003;30:353–377.
58. Serdula MK, Mokdad AH, Williamson DF, et al. Prevalence of attempting weight lost and strategies for controlling weight. J Am Med Assoc. 1999;282:1353–1358.
59. Silvestre R, West C, Maresh CM, et al. Body composition and physical performance in men's soccer: a study of a National Collegiate Athletic Association Division I team. J Strength Cond Res. 2006;20:177–183.
60. Siri WE. The gross composition of the body. Adv Biol Med Physiol. 1956;4:239–280.
61. Slyper AH. Low density lipoprotein and atherosclerosis. Unraveling the connection. J Am Med Assoc. 1994;272:305–308.
62. Stallknecht B, Dela F, Helge JW. Are blood flow and lipolysis in subcutaneous adipose tissue influenced by contractions in adjacent muscles in humans? Am J Physiol Endocrinol Metab. 2007;292: E394–E399.
63. Stoving RK, Hangaard J, Hansen-Nord M, et al. A review of hormonal changes in anorexia nervosa. J Psychiatr Res. 1999;33:139–152.
64. Stuempfle KJ, Katch FI, Petrie DE. Body composition relates poorly to performance tests in NCAA Division III football players. J Strength Cond Res. 2003;17:238–244.

65. Tumilty D. Physiological characteristics of elite soccer players. Sports Med. 1993;16:80–96.
66. Ugarkovic D, Matavulj D, Kukolj M, et al. Standard anthropometric, body composition, and strength variables as predictors of jumping performance in elite junior athletes. J Strength Cond Res. 2002;16:227–230.
67. Ukkola O, Pöykkö S. Ghrelin, growth and obesity. Ann Med. 2002;34:102–108.
68. Utter AC, Goss FL, Swan PD, et al. Evaluation of air displacement for assessing body composition of collegiate rowers. Med Sci Sports Exerc. 2003;35:500–505.
69. van Someren KA, Plamer GS. Prediction of 200-m sprint kayaking performance. Can J Appl Physiol. 2003;28:505–517.
70. Vescovi JD HL, Miller W, Hammer R, et al. Evaluation of the BOD POD for estimating percent fat in female college athletes. J Strength Cond Res. 2002;16:599–605.
71. Volek JS, Forsythe CE. The case for not restricting saturated fat on a low carbohydrate diet. Nutr Metab (Lond). 2005;2:21.
72. Volek JS, Fernandez ML, Feinman RD, et al. Dietary carbohydrate restriction induces a unique metabolic state positively affecting atherogenic dyslipidemia, fatty acid partitioning, and metabolic syndrome. Prog Lipid Res. 2008;47:307–318.
73. Wang Z, Heshka S, Wang J, et al. Magnitude and variation of fat-free mass density: a cellular-level body composition modeling study. Am J Physiol Endocrinol Metab. 2003;284:E267–E273.
74. Wardle J, Cooke L. The impact of obesity on psychological well-being. Best Pract Res. 2005;19:421–440.
75. Weinsier RL, Schutz Y, Bracco D. Reexamination of the relationship of resting metabolic rate to fat-free mass and to the metabolically active components of fat-free mass humans. Am J Clin Nutr. 1992;55:790–794.
76. Weyer C, Walford RL, Harper IT, et al. Energy metabolism after 2 y of energy restriction: the biosphere 2 experiment. Am J Clin Nutr. 2000;72:946–953.
77. Weyers AM, Mazzetti SA, Love D, et al. Comparison of methods for assessing body composition changes during weight loss. Med Sci Sports Exerc. 2002;34:497–502.
78. Whaley MH, Brubaker PH, Otto RM, eds. ACSM's Guidelines for Exercise Testing and Prescription, 7th ed. Philadelphia, PA: Lippincott Williams & Wilkins, 2006.
79. Whitney E, Rolfes SR. Understanding Nutrition, 10th ed. Belmont, CA: Thomson/Wadsworth, 2005.
80. Wong SL, Katzmarzyk P, Nichaman MZ, et al. Cardiorespiratory fitness is associated with lower abdominal fat independent of body mass index. Med Sci Sport Exerc. 2004;36:286–291.

Suggested Readings

Berkman ND, Lohr KN, Bulik C. Outcomes of eating disorders: a systematic review of the literature. Int J Eat Disord. 2007;40:293–309.
Burnett M. Female athlete triad. Clin Sports Med. 2005;**21**:623–636.
Fairburn CG, Harrison PJ. Eating disorders. Lancet. 2003;361:407–416.
Fulton JE, McGuire MT, Casoersen CJ, et al. Interventions for weight loss and weight gain prevention among youth current issues. Sports Med. 2001;31:153–165.
Heyward VH, Wagner DR. Applied Body Composition Assessment, 2nd ed. Champaign, IL: Human Kinetics, 2004.
Kannel WB, Cupples LA, Ramaswami R, et al. Regional obesity and risk of cardiovascular disease: the Framingham study. J Clin Epidemiol. 1991;44:183–190.
Kostek MA, Pescatello LS, Seip RL, et al. Subcutaneous fat alterations resulting from an upper-body resistance training program. Med Sci Sports Exerc. 2007;39:1177–1185.
Lemmer JT, Ivey FM, Ryan AS, et al. Effect of strength training on resting metabolic rate and physical activity: age and gender comparisons. Med Sci Sports Exerc. 2001;33:532–541.
Melanson EL, Sharp TA, Seagle HM, et al. Resistance and aerobic exercise have similar effects on 24-h nutrient oxidation. Med Sci Sports Exerc. 2002;34:1793–1800.
Serdula MK, Mokdad AH, Williamson DF, et al. Prevalence of attempting weight lost and strategies for controlling weight. J Am Med Assoc. 1999;282:1353–1358.
Wong SL, Katzmarzyk P, Nichaman MZ, et al. Cardiorespiratory fitness is associated with lower abdominal fat independent of body mass index. Med Sci Sports Exerc. 2004;36:286–291.

Classic References

Brozek J. Physical activity and body composition. Arh Hig Rada. 1954;5(2):193–212.
Jackson A, Pollock ML. Generalized equations for predicting body density of men. Br J Nutr. 1978;40:497–504.
Jackson AS, Pollock ML, Ward A. Generalized equations for predicting body density of women. Med Sci Sports Exerc. 1980;12:175–182.
Katch F, Michael ED, Horvath SM. Estimation of body volume by underwater weighing: description of a simple method. J Appl Physiol. 1967;23(5):811–813.
Lohman TG. Biological variation in body composition. J Anim Sci. 1971;32(4):647–653.

12

Aerobic and Strength Training Prescription for Health and Performance

After reading this chapter, you should be able to:

1. Discuss training for health benefits
2. Explain and differentiate types of cardiovascular disease
3. Identify risk factors for coronary artery disease (CAD)
4. Recognize when it is important to obtain medical clearance
5. Explain and apply aerobic training guidelines for health
6. Explain and apply resistance training guidelines for health
7. Design a training session
8. Discuss the effects of detraining
9. Apply the principles of periodization

A thletes train to increase performance in their respective sports. Many people, however, train not just for increased physical performance, but for the health benefits associated with physical activity. A **fitness benefit** is a physiological adaptation, such as increased lactate threshold, vertical jump ability, and maximal strength, that potentially increases performance in a sport or activity. A **health benefit** is a physiological adaptation, such as decreased resting blood pressure, that reduces the risk of developing a disease, such as cardiovascular disease. Some physiological adaptations may bring about both fitness and health benefits. Increased peak oxygen consumption is associated not only with the fitness benefit of increased performance in endurance sports such as 800- and 1500-m running,[30] but also with health benefits related to decreased overall mortality.[8,46] Training **intensity** is a measure of how difficult the exercise is, whereas **volume** is a measure of how much work or exercise is performed. The physical training necessary to bring about health benefits is lower in intensity and volume than that needed to bring about fitness benefits. In this chapter, we will focus on both aerobic and resistance training guidelines for the general population with the goal of causing health benefits particularly related to cardiovascular disease, as well as general fitness benefits. We also consider several topics critical to training, including medical clearance, structure of a training session, detraining, and periodization.

EXERCISE AND PREVENTION OF CARDIOVASCULAR DISEASE

One of the greatest health benefits of exercise, for both athletes and the general population, is the prevention of cardiovascular disease. In this section, we consider the prevalence of cardiovascular disease in the United States, the types of cardiovascular disease, and risk factors related to cardiovascular disease, including physical inactivity.

Prevalence of Cardiovascular Disease

In the 1970s, cardiovascular diseases were the leading cause of death and accounted for more than 50% of all deaths in the United States. In 2004, cardiovascular diseases were still the leading cause of death but accounted for only 36.3% of all deaths. However, even this rate equates to an average of 1 death every 37 seconds.[4] The long-term trend of decreased deaths due to cardiovascular disease is not related to one particular factor, but probably to the interaction of several factors related to cardiovascular disease prevention and treatment:

- Changes in lifestyle, such as improved nutrition, smoking cessation, and regular exercise, that help prevent cardiovascular disease
- Development of medical techniques that allow earlier and better diagnosis
- Improved emergency care and treatment for heart attack and stroke victims
- Improved medical techniques for treatment (bypass surgery, angioplasty, and drug-coated stints)
- Improved drugs for long-term treatment

All these factors have resulted in decreased deaths from the various types of cardiovascular disease.

Types of Cardiovascular Disease

Several different types of cardiovascular disease exist, with coronary heart disease accounting for more than 50% of all deaths associated with cardiovascular problems (Fig. 12-1). Here, we will focus only on coronary artery disease (CAD), stroke, heart failure, hypertension, and peripheral artery disease (PAD), all of which are affected by lifestyle choices.

Coronary Artery Disease

The coronary arteries supply the cardiac tissue with blood. If a coronary artery is blocked, the cardiac tissue it supplies with blood does not receive needed oxygen and nutrients. A minor or partial blockage of a coronary artery results in **ischemia**, or insufficient blood supply to the tissue supplied by the artery (Fig. 12-2). Ischemia can occur at anytime, but cardiac tissue is especially vulnerable to ischemia during physical activity or times of stress, when the oxygen needs of the heart are increased. Ischemia can result in severe chest pain, or **angina pectoris**. If a coronary artery is severely or totally blocked, ischemia becomes severe enough to result in a **myocardial**

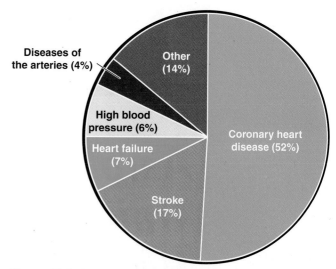

Figure 12-1. Percentage breakdown of deaths in the United States (2004) due to various types of cardiovascular diseases. CAD, stroke, heart failure, hypertension, diseases of the arteries, and other causes, such as congenital heart problems, are all causes of a substantial number of deaths in the United States. Note that heart failure is not a true underlying cause of death. (From the American Heart Association. Heart Disease and Stroke Statistics—2010 Update. Available at http://www.americanheart.org/downloadable/heart/12626426574432010%20Stat%20charts%20FINAL.ppt#484,2,Slide 9. Original data from the CDC, National Center for Health Statistics.)

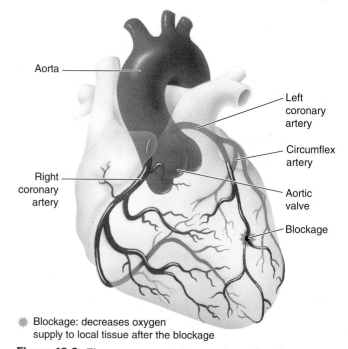

❋ Blockage: decreases oxygen supply to local tissue after the blockage

Figure 12-2. The coronary arteries supply cardiac tissue with needed oxygen and nutrients. Blockage of a coronary artery due to atherosclerosis results in ischemia to the cardiac tissue supplied by the artery. (Adapted from an asset provided by Anatomical Chart Co.)

infarction, more commonly known as a heart attack. During myocardial infarction, a lack of blood and oxygen for several minutes results in death, or necrosis, of myocardial cells. Depending on the extent of myocardial cell necrosis (i.e., cell death), mild, moderate, or severe disability will result. In minor cases of myocardial infarction, the person affected may not know he or she has had a minor heart attack until weeks or months later. The longer ischemia lasts, the greater the amount of myocardial necrosis. This is why it is important for a person suffering a myocardial infarction to receive medical attention as soon as possible.

CAD is the disease process causing eventual blockage and hardening of arteries supplying cardiac tissue with blood, as just discussed. The blockage is caused by **atherosclerosis**: a progressive narrowing of an artery due to the formation of fatty plaque on the interior wall of the artery. Atherosclerosis can occur within any blood vessel, but when it occurs within a coronary artery it is termed CAD. As the narrowing progresses, so does the extent of ischemia, eventually resulting in myocardial infarction. Atherosclerosis and **arteriosclerosis**, or thickening and loss of elasticity of the arterial wall, are the result of chronic low-grade inflammation of the blood vessel walls. Because of the inflammation, a plaque or buildup consisting of muscle cells from the middle layer of the arterial wall, blood lipids, and connective tissue develops on the interior arterial wall (Box 12-1). The buildup of plaque results in narrowing of the artery (atherosclerosis) and arteriosclerosis because the plaque is less elastic than normal arterial wall tissue. The presence of cardiovascular disease also increases the chance that a **thrombus** or blood clot will partially or completely block an artery.

Stroke

Stroke is a lack of blood supply to a portion of the brain. Similar to myocardial infarction, a stroke results in necrosis of brain tissue. What portion of the brain is damaged dictates the resulting symptoms. Stroke can affect the senses,

---

Box 12-1 DID YOU KNOW?
Development of Plaque

Plaque development resulting in atherosclerosis and arteriosclerosis is caused by a chronic low-grade infection of the arterial walls.[1] This process starts with monocytes, a type of white blood cell, attaching to the area between endothelial cells that line the interior of the arterial wall. The monocytes differentiate into macrophages, which are capable of enzymatically destroying cellular matter. The macrophages engulf oxidized LDL-C and slowly become foam cells underneath the endothelial lining, forming fatty streaks.[2] Smooth muscle cells from the middle layer of the arterial wall also gradually accumulate underneath the endothelial wall. The endothelial cells eventually are sloughed off of the arterial wall, exposing the underlying connective tissue. Platelets are attracted to the exposed arterial wall tissue, and LDL-C is deposited in the plaque.

As the plaque builds up, the vessel becomes increasingly narrow. Plaque has a fibrous cap, which can help to make the plaque buildups either stable or prone to rupture. Plaque buildups prone to rupture have a thin fibrous cap, a large amount of foam cells, and a low density of smooth muscle cells. If a plaque ruptures, proteolytic enzymes are released, breaking down the cellular structure, resulting in a blood clot or thrombus. The thrombus, if large enough, can block the artery. Thus, plaque development results in atherosclerosis (narrowing of the artery) and arteriosclerosis (hardening of the artery because the plaque is less elastic than a healthy arterial wall) and increases the chance of thrombus development.

References
1. Romero FI, Khamashta MA, Hughe GRV. Lipoprotein(a) oxidation and autoantibodies: a new path in atherothrombosis. Lupus 2000;9:206–209.
2. Ross R. Atherosclerosis—an inflammatory disease. N Eng J Med. 1999;340:115–126.

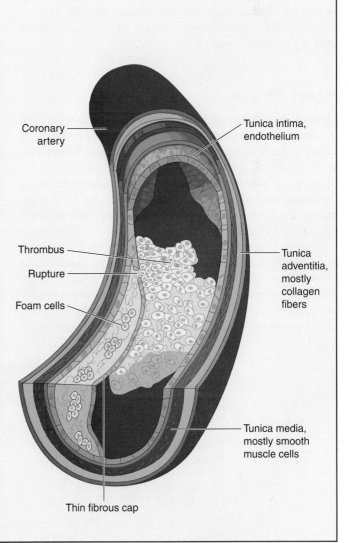

short- and long-term memory capabilities, and speech patterns. Paralysis on one side of the body is also a common symptom of stroke.

Ischemic stroke, similar to cardiac ischemia, results in a lack of blood supply to a particular area of brain due to a blockage of a blood vessel. Ischemic stroke can be the result of cerebral thrombosis (a thrombus developing in a cerebral vessel). A common site of thrombus development is where atherosclerosis has developed. A cerebral embolism is the result of fat globules, a small piece of tissue, or a blood clot breaking loose from another area of the body, being carried by the blood to the brain, and eventually blocking a cerebral blood vessel.

Blood flow interruption can also result from the rupture of a blood vessel, termed a *hemorrhagic* stroke. If a cerebral *artery* ruptures, it is termed a *cerebral hemorrhage*. If a blood vessel on the surface of the brain ruptures, it is termed a *subarachnoid hemorrhage*. Hemorrhages not only interrupt blood flow to the area of the brain the vessel supplies but also result in an accumulation of blood within the cranial cavity, resulting in an increase in pressure. The increase in pressure can do further damage to brain tissue. Predisposing factors for a hemorrhage are hypertension (increased blood pressure) and atherosclerotic damage that creates a weak spot in the blood vessel's wall.

Heart Failure

Heart failure is impairment in the ability of the ventricles to contract to the point that cardiac output is insufficient to meet the body's oxygen needs. Acute heart failure can be the result of a heart attack caused by a toxic substance, drug, or coronary artery blockage. Chronic heart failure is the impairment of cardiac function due to the long-term effects of such things as hypertension, multiple minor heart attacks, or a viral infection.

One response to a gradual decrease in cardiac output resulting from chronic heart failure is an increase in blood volume due to fluid retention by the kidneys. With moderate heart failure, the increase in blood volume results in maintenance of normal cardiac output but at a higher blood pressure, which increases the work the ventricles

must perform to maintain cardiac output. The increase in work the ventricles must perform results in ventricular hypertrophy (see Chapter 5). The higher blood pressure also results in fluid accumulation or edema. The edema can take place within the ankles and legs or the lungs, the latter being referred to as pulmonary edema. Unless properly treated, chronic heart failure progresses. Even with ventricular hypertrophy and an increase in blood volume, eventually the ventricles cannot develop enough pressure to maintain cardiac output.

Hypertension

Hypertension is chronic high blood pressure at rest. It is defined as resting arterial blood pressure equal to or greater than 140 and 90 mm Hg for systolic and diastolic blood pressure, respectively. As blood pressure increases, the work the heart must perform to pump blood throughout the body increases, which increases the oxygen demand of the cardiac tissue. Chronic hypertension also increases the strain on arteries and arterioles. As resting blood pressure increases, the risk increases not only for heart failure and atherosclerosis but also for peripheral vascular disease and kidney failure. Thus, it is not surprising that hypertension is an important consideration for cardiovascular health. Guidelines for defining hypertension in adults have been developed. As might be expected, as resting blood pressure increases, so does the severity of hypertension (Table 12-1).

Resting blood pressure in part depends on body size. Thus, children and young adolescents typically have lower resting blood pressures than do adults. Furthermore, approximately 65% and 75% of hypertension cases in women and men, respectively, are due to a person being overweight or obese.[24] Hypertension affects a large percentage of people. Overall, approximately one in three adult Americans is hypertensive, but hypertension and heart disease are more prevalent in certain segments of the American population. African-Americans have a greater incidence of hypertension than either Mexican-Americans or Caucasian-Americans.[4] Consequently, African-Americans have a higher incidence of deaths

Table 12-1. Classification of Adult Resting Blood Pressure		
Classification	**Systolic Pressure (mm Hg)**	**Diastolic Pressure (mm Hg)**
Normal	<120	<80
Prehypertension	120–139	80–89
Stage 1 hypertension	140–159	90–99
Stage 2 hypertension	≥160	≥100

Reprinted with permission from the Seventh Report of the Joint National Committee on Prevention, Detection, Evaluation, and Treatment of High Blood Pressure. Hypertension. 2003;42:1206–1252.

from heart disease, fatal strokes, nonfatal strokes, and end-stage renal disease.

Despite the prevalence and severe consequences of hypertension, its causes are not well understood. Most hypertensive cases are defined as essential or idiopathic hypertension, meaning the exact cause of the increase in blood pressure is not known. However, there are known risk factors associated with hypertension[4]:

- Physical inactivity
- Overweight and obesity
- Heredity, including racial ancestry
- Being of male sex
- Increasing age
- Sodium sensitivity
- Use of tobacco products
- Excessive alcohol consumption
- Psychological stress
- Diabetes
- Use of oral contraceptives
- Pregnancy

Peripheral Artery Disease

PAD is the presence of atherosclerosis in the peripheral circulation. The development of PAD is similar to that of CAD. PAD many times results in diminished blood flow to the legs, resulting in decreased oxygen delivery. Blood clotting is also a primary symptom of PAD. The calves are primarily affected, but the entire leg and buttocks can also be stricken. PAD results in pain in one or both legs while walking, but it usually goes away with rest. Some people with PAD become so deconditioned that they are housebound, and in severe cases, ischemia occurs even at rest, requiring surgery or in severe cases amputation.[2] Because the mechanisms of atherosclerotic development in the periphery, including the legs, are the same as for CAD, it is not surprising that the risk factors for both are similar. Research has revealed that a walking (Pole Striding) exercise program can reduce the perceived pain and increase exercise tolerance in people with PAD.[10] Both aerobic and resistance training are generally prescribed as part of the treatment for PAD.[2]

Quick Review

- Cardiovascular diseases are the leading cause of death in the United States.
- Atherosclerosis and arteriosclerosis of the coronary vessels can result in an ischemic response, heart attack, stroke, or PAD.
- Hypertension is a contributing factor to atherosclerosis and arteriosclerosis.

CAD: Risk Factors

Major or primary risk factors are those that are strongly associated with CAD. The American Heart Association (www.americanheart.org) classifies major risk factors into two categories: those that can be affected by lifestyle changes and those that you have no control over. Uncontrollable major risk factors are increasing age, being of the male sex, and heredity. Increasing age is a risk factor because it takes years or even decades for CAD to develop to the severity at which symptoms are apparent. Thus, about 82% of people who die from CAD are 65 years or older. Being male is a risk factor because generally men have a greater risk of heart attack than women and have heart attacks earlier in life. This is true even after women experience menopause, at which point the death rate of women due to heart disease increases but is still less than that of men. If there is a history of CAD, heart attacks, or stroke in your family, you will be at greater risk for these same diseases; thus, heredity is a risk factor. Heredity is also a risk factor because, as previously discussed, some races have a higher risk of heart disease and hypertension than other races. Controllable major risk factors, which are linked to undesirable behavior, include the following:

- Smoking tobacco
- Blood lipid profile
- Hypertension
- Obesity and overweight
- Diabetes mellitus
- Physical inactivity

Other controllable factors that contribute to increased risk for CAD include psychological stress, alcohol consumption, as well as diet and nutrition. Psychological stress may be a contributing factor to CAD risk because it may affect other risk factors. People under stress may overeat (resulting in increased weight gain), start to smoke, or smoke more (if they are already smokers). Although moderate alcohol consumption of one drink (one drink = 4 fluid ounces of wine or 12 fluid ounces of beer) per day for women or two drinks per day for men may reduce cardiovascular risk, excessive alcohol consumption increases blood pressure, increases blood triglycerides, and contributes to heart failure. A diet low in saturated fats, not excessive in total calories, and that supplies all the essential macro- and micronutrients helps to reduce CAD risk. The above factors, although they contribute to CAD risk, are not considered major risk factors. In the following section, we will focus on major risk factors that can be directly affected by physical activity.

Blood Lipid Profile

Lipids, including cholesterol and triglycerides, are insoluble in blood. To make them soluble in blood so that they can be transported throughout the body, lipids are clustered with protein. **Lipoprotein** refers to clusters of lipids and proteins that are found in the blood. **Low-density lipoprotein cholesterol (LDL-C)** is produced by the liver to transport cholesterol and triglycerides to the body's tissues for their use. The liver also produces **high-density lipoprotein cholesterol (HDL-C)**, but the purpose of HDL-C is to transport lipids from the cells of the body back to the liver. LDL-C and HDL-C, as their names imply, differ in density. Protein is denser than lipids. LDL-C has a lower density than HDL-C because it contains greater amounts of cholesterol and triglycerides and smaller amounts of protein than does HDL-C. The cholesterol molecule or type of cholesterol does not differ between LDL-C and HDL-C.

Increased blood cholesterol, increased LDL-C, and decreased HDL-C are all associated with a higher risk of CAD (Table 12-2). High concentrations of cholesterol and LDL-C are associated with the development of atherosclerosis because they are involved in the development of plaque and are deposited into plaque. HDL-C, however, tends not be deposited into plaque, and so high levels of HDL-C are not associated with atherosclerosis development. Very low–density lipoprotein cholesterol (VLDL-C) is also produced by the liver and is associated with an increased cardiovascular risk.

The ratio of total cholesterol to HDL-C (total cholesterol/HDL-C) is also used as an indicator of cardiovascular risk. A low ratio is indicative of less cardiovascular risk and could be the outcome of decreased total cholesterol, increased HDL-C, or both. A total cholesterol to HDL-C ratio of 3.0 or less indicates low risk, whereas a ratio of 5.0 or greater indicates high risk. Thus, it is not only the values of cholesterol and HDL-C, but also their ratio that indicate increased risk of CAD.

Hypertension

Resting hypertension increases the work and oxygen needs of the heart to eject blood into the peripheral circulation.

Hypertension is also associated with the development of atherosclerosis and, so, the development of CAD. Hypertension not only increases the oxygen needs of the heart at rest, but also results in increased blood pressure and cardiac oxygen needs during exercise. It is also associated with CAD, which decreases oxygen delivery to cardiac tissue. All these factors set the stage for a heart attack. So, hypertension is associated with several factors that result in increased cardiovascular risk.

Obesity and Overweight

Excess body fat (see Chapter 11) resulting in obesity or being overweight increases the risk of a heart attack or stroke even if other risk factors are not present. Increased body mass due to excess body fat increases the heart's work, raises blood pressure, raises cholesterol, decreases HDL-C, and makes the development of diabetes mellitus more likely. Thus, obesity and being overweight affect other major risk factors, increasing overall cardiovascular risk and the development of CAD. Obesity and overweight can generally be defined using body mass index (BMI). However, BMI does not account for body composition (see Chapter 11).

Diabetes Mellitus

Diabetes increases the risk of developing CAD and the risk of a heart attack or stroke. This is true even if blood glucose levels are controlled by diet, exercise, or drugs. If blood glucose levels are not controlled, cardiovascular risk increases even more. This results in at least 65% of people with diabetes dying from some form of blood vessel or heart disease.

Physical Inactivity

Physical inactivity is a major CAD risk factor. Physical activity, on the other hand, decreases CAD risk because it results

Table 12-2. Risk Level of CAD due to Selected Risk Factors			
Risk Factor	**Little Risk**	**Some Risk**	**Serious Risk**
Blood lipid profile			
Total cholesterol (mg·dL^{-1})	<200	200–239	≥240
LDL-C (mg·dL^{-1})	<130	130–159	≥160
HDL-C (mg·dL^{-1})	≥60	40–59	<40
Triglycerides (mg·dL^{-1})	<150	150–199	≥200
Resting hypertension			
Systolic pressure (mm Hg)	<120	120–139	≥140
Diastolic pressure (mm Hg)	<80	80–89	≥90
Overweight and obesity (BMI [kg·m$^{2-1}$])	<25	25–29.9	≥30
Fasting plasma glucose (mg·dL^{-1})	<100	100–125	≥126
Physical activity (min·day^{-1}; moderate to vigorous most days of the week)	30–60	15–29	<15

Reprinted with permission from the American Heart Association 2008 (www.americanheart.org).

in many positive physiological adaptations that control the onset and/or severity of CAD. Many physiological adaptations to the circulatory system and skeletal muscle have already been discussed in previous chapters. Here, we will focus on adaptations that affect major CAD risk factors. Both aerobic and weight training reduce not only CAD, but total cardiovascular risk. Men who run 1 hour or more per week, or who weight train 30 minutes or more per week, or who row for 1 hour or more per week show an overall reduction in cardiovascular risk of 42%, 23%, and 18%, respectively.[55]

Both aerobic and weight training can positively affect the blood lipid profile. The most common blood lipid adaptation due to aerobic training (occurring in approximately 40% of training studies) is a 4.6% increase in HDL-C. Less frequently, approximate decreases of 5.0% in LDL-C, 3.7% in triglycerides, and 1.0% (not statistically significant) in total cholesterol occur.[38] Positive blood lipid profile changes occur due to some but not all weight training programs.[18,49,51] For example, during 14 weeks of resistance training, 27-year-old women demonstrated significant decreases in total cholesterol of 9.0%, LDL-C of 14%, and total cholesterol to HDL-C ratio of 14%, but no significant change in HDL-C and triglyceride.[49] Changes in blood lipid profile may be more apparent when training is accompanied by dietary counseling emphasizing decreasing total fat and saturated fat ingestion while increasing unsaturated fat ingestion. Reasons for the inconsistent changes in the blood lipid profile due to training include initial blood lipid measures (if they are normal at the start of training, positive adaptations may be less evident), duration of the training program, and intensity and volume of the training program. Even though changes in the blood lipid profile do not occur with all aerobic or resistance training programs, it is well accepted that both types of programs can potentially have a positive impact on blood lipid profile and so reduce CAD risk.

The American College of Sports Medicine recommends that to prevent and treat hypertension, one should perform primarily endurance training, supplemented by resistance training.[46] Meta-analyses show that aerobic training programs reduce resting systolic and diastolic blood pressures on average by 3 to 4 mm Hg and 2 to 3 mm Hg, respectively.[15,61] Likewise, meta-analyses show that resistance training programs reduce both resting systolic and diastolic blood pressure on average by about 3 mm Hg.[11,35] So, both aerobic and resistance training can reduce resting blood pressures. It is important to note that these decreases may be more apparent in people who are hypertensive at the start of the training program.

Overweight and obesity are at epidemic proportions in the American population. Both aerobic and resistance training increase caloric expenditure during and after a training bout (see Chapter 11). Both types of training also can result in decreased % body fat and increased fat-free mass, with the latter especially apparent with resistance training. So, both types of training can decrease obesity mainly by decreasing body fat.

Diabetes drastically increases the risk of developing CAD. The American College of Sports Medicine recommends that both aerobic and low-volume resistance training be performed to help control diabetes. Both aerobic[1,34] and resistance training[17,58] can increase insulin sensitivity and decrease fasting blood glucose levels. So, both types of training have been recommended by health experts to help control blood glucose levels. Overall then, research has shown that physical activity can positively affect virtually all controllable major CAD risk factors.

MEDICAL CLEARANCE

Although perceived by some as a hindrance to beginning an exercise program, medical clearance is recommended before starting an exercise program. It is important, especially for anyone having contraindications to exercise, for the following reasons:

- Some people have severe medical contraindications to exercise and should not exercise at all.
- Some people have increased risk for diseases such as cardiovascular disease, due to age, symptoms, or risk factors, and they should undergo exercise testing before beginning an exercise program.
- Some people have been diagnosed to have certain diseases and should only exercise in a medically supervised setting.
- Information obtained from the medical evaluation is useful in prescribing the appropriate type of exercise.
- Some clinical measures, such as blood pressure, blood lipid profile, and body composition, can be used to determine initial health status and determine progress in health status.
- For some people, clinical measures of health status may be motivational and increase adherence to an exercise program.
- Periodic medical evaluations are useful for early diagnosis of diseases, such as cardiovascular disease, cancer, and diabetes, when chances of successful treatment are at their highest.

Table 12-3. CAD Risk Factors Indicating the Need for Medical Clearance

Positive Risk Factors	Criteria
Family history	Myocardial infarction, coronary revascularization, or sudden death before 55 years of age in father or other male first-degree relative or before 65 years of age in mother or other female first-degree relative
Cigarette smoking	Current cigarette smoker or those who have quit within the previous 6 months
Hypertension	Systolic blood pressure ≥140 mm Hg or diastolic pressure ≥90 mm Hg (confirmed by measurements on at least two separate occasions), or on antihypertensive medication
Dyslipidemia	LDL-C >130 mg·dL^{-1} (3.4 mmol·L^{-1}) or HDL-C <40 mg·dL^{-1} (1.03 mmol·L^{-1}), or on lipid-lowering medication. If total serum cholesterol is all that is available, use >200 mg·dL^{-1} (5.2 mmol·L^{-1}) rather than LDL >130 mg·dL^{-1}
Impaired fasting glucose	Fasting blood glucose ≥100 mg·dL^{-1} (5.6 mmol·L^{-1}) confirmed by measurements on at least two separate occasions
Obesity	BMI >30 kg/m, waste girth >102 cm for men and >88 cm for women, or waste/hip ratio ≥0.95 for men and ≥0.86 for women
Sedentary lifestyle	Persons not participating in a regular exercise program or not meeting the minimal physical activity (≥30 min·day^{-1}) recommendations from the U.S. Surgeon General's Report
Negative Risk Factor	**Criteria**
High-serum HDL-C	≥60 mg·dL^{-1} (1.6 mmol·dL^{-1})

Notes: It is common to sum risk factors in making clinical judgments. If HDL is high, subtract one risk factor from the sum of positive risk factors because high HDL decreases CAD risk.

Adapted with permission from the American College of Sports Medicine. ACSM's Guidelines for Exercise Testing and Prescription, 7th ed. Philadelphia, PA: Lippincott Williams & Wilkins, 2006:22.

Medical Evaluation

It is generally accepted that many apparently healthy, sedentary people can begin a low- to moderate-intensity exercise program without an extensive medical evaluation.[2] Moreover, it has not been conclusively demonstrated that a medical evaluation reduces medical risks due to exercise. Therefore, recommendations have been developed to identify people who should have a medical evaluation before exercising.[2] People considered at moderate to high risk should undergo a medical evaluation before exercise. Two or more risk factors for CAD indicate moderate risk (Table 12-3), whereas one or more signs or symptoms of cardiovascular, pulmonary, or metabolic disease indicate high risk (Box 12-2). A very detailed description of medical evaluation procedures and tests has been published by the American College of Sports Medicine and should be consulted to determine who should undergo a complete medical evaluation before exercise and what tests should be included in the evaluation.[2]

Box 12-2 APPLYING RESEARCH

The Major Signs or Symptoms Suggestive of Cardiovascular, Pulmonary, or Metabolic Disease

- Pain or discomfort (or other anginal equivalent) in the chest, neck, arms, or other areas resulting from ischemia
- Shortness of breath at rest or with mild exertion
- Dizziness or syncope
- Orthopnea (breathlessness relieved by an upright sitting position) or paroxysmal nocturnal dyspnea
- Ankle edema
- Palpitations or tachycardia
- Intermittent claudication

- Known heart murmur
- Unusual fatigue or shortness of breath with usual activities

These signs or symptoms must be interpreted within the clinical context in which they appear because they are not all specific to cardiovascular, pulmonary, or metabolic disease.

Adapted with permission from American College of Sports Medicine. ACSM's Guidelines for Exercise Testing and Prescription, 7th ed. Philadelphia, PA: Lippincott Williams & Wilkins, 2006:24.

Electrocardiogram

An **electrocardiogram (ECG)**, which measures cardiac electrical conductivity, is used to determine cardiac rhythm or contraction and relaxation. Electrical conductivity is the movement of ions during contraction and relaxation of the cardiac tissue (Fig. 12-3). The normal ECG consists of atrial contraction (P wave), ventricular contraction (QRS complex), and ventricular relaxation (T wave). Relaxation of the atria takes place during ventricular contraction and so is not generally seen on an ECG. The combination of the height and length (area under the curve) of a wave indicates the total amount of ions moving and, so, the total amount of cardiac tissue contracting or relaxing. This is why the QRS complex, representing ventricular contraction (more muscle mass), is taller than the P wave, representing atrial contraction (less muscle mass). This is also the reason why if physical training results in ventricular hypertrophy (see Chapter 5), the QRS complex becomes taller. Horizontal distance of a wave or horizontal distance between two waves indicates time. In a normal ECG, it can be seen that it takes a shorter period of time for ventricular contraction than for ventricular relaxation (QRS complex is not as wide as the T wave). Horizontal distance between the end of the P wave and the beginning of the QRS complex indicates the time between the end of atrial contraction and the beginning of ventricular contraction. This timeframe is controlled by the

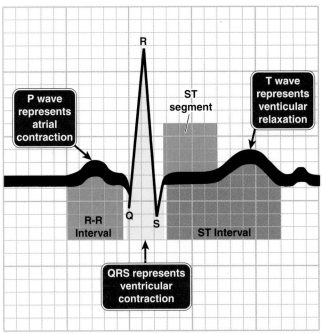

Figure 12-3. The waveforms in an ECG represent contraction and relaxation of the atria and ventricles. The combination of height and length (area under the curve) represent total ionic movement and so total amount of cardiac muscle contracting or relaxing. Horizontal length represents time. Some portions of the ECG are labeled using the letters representing the waveforms of atrial contraction, ventricular contraction, and ventricular relaxation. (Adapted from Nursing Procedures, 4th ed. Ambler: Lippincott Williams & Wilkins, 2004.)

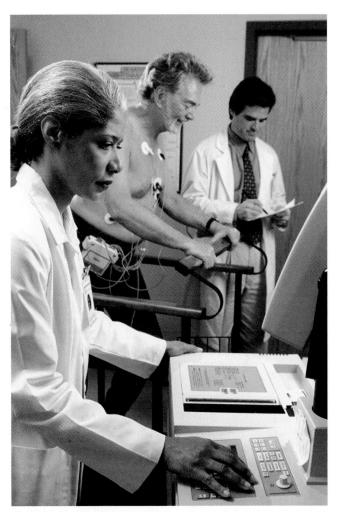

Figure 12-4. During a graded exercise test, an ECG is typically monitored. Abnormal responses in the ECG can represent presence of a disease.

atrioventricular (AV) node (see Chapter 5) and so indicates whether the AV node is holding the impulse for ventricular contraction shorter or longer than normal.

An ECG is a normal part of a graded exercise test, which is part of the medical evaluation before exercise (Fig. 12-4). During a graded exercise test, the speed and elevation of a motorized treadmill or the workload on a bicycle ergometer are gradually increased. During the test, the ECG and blood pressure are observed for abnormal responses to exercise.

Possible abnormalities in the ECG include cardiac arrhythmias (irregular heart rhythms) and ST-segment depression (Fig. 12-5). Many portions of the ECG are denoted by the letters representing the cardiac waveforms. So, the ST segment begins at the end of the QRS complex and ends at the start of the T wave. The ST segment is normally flat or horizontal. If the ST segment slopes down 1.0 mm or greater below the isoelectric line for 80 ms or longer, this indicates insufficient blood supply to the cardiac tissue or myocardial ischemia. In turn, myocardial ischemia indicates the presence of CAD.

Blood pressure will increase during any physical activity, including a graded exercise test. However, abnormal

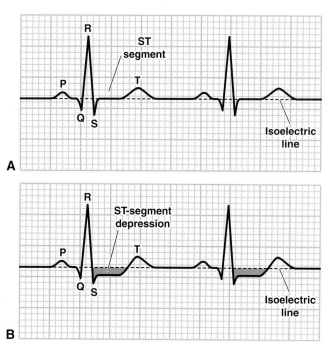

Figure 12-5. ST-segment depression indicates CAD. (A) In a normal ECG, the ST segment is flat. **(B)** ST-segment depression indicates myocardial ischemia due to the presence of CAD.

increases in systolic or diastolic blood pressure or both signal the presence of CAD. During a graded exercise test, medical personnel should talk to the person performing the test and look for other signs and symptoms during and after the test indicative of cardiovascular, pulmonary, or metabolic disease, such as shortness of breath, dizziness, angina (chest pain), or pain in the neck, jaw, or arms. Such signs and symptoms may result in termination of the exercise test.

Although an ECG can indicate CAD, the test is not 100% accurate. Exercise ECG results correctly identify about 66% of people with CAD, whereas approximately 34% who actually have CAD are diagnosed as free from disease.[20] These types of inaccuracies are the reasons why a graded exercise test is not recommended before beginning an exercise program until men are past the age of 45 years and women past the age of 55 years, except in cases where moderate or high risk for disease is present. It takes years for CAD to develop, and so it is much more likely after these ages.

Quick Review

- A medical evaluation before beginning an exercise program is recommended for men past the age of 45 years, women past the age of 55 years, and those with signs and symptoms of cardiovascular or other diseases.
- The ECG represents the electrical conductivity of cardiac tissue and can be used to determine cardiac rhythm as well as abnormal cardiac function.

AEROBIC TRAINING GUIDELINES

Aerobic fitness training guidelines have been developed to improve aerobic capabilities in people who have little or no history of performing endurance exercise. It should be noted that in improving aerobic fitness, health benefits—such as protection from cardiovascular disease, osteoporosis, and certain cancers—will also be accrued. However, the following guidelines are not appropriate for those individuals whose main interest is to increase their health status with only a minimal commitment to exercise training (such health focused programs should include 30 minutes a day—in a single session or additive over 3 sessions—of moderate intensity activity, e.g. brisk walking, on most, if not all days of the week). Nor are they applicable for competitive endurance athletes who already possess high levels of fitness. These guidelines may, however, be applicable to strength and power athletes, such as Olympic weightlifters and shot putters, who wish to maintain some level of aerobic fitness and reduce body fat, which can have a negative effect on performance (e.g., reduce speed, decrease vertical power production).

The aerobic training exercise prescription involves four basic components:

1. Type of exercise
2. Duration of each exercise session
3. Frequency of training
4. Intensity of exercise

The lower limit of the last three components defines a minimal threshold, or the lowest duration, frequency, and intensity of exercise that must be reached to bring about aerobic fitness gains. Even though a minimal threshold is given, there is substantial individual variation in that threshold necessary to bring about aerobic fitness gains. Thus, the minimal thresholds vary from person to person, meaning that although some people may increase their aerobic fitness by exercising less than what it suggested here, others will have to exceed the stated minimal threshold of exercise to improve their fitness. And as aerobic fitness improves, it is also likely that the prescribed minimal threshold will need to be exceeded to bring about continued aerobic fitness gains. As mentioned above, the guidelines for those who are interested only in gaining significant health benefits with a minimal investment in an exercise program are less robust. Specifically, a health related activity program should encompass 30 minutes of physical activity of moderate intensity (e.g., brisk walking) on most, if not all days of the week. The 30 minutes can be completed in a single session, or even accumulated over 3 brief sessions daily.

Type of Exercise

Different types of aerobic exercise bring about similar aerobic fitness gains with all types usually involving several large muscle groups.[47] Thus, the most frequently prescribed exercises are as follows:

- Jogging
- Running
- Cycling
- Spinning
- Elliptical machines
- Swimming
- Aerobic dance
- Rowing

The type of exercise selected should be enjoyable. If the person enjoys the exercise, he or she is more likely to continue to exercise for life. Continued exercise performance is important because no matter a person's age, cessation of exercise will result in loss of fitness gains. Another popular type, or mode, of exercise is **cross-training**, or the inclusion of several types of aerobic exercise in the training program. Cross-training may be useful to maintain exercise motivation and to minimize the chance of an overuse injury. Additionally, due to seasonal climate changes, weather conditions, and travel time to a gym, performing several types of activity may make it easier to comply with an exercise program.

Duration of Each Exercise Session

Similar aerobic fitness gains are achieved with short-duration, high-intensity exercise and long-duration, low-intensity exercise sessions, as long as the minimal thresholds for both frequency and intensity of training are met. Thus, multiple short exercise sessions, such as three 10-minute exercise bouts, or one long exercise bout, such as a 30-minute exercise bout, will result in similar fitness gains. However, longer sessions of moderate intensity are typically recommended for most adults because high-intensity exercise is associated with greater cardiovascular risk, greater chance of orthopedic injury, and lower adherence to training than moderate-intensity exercise.[47] Thus, the minimal duration threshold is 20 to 30 minutes per session.

Frequency of Training

The minimal threshold for frequency is 3 days·week^{-1}.[47] The majority of increases in peak oxygen consumption occur with a frequency of 3 days·week^{-1}, with increasing frequency up to 5 days·week^{-1} bringing about increased aerobic capabilities. However, the additional time spent training to achieve a slightly greater increase in peak oxygen consumption relative to a frequency of 3 days·week^{-1} may not be important to some people. If a major training goal is to decrease body fat, then additional training sessions to increase caloric expenditure may be beneficial. Although endurance athletes may train more than 5 days·week^{-1} to gain additional small increases in aerobic fitness, training frequencies greater than 5 days·week^{-1} do increase the incidence of injury.[47]

Intensity of Exercise

The intensity or stressfulness of exercise is the most important training variable to bring about increased aerobic fitness. The minimal intensity threshold is 55% to 65% of maximal heart rate (HR_{max}).[47] This range is based on individual variability in the exercise intensity necessary to bring about aerobic fitness gains. Those with low aerobic fitness will achieve fitness improvements by training at the lower end of this range. Competitive athletes will need to train at higher intensities than will people interested only in health and fitness gains. The upper end of the range of training intensity for health and fitness gains is approximately 94% of HR_{max}.[2] However, for most people, intensities between 77% and 90% HR_{max} are sufficient to bring about near-optimal gains in aerobic fitness.[2]

Exercise Heart Rate

Exercise or training heart rate (HR) is widely used to determine intensity. HR has a linear relationship with increasing workload and oxygen consumption, with HR plateauing at maximal oxygen consumption (see Chapter 5). Because of these relationships, HR, as measured by a HR monitor, can be used to determine exercise intensity.

To calculate the intensity range needed to increase aerobic fitness using a percentage of HR_{max}, one must first know his or her HR_{max}. A common equation used to estimate HR_{max} is as follows:

$$HR_{max} = 220 - \text{age in years} \qquad (1)$$

This equation indicates that HR_{max} decreases by approximately 5% to 7% per decade. However, HR_{max} actually decreases by approximately 3% to 5% per decade. Thus, this equation results in error when estimating HR_{max}.[25] Although this equation does give a viable estimate of HR_{max}, the following equation results in a more accurate estimate of HR_{max}:

$$HR_{max} = 207 - (0.7 \times \text{age in years}) \qquad (2)$$

Using this second equation to estimate HR_{max} results in the following HR range needed to achieve aerobic fitness benefits for most 20-year-olds:

$$HR_{max} = 207 - (0.7 \times 20 \text{ years})$$
$$HR_{max} = 193 \text{ beats per minute (bpm)}$$
$$77\% \text{ of } HR_{max} = 193 \text{ bpm} \times 0.77$$
$$77\% \text{ of } HR_{max} = 148.6 \text{ bpm}$$
$$90\% \text{ of } HR_{max} = 193 \text{ bpm} \times 0.90$$
$$90\% \text{ of } HR_{max} = 173.7 \text{ bpm} \qquad (3)$$

So, for most 20-year-olds, performing aerobic exercise at a HR between 149 and 174 bpm would result in aerobic fitness gains. HR does have a good relationship to oxygen consumption. However, when exercising at a specific percentage of HR_{max}, you are actually exercising at a substantially lower percentage of peak oxygen consumption (Fig. 12-6). The HR reserve (HRR) method of determining exercise intensity described in the next section estimates the HR at a specific percentage of peak oxygen consumption,

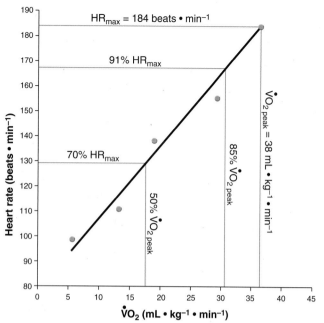

Figure 12-6. A specific percentage of HR$_{max}$ represents a lower percentage of peak oxygen consumption. In the figure, 91% and 70% of HR$_{max}$ are equivalent to 85% and 50% of peak oxygen consumption (V̇O$_{2peak}$), respectively. (Adapted with permission from American College of Sports Medicine. ACSM's Guidelines for Exercise Testing and Prescription, 8th ed. Baltimore: Lippincott Williams & Wilkins, 2010:159.)

which results in a different training HR than training at a specific percentage of HR$_{max}$ (Box 12-3).

HRR Method

The HRR method, or Karvonen method, can be used to estimate the HR needed to exercise at a specific percentage of peak oxygen consumption. To elicit aerobic fitness gains, most people need to train from 40% to 50% up to 85% of peak oxygen consumption, although significant individual differences exist. HRR method refers to the difference

between resting HR (HR$_{rest}$) and HR$_{max}$. Target HR (THR) refers to the HR needed to be exercising at a specific percentage of peak oxygen consumption. The following equations can be used to estimate the THR at any percentage of peak oxygen consumption. The example given estimates the THR needed to be exercising at 70% of peak oxygen consumption.

$$HRR = HR_{max} - HR_{rest}$$

$$HRR = 190 \text{ bpm} - 75 \text{ bpm}$$

$$HRR = 115 \text{ bpm}$$

THR at 70% of peak oxygen consumption = HR$_{rest}$ + 0.70 (HRR)

THR at 70% of peak oxygen consumption = 75 bpm + 0.70 (115 bpm)

THR at 70% of peak oxygen consumption = 155.5 bpm   (4)

This calculation estimates that a THR of approximately 155 bpm would result in exercising at 70% of peak oxygen consumption. To estimate the THR for any other percentage of peak oxygen consumption, merely substitute the desired percentage into the equation. Whether using a percentage of HR$_{max}$ or the HRR method to determine exercise intensity, as a person gains aerobic fitness, he or she will be able to perform (jog, run, or cycle faster) more work at any given HR. This is in part because as aerobic condition improves, HR at any given workload decreases and HR at rest may also decrease slightly. Thus, using HR as an estimate of intensity allows for improvement in aerobic ability with training. Similar calculations can be used to calculate training intensity using peak oxygen consumption reserve (Box 12-4).

Perceived Exertion

Rating of perceived exertion (RPE) involves subjectively rating how hard one is working. The classical Borg RPE

Box 12-3 PRACTICAL QUESTIONS FROM STUDENTS

Is There Really a Difference Between Prescribing Aerobic Exercise Intensity Using HR$_{max}$ or Percentage of Peak Oxygen Consumption?

Both ways of prescribing aerobic exercise intensity can be used. However, it is important to understand there is a difference between the two methods. For example, a 20-year-old using the formula HR$_{max}$ = 207 − (0.7 × age in years) has an HR$_{max}$ of approximately 193 bpm. If the desired training intensity is 60% of HR$_{max}$, this would result in a training HR of 116 bpm (193 bpm × 0.6). If the HRR method is used to determine a 60% of peak oxygen consumption training HR for this individual with an HR$_{rest}$ of

70 bpm, a substantially different HR is obtained. The HRR would be 123 bpm (HRR = 193 bpm − 70 bpm). The training HR at 60% of peak oxygen consumption would be 144 bpm (THR 60% of peak oxygen consumption = 70 bpm + [123 bpm × 0.6]). So, the training HR at 60% of peak oxygen consumption and 60% of HR$_{max}$ are 144 and 116 bpm, respectively. This is a substantial difference, even though both would fall within the prescribed training zone to increase aerobic fitness.

Box 12-4 PRACTICAL QUESTIONS FROM STUDENTS

Can the Percentage of Peak Oxygen Consumption Be Used to Prescribe Aerobic Training?

If a person's peak oxygen consumption has been determined, such as during a treadmill or cycling oxygen consumption test, it can be used to prescribe training intensity. Recall that the HRR, or the Karvonen method, uses a calculation to prescribe a training intensity equivalent to a specific percentage of peak oxygen consumption. Determining exercise intensity using oxygen consumption involves a similar calculation. The training guidelines for exercise intensity are the same as those for the HRR method: training should occur from the minimum threshold, 40% to 50%, up to 85% of oxygen uptake reserve ($\dot{V}O_2R$) or $\dot{V}O_{2max} - \dot{V}O_{2rest}$. Calculating a target $\dot{V}O_2$ using $\dot{V}O_2R$ is done using the following equation:

$$\text{Target } \dot{V}O_2 \ (\text{mL·kg}^{-1}\text{·min}^{-1}) = (\dot{V}O_{2max} - \dot{V}O_{2rest}) \text{ (exercise intensity)} + \dot{V}O_{2rest}$$

$\dot{V}O_{2rest}$ is generally assumed to be 3.5 mL·kg^{-1}·min^{-1} (1 MET). If a person's measured peak oxygen consumption is 50 mL·kg^{-1}·min^{-1}, the training zone between 50% and 85% of peak oxygen consumption can be estimated with the following calculations:

50% Target $\dot{V}O_2$ (mL·kg^{-1}·min^{-1}) = (50 mL·kg^{-1}·min^{-1} − 3.5 mL·kg^{-1}·min^{-1}) (0.50) + 3.5 mL·kg^{-1}·min^{-1}

50% Target $\dot{V}O_2$ (mL·kg^{-1}·min^{-1}) = 26.7 mL·kg^{-1}·min^{-1}

85% Target $\dot{V}O_2$ (mL·kg^{-1}·min^{-1}) = (50 mL·kg^{-1}·min^{-1} − 3.5 mL·kg^{-1}·min^{-1}) (0.85) + 3.5 mL·kg^{-1}·min^{-1}

85% Target $\dot{V}O_2$ (mL·kg^{-1}·min^{-1}) = 43.0 mL·kg^{-1}·min^{-1}

To stay within the recommended training zone, this person would need to perform training between 26.7 and 43 mL·kg^{-1}·min^{-1}. Typically, during a test to determine peak oxygen consumption, workload, such as running pace, is gradually increased while oxygen consumption and HR are constantly monitored. Using the information from the peak oxygen consumption test, it is easy to determine the running pace necessary to consume oxygen within the recommended zone for aerobic training. It is also easy to determine the HR necessary to consume oxygen within the recommended training zone. One limitation of this and other methods is that other factors, such as the environment and type of terrain, can affect oxygen consumption.

Table 12-4.   MET Values of Selected Activities

Activity	MET	Activity	MET
Home activities			
Sitting on a couch	1.0	Dressing and undressing	2.0
Eating	1.0	Washing hands and face	2.0
Talking	1.0	Washing dishes	2.3
Standing quietly	1.2	Putting away groceries	2.5
Making bed	2.0	Scrubbing floors	3.8
Working			
Sitting at desk	1.5	Orange grove work	4.5
Typing	2.0	Loading and unloading a truck	6.5
Farming, driving tractor	2.5	Shoveling 4.5–6.8 kg	7.0
General carpentry	3.5	Fire fighter hauling hoses on ground	8.0
Electrical, plumbing work	3.5	Digging ditches	8.5
Sports and recreation			
Golf, using a cart	3.5	Running 5 mph	8.0
Hacky sack	4.0	Volleyball, competitive	8.0
Aerobic dancing, low impact	5.0	Rowing 150 W	8.5
Boxing, punching bag	6.0	Inline skating	12.5
Broomball	7.0	Running 10.9 mph	18.0

Data from: Ainsworth BE, Haskell WL, Whitt MC, et al. Compendium of physical activities: an update of activity codes and met intensities. Med Sci Sports Exerc. 2000;32:S498–S516.

RPE Scale	% $\dot{V}O_{2\,peak}$	% Maximal Heart Rate	% $\dot{V}O_{2\,peak}$ or Heart Rate Reserve
6	Rest		
7 Very, Very Light			
8			
9 Very light		<35%	<20%
10		35%–54%	20%–39%
11 Fairly light	31%–50%		
12	51%–75%	55%–69%	40%–59%
13 Somewhat Hard			
14	76%–85%		
15 Hard		70%–89%	60%–84%
16	>85%		
17 Very Hard			
18		>90%	>85%
19 Very, Very Hard			
20	100%	100%	100%

Figure 12-7. The Borg scale can be used to estimate aerobic exercise intensity. Different RPEs correlate to different percentages of peak oxygen consumption ($\dot{V}O_{2peak}$), HR_{max}, $\dot{V}O_{2peak}$ reserve, and HRR. (Modified with permission from Borg GA. Psychological basis of physical exertion. Med Sci Sports Exerc. 1982;14:377–381 and Pollock ML, Gaesser GA, Butcher JD, et al. The recommended quantity and quality of exercise for developing and maintaining cardiorespiratory and muscular fitness, and flexibility in healthy adults. Med Sci Sports Exerc. 1998;30:975–991.)

scale (Fig. 12-7) begins at 6, with the first descriptive anchor at 7 ("very, very light"), and progresses to 20, with the last descriptive anchor at 19 ("very, very hard").[45] The average RPE associated with aerobic adaptations to exercise is 12 to 16.[2] The same RPE may not consistently indicate the same intensity during an exercise session or the same intensity for different types of exercise.[2] However, generally a specific RPE does represent percentages of peak oxygen consumption, HR_{max}, peak oxygen consumption reserve, and HRR. Thus, the scale can be used to estimate the workload needed to achieve aerobic fitness gains.

Metabolic Equivalents

One **MET**—or metabolically equivalent task—is equal to the rate of oxygen consumption at rest. With the MET

system, intensity of an activity is expressed as how many times greater than resting oxygen consumption is required to perform the activity. If an activity is equivalent to 3 METS, to perform the activity requires three times resting oxygen consumption. Resting oxygen consumption is typically assumed to be 3.5 mL·kg^{-1}·min^{-1}, so an activity equivalent to 3 METs requires 10.5 mL·kg^{-1}·min^{-1} (3 METs × 3.5 mL·kg^{-1}·min^{-1}) of oxygen to be performed. The greater the METs, the more intense the activity. Moderate-intensity activity is generally defined as 3 to 6 METs, whereas vigorous activity is greater than 6 METs (Table 12-4).

Use of METs to determine intensity does have limitations.[2] The use of the standard 3.5 mL·kg^{-1}·min^{-1} equals 1 MET introduces error because resting oxygen consumption varies between 1.6 and 4.1 mL·kg^{-1}·min^{-1}. The MET value of activity can vary substantially depending on the skill of the person performing the activity. The MET value of activity can also vary substantially depending on the environmental conditions, altitude, and hydration status. If METs are used to determine intensity of activity, the estimate should be viewed as a guideline and not an absolute value.

Talk Test

The talk test is a simple and convenient method to determine the minimum intensity level to bring about aerobic fitness gains. It is based on the idea that the lower end of the intensity range necessary to bring about fitness gains is marked by the ability to still hold a normal conversation while exercising.[22] This test is typically used as an intensity guideline for people just beginning an aerobic fitness program or who wish to train predominantly at the minimum intensity necessary.

Progression of Aerobic Fitness Training

Progression, or increasing the difficulty, of aerobic training is necessary if continued gains in fitness are desired. If a person has achieved an aerobic fitness level sufficient to meet his or her daily life, recreation, or sport needs, the difficulty of aerobic training need not be increased and a plateau in aerobic fitness will occur.

All the aerobic fitness guidelines do allow for a progression in training. The type of exercise can be progressed from low impact, such as walking, cycling, or elliptical training, to higher impact, such as jogging or running, if desired. This type of progression may be especially appropriate for people just beginning a training program or for those who are overweight. Training duration can be progressed from the minimal threshold of 20 to 30 min·day^{-1} to longer time periods. Normally, the upper limit for aerobic fitness is 60 min·day^{-1}. Duration can also be progressed by initially performing shorter (three 10-minute bouts per day) but more frequent training, totaling 20 to 30 min·day^{-1}, and gradually decreasing the number of training bouts per day and increasing the length of each training bout (two 15-minute bouts or one 30-minute bout per day). Intensity can be progressed from the minimum threshold value (55% HR$_{max}$) up to the upper end of intensity guidelines (90% HR$_{max}$). As training progresses, each training session or week of training need not be more difficult than the previous session or week. Having training sessions or weeks of training that are less difficult than previous sessions or weeks can be used to allow for recovery and decrease the chance of injury. During short periods of less difficult training, aerobic fitness gains will be maintained and detraining, or loss of fitness gains, will be minimal or nonexistent (see the following section on detraining). However, it is important to have some type of progress if increased fitness is desired.

RESISTANCE TRAINING GUIDELINES

As with aerobic training, guidelines have also been developed for resistance or weight training. Guidelines have been developed for novice trainers or people with little or no resistance training experience, intermediate trainers or individuals with some training experience, and advanced trainers, who have a long history of resistance training experience.[1,3] These guidelines are meant to bring about both health and fitness benefits.

Similar to that for aerobic training, resistance training exercise prescription involves several basic components:

1. Type of exercise
2. Volume of an exercise session
3. Rest period length between sets and exercises
4. Frequency of training
5. Intensity of exercise

Resistance training programs can emphasize one major physiological adaptation, such as increased maximal strength, over other adaptations, such as muscle hypertrophy.[3] Although such emphasis may not be necessary for the novice resistance trainer, more advanced trainers may desire it.

Similar to aerobic training guidelines, individual response to a resistance training program can vary substantially. Thus, the guidelines contain considerable ranges in the exercise prescription and should be viewed as a starting point from which to develop individualized training programs.

Type of Exercise

Different types of resistance training exercise equipment can bring about increases in maximal strength and muscle hypertrophy. The most frequently prescribed types of resistance training exercises can be performed with:

1. Free weights or barbells and dumbbells
2. Resistance training machines

There are, however, many other types of resistance training exercises, such as rubber cord and body weight exercises, that can increase strength and hypertrophy.[1,19] General health and fitness programs typically include at least one exercise for each major muscle group of the body. **Multi–muscle group,** or multi-joint exercises, involve movement at more than one joint and force development by more than one muscle group, such as a bench press or leg press. **Single–muscle group,** or single-joint exercises, predominantly involve movement at one joint and force development by one muscle group, such as arm curls or leg extensions. Multi–muscle group or multi-joint exercises are also referred to as major or core exercises, whereas single–muscle group or single-joint exercises are referred to as assistance exercises. The goals of most training programs can be met using an exercise order in which the multi-joint exercises are performed before the single-joint exercises.

Volume of an Exercise Session

Resistance training volume is a measure of the total amount of work performed and is determined by the number of exercises performed, number of sets of each exercise (see Box 12-5), and number of repetitions per set. Changes in training volume as well as other training variables can be used to emphasize maximal strength, hypertrophy, power, or local muscular endurance (Table 12-5). The novice resistance trainer typically begins by performing one set of each exercise and then progresses to multiple sets of each exercise as training experience increases. The number of repetitions per set varies depending on the adaptation being emphasized and training experience. Typically, higher numbers of repetitions are used to emphasize local muscular endurance, whereas lower numbers of repetitions are used when emphasizing maximal power and strength, especially as training experience increases. Also, as experience increases, so does the repetition range used to emphasize a training outcome. This allows greater variation in training as experience increases, which appears to be important to bring about continued fitness gains in those with greater training experience.[3]

Rest Period Length Between Sets and Exercises

The longer the rest period between sets and exercises, the greater the opportunity for physiological recovery of the anaerobic energy stores (intramuscular adenosine triphosphate [ATP] and phosphocreatine, or PC) and the more time available to decrease blood and muscle acidity (see Chapter 3). Short rest periods allow little time for

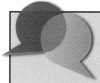

Box 12-5   EXPERT VIEW
The Dose–Response for Strength Development

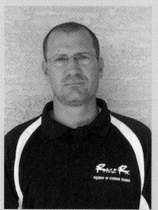

Matthew Rhea, PhD
Director of Research and Development,
RACE Rx Academy of Exercise Sciences

For decades, arguments persisted between exercise professionals and researchers regarding the appropriate prescription of resistance training for achieving maximal strength gains. The focal point of this debate has centered on the number of sets per workout needed to develop maximal strength (single set vs. multiple sets). Resolving this debate, by identifying research-based guidelines for prescribing resistance exercise, is of critical importance. One challenge in drawing conclusions from a body of research is accurately identifying what the whole of the research supports. While each individual study is important, its greatest value is only exhibited when it is properly combined with all other studies examining resistance training for strength improvements. Many researchers and professionals have read some, or even all, of the existing literature and drawn their own conclusions regarding what the body of research concerning the optimal number of sets supports. Unfortunately, this has not ended the debate because individuals on both sides of the argument claim that the body of research supports their views. What is needed is a procedure for quantitatively combining related studies utilizing statistical procedures to combine and evaluate the data in each study rather than an opinion based on a qualitative review of the literature. Such a procedure, the meta-analysis, exists, and several such analyses have been conducted, shedding significant light on the matter.

A number of meta-analyses have been published in recent years.[1-4] These analyses individually, and collectively, demonstrate that multiple-set training programs elicit greater strength improvements than single-set training. Based on the meta-analyses completed by me and a group of colleagues,[1-3] four sets per muscle group, per workout, result in maximum strength gains among untrained and trained populations, while athletes (more highly trained) saw the greatest benefits with six sets of training. In untrained and trained exercisers, single-set training did result in some strength improvement, but this improvement was only a fraction of the maximal gains achieved with multiple sets.

These data support the principle of progression. For beginners, single-set training may be appropriate at the initial stages of development. Over time, volume of training must increase to continue to overload the neuromuscular system. For those accustomed to training, a higher level of training volume is needed to elicit maximal gains. However, if an experienced exerciser does not need or desire maximum strength gains, or time limitations prevent them from being able to perform high-volume training, one or two sets per muscle group is sufficient to maintain or even improve strength, whereas athletes, or those seeking maximal strength improvements for performance enhancement, must follow a higher volume training program to achieve this goal.

Though the volume of training is an important variable, other factors, such as intensity and frequency, should also be considered. These other training variables were also examined in our meta-analyses and were found to exhibit a dose–response relationship. For untrained exercisers, maximal strength gains were achieved when the average training intensity was set at 65% of 1-RM, while trained populations and athletes achieved maximum strength at 85% or higher of 1-RM. Untrained populations benefit from three light training sessions per week, whereas trained populations respond best to two heavy workouts per week.

The significance of these analyses is found in the details that they provide the exercise professional with regards to appropriate exercise prescription. The goal of the trainer should be to help their clients to achieve a desired goal by applying the necessary stimulus. Too little stimulus and the client will fail to achieve the goal. Too much stimulus can result in overtraining and/or overstress injury. While more research may be needed to further clarify the optimal dose of training, these analyses have at least helped to point us in the right direction and resolve decades of debate regarding the difference in strength gains following single- versus multiple-set training.

References

1. Peterson MD, Rhea MR, Alvar BA. Maximizing strength development in athletes: a meta-analysis to determine the dose–response relationship. J Strength Cond Res. 2004;18:377–382.
2. Rhea M, Alvar BA, Burkett LN. Single versus multiple sets for strength: a meta-analysis to address the controversy. Res Q Exerc Sport. 2002;73:485–488.
3. Rhea M, Alvar BA, Burkett LN, et al. A meta-analysis to determine the dose–response relationship for strength development: volume, intensity, and frequency of training. Med Sci Sport Exerc. 2003;35:456–464.
4. Wolfe BL, LeMura LM, Cole PJ. Quantitative analysis of single- vs. multiple-set programs in resistance training. J Strength Cond Res. 2004;18:35–47.

physiological recovery and therefore result in greater fatigue levels as the training session progresses. Additionally, short rest periods result in acute hormonal responses, such as increased serum growth hormone, that may be important for long-term muscle hypertrophy. Longer rest periods are typically used when emphasizing maximal strength and maximal power, especially when performing multi-

joint exercises. Short rest periods are typically used when emphasizing local muscular endurance and hypertrophy.

Frequency of Training

In resistance training, frequency refers to the number of times per week a particular exercise is performed or muscle group is trained. With a **total body resistance training**

Table 12-5. Resistance Training Guidelines

Frequency per Week	Number of Sets per Exercise	Number of Repetitions per Set	Intensity Percentage of 1-RM	Rest Between Sets
Emphasize Maximal Strength				
Novice trainer				
2–3 total body sessions	1–3	8–12	60%–70%	2–3 min major exercises 1–2 min assistance exercises
Intermediate trainer				
3 total body sessions and 4 split routines	Multiple	8–12	60%–70%	2–3 min major exercises 1–2 min assistance exercises
Advanced trainer				
4–6 split routines	Multiple	1–12	Up to 80%–100% in a periodized manner	2–3 min major exercises 1–2 min assistance exercises
Emphasize Hypertrophy				
Novice trainer				
2–3 total body sessions	1–3	8–12	70%–85%	1–2 min
Intermediate trainer				
3 total body sessions and 4 split routines	1–3	8–12	70%–85%	1–2 min
Advanced trainer				
4–6 split routines	3–6	1–12 (mostly 6–12)	70%–100% in a periodized manner	2–3 min major exercises 1–2 min assistance exercises
Emphasize Power				
Novice trainer				
2–3 total body sessions	Maximal strength training + 1–3 power-type exercises	3–6 (not to failure)	Upper body: 30%–60% Lower body: 0%–60%	2–3 min for major exercises with high intensity 1–2 min assistance and major exercises with low intensity
Intermediate trainer				
3–4 total body or split routines	Novice + progression to 3–6 power-type exercises	Novice + progression to 1–6	Novice + progression to 85%–100%	2–3 min for major exercises with high intensity 1–2 min assistance and major exercises with low intensity
Advanced trainer				
4–5 total body or split routines	novice + progression to 3–6 power-type exercises	Novice + progression to 1–6	Novice + progression to 85%–100%	2–3 min for major exercises with high intensity 1–2 min assistance and major exercises with low intensity
Emphasize Local Muscular Endurance				
Novice trainer				
2–3 total body sessions	Multiple	10–15	Low	1 min or less
Intermediate trainer				
3 total body sessions and 4 split routines	Multiple	10–15	Low	1 min or less
Advanced trainer				
4–6 split routines	Multiple	10–25	Various percentages	1 min or less 10–15 reps 1–2 min 15–25 reps

Adapted from Ratamess NA, Alvar BA, Evetoch TK, et al. Progression models in resistance training for healthy adults. Med Sci Sports Exer. 2009;42:687–708.

program, all major muscle groups are trained during each training session. With a **split routine**, the body is divided into different areas, with each area being trained with a separate resistance training session. For example, in an upper and lower body split, the upper body and lower body are trained with two different training sessions. In a body part program, a particular body part, such as the legs or upper back, is trained with a different training session. Note that with a split or body part routine, a particular muscle group is trained with a lower frequency than the total number of training sessions. Typically, with split or body part routines, more exercises for a particular muscle group are performed per training session, resulting in a greater training volume for a particular muscle group per training session than with a total body program. Normally, as training experience increases, the total number of training sessions per week increases. However, the increase in training frequency per muscle group is less than that indicated by the increased total number of training sessions per week.

Intensity of Exercise

Resistance training exercise intensity is represented by a percentage of the maximal weight possible for one complete repetition of an exercise or one-repetition maximum (1-RM). The higher the percentage of 1-RM, the fewer the number of repetitions possible in a set.

Another consideration when performing a set is whether the set is performed to the point at which no more repetitions are possible, also known as momentary failure or failure. Failure typically occurs in the concentric portion of the repetition. Fitness gains have occurred both when performing sets to failure and when sets are not performed to failure.[3] Training to failure in advanced lifters may be appropriate when attempting to break through a training plateau,[62] yet care must be taken as training to failure has been shown to promote overtraining and increase joint stresses.[32] In any case, normally, sets are performed at least to a point close to failure (one or two repetitions more would be possible in a set).

Resistance training intensity varies depending on the physiological adaptation being emphasized, and training guidelines allow for this. The training intensity and volume are related. To perform higher training volumes, one must lower training intensities. This interrelationship is key when emphasizing different training outcomes, such as maximal strength, hypertrophy, power, and local muscular endurance.

Progression of Resistance Training

Training progression requires systematically increasing the demands placed on the body and is necessary to bring about continued fitness gains, especially as training experience increases. Training progression typically includes one or more of the following, in gradual increments: increasing training intensity, increasing training volume, or shorten-

ing and lengthening rest periods to emphasize local muscular endurance and hypertrophy or maximal strength and power, respectively. The most common way of progressing training is to increase training intensity by increasing the resistance used for a specified number of repetitions as strength, local muscular endurance, or power capabilities increase. Long-term training progression is discussed in a following section and is necessary for both resistance and aerobic training if continued fitness gains are to be achieved (Box 12-6).

INTERVAL TRAINING

Interval training was used by sprint and endurance athletes to improve performance beginning as early as the 1930s. More recently, ball game (basketball, volleyball, and soccer) and other types of athletes have also used interval training. The concept of interval training that is a greater amount of intense training can be performed if the training is interspaced with rest periods, with the greater amount of intense training resulting in greater fitness gains. This concept is supported by research. Moderately trained men (pretraining mean peak oxygen consumption 55–60 mL·kg^{-1}·min^{-1}) who performed long slow distance running at 70% of HR_{max} for 45 minutes or running at 85% of HR_{max} for 24 minutes showed no significant increase in peak oxygen consumption.[27] But performing 47 repetitions of 15-second intervals at 90% to 95% HR_{max} with 15-second rest periods between intervals or four intervals at 90% to 95% HR_{max} of 4 minutes separated by 3-minute rest periods significantly increased peak oxygen consumption by 5.5% and 7.2%, respectively. The interval groups also showed a significant increase in left ventricular stroke volume, while the other two groups showed

Box 12-6 AN EXPERT VIEW
Working as a Strength Coach in the National Football League

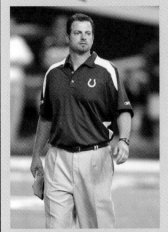

Jon Torine
Head Strength and Conditioning Coach
National Football League—
Indianapolis Colts

I have been a Strength and Conditioning Coach in the National Football League for 16 years. It is a job that encompasses a vast array of duties and responsibilities. I have always believed that it is a privilege to work with the players, and with that comes an enormous set of obligations to the organization, the team as a whole, and the individuals with whom you work with on a day-to-day basis.

The multipronged approach to this philosophy is to improve durability, increase performance, and take the players' genetic gifts to the appropriate maximal attainable level. This is first accomplished with baseline findings such as movement screening, mobility, stability, strength, power, change of direction, anaerobic endurance, and body composition testing. Baseline findings allow us to establish a direction and purpose in our training with the individual. We then strive to achieve gains and have a working knowledge, both practically and scientifically, in the areas of corrective exercise, mobility and stability training, neuromuscular training, strength training, power training, anaerobic endurance training, position-specific conditioning, game-specific conditioning, speed, start, acceleration, deceleration and change of direction training, plyometrics, and nutrition. The end goal in mind is to support what is needed for the game. There is no other goal or agenda. We are not training bodybuilders, power lifters, or Pilates instructors. Those are examples of different sports requiring different physical characteristics. We are training to be able to compete at the highest level in the National Football League.

It seems most people in the sports and exercise arena have some comprehension of what a strength and conditioning coach is asked to do. However, there are several other areas in which we support and work with the organization. During the season, we are involved in the weekly medical meetings to discuss players in terms of injury status, rehabilitation, conditioning, and date of return. We closely work with our medical staff, athletic trainers, and physical therapists in return to play criteria and readiness. Nutrition plays a major role; we plan meals and work closely with our in-house chef on daily meals and supplementation. We plan the pregame meals and snacks at both our home and road hotels as well as with the airline on departure and return flights. All drinks and supplementation in the locker room during the week and during games is approved by the strength and conditioning and medical staffs. During training camp, we work closely with the food service people in the menu planning as well.

Player recovery and rest is another area that we are involved in. This can be simple things such as stretching and aquatic recovery programs or as complex as circadian rhythm and planning of sleep and wake cycles as they pertain to our daily schedule as well as night game and afternoon game times.

Another role we participate in is helping the personnel staff with player physical evaluations from the combine or other workouts. This can include evaluating flexibility, body composition, or even potential injury risk. Individual goal planning for our players is done with the entire coaching staff, personnel staff, and medical staff so that each player can achieve maximum efficiency. Finally, the ability to handle budgeting, payroll, writing, computer proficiency, communication, and studying all play a vital role in this profession.

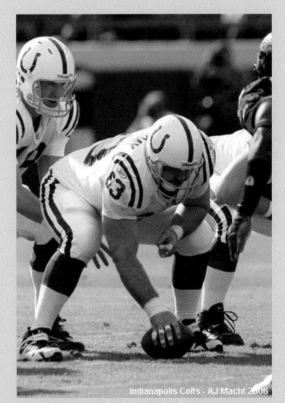

(Photos by AJ Macht, 2006. Courtesy of the Indianapolis Colts.)

Table 12-6.   Typical General Fitness Interval Training Sessions

Session	Beginner	Intermediate	Advanced
High intensity	5-min warm-up 5×1-min at 70%–75% HR_{max} 2-min rest period at 50%–60% HR_{max} 5-min cool-down	5-min warm-up 5×2-min at 75%–85% HR_{max} 3-min rest period at 55%–65% HR_{max} 5-min cool-down	10-min warm-up 5×2-min at 85%–90% HR_{max} 3-min rest period at 60%–65% HR_{max} 10-min cool-down
Low intensity	5-min warm-up 3×5-min at 60%–65% HR_{max} 5-min walk rest periods 5-min cool-down	5-min warm-up 2×10-min at 65%–70% HR_{max} 5-min walk rest periods 5-min cool-down	5-min warm-up 5×5-min at 75%–80% HR_{max} 3-min rest periods at 60%–70% HR_{max} 10-min cool-down

no significant change. All groups trained 3 days·week^{-1} for 8 weeks. It is also important to note that the total amount of work performed during each type of training was equated.

Although historically athletes have predominantly used interval training, it is also gaining popularity for fitness enthusiasts. Although interval training programs can be developed for swimming, running, elliptical training, and rowing, running programs seem to be the most popular for general fitness. Typical general fitness interval training sessions are presented in Table 12-6. Training variables that can be manipulated during interval training include distance or duration of the interval, training intensity, duration and type of rest periods between intervals, number of interval repetitions performed per set of intervals, and frequency of training. These training variables affect each other. For example, an athlete wishing to improve sprint ability might perform short-duration, high-intensity intervals interspaced with relatively long rest periods. However, as shown by the study referenced earlier, if short-duration, high-intensity intervals interspaced with relatively short rest periods are performed, peak oxygen consumption can also be improved. Thus, the interval training prescription is dependent upon the training goals.

Training Intensity

Training intensity of an interval is normally defined as either a percentage of the best time for the length of the interval or a percentage of HR_{max}. For shorter distances, it is more practical to define intensity as a percentage of the best time for the length of the interval or a specific time in which to perform the interval, for example, running 200 m in 30 seconds. To train maximal sprint ability or the ATP–phosphocreatine (PCr) energy source, typically high-intensity training is performed (e.g., 90%–100% of the best time or of HR_{max}). To develop the anaerobic glycolytic system or intermediate sprint distances, such as running 400 m, high intensities are also typically used (e.g., 80%–95% of the best time or 85%–100% of HR_{max}), whereas when training to develop aerobic or endurance capabilities, moderate-to-high intensities are utilized (75%–85% of the best time or 70%–90% of HR_{max}). These intensities are meant to be guidelines

and need to be adjusted to the fitness level of the trainee. Training intensity is also dependent upon the duration of the interval and the number of intervals to be performed.

Interval Duration

Typically short-duration (5–10 seconds) intervals are used to train short-term sprint ability, or the ATP–PCr energy source.[33] Longer duration intervals of 30 seconds to 2 minutes are used to train the anaerobic glycolytic system or intermediate sprint ability, and intervals greater than 2 minutes are used to train aerobic or endurance capabilities. However, the length of the interval is also dependent upon the goal of a training session. For example, a basketball player might utilize short intervals of 30 m to increase sprint speed while 150- to 200-m intervals may be utilized to improve local muscular endurance or the capabilities of the anaerobic glycolytic system.

Number of Intervals

The total number of intervals performed is dependent upon the number of intervals performed in a set, or repetitions per set, and the number of sets performed. It is also important to note that the duration of intervals may be varied during different sets of an interval training program. For example, a sprint athlete might perform one set of six repetitions of 100 m in length followed by one set of three repetitions of 200 m, whereas someone training for fitness might perform one set of five repetitions of 1-minute intervals running on a treadmill followed by one set of three repetitions 2 minutes in length. The total number of intervals per set and number of sets is dependent upon the training goals and fitness level of an individual.

For general fitness training, a beginning program might consist of 5- to 10-second high-intensity intervals repeated five to ten times,[33] whereas moderately high intensity intervals 30 seconds to 2 minutes in length might be repeated a minimum of three times, with more advanced individuals performing six to eight repetitions. Longer duration intervals of greater than 2 minutes should be performed for somewhere between 3 to 5 and 8 to 12 interval repetitions.

Rest Period Length

Recovery HR can be used to determine the rest period length between intervals. With this method of determining rest period length, the next interval is not started until the HR is at the desired recovery rate. Suggested recovery HRs are 140 bpm for 20- to 29-year-olds, 130 bpm for 30- to 39-year-olds, 120 bpm for 40- to 49-year-olds, 115 bpm for 50- to 59-year-olds, and 105 bpm for 60- to 69-year-olds.[23]

Rest period length can also be determined based on a work-to-rest ratio. For example, for short-term, high-intensity intervals, a work-to-rest ratio of approximately 1:3 to 1:6 is used.[33] This means if an interval was 10 seconds in length, the rest period is between 30 and 60 seconds in length. For intervals ranging from 30 seconds to 2 minutes in length, a work-to-rest ratio of approximately 1:2 is used, whereas for intervals greater than 2 minutes in length, the work-to-rest ratio is approximately 1:1.

Type of Rest Interval

Generally passive (little or no activity) rest periods are used when high-intensity, short-duration intervals are performed.[33] This allows for resynthesis of intramuscular ATP–PCr so that it is available to perform the next high-intensity interval (see Chapter 2, excess postexercise oxygen consumption (EPOC)). Active recovery periods (activity lower than lactate threshold) are utilized with intervals 30 seconds and longer.

All the aforementioned recommendations must be viewed within the context of the training goals, fitness level, and training history of the individual or athlete performing interval training. Additionally, if an athlete is performing interval training during the competitive season, the other training needs, team or race strategy, conditioning due to sport-specific technique drills, and other types of training being performed need to be considered.

Training Frequency

Interval training is a high-intensity type of training. Therefore, initially low training frequencies are used to allow recovery between training sessions. For general fitness, initially, one to two interval training sessions per week may be performed. Athletes using interval training as part of their total training program typically perform two to four interval training sessions per week. However, some types of athletes, such as swimmers, almost exclusively use interval training, but different interval durations; total number of interval repetitions and length of rest periods are varied during each training session.

All the aforementioned guidelines must be viewed within the context of the training goals, fitness level, and training history of the individual or athlete performing interval training. As with other types of training, all training variables need to be adjusted to meet specific training goals and fitness level of the trainee.

Quick Review

- Interval training can be used to increase fitness of athletes and fitness enthusiasts.
- Intensity can be determined as either a percentage of the best time to cover a certain distance or a percentage of HR_{max}.
- Interval duration, number of intervals, rest period length, and training frequency all need to be adjusted to meet the training goals and fitness level of the trainee.

STRUCTURE OF A TRAINING SESSION

Any training session typically consists of a warm-up, body of the session, and cool-down. The body of the session refers to the training performed in the session. A considerable amount is known concerning the effects on performance of a warm-up including flexibility training or stretching. Less is known concerning the possible benefits of a cool-down after a training session.

Stretching

Many warm-up and cool-down portions of a training session include flexibility training or stretching. When included in a warm-up, stretching should be performed at the end of the warm-up, after body temperature has been increased slightly. There are several different stretching techniques in common use. **Proprioceptive neuromuscular facilitation (PNF)** techniques, of which there are several types, involve contraction of a muscle before stretching. The contraction causes a reflex relaxation of the muscle being stretched so that a greater range of motion is achieved during the stretch. **Ballistic stretching** involves a dynamic movement. The momentum of the body part involved in the stretch causes stretching of muscle at the end of the range of motion of the dynamic movement. The most popular form of flexibility training is **static stretching**. This type of stretch is performed by slowly moving through the range of motion of a muscle and holding it near the end of the range of motion, where a stretch is felt in the muscle. All three types of stretching will increase flexibility. However, a meta-analysis found no significant difference in flexibility increases between them.[13]

Extreme ranges of motion or flexibility at some joints is necessary for performance of some sports, such as gymnastics and high hurdling. Athletes involved in these types of sports need to perform flexibility training. Another reason stretching is performed is to prevent injury. It is purported that some types of injuries may be prevented by stretching, due to an increase in the range of motion of a joint. However, a meta-analysis found that stretching was not significantly associated with reduction in injury, but concluded that there's not sufficient evidence to either endorse or discontinue stretching before or after exercise to prevent injury among competitive or recreational athletes.[56] A study, involving army recruits, also concluded that stretching added to a warm-up does not significantly change the risk of injury.[48] There is little evidence to substantiate that stretching significantly reduces the chance of injury in most situations.

Stretching immediately before a maximal effort may actually decrease maximal force or power. Five ballistic stretches for the knee extensors and flexors performed 10 to 25 minutes before determining 1-RM decreased maximal values by 7% in knee flexion and 5% in knee extension.[44] Four static stretches for the knee extensors performed approximately 4 minutes before determining isokinetic peak torque decreased peak torque by 3% at both 60 and $240°·sec^{-1}$.[12] Static stretching and ballistic stretching of the lower body in rugby players significantly increased (3.23 vs. 3.27 sec) and decreased (3.24 vs. 3.18 sec), respectively, the 20-m sprint time compared with the sprint time without stretching.[21] This finding indicates that static stretching decreases whereas ballistic stretching increases sprint performance. In a very interesting study using elite collegiate track performers, it was shown that static stretching before a 100-m sprint decreased performance.[63] However, not all studies show a significant effect of stretching on performance. If one allows enough rest after a stretching bout, negative effects might not be as dramatic and allow the elastic component of muscle to recover. This was observed in collegiate field performers in upper body throwing and power tasks when stretching was delayed over 10 minutes before the test.[59] Neither static nor ballistic stretching in women collegiate basketball players significantly affected vertical jump performance.[60] When they do occur, decreases in maximal force and power after stretching appear to be related to an inability to fully activate the stretched muscle[5] or to a central nervous system inhibitory mechanism on the muscle stretched.[12]

Although not shown in all studies, stretching induced decreases in performance involving maximal force or power output in a variety of tasks have been shown in both untrained and trained subjects. Decreases in performance due to stretching immediately before a maximal effort may not be important to someone training for general health and fitness. However, such decreases would be important to athletes. Therefore, it would seem prudent for people interested in truly developing maximal force and power not to stretch immediately before trying to develop maximal force and power, either in training or in competition.

Effects of a Warm-Up and Cool-Down

An **active warm-up** consists of physical activity performed before training. Active warm-ups can be divided into general types. A **general warm-up** consists of activity not specifically related to the task or training to follow. A general warm-up could consist of low-intensity (60% $\dot{V}o_2$ peak) aerobic activity for 10 to 15 minutes, stretching, and calisthenics. A **sport-specific warm-up** includes activity that is specifically related to the task or training to follow, such as swinging a baseball bat before batting, shooting a basketball before a basketball game, and sprinting before a sprint test.

It has been suggested that warming up may increase performance due to several mechanisms.[6,7,14] The warm-up may allow an athlete time to mentally prepare and concentrate on the upcoming event. Thus, psychological factors may be an aspect of a warm-up. Warm-ups may also increase body temperature, which could positively affect performance due to the following:

- Decreased muscle and tendon stiffness
- Increased nerve conduction velocity
- Altered force–velocity relationship of muscle
- Increased anaerobic (glycogen) energy availability

However, increased body temperature due to a warm-up may decrease the ability to maintain thermoregulation and may decrease performance, especially during long-term activity. Nontemperature related physiological mechanisms that may increase performance include the following:

- Increased oxygen delivery to tissue due to increased blood flow
- Increased preactivity oxygen consumption, which may decrease reliance on anaerobic energy sources
- Increased force capabilities due to previous muscle activity (postactivation potentiation)

These different mechanisms may affect performance, depending on the activity for which the warm-up is meant. Decreased muscle and tendon stiffness and increased nerve conduction velocity may be especially important for strength and power activities. Increased oxygen delivery to tissue and decreased ability to maintain thermoregulation may affect performance more in long-term endurance events.

Do warm-ups actually increase performance? A review of the literature indicates that the answer to this question is "yes."[7] Active warm-ups increase performance in short-term, high-power activities. Vertical jump performance is increased approximately 3% to 4% due to an active warm-up of moderate intensity. Performance in short-term, high-power activities may, however, decrease if the warm-up is too intense or there is not sufficient recovery time between the warm-up and the activity, resulting in decreased availability of intramuscular phosphates (ATP and PC). Active warm-ups may slightly improve performance in intermediate-length tasks (10 seconds to 5 minutes) and long-term tasks (more than 5 minutes) if the warm-up allows the person to start the event in a nonfatigued state, but with increased oxygen consumption. The warm-up for these types of tasks, therefore, can either be of low intensity or of higher intensity if sufficient recovery is allowed between the end of the warm-up and the beginning of the event. So, an active warm-up can increase performance slightly if it is correctly structured for the specific event.

Quick Review

- Training sessions generally consist of an active warm-up, a body of the session, and a cool-down.
- An active warm-up can increase physical performance.
- A general warm-up consists of activity not related to the task or training to follow.
- A sport-specific warm-up consists of activity specifically related to the task or training to follow.
- Stretching immediately before physical activity can decrease maximal strength and power in both trained and untrained people.

A cool-down period consisting of light aerobic activity (below lactic acid threshold) for approximately 10 to 15 minutes is performed after many training sessions. One goal of a cool-down is to prevent blood from pooling in the legs, which can cause lightheadedness, dizziness, or even fainting after a strenuous training session. A cool-down can also aid in the lowering of blood acidity (see Chapter 2, "Maximizing Recovery"). Although not related to muscle soreness after a training session (delayed-onset muscular soreness), removal of blood lactate or lowering blood and muscle acidity will aid in recovery immediately following a training session.

DETRAINING

Detraining refers to the loss of physiological adaptations that occurs with complete cessation of training or a reduction in the volume and intensity of training. This process can occur after either endurance or resistance training. Loss of physiological adaptations during detraining is an important consideration for athletes during the off-season and for the fitness enthusiast who goes on a 2-week vacation. Here, we will focus primarily on changes in physical performance during detraining. However, health benefits also decrease because of detraining. After 6 months of aerobic training resulting in positive lipoprotein changes, a 15-day period of inactivity results in increased LDL-C, but no significant change in HDL-C.[53] Different adaptations, such as changes in LDL-C and HDL-C just noted, can follow different patterns of change during detraining. The loss of physiological adaptations during detraining is also affected by age, length of training period before detraining, and volume and intensity of training before detraining. Thus, although different physiological adaptations decrease at different rates during detraining, eventually all physiological adaptations brought about by training will decrease.

Cessation of Strength Training

Complete cessation of strength training results in loss of both strength and power, but the loss can be quite variable.[19] Type I muscle fiber cross-sectional area may be maintained

during short (6 weeks) detraining periods, but type II fiber area significantly decreases.[54] Interestingly, retraining after extensive prior training can bring back the muscle fiber size at a faster rate than that which occurs during initial fiber hypertrophy, supporting the term "muscle memory" that is commonly used in training vernacular.[54] Generally, there is a relatively quick loss of strength and power in the first several weeks of detraining, followed by a more gradual loss of ability as the detraining duration increases.

After periods of detraining as long as 30 weeks, strength decreases significantly from trained values but is still significantly greater than it was before training.[19] For example, after 14 weeks of detraining following 10 weeks of training, concentric and eccentric isokinetic knee extensor peak torques had decreased from trained values by 6% and 11%, respectively; however, they were still 14% and 18%, respectively, above prior-to-training values.[9]

Physical performance, in part determined by maximal strength and power, also decreases during detraining periods. Team handball players showed significant increases in ball-throwing velocity and jumping ability during 12 weeks of training. However, during 7 weeks of detraining, ball-throwing velocity decreased significantly by 2.6% and jumping ability decreased nonsignificantly by 1.6%.[39]

As noted by the differences between concentric and eccentric peak torque changes, ball-throwing velocity, and vertical jump ability, how strength or power is determined will affect the rate of change and amount of change in a detraining period. Generally, muscular power decreases at a faster rate than maximal strength with cessation of training.[19,31] Age also affects the rate of strength change during detraining, with older people generally showing more rapid decreases.[37] Intensity of training may also affect the rate of strength loss with cessation of training. During 24 weeks of detraining following low-intensity (40% of 1-RM), moderate-intensity (60% of 1-RM), or high-intensity (80% of 1-RM) training, men aged 65 to 78 years all showed significant decreases in strength.[16] However, strength loss in the upper and lower body during detraining was intensity related, with low-intensity training showing the greatest decreases (70%–98%), followed by the moderate-intensity training (44%–50%) and high-intensity training (27%–29%). Many factors may affect the rate and magnitude of strength and power changes during detraining, but strength and power will eventually decrease with cessation of strength training.

Reduced Volume of Strength Training

Strength training volume can be reduced by decreasing the number of sets performed, number of repetitions per set, and/or frequency of training (Box 12-7). Studies examining the effect of reduced strength training volume have, for the most part, involved reduced training frequency. After 12 weeks of concentric isokinetic training, maximal strength was maintained for 12 weeks with a training

Box 12-7   AN EXPERT VIEW
Strength and Conditioning for Collegiate Basketball Players

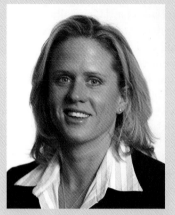

Andrea Hudy, MS
Assistant Athletic Director for Sport
Performance
University of Kansas Athletics
Lawrence, KS

With the rich traditions and the unlimited support that the University of Kansas, its community, and its alumni provide, we are able to train in one of the best facilities in the country. Athletes come to Kansas to follow the footsteps of the people before them. Basketball legends such as Wilt Chamberlain, Danny Manning, and Paul Pierce have laid the groundwork of hard work and dedication for the athletes of today. Therefore, it is imperative that we as coaches help instill those qualities in our training program and adhere to the best training philosophies that research provides.

As a strength and conditioning coach, it is my mission to physically and mentally prepare our student-athletes for the rigors of intercollegiate athletics with integrity and excellence. Two primary goals of our strength and conditioning program are to enhance sport performance and increase injury prevention through our various training and recovery techniques.

My lifting philosophy consists of ground-based explosive style resistance training. Weightlifting, power lifting, and resistance training are utilized.

My philosophy for programming is a nonlinear periodization model with periodization trends. Throughout the mesocycles, there is an increase in load and a decrease in volume. There are two types of nonlinear periodization. The first type is planned nonlinear periodization. Planned nonlinear periodization occurs in the postseason, summer, and preseasons. Percentages for most core lifts are used, and each day has a specific goal. For example, Day 1 is a high-volume circuit with work capacity (hormone response) as the main goal. Day 2 is a strength/speed training session with mainly high loads and low volume with increased neuromuscular recruitment as a main goal. Day 3 is a typical strength day designed with protein synthesis and neuromuscular recruitment as a main goal. Day 4 is a speed/strength day with mainly low-to-medium loads with an emphasis on speed of movement under a load.

The second type is flexible nonlinear periodization that occurs during the sports season. The weight training sessions are solely based on what occurs during the specific sport session, in this case, basketball practice. If the on-court practice is completed with powerful high-intensity synchronous running and jumping activities, then the weight training session is less intense and would usually have asynchronous qualities such as a circuit. If the on-court practice is not intense, i.e., a shoot-around, then the weight training session is more powerful and intense and filled with more synchronous activities such as a strength/speed session or a speed/strength session. Most of the core lifts have a percentage range, but not a specific percentage that is used. During the in-season, as long as the percentage range is used, the specific loads per person are self-regulated.

It is important that we have a yearly template that serves as a solid foundation for our program, but it also needs to be one that we can change on a moment's notice due to practice or sport coaching constraints. In other words, we provide a solid framework but tailor to the team time constraints and/or individual needs of someone with an injury or specific goals.

---

frequency of one or two times per week.[41] After 21 weeks of training two times per week, maximal leg press strength (1-RM) did not show a significant decrease during 21 weeks of training with only three sessions every 2 weeks.[52] In fact, leg strength actually increased an additional 5% during the first half of the 21 weeks of detraining and then decreased slightly (2%) during the last half of detraining. It appears that reducing training frequency to one or two sessions per week after training with a higher frequency does maintain strength levels for relatively long periods of time if training intensity is maintained.

The effect of reduced training volume is also important during in-season programs for athletes. Similar to the information presented earlier, it appears that one or two strength training sessions will maintain strength levels for relatively long periods of time in-season if training intensity is maintained.[19] Basketball players during a 20-week season showed no significant decrease in maximal strength levels and vertical jump ability (−1% to +5%), but short-sprint ability declined significantly by 3%.[29] It appears that maximal strength levels in athletes can be maintained in-season with training frequencies of one or two times per week, but some decrements in other performance measures may occur. One important aspect of reduced strength training volume for athletes in-season is that other types of training are performed, which may help to reduce any decrease in maximal strength or performance levels. **Tapering**, a planned reduction in training volume and possibly intensity (see Refs. 56 and 57), is used by many athletes to peak or maximize performance immediately after the taper (Box 12-8).

Box 12-8 DID YOU KNOW?

A Taper Can Increase Performance

Both endurance and anaerobic athletes use tapering to maximize performance for a specific competition. Reduction in training volume and/or intensity for a short period of time results in recovery from the previous training and, ideally, supercompensation or an increase in performance capabilities. Tapering is used by many athletes, including Olympic weightlifters, swimmers, triathletes, runners, and cyclists. Tapering can result in the following increases:

- 5% to 6% in cycling criterion performance
- up to 20% in power and strength
- 1% to 9% in $\dot{V}O_{2peak}$
- 15% in red blood cell volume
- 5% in serum testosterone
- 10% in anti-inflammatory immune cells
- improvement in mood states[2]

All these factors could result in increased performance. The performance gains from a taper can be quite variable, but even small gains may be important for an athlete, especially at a major competition. A taper can last from 7 to 30 days and normally involves a maintenance of or a slight increase in training intensity. Training volume is normally reduced from 40% to as much as 90%, depending on the athlete's fatigue level, type of athlete, and length of taper. An example taper used by handball players after performing higher volume weight training lasted 4 weeks and consisted of strength training using 90% to 95% of 1-RM for two to three sets of each exercise for two to four repetitions per set.[1] The taper resulted in gains of 2% in bench press 1-RM, 3% in squat 1-RM, significant gains in both bench press and squat power, but no significant increase in jumping ability. A taper can be an important part of planning an athlete's training.

References

1. Izquierdo J, Ibanez J, Gonzalez-Badillo JJ, et al. Detraining and tapering effects on hormonal responses and strength performance. J Strength Cond Res 2007;21:768–775.
2. Wilson JM, Wilson GJ. A practical approach to the taper. Strength Cond J 2008;30(2):10–17.

Cessation of Endurance Training

Cessation of endurance training results in a relatively rapid decrease in $\dot{V}O_{2peak}$. Peak oxygen consumption decreases approximately 14% in male basketball players who stop training for 4 weeks at the end of a season.[26] The decrease in $\dot{V}O_{2peak}$ can be quite variable and, in part, dependent on length of training and aerobic capabilities before cessation of training. Highly trained athletes with high $\dot{V}O_{2peak}$ within the first 8 weeks of training cessation show decreases in $\dot{V}O_{2peak}$, ranging from 4% to 20%.[42] However, those with lower $\dot{V}O_{2peak}$ values or shorter training periods (4–8 weeks) before training cessation show much smaller decreases in $\dot{V}O_{2peak}$, ranging from 0% to 6% within 2 to 4 weeks of training cessation.[42] In both cases, $\dot{V}O_{2peak}$ remains above untrained values.

Many factors contribute to the decrease in aerobic capabilities with training cessation. The initial decrease in $\dot{V}O_{2peak}$ is due to a rapid decline in blood volume, resulting in a decrease in stroke volume, which cannot be offset by increases in HR during exercise.[42] This results in a decrease in maximal cardiac output (cardiac output = HR × stroke volume) and, so, a decrease in blood supply and oxygen delivery to tissue. Cardiac end-diastolic volume also decreases, which contributes to the decrease in stroke volume (stroke volume = end-diastolic volume – end-systolic volume; see Chapter 5). Left ventricular mass may also decrease with training cessation. Aerobic enzyme activity decreases, but specific enzymes show variable responses to cessation of training. Mitochondrial density decreases, whereas capillary density remains unchanged. Respiratory exchange ratio within 3 weeks of training cessation increases substantially (0.89–0.95) during exercise at 60% of $\dot{V}O_{2peak}$, indicating an increased reliance on carbohydrate for metabolic fuel (see Chapter 2). Remember that, per liter of oxygen, aerobic metabolism of carbohydrates generates more energy (ATP) than does aerobic metabolism of fats. Muscle glycogen stores decrease rapidly (up to 20% in 4 weeks), and insulin sensitivity is reduced, compromising the ability to use carbohydrate as a metabolic substrate.[42] All these factors compromise the ability to perform aerobic metabolism, resulting in a decreased ability to perform maximal aerobic activity.

Reduced Volume of Endurance Training

Reduction in endurance training volume can either be accomplished by reducing the volume of training performed in a training session or the frequency of training. The interaction between training intensity and volume is important when endurance training volume is reduced. Reductions in training intensity, even if training frequency and volume are maintained, result in decreased aerobic capabilities in people who aerobically trained for short periods of time (10 weeks) or in highly trained athletes.[43] To maintain aerobic capabilities during periods of reduced training volume, training intensity must be maintained. Moderately aerobically trained people (10 weeks of training) maintain endurance capabilities for up to 15 weeks with training volume reduced one-third or two-thirds, if training intensity is maintained.[28] Similarly, aerobic capabilities in trained athletes can be maintained with reductions of 50% to 70% in training volume for short periods of time.[43] Similar to maintenance of strength capabilities, to maintain aerobic capabilities with a reduction in training volume, training intensity must be maintained.

PERIODIZATION

Periodization refers to planned variation in training, with the goal of optimizing physical performance over long training periods. Endurance and strength-power athletes and fitness enthusiasts alike use periodized training. Periodized programs use changes in training volume and intensity to create training variation. For athletes, changes in the amount of skill and game or event strategy training are also varied throughout a competitive season. A meta-analysis concludes that periodized resistance training results in greater strength gains than nonperiodized programs in both genders, people younger and older than 55 years of age, and in untrained and trained weight trainers.[50] Indeed, periodization of strength training has been recommended for both untrained and trained people.[3] A substantial amount of research has been performed on periodized strength training, demonstrating it to be superior to nonperiodized programs in causing strength gains, changes in body composition, and motor performance (short sprints, maximal cycling power, and vertical jump ability). For a more detailed discussion of periodized strength training, see Fleck and Kraemer, 2004, and Kraemer and Fleck, 2007, in the Suggested Readings list. All types of training can be periodized; here, we will examine concepts of strength and aerobic training periodization.

Classic Strength-Power Periodized Training

With a classic strength-power or linear periodized strength program, training begins with high-volume, low-intensity training and progresses toward low-volume, high-intensity training (Table 12-7). Several training phases make up the entire training cycle, each lasting typically 4 to 6 weeks and having different major training goals. In many programs, an active recovery phase of 1 to 2 weeks, consisting of light resistance training, follows the last training phase. Also, in many programs, only multi-joint exercises follow the periodized program.

One goal of the active recovery phase is to allow physiological and psychological recovery from the preceding high-intensity training. Training volume and intensity predominantly change due to changes in the number of sets and repetitions per set. This type of training is meant to peak, or maximize, maximal strength and power after the last, or peaking, training phase. After the active recovery phase, the entire training cycle is repeated. Ideally, heavier weights can be used in the new cycle due to an increase in strength brought about by the preceding training cycle. Training variation can also be introduced by changes in the type of resistance exercises performed. Typically, this means greater emphasis on maximal strength in the initial training phases by performing strength exercises, such as squats and dead lifts. Then, trainees would switch to power-oriented exercises, such as power cleans and power snatches, toward the end of the training cycle. Note that the range in the number of sets and repetitions in each training phase also allow for variation in volume and intensity on a weekly or training session basis.

Nonlinear Periodized Training

Nonlinear periodization consists of performing successive training sessions in a recurring pattern of very different training volume and intensity. A typical training pattern might be performing exercises using 4 to 6, 8 to 10, and 12 to 15 repetitions per set for 2 to 3 sets per exercise on each of three training sessions in a week. This results in substantial changes in training volume and intensity in a week of training, due predominantly to the number of

	Training Phase			
Table 12-7. Classic Strength-Power Periodized Strength Training				
Training Variable	**Hypertrophy**	**Strength**	**Power**	**Peaking**
Sets	3–5	3–5	3–5	1–5
Repetitions/set	8–12	2–6	2–3	1–3
Volume	Very high	High	Moderate	Low
Intensity	Low	Moderate	High	Very high

repetitions performed per set. The pattern of changes in the number of repetitions per set is repeated on a weekly basis. In some nonlinear programs, all exercises follow the nonlinear pattern. In other programs, only the multi-joint exercises follow the nonlinear pattern. After a month or several months of training, an active recovery phase can take place, with nonlinear periodization resumed after the active recovery phase. With the use of "flexible" nonlinear training, one can test and determine what workout might work best that day based upon an athlete's fatigue level, practice demands, game schedule, or illness and match the type of workout that can be most optimally performed on that given day. Nonlinear periodization has been shown to be superior to nonperiodized programs in strength gains, body composition changes, and motor performance in untrained subjects as well as athletes.[36,40]

Aerobic Training Periodization

The concepts used to periodize aerobic training are similar to those used for strength training. Training volume is typically measured as total distance swam, run, or rowed. In many programs, percentage of HR_{max} is used to determine training intensity; however, intensity can also be determined as the percentage of the best time to cover a certain distance. A typical periodized program for a distance runner is depicted in Figure 12-8. In this training plan, weekly training volume is gradually increased during several weeks (weeks 1–6, 8–10, 12–14) of training followed by a 1-week recovery period of training during which volume and intensity are reduced. Although training intensity varied daily and within a training session, generally, during the first 10 weeks of training, intensity as a percentage of HR_{max} is also gradually increased from an HR below lactate threshold to an HR substantially above lactate threshold. Weeks 11, 15, and 19 are recovery weeks with a decrease in both the training volume and intensity. Several weeks of training (12, 14, 16, and 18) are difficult because both training volume and overall training intensity remain high. In the last several weeks of training (weeks 22–24), a taper

is used in the training plan. Both volume and intensity are reduced in this phase of the training plan with intensity being maintained at higher levels longer than volume.

Fitness aerobic training plans can also vary and progress training in a periodized manner and remain within the guidelines for aerobic fitness training (see "Aerobic Training Guidelines"). This can be accomplished by gradually progressing the percentage of HR_{max}, varying the training duration or distance and increasing the frequency of training. For example, intensity could be gradually increased from 60% HR_{max} to 80% as aerobic fitness increased, training duration could be increased from 20 minutes up to 60 minutes, and training frequency could be gradually progressed from 3 to 5–6 times per week. However, it is not necessary in a periodized plan that training intensity, duration, and frequency always progress to make the training more difficult. It is possible to have higher-intensity, shorter-duration sessions (80% HR_{max}, 20-minute session) within a week of training with other sessions of lower intensity but longer duration (65% HR_{max}, for 5-minute session). It is also possible within a fitness focused aerobic training plan to have recovery weeks of training as depicted in Fig. 12-8. Within the fitness training program, different modes of exercise, such as running, cycling, and elliptical training also can be incorporated on a session-by-session or in any other variation pattern to avoid boredom and possibly an overuse injury. Manipulation of training variables allows virtually a limitless number of different types of aerobic training sessions.

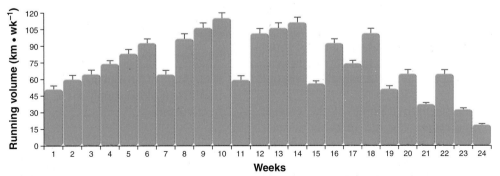

Figure 12-8. An endurance training periodization training plan. Training volume of well-trained endurance runners (68 mL $O_2 \cdot kg^{-1} \cdot min^{-1}$) is depicted during 24 weeks of training. Training intensity was also varied (see text for explanation). (Figure courtesy of Alejandro Lucia's laboratory, European University of Madrid.)

CASE STUDY

Scenario

You are designing the resistance training program for a shot putter in preparation for an upcoming major competition. What type of resistance training program will you design, and what type of changes will you make as a shot putter prepares for the competition?

Options

I would design a classic strength/power periodized resistance training program. Thus, the training would move from high-volume, low-intensity to low-volume, high-intensity training as the training phases progress. The hypertrophy, strength, power, and peaking training phases would all be approximately 4 weeks in length. They would be scheduled so that immediately before the competition a peaking phase occurs. In addition to moving toward high-intensity, low-volume training as the training progressed, several other changes would be made. The hypertrophy phases would consist of a mixture of single- and multi-joint exercises. However, as the training progressed toward the peaking phase, to help reduce total training volume, the number of single-joint exercises would be gradually reduced. Also, as training progressed toward the peaking phase, power-type exercises, such as power cleans and snatch pulls, would be emphasized. I would also be cautious not to perform static stretching exercises in a warm-up preceding resistance training sessions. This type of flexibility training has been shown to reduce maximal strength and power immediately after stretching. However,

I would include stretching, including static stretching, in the cool-down period after resistance training sessions. Immediately before the competition, a peaking phase of 7 to 10 days would be performed to help maximize power development.

Scenario

A friend has asked you to design a beginning aerobic training program for him. What type of training session will you recommend, and what types of training progression will be utilized in the program?

Options

The initial training sessions would consist of 20 to 30 minutes of exercise at an intensity of 60% to 65% of HR_{max}. Training frequency would be 3 days·week^{-1} with 1-day rest between sessions. As the training progressed, training intensity would be gradually increased to approximately 90% of HR_{max}, with the training session duration increased to 60 minutes and training frequency gradually increased to 5 or 6 days·week^{-1}. I would be cautious as training progressed not to initially include higher intensity and higher volume training in the same session. Thus, as training is progressed when training intensity was increased I would not increase training volume in the same session and vice versa. As training frequency is increased, I would recommend a mixture of running, elliptical training, and cycling to help avoid any overuse injury.

CHAPTER SUMMARY

Although deaths associated with cardiovascular diseases are declining, they still account for 36.3% of all deaths in the United States. Cardiovascular diseases include CAD, stroke, hypertension, and diseases of the arteries. Noncontrollable risk factors associated with cardiovascular disease include being male, advancing age, and heredity. Controllable risk factors include smoking tobacco, blood lipid profile, hypertension, obesity, diabetes, and physical activity. These factors are all interrelated, with physical activity resulting in positive adaptations of virtually all other controllable risk factors.

Both aerobic and strength training of the correct intensity and volume reduce the risk of cardiovascular disease. The volume and intensity of physical activity necessary to bring about health benefits is less than those needed to bring about fitness benefits. However, if fitness benefits occur, health benefits will also occur. Detraining results in loss of physiological adaptations due to training, although the pattern and magnitude of loss vary depending

on the adaptation. Thus, both athletes and those interested in health or fitness benefits of training should avoid long periods of detraining. Nonperiodized training does increase fitness; however, periodized training is recommended for both fitness enthusiasts and athletes because it results in greater fitness benefits than nonperiodized training.

REVIEW QUESTIONS

Fill-in-the-Blank

1. A blockage of a coronary artery results in _____, or insufficient blood supply to the cardiac tissue supplied by the artery.

2. If a coronary artery is severely or totally blocked, ischemia becomes severe enough to result in a _____, more commonly known as a heart attack.

3. Individuals considered to have moderate-to-high risk for cardiovascular disease should undergo a _____ before exercise participation.

4. If physical training results in ventricular hypertrophy, the QRS complex in an ECG becomes _____.

5. _____ involves a person subjectively rating how hard he or she is working.

Multiple Choice

1. Which of the following can be affected by a stroke?
   a. Senses
   b. Short-term memory capabilities
   c. Long-term memory capabilities
   d. Speech patterns
   e. All of the above

2. What type of heart failure is a result of a toxic substance or drug or due to coronary artery blockage resulting in a heart attack?
   a. Acute
   b. Chronic
   c. Stroke
   d. Arteriosclerosis
   e. Artery disease

3. What type of heart failure results from the impairment of cardiac function due to the long-term effects of such factors as hypertension, multiple minor heart attacks, or a viral infection?
   a. Acute
   b. Chronic
   c. Stroke
   d. Arteriosclerosis
   e. Artery disease

4. Hypertension is the medical term for chronically high resting blood pressure. It is defined as resting arterial blood pressure equal to or greater than which of the following?
   a. 120 and 80 mm Hg for systolic and diastolic blood pressure, respectively
   b. 100 or 60 mm Hg for systolic and diastolic blood pressure, respectively
   c. 140 or 90 mm Hg for systolic and diastolic blood pressure, respectively
   d. 160 or 110 mm Hg for systolic and diastolic blood pressure, respectively
   e. None of the above

5. Which controllable cardiovascular risk factor can negatively impact all other controllable cardiovascular risk factors?
   a. Blood lipid profile
   b. Hypertension
   c. Obesity or overweight
   d. Diabetes mellitus
   e. Physical inactivity

True/False

1. Atherosclerosis can occur within any blood vessel.
2. Atherosclerosis and arteriosclerosis, or thickening and loss of elasticity of the arterial wall, are the result of a chronic low-grade inflammation of the blood vessel walls.
3. As blood pressure increases, the force the left ventricle must develop to pump blood throughout the body decreases, which increases the oxygen demand by the cardiac tissue.
4. Decreased blood cholesterol, decreased LDL-C, and decreased HDL-C are all associated with increased CAD risk.
5. One MET is equal to oxygen consumption at rest.

Short Answer

1. What are the typical parts of a resistance or aerobic training session?
2. Explain how chronic low-grade inflammation leads to artery blockage or atherosclerosis and arteriosclerosis.
3. Explain why hypertension is an important consideration for cardiovascular health.
4. Explain why the QRS complex of an ECG is taller than the P wave.
5. What types of signs and symptoms will medical personnel look for during and after a graded exercise test?

KEY TERMS

active warm-up: activity performed before training
angina pectoris: chest pain due to ischemia to cardiac tissue
arteriosclerosis: progressive thickening and loss of elasticity of an arterial wall due to a chronic low-grade inflammation
atherosclerosis: progressive narrowing of an artery due to the formation of fatty plaque on the interior wall of an artery
ballistic stretch: flexibility training involving a dynamic movement, in which the momentum of the body part involved in the stretch causes a muscle to be stretched at the end of the range of motion of the dynamic movement
coronary artery disease (CAD): disease process causing eventual blockage and hardening of the arteries that supply cardiac tissue with blood
cross-training: performance of several types of aerobic exercise in a period of training
detraining: loss of physiological adaptations with complete cessation of training or a reduction in the volume or intensity of training
electrocardiogram (ECG): a measurement of cardiac electrical conductivity; used to determine cardiac rhythm or contraction and relaxation
fitness benefit: physiological adaptation resulting in increased physical performance
general warm-up: a type of warm-up consisting of activity not specifically related to the training to follow
health benefit: physiological adaptation that reduces the risk of developing a disease

heart failure: impairment of the ventricles' ability to contract to the point that cardiac output is insufficient to meet the body's oxygen needs

high-density lipoprotein cholesterol (HDL-C): lipoprotein produced by the liver to transport lipids from the cells of the body back to the liver

hypertension: chronic, resting high blood pressure

intensity of exercise: measure of how difficult exercise is or the stressfulness of exercise

interval training: repeated exercise bouts separated by rest periods

ischemia: insufficient blood supply to a tissue

lipoprotein: a cluster of lipids and proteins that is transported in the blood

low-density lipoprotein cholesterol (LDL-C): a lipoprotein produced by the liver to transport cholesterol and triglycerides to the body's tissues for their use

major or primary risk factors: factors that are strongly associated with CAD

metabolic equivalent (MET): a measure of oxygen consumption relative to rest; 1 MET equals approximately 3.5 mL·kg^{-1}·min^{-1}; exercising at 4 METS is equivalent to an oxygen consumption four times resting oxygen consumption

multi–muscle group exercise: resistance training exercise that involves movement at more than one joint and force development by more than one muscle group, such as a bench press or leg press; also termed *multi-joint exercise*

myocardial infarction: severe ischemia to cardiac tissue; commonly known as a heart attack

periodization: planned variation in training with the goal of optimizing physical performance over long training periods

peripheral artery disease (PAD): development of atherosclerosis in the peripheral circulation

proprioceptive neuromuscular facilitation (PNF): flexibility training technique involving contraction of a muscle before stretching to cause a reflex relaxation of the muscle being stretched so that a greater range of motion is achieved during the stretch

rating of perceived exertion (RPE): subjective rating of how hard a person is working

single–muscle group exercise: resistance training exercise that predominantly involves movement at one joint and force development by one muscle group, such as arm curls or leg extensions; also termed *single-joint exercise*

split routine: resistance training program in which the body is divided into different areas, with each area being trained with a separate resistance training session

sport-specific warm-up: a type of active warm-up consisting of activity that is specifically related to the training to follow

static stretch: flexibility training that is performed by slowly moving through the range of motion of a flexibility exercise and holding the exercise near the end of the range of motion, where a stretch is felt in the muscle being stretched

stroke: lack of blood supply to a portion of the brain

tapering: a planned reduction in training volume and possibly intensity

thrombus: blood clot that partially or completely blocks an artery

total body resistance training program: resistance training program in which all the major muscle groups are trained each training session

volume of training: measurement of how much total work or training is performed

REFERENCES

1. Albright A, Franz M, Hornsby G, et al. Position stand: exercise and type 2 diabetes. Med Sci Sports Exerc. 2000;32:1345–1360.
2. American College of Sports Medicine. ACSM's Guidelines for Exercise Testing and Prescription, 7th ed. Philadelphia, PA: Lippincott Williams & Wilkins, 2006.
3. American College of Sports Medicine. American College of Sports Medicine position stand. Progression models in resistance training for healthy adults. Med Sci Sports Exerc. 2009;42:687–708.
4. American Heart Association. Heart disease and stroke statistics —2008 uptake. A report from the American Heart Association Statistics Committee and Stroke Statistics Subcommittee. Circulation. 2008;117:e25–e146.
5. Behm DG, Button DC, Butt JC. Factors affecting force loss with prolonged stretching. Can J Appl Physiol. 2001;26:261–272.
6. Bishop D. Warm up I: potential mechanisms and the effects of passive warm up on exercise performance. Sports Med. 2003;33: 439–454.
7. Bishop D. Warm up II: performance changes following active warm up and how to structure the warm up. Sports Med. 2003;33: 483–498.
8. Blair SN, Kampert JB, Kohl HW III, et al. Influences of cardiorespiratory fitness and other precursors on cardiovascular disease and all-cause mortality in men and women. JAMA. 1996;276: 205–210.
9. Blazevich AJ, Cannavan D, Coleman DR, et al. Influence of concentric and eccentric resistance training on architectural adaptation in human quadriceps muscles. J Appl Physiol. 2007;103:1565–1575.
10. Collins EG, Edwin Langbein W, Orebaugh C, et al. PoleStriding exercise and vitamin E for management of peripheral vascular disease. Med Sci Sports Exerc. 2003;35:384–393.
11. Cornelissen VA, Fagard RH. Effect of resistance training on resting blood pressure: a meta-analysis of randomized controlled trials. J Hypertens. 2005;23:251–259.
12. Cramer JT, Housh TJ, Weir JP, et al. The acute effects of static stretching on peak torque, mean power output, electromyography, and mechanomyography. Eur J Appl Physiol. 2005;93:530–539.
13. Decoster LC, Cleland J, Altieri C, et al. The effects of hamstring stretching on range of motion: a systematic literature review. J Orthop Sports Phys Ther. 2005;35:377–387.
14. DeLorey DS, Kowalchuk JM, Heenan AP, et al. Prior exercise speeds pulmonary O$_2$ uptake kinetics by increases in both local muscle O$_2$ availability and O$_2$ utilization. J Appl Physiol. 2007;103:771–778.
15. Fagard RH. Exercise characteristics and the blood pressure response to dynamic physical training. Med Sci Sports Exerc. 2001;33: S484–S492; discussion S493–S484.
16. Fatouros IG, Kambas A, Katrabasas I, et al. Resistance training and detraining effects on flexibility performance in the elderly are intensity-dependent. J Strength Cond Res. 2006;20:634–642.
17. Ferrara CM, Goldberg AP, Ortmeyer HK, et al. Effects of aerobic and resistive exercise training on glucose disposal and skeletal muscle metabolism in older men. J Gerontol A Biol Sci Med Sci. 2006;61:480–487.
18. Fleck SJ. Cardiovascular response to strength training. In: Komi PV, ed. Strength and Power in Sport: Olympic Encyclopedia of Sports Medicine, 2nd ed., Vol. III. Oxford, England: Wiley-Blackwell, 2002:387–406.
19. Fleck SJ, Kraemer WJ. Designing Resistance Training Programs, 3rd ed. Champaign, IL: Human Kinetics, 2004.
20. Fletcher GF, Balady GJ, Amsterdam EA, et al. Exercise standards for testing and training: a statement for healthcare professionals from the American Heart Association. Circulation. 2001;104:1694–1740.
21. Fletcher IM, Jones B. The effect of different warm-up stretch protocols on 20 meter sprint performance in trained rugby union players. J Strength Cond Res. 2004;18:885–888.
22. Foster C, Porcari JP, Gibson M, et al. Translation of submaximal exercise test responses to exercise prescription using the talk test. J Strength Cond Res. 2009;23:2425–2429.
23. Fox EL. Interval training. Bull Hosp Joint Dis. 1979;40:64–71.
24. Garrison RJ, Kannel WB, Stokes J III, et al. Incidence and precursors of hypertension in young adults: the Framingham Offspring Study. Prev Med. 1987;16:235–251.

25. Gellish RL, Goslin BR, Olson RE, et al. Longitudinal modeling of the relationship between age and maximal heart rate. Med Sci Sports Exerc. 2007;39:822–829.

26. Ghosh AK, Paliwal R, Sam MJ, et al. Effect of 4 weeks detraining on aerobic & anaerobic capacity of basketball players & their restoration. Indian J Med Res. 1987;86:522–527.

27. Helgerud J, Hoydal K, Wang E, et al. Aerobic high-intensity intervals improve $\dot{V}O_{2max}$ more than moderate training. Med Sci Sports Exerc. 2007;39:665–671.

28. Hickson RC, Kanakis C Jr, Davis JR, et al. Reduced training duration effects on aerobic power, endurance, and cardiac growth. J Appl Physiol. 1982;53:225–229.

29. Hoffman JR, Fry AC, Howard R, et al. Strength, speed and endurance changes during the course of a division I basketball season. J Appl Sport Sci Res. 1991;3:144–149.

30. Ingham SA, Whyte GP, Pedlar C, et al. Determinants of 800-m and 1500-m running performance using allometric models. Med Sci Sports Exerc. 2008;40:345–350.

31. Izquierdo M, Ibanez J, Gonzalez-Badillo JJ, et al. Detraining and tapering effects on hormonal responses and strength performance. J Strength Cond Res. 2007;21:768–775.

32. Izquierdo M, Ibanez J, Gonzalez-Badillo JJ, et al. Differential effects of strength training leading to failure versus not to failure on hormonal responses, strength, and muscle power gains. J Appl Physiol. 2006;100:1647–1656.

33. Karp JR. Interval training for the fitness professional. Strength Cond J. 2000;22:64–69.

34. Kavouras SA, Panagiotakos DB, Pitsavos C, et al. Physical activity, obesity status, and glycemic control: the ATTICA study. Med Sci Sports Exerc. 2007;39:606–611.

35. Kelley GA, Kelley KS. Progressive resistance exercise and resting blood pressure: a meta-analysis of randomized controlled trials. Hypertension. 2000;35:838–843.

36. Kraemer WJ, Ratamess N, Fry AC, et al. Influence of resistance training volume and periodization on physiological and performance adaptations in collegiate women tennis players. Am J Sports Med. 2000;28:626–633.

37. Lemmer JT, Hurlbut DE, Martel GF, et al. Age and gender responses to strength training and detraining. Med Sci Sports Exerc. 2000;32:1505–1512.

38. Leon AS, Sanchez OA. Response of blood lipids to exercise training alone or combined with dietary intervention. Med Sci Sports Exerc. 2001;33:S502–S515; discussion S528–S509.

39. Marques MC, Gonzalez-Badillo JJ. In-season resistance training and detraining in professional team handball players. J Strength Cond Res. 2006;20:563–571.

40. Marx JO, Ratamess NA, Nindl BC, et al. Low-volume circuit versus high-volume periodized resistance training in women. Med Sci Sports Exerc. 2001;33:635–643.

41. McCarrick MJ, Kemp JG. The effect of strength training and reduced training on rotator cuff musculature. Clin Biomech (Bristol, Avon). 2000;15(Suppl 1):S42–S45.

42. Mujika I, Padilla S. Cardiorespiratory and metabolic characteristics of detraining in humans. Med Sci Sports Exerc. 2001;**33**:413–421.

43. Mujika I, Padilla S. Scientific bases for precompetition tapering strategies. Med Sci Sports Exerc. 2003;35:1182–1187.

44. Nelson AG, Kokkonen J. Acute ballistic muscle stretching inhibits maximal strength performance. Res Q Exerc Sport. 2001;72:415–419.

45. Noble BJ, Robertson RJ. Perceived Exertion. Champaign, IL: Human Kinetics, 1996.

46. Pescatello LS, Franklin BA, Fagard R, et al. American College of Sports Medicine position stand. Exercise and hypertension. Med Sci Sports Exerc. 2004;36:533–553.

47. Pollock ML, Gaesser GA, Butcher JD, et al. The recommended quantity and quality of exercise for developing and maintaining cardiorespiratory and muscular fitness, and flexibility in healthy adults. Med Sci Sports Exerc. 1998;30:975–991.

48. Pope RP, Herbert RD, Kirwan JD, et al. A randomized trial of preexercise stretching for prevention of lower-limb injury. Med Sci Sports Exerc. 2000;32:271–277.

49. Prabhakaran B, Dowling EA, Branch JD, et al. Effect of 14 weeks of resistance training on lipid profile and body fat percentage in premenopausal women. Br J Sports Med. 1999;33:190–195.

50. Rhea MR, Alderman BL. A meta-analysis of periodized versus nonperiodized strength and power training programs. Res Q Exerc Sport. 2004;75:413–422.

51. Sallinen J, Fogelholm M, Pakarinen A, et al. Effects of strength training and nutritional counseling on metabolic health indicators in aging women. Can J Appl Physiol. 2005;30:690–707.

52. Sallinen J, Fogelholm M, Volek JS, et al. Effects of strength training and reduced training on functional performance and metabolic health indicators in middle-aged men. Int J Sports Med. 2007;28:815–822.

53. Slentz CA, Houmard JA, Johnson JL, et al. Inactivity, exercise training and detraining, and plasma lipoproteins. STRRIDE: a randomized, controlled study of exercise intensity and amount. J Appl Physiol. 2007;103:432–442.

54. Staron RS, Leonardi MJ, Karapondo DL, et al. Strength and skeletal muscle adaptations in heavy-resistance-trained women after detraining and retraining. J Appl Physiol. 1991;70:631–640.

55. Tanasescu M, Leitzmann MF, Rimm EB, et al. Exercise type and intensity in relation to coronary heart disease in men. JAMA. 2002;288:1994–2000.

56. Thacker SB, Gilchrist J, Stroup DF, et al. The impact of stretching on sports injury risk: a systematic review of the literature. Med Sci Sports Exerc. 2004;36:371–378.

57. Thomas L, Busso T. A theoretical study of taper characteristics to optimize performance. Med Sci Sports Exerc. 2005;37:1615–1621.

58. Tokmakidis SP, Zois CE, Volaklis KA, et al. The effects of a combined strength and aerobic exercise program on glucose control and insulin action in women with type 2 diabetes. Eur J Appl Physiol. 2004;92:437–442.

59. Torres EM, Kraemer WJ, Vingren JL, et al. Effects of stretching on upper-body muscular performance. J Strength Cond Res. 2008;22:1279–1285.

60. Unick J, Kieffer HS, Cheesman W, et al. The acute effects of static and ballistic stretching on vertical jump performance in trained women. J Strength Cond Res. 2005;19:206–212.

61. Whelton SP, Chin A, Xin X, et al. Effect of aerobic exercise on blood pressure: a meta-analysis of randomized, controlled trials. Ann Intern Med. 2002;136:493–503.

62. Willardson JM. The application of training to failure in periodized multiple-set resistance exercise programs. J Strength Cond Res. 2007;21:628–631.

63. Winchester JB, Nelson AG, Landin D, et al. Static stretching impairs sprint performance in collegiate track and field athletes. J Strength Cond Res. 2008;22:13–19.

Suggested Readings

Albright A, Franz M, Hornsby G, et al. Position stand: exercise and type 2 diabetes. Med Sci Sports Exerc. 2000;32:1345–1360.

American College of Sports Medicine. American College of Sports Medicine position stand. Progression models in resistance training for healthy adults. Med Sci Sports Exerc. 2009;42:687–708.

Behm DG, Button DC, Butt JC. Factors affecting force loss with prolonged stretching. Can J Appl Phy. 2001;26:261–272.

Bishop D. Warm up I: potential mechanisms and the effects of passive warm up on exercise performance. Sports Med. 2003;33:439–454.

Bishop D. Warm up II: performance changes following active warm up and how to structure the warm up. Sports Med. 2003;33:483–498.

Cornelissen VA, Fagard RH. Effect of resistance training on resting the pressure: a meta-analysis of randomized controlled trials. J Hypertens. 2005;23:251–259.

Fleck SJ. Cardiovascular response to strength training. In: Komi PV, ed. Strength and Power in Sport: Olympic Encyclopedia of Sports Medicine, 2nd ed., Vol. III. Oxford, England: Wiley-Blackwell, 2002:387–406.

Fleck SJ, Kraemer WJ. Designing Resistance Training Programs, 3rd ed. Champaign, IL: Human Kinetics, 2004.

Fletcher GF, Balady GJ, Amsterdam EA, et al. Exercise standards for testing and training: a statement for healthcare professionals from the American Heart Association. Circulation. 2001;104:1694–1740.

Kraemer WJ, Fleck SJ. Optimizing Strength Training: Designing Nonlinear Periodization Workouts. Champaign, IL: Human Kinetics, 2007.

Mujika I, Padilla S. Cardiorespiratory and metabolic characteristics of detraining in humans. Med Sci Sports Exerc. 2001;33:413–421.

Mujika I, Padilla S. Scientific basis for precompetition tapering strategies. Med Sci Sports Exerc. 2003;35:1182–1187.

Pescatello LS, Frankilin BA, Fagard R, et al. American College of Sports Medicine position stand. Exercise and hypertension. Med Sci Sports Exerc. 2004;36:533–553.

Plisk SS, Stone MH. Periodization strategies. Strength Cond J. 2003;25(6):19–37.

Pollock ML, Gaesser GA, Butcher JD, et al. The recommended quantity and quality of exercise for developing and maintaining cardiorespiratory and muscular fitness, and flexibility in healthy adults. Med Sci Sports Exerc. 1998;30:975–991.

Thacker SB, Gilchrist J, Stroup DF, et al. The impact of stretching on sports injury risk: a systematic review of literature. Med Sci Sports Exerc. 2004;36:371–378.

Thomas L, Busso T. A theoretical study of paper characteristics to optimize performance. Med Sci Sports Exerc. 2005;37:1615–1621.

Wallmann H. An introduction to the periodization training for the triathlete. Strength Cond J. 2001;23:55–64.

Wilson JM, Wilson GJ. A practical approach to the taper. Strength Cond J. 2008;30:10–17.

Classic References

DeLorme TL. Watkins AL. Techniques of progressive resistance exercise. Arch Phys Med. 1948;29:263–273.

Dexter L, Lewis BM, Houssay HE, et al. The dynamics of both right and left ventricles at rest and during exercise in patients with heart failure. Trans Assoc Am Physicians. 1953;66:266–274.

Komi PV. Factors affecting muscular strength and principles of training. Duodecim. 1974;90(7):505–516.

Matoba H, Gollnick PD. Response of skeletal muscle to training. Sports Med. 1984;1(3):240–251.

Matveyev L. Fundamentals of Sports Training. Moscow: Progress, 1981.

Maud PJ, Pollock ML, Foster C, et al. Fifty years of training and competition in the marathon: Wally Hayward, age 70—a physiological profile. S Afr Med J. 1981;59(5):153–157.

O'Shea P. Quantum Strength and Power Training: Gaining the Winning Edge. Corvallis, OR: Patrick's Books, 1995.

Shaffer CF, Chapman DW. The exercise electrocardiogram; an aid in the diagnosis of arteriosclerotic heart disease in persons exhibiting abnormally large Q3 waves. Am J Med. 1951;11(1):26–30.

13

Exercise Testing for Health, Physical Fitness, and Predicting Sport Performance

After reading this chapter, you should be able to:

1. Explain the role that testing of physical fitness and physiological functional capacity plays, not only for competitive athletes, but also for those interested in improving their health.

2. Describe how the specific parameters of fitness to be tested depend on the individual and his or her training objectives.

3. Discuss the importance of selecting population-specific norms in assessing an individual's test results.

4. Explain why certain popular fitness tests are performed and understand how to perform them.

5. Describe the physiological systems evaluated in various tests.

Exercise scientists, athletic trainers, and others perform testing of a person's physiological response or ability for many reasons, including determining initial fitness levels, tracking changes in fitness levels, or for diagnostic purposes. The type of test chosen greatly depends on the individual or individuals being tested and the physiological characteristic for which information is desired. For example, the maximal amount of weight possible for one repetition in a power clean may be important for tracking training progress in some types of athletes, such as American football players or shot putters. However, this would not be important for most people interested in general fitness. Directly measuring endurance capabilities (maximal oxygen consumption, lactate threshold) would be important for an endurance athlete to track training progress. However, an estimate of maximal oxygen consumption would probably suffice for most fitness enthusiasts to track training progress.

As with the tests, the norms used to assess a person's fitness level vary depending on whether the person just exercises for health or wants to achieve optimal athletic performance. Indeed, when evaluating anyone's fitness, you must use appropriate tests and norms for that person's age, sex, medical status, and training objectives. For example, the tests and norms selected to gauge the fitness of a professional athlete would be far more rigorous than those used to evaluate the success of a health-related fitness program for a 50-year-old business executive.

Moreover, it also must be considered that some tests have specific limitations. For example, tests used to estimate maximal oxygen consumption have not been validated to determine the extremely high maximal oxygen consumption of endurance athletes. Use of these tests to estimate maximal oxygen consumption in endurance athletes results in a substantial amount of error. Additionally, these tests are not accurate enough to track the small changes in maximal oxygen consumption throughout a training year or season in endurance athletes. Some tests, due to the type of information obtained, are not appropriate for certain populations. Performing a stress test involving an electrocardiogram (ECG) in an apparently healthy competitive athlete would typically provide little useful information. An ECG would be appropriate, however, in an elderly person with a history of chest pain. All tests have an inherent risk of injury. This is especially true when testing requires maximal effort testing of individuals at increased risk for disease or individuals recovering from a previous injury. Thus, appropriate safety precautions need to be taken during physical testing. Information concerning test selection and chance of injury should be considered when choosing tests for a specific person or population. The purpose of this chapter is not to provide an exact test protocol or testing procedure for the tests discussed, but rather to provide information concerning the types of tests typically performed and interpretation of test results.

MUSCULAR WORK VERSUS POWER

The terms *work* and *power* are often times used interchangeably among laypersons, and even athletes and coaches, but they should not be. They represent different functional capacities of skeletal muscle and can translate into different athletic abilities.

Work

The term **work** is defined as force exerted over a distance; as a formula, it is presented as follows:

$$\text{work} = \text{force} \times \text{distance} \tag{1}$$

Thus, work necessarily includes movement of an object over a distance and, typically, the movement of body parts through a range of motion. Technically, because work requires movement over a distance (see Box 13-1), no work is performed during a muscle action when no movement occurs (isometric action), although energy (adenosine triphosphate [ATP]) is being expended.

The proper units used to quantify the amount of work done are joules (J). A single joule represents 1 Newton (N, 1 kgm = 9.81 N) of force exerted over a distance of 1 meter. Many times in exercise science, however, work is expressed in units such as the kilopond (Kp) or the kilogram-meter (kg × m). These terms are derived from standard mechanically braked cycle ergometers, which traditionally have been used to quantify exercise performance. With these ergometers, a single complete revolution of the flywheel covers a distance of 6 meters. Many cycle ergometry tests are conducted at a pedaling rate of 50 revolutions per minute (rpm); so if 1 kilogram of resistance is applied to the flywheel, the work produced during 1 minute is 300 kg·m·min^{-1} (i.e., 50 rpm × 6 m × 1 kg). This work rate of 300 kg·m·min^{-1}, or 300 kgm, is also quantified as a single kilopond or 1 Kp. Although steeped in tradition and still regularly reported, these units are inconsistent with the terminology put forth in the Système International d'Unités (SI), which has been adopted internationally by the scientific community to standardize units of measurement. As with scientists from other academic disciplines, exercise scientists should express work in joules.

Power

Unlike work, the assessment of **power** involves a time factor; thus, the rate at which work is performed indicates power. The formula used to define power is as follows:

$$\text{power} = \frac{\text{force} \times \text{distance}}{\text{time}} \text{ or, alternatively,}$$
$$\text{power} = \text{force} \times \text{velocity} \tag{2}$$

Thus, the more rapidly a given amount of work can be performed, the greater the power exhibited. According to the SI, the units in which power is expressed are watts (W, 1 W = 1 J·s^{-1}).

For a real-life example of the difference between work and power, consider the following: two people lifting the same weight off the ground for the same distance have performed an identical amount of work. However, if one person was able to complete the task in less time, then

Box 13-1 PRACTICAL QUESTIONS FROM STUDENTS

How are Work and Power Calculated during a Physical Task Like Lifting a Weight or Running Up a Hill?

To calculate work and power the resistance moved, the distance the resistance is moved and time needed to perform the task must be known. First let us calculate the work and power when performing an arm curl when an individual lifts 20 kilograms (44 lb) 63 centimeters vertically (0.63 meters, 25 inches) in 3 seconds. Note that this calculation ignores the mass of the person's forearm.

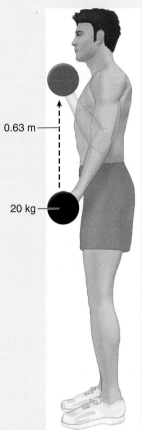

$1\ kgm = 9.81\ joules\ (J)$
$work = force \times distance$
$work = 20\ kg \times 0.63\ m$

$work = 12.6\ kgm$
$work = 12.6\ kgm \times 9.81\ J \cdot kg \cdot m^{-1}$
$work = 123.6\ J$
$1\ watt = 1\ J \cdot s^{-1}$

$$power = \frac{force \times distance}{time} = \frac{work}{time}$$

$$power = \frac{123.6\ J}{3\ sec}$$

$power = 41.2\ watts$

When someone runs, uphill force is equivalent to their body mass, and the vertical distance uphill needs to be known. For example, if a 75-kilogram (165 lb) person runs uphill a vertical distance of 3.67 meters (4 yards, 1 meter = 1.09 yards) in 10 seconds, work and power would be calculated as follows:

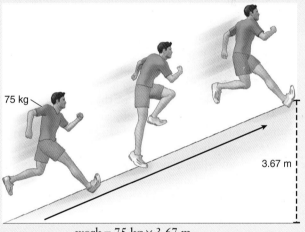

$work = 75\ kg \times 3.67\ m$
$work = 275.25\ kgm$
$work = 275.25\ kgm \times 9.81\ J \cdot kg \cdot m^{-1}$
$work = 2700.2\ J$

$$power = \frac{2700.2\ J}{10\ sec}$$

$power = 270.02\ watts$

that individual demonstrated a greater degree of power. In most sports and athletic events, power is considered to be more critical to success than strength or ability to do work. For example, all competitors at a shot put event are strong enough to do the work of moving the weight of the shot the distance from the starting point, where it is lodged under the chin with a flexed arm, to the point of release, where the arm is fully extended. But it is the athlete who can do that work most rapidly who will ultimately propel the shot the farthest distance before it lands. Power is sometimes referred to as "explosive strength," and in sports

and activities that feature dynamic movements, it is typically valued more than strength.

Although some of the determinants of power are genetically derived—those with a high percentage of fast-twitch muscle fibers (type II) tend to be better power athletes—training can also be used to enhance the power capacity of muscle. Yet, athletes and their conditioning coaches must bear in mind that developing power generally requires different strategies than strength training. That is, strength training entails lifting heavy resistances of 70% to 100% of one's maximum voluntary contraction,

Quick Review

- Testing of a physiological response or ability is performed for many reasons, including determining initial fitness levels, tracking changes in fitness levels, or for diagnostic purposes.
- The type of test chosen depends greatly on the person being tested and the physiological characteristic for which information is desired.
- The terms *work* and *power* represent different functional capacities of skeletal muscle and can translate into different athletic abilities.
- The term *work* is defined as force exerted over a distance; as a formula, it is presented as work = force × distance.
- The assessment of power involves a time factor; thus, the rate at which work is performed indicates power. The formula used to define power is:

$$power = \frac{force \times distance}{time}$$

or, alternatively,

$$power = force \times velocity$$

or the 1-repetition maximum (1-RM). On the other hand, training for power uses lighter resistances—30% to 60% of 1-RM—allowing for faster movements that should not include opposing or braking contractions to slow down movement toward the end of the range of motion. To reiterate: when testing the efficacy of conditioning programs to enhance the functional capacity of muscle, it is essential to distinguish between the ability of the muscle to perform work and display power. Similarly, it is important to use proper units of measurement, as defined by the SI, for those two parameters: joules to quantify work and watts to quantify power.

CARDIOVASCULAR ENDURANCE TESTS

Cardiovascular endurance is one of the oldest and most commonly measured physiological parameters in exercise science. It is normally quantified as the maximal amount of oxygen consumed in mitochondrial respiration during prolonged maximal exercise. The measure most commonly associated with cardiovascular endurance is maximal oxygen consumption ($\dot{V}O_{2max}$), also referred to as maximal aerobic power or aerobic capacity. It is an important measure because it is an indicator of not only endurance capabilities for athletes but also for health status, and it is a predictor of mortality in both healthy and diseased populations.[8,31] For example, even a slight a reduction (3.5 mL·kg^{-1}·min^{-1}) in diseased people decreases survival rates by approximately 12%.[31] There also appears to be a minimal $\dot{V}O_{2max}$ (13 mL·kg^{-1}·min^{-1}) necessary to maintain independent living.[40] Because of its relationship to not only endurance

performance, but also mortality and ability to maintain independent living, $\dot{V}O_{2max}$ is tested in a wide variety of people, from elite endurance athletes to diseased populations and seniors.

Although $\dot{V}O_{2max}$ does represent maximal ability of the cardiorespiratory system, other measures, including heart rate, blood pressure, ECG, and oxygen consumption at submaximal workloads, also represent cardiorespiratory function. So, these measures are many times also determined when testing cardiovascular endurance, especially if the test is being performed for diagnostic purposes, such as determination or treatment of cardiovascular disease. The type of test performed depends on the purpose of the test, the person being tested, and the equipment, facilities, and personnel available to perform the test.

In a laboratory setting, the **graded exercise test (GXT)** is most commonly used to determine both $\dot{V}O_{2max}$ and submaximal values of any desired cardiovascular variable, but it can also be estimated (Box 13-2). In this test, the workload performed is gradually increased, typically using a treadmill or bicycle ergometer. There are also field tests of cardiovascular endurance, which require substantially less equipment and are therefore less expensive than laboratory tests. Results of cardiovascular endurance tests are used to judge initial fitness levels, monitor fitness levels or physiological changes due to training or a disease state, and to prescribe physical training. In the following sections, common protocols and variables determined during both laboratory and field tests of cardiovascular endurance will be discussed.

Laboratory Tests

Cardiovascular endurance or GXT laboratory tests are typically performed using either a bicycle ergometer or a motorized treadmill. Generally, $\dot{V}O_{2max}$ values are approximately 10% higher during treadmill running compared with bicycle ergometry.[17]

With some populations, other equipment can be used. For example, rowers and swimmers may use a rowing ergometer or a swim flume, respectively. This alternative equipment is used because a person who has trained using a particular mode of exercise may achieve a higher $\dot{V}O_{2max}$ using that mode of exercise compared with other types of exercise. Additionally, information from the test (heart rate at a specific workload) that can be used for prescribing training will be more accurate if obtained using the person's typical form of exercise.

Another consideration is contraindications to a certain type of exercise. A senior may have orthopedic problems, such as arthritic knees, contraindicating treadmill exercise. In this case, the exercise scientist may choose bicycle ergometry. Or, if the arthritic problems are very severe, the person may perform some type of arm ergometry. Bicycle ergometry may also be appropriate if the person has postural instability while walking or running, or a neuromuscular disease. Treadmill protocols are generally more appropriate

Box 13-2 PRACTICAL QUESTIONS FROM STUDENTS

Can $\dot{V}O_{2max}$ *Be Predicted Without Doing Any Physical Test?*

$\dot{V}O_{2max}$ of college-age people can be predicted using nonexercise data. Using nonexercise data to predict $\dot{V}O_{2max}$ is useful when screening large groups of people. The prediction involves using information obtained by a questionnaire to estimate physical activity levels, which is then used to predict $\dot{V}O_{2max}$. Participants are asked to complete the following questionnaire.

A. Physical Activity Rating (PA-R)

Select the number that best describes your overall level of physical activity for the previous 6 months:

0. **inactive:** avoid walking or exertion, always use elevator, drive when possible instead of walking
1. **light activity:** walk for pleasure, routinely use stairs, occasionally exercise sufficiently to cause heavy breathing or perspiration
2. **moderate activity:** 10 to 60 minutes per week of moderate activity such as golf, horseback riding, calisthenics, table tennis, bowling, weightlifting, yard work, cleaning house, walking for exercise
3. **moderate activity:** over 1 hour per week of moderate activity described above
4. **vigorous activity:** run less than 1 mile per week, or spend less than 30 minutes per week in comparable activity such as running or jogging, lap swimming, cycling, rowing, aerobics, skipping rope, running in place, or engaging in vigorous aerobic-type activity such as soccer, basketball, tennis, racquetball, or handball
5. **vigorous activity:** run 1 mile to less than 5 miles per week, or spend 30 minutes to less than 60 minutes per week in comparable physical activity as described above
6. **vigorous activity:** run 5 miles to less than 10 miles per week, or spend 1 hour to less than 3 hours per week in comparable activity as described above
7. **vigorous activity:** run 10 miles to less than 15 miles per week, or spend 3 hours to less than 6 hours per week in comparable activity as described above
8. **vigorous activity:** run 15 miles to less than 20 miles per week, or spend 6 hours to less than 7 hours per week in comparable activity as described above
9. **vigorous activity:** run 20 to 25 miles per week, or spend 7 hours to less than 8 hours per week in comparable activity as described above
10. **vigorous activity:** run over 25 miles per week, or spend over 8 hours per week in comparable physical activity as described above

B. Perceived Functional Ability (PFA) Questions

Suppose you exercise continuously on an indoor track for 1 mile. Which exercise pace is right for you: not too easy or not too hard? Circle the appropriate number from 1 to 13.

1. Walking at a slow pace (18-minute mile or more)
2.
3. Walking at a medium pace (16-minute mile)
4.
5. Walking at a fast pace (14-minute mile)
6.
7. Jogging at a slow pace (12-minute mile)
8.
9. Jogging at a medium pace (10-minute mile)
10.
11. Jogging at a fast pace (8-minute mile)
12.
13. Running at a fast pace (7-minute mile or less)

How fast could you cover a distance of 3 miles and **not** become breathless or overly fatigued? Be realistic. Circle the appropriate number from 1 to 13.

1. I could walk the entire distance at a slow pace (18-minute mile or more)
2.
3. I could walk the entire distance at a medium pace (16-minute mile)
4.
5. I could walk the entire distance at a fast pace (14-minute mile)
6.
7. I could jog the entire distance at a slow pace (12-minute mile)
8.
9. I could jog the entire distance at a medium pace (10-minute mile)
10.
11. I could jog the entire distance at a fast pace (8-minute mile)
12.
13. I could run the entire distance at a fast pace (7-minute mile or less)

In addition to the answers to the above questionnaire, several other pieces of information are needed:

Sex (female = 0; male = 1)
Body mass index (BMI): BMI = body mass (kg)·body height^{-1} (m^2)

The following equation is then used to predict $\dot{V}O_{2max}$:

$$\dot{V}O_{2max} \ (mL \cdot kg^{-1} \cdot min^{-1}) = 44.895 + (7.042 \times sex) - (0.823 \times BMI) + (0.738 \times PFA) + (0.688 \times PA\text{-}R)$$

For example, a male, 165 lb (75 kilograms), 5 feet, 10 inches tall (1.79 meters) with a PA-R of 6 and PFA of 18 (9 + 9) would have a predicted $\dot{V}O_{2max}$ of

$$BMI = 75/(1.79 \times 1.79)$$
$$BMI = 24.6$$
$$\dot{V}O_{2max} \ (mL \cdot kg^{-1} \cdot min^{-1}) = 44.895 + (7.042 \times 1)$$
$$- (0.823 \times 24.6) + (0.738 \times 18) + (0.688 \times 6)$$
$$\dot{V}O_{2max} \ (mL \cdot kg^{-1} \cdot min^{-1}) = 49.10 \ mL \cdot kg^{-1} \cdot min^{-1}$$

Reprinted with permission from George LD, Stone WJ, Burkett LN. Nonexercise $\dot{V}O_{2max}$ estimation for physically active college students. Med Sci Sports Exerc. 1997;29:415–423.

because most people are more familiar with walking and running than with cycling exercise. Additionally, if a person is not familiar with or trained in cycling, cycling exercise may result in local muscular fatigue of the legs prior to reaching $\dot{V}O_{2max}$ or prior to adequately stressing the cardiovascular system for diagnostic purposes.

Besides the type of exercise to perform during a GXT, one must consider the protocol or manner in which exercise intensity is increased during the test. During a **continuous protocol** exercise test, intensity is increased in stages with no rest or break between stages. Continuous protocols are the most widely used. During a **discontinuous protocol**, exercise intensity is increased in stages, but with a short rest period between stages. Discontinuous protocols are useful in some situations, such as among patient populations who cannot tolerate continued exercise at ever increasing intensities. If patients can tolerate continuous protocols, however, they are preferred.

Whether a continuous or discontinuous protocol is used, the initial workload will vary depending on who is being tested. For example, a cardiovascular patient may achieve a final workload that is less than the initial workload of a trained athlete. Each workload in a continuous or discontinuous protocol is generally 2 to 3 minutes in length. This time frame is usually long enough for the cardiovascular system to achieve a steady state (see Chapter 5), if possible. Achievement of steady state is necessary if the test is to be used in the prescription of training intensity for either an athlete or a patient. However, if the major goal of the test is determining $\dot{V}O_{2max}$, achieving steady state at submaximal workloads is not a necessity.

How much the workload is increased during each stage of a test is also a consideration. For healthy individuals or athletes one can increase the workload in larger increments than for those with a disease, such as cardiovascular disease or diabetes, or who are involved in a cardiac rehabilitation program. Large increments in workload with each stage, or per minute, result in fast protocols, and small increments in workload result in slow protocols. Both fast and slow protocols may decrease $\dot{V}O_{2max}$ compared with intermediate protocols, which are 8 to 12 minutes in length. Fast protocols have been suggested to result in early termination of a GXT due to insufficient muscular strength to tolerate the large work rate increases during the final stages of a test. This results in an underestimation of $\dot{V}O_{2max}$.[12] On the other hand, slow protocols may result in increased core temperature and decreased motivation to continue the test. Increased core temperature results in redistribution of blood flow to the skin as opposed to active muscle. These factors may also result in a decreased $\dot{V}O_{2max}$. Thus, tests to elicit $\dot{V}O_{2max}$ should be between 8 and 12 minutes in length. However, $\dot{V}O_{2max}$ cycle ergometry tests lasting between 7 and 26 minutes and treadmill tests lasting between 5 and 26 minutes result in valid $\dot{V}O_{2max}$ determinations.[32] A caveat of these test time frames is that short tests are preceded by an adequate warm-up and that treadmill grades do not exceed 15%.

The choice of exercise mode and test protocol for either submaximal or maximal cardiovascular endurance determination can vary depending on the major goals of the test. The choice of mode of exercise and test protocol needs to be made based on the population being tested (cardiac patients, athletes), major purpose ($\dot{V}O_{2max}$, diagnose cardiovascular disease), equipment, and testing personnel available. In the next sections, typical protocols for cycle ergometry and treadmill tests, the two most common types of tests, are described.

Treadmill Protocols

Many treadmill protocols have been developed for various populations. Treadmill protocols increase workload by increasing velocity, grade, or a combination of these two factors (Fig. 13-1). Graded running tests give the highest $\dot{V}O_{2max}$, followed by running tests at 0% grade, and then walking tests. During running treadmill tests, it can be difficult to obtain valid measures of blood pressure and

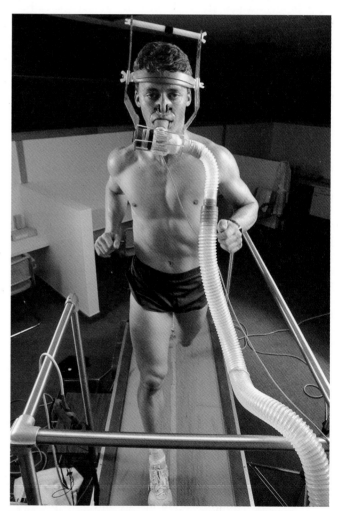

Figure 13-1. Treadmill protocols increase the workload by either increasing velocity or the percent grade. The increment in workload and how quickly workload is elevated depends on the purpose of the test.

Table 13-1.	**Balke Treadmill Protocol**			
Stage	**Speed (miles·hr⁻¹)**	**Speed (km·hr⁻¹)**	**Grade (%)**	**Duration (min)**
1	3.3	5.3	0	1
2	3.3	5.3	2	1
3–25	3.3	5.3	Increase 1%/min	1 at each % grade
26	3.5	5.62	25	1
27 and higher	Increase 0.2 each stage	Increase 0.32 each stage	25	1 at each speed increase

Table 13-2.	**Bruce Treadmill Protocol**			
Stage	**Speed (miles·hr⁻¹)**	**Speed (km·hr⁻¹)**	**Grade (%)**	**Duration (min)**
0	1.7	2.7	0	3
0.5	1.7	2.7	5	3
1	1.7	2.7	10	3
2	2.5	4.0	12	3
3	3.4	5.4	14	3
4	4.2	6.7	16	3
5	5.0	8.0	18	3
6	5.5	8.8	20	3
7	6.0	9.6	22	3

Stages 0 and 0.5 are additions to the original protocol and are termed the modified Bruce treadmill protocol.

artifact in an ECG is increased. These factors limit the use of running tests for some diagnostic procedures. Holding onto the hand rails of a treadmill should not be allowed during testing, unless needed to maintain balance, as this significantly lowers physiological stress, which is indicated by a significant decrease in heart rate.

The Balke test[4] is a widely used walking GXT (Table 13-1), especially in clinical settings in which patients have low cardiovascular and functional capabilities. Its popularity in clinical settings is due to its initial low workload and gradual increase in workload. The speed is 3.3 miles·hr⁻¹ (5.3 km·hr⁻¹) and the initial grade 0%. The speed is held constant, but the grade is increased to 2% after the first minute and increased 1% every 2 minutes until a grade of 25% is reached. Thereafter, the grade is held at 25% with speed increased 0.2 miles·hr⁻¹ (0.32 km·hr⁻¹) each minute. This protocol yields valid $\dot{V}o_{2max}$ values for people who are less fit cardiovascularly, but for those who have greater cardiovascular fitness, the test duration becomes very long. Some patients also complain about local muscular discomfort, especially of the lower back and calf muscles, which may limit their ability to achieve a true $\dot{V}o_{2max}$.

Another GXT, the Bruce protocol, is perhaps the most widely used treadmill testing procedure (Table 13-2).[41] With this protocol, both speed and grade are changed every 3 minutes (stages 1–7). This results in a relatively quick and large increase in workload, resulting in volitional fatigue in a short period of time. The relatively large initial worked and fast increase in workload makes the test inappropriate for those who are less fit cardiovascularly, such as those suffering from chronic diseases. To make the test more appropriate for those who are less fit, it was modified by adding lower initial workloads (stages 0 and 0.5). Both versions of the Bruce protocol are appropriate for normal, healthy, or moderately fit people.

Many treadmill protocols have been developed, and no doubt more will be developed in the future for specific populations and purposes. The initial workload, elevation in workload, and whether increased workload is achieved by an increase in speed or grade depend on the population being tested and purpose of the test. A commonly used treadmill protocol to establish maximal oxygen uptake in healthy individuals is presented in Table 13-3.

Cycle Ergometry Protocols

$\dot{V}o_{2max}$ is typically 5% to 25% lower during cycle ergometry compared with treadmill running.[41] However, testing specificity for cyclists and triathletes may be important if the goal of the test is to monitor sport-specific fitness or assist with training program design (Fig. 13-2). Cycle ergometry is also more appropriate for those with postural instability or other contraindications to treadmill exercise, such as arthritic problems of the legs. Furthermore, cycle ergometry also offers some other advantages over treadmill protocols, such as ability to monitor blood

Table 13-3. Treadmill Testing Protocol to Determine $\dot{V}o_{2max}$ in Healthy Young Adults					
Time (min)	**Grade (%)**	**Speed (males) (mph)**	**Speed (male runners) (mph)**	**Speed (females) (mph)**	**Speed (female runners) (mph)**
0–2	0	8.0	8.5	7.0	7.5
2–4	2	8.0	8.5	7.0	7.5
4–6	4	8.0	8.5	7.0	7.5
6–8	6	8.0	8.5	7.0	7.5
8–10	8	8.0	8.5	7.0	7.5
10–12	10	8.0	8.5	7.0	7.5
12–14	12	8.0	8.5	7.0	7.5

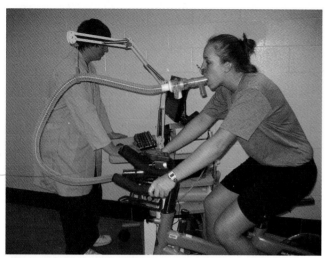

Figure 13-2. Cycle ergometry typically results in lower V̇o₂max values than treadmill exercise. However, it offers several advantages compared to treadmill exercise, such as testing specificity for cycling athletes and small increments in workload, as well as being more appropriate for people with postural instability.

Table 13-4.	Cycle Ergometer Testing Protocol to Determine $\dot{V}O_{2max}$ in Healthy Young Adults			
Time (min)	**Power Output (Untrained)**		**Power Output (Trained)**	
	kpm	**W**	**kpm**	**W**
0–2	300	50	600	100
2–4	600	100	900	150
4–6	900	150	1200	200
6–8	1100	180	1500	250
8–10	1300	215	1800	300
10–12	1500	250	2100	350
12–14	1700	280	2400	400

pressure easily, less ECG artifact, and small increments in workload.

During treadmill exercise, a person must carry his or her body mass; thus, body mass does affect the workload. However, during cycle ergometry, the workload depends on the resistance to peddling and the revolutions per minute of peddling and is independent of a person's body mass. For example, if the workload requires a $\dot{V}O_2$ of 2000 mL O_2 per minute, this represents a $\dot{V}O_{2max}$ of 40 mL·kg⁻¹·min⁻¹ for a 50-kilogram person, but only 26.6 mL·kg⁻¹·min⁻¹ for a 75-kilogram person. Workload during ergometry can be increased in small increments, but the increment in workload may be large for an unfit or lighter person relative to a fit or heavier person. If the workload was increased 25 Watts (150 kg·m·min⁻¹), it would require a change in $\dot{V}O_2$ of 27 mL·min⁻¹. The better a person's cardiovascular fitness, the smaller the cardiovascular adjustments necessary to accommodate the increase in workload. Conversely, the more unfit a person is, the greater the cardiovascular adjustments necessary to accommodate the increase in workload.

During ergometry tests for nonathletes, the peddling rate is typically 50 to 60 rpm and the workload is increased in increments of 25 Watts (150 kg·m·min⁻¹) every 2 to 3 minutes. For athletes, the rpm is typically higher (70–100 rpm) and the increments in workload can be greater. If the test is performed using a mechanical ergometer, the rpm must be held constant. However, if an electronically braked ergometer is used, rpm can vary at a particular workload as the ergometer will adjust the resistance to maintain a constant workload. Arm ergometry can be performed by those who cannot perform leg exercise, such as disabled people. During arm ergometry tests, $\dot{V}O_{2max}$ is generally 20% to 30% less than during treadmill exercise and workloads are increased in smaller increments (12.5 Watts,

75 kg·m·min⁻¹) because of the smaller muscle mass involved in arm ergometry compared with leg exercise.[41]

Cycle ergometry can also be used to determine submaximal and maximal cardiovascular and other responses. Similar to treadmill protocols, cycle ergometry protocols can be developed to meet the testing needs of various populations. Cycle ergometry does offer some advantages (e.g., greater safety, small increments in workload) over treadmill exercise that make cycle ergometry a better testing mode for some populations. Table 13-4 depicts protocols using cycling ergometry to determine maximal oxygen uptake in both healthy untrained and trained people.

Typical Maximal Oxygen Consumption Values

Maximal oxygen consumption typically is expressed relative to a person's body mass (mL·kg⁻¹·min⁻¹). $\dot{V}O_{2max}$ relative to body mass is important for performance to most athletes because they must carry their body mass during competition and training. Relative to body mass, international-class endurance athletes have the highest $\dot{V}O_{2max}$ values. Female and male international-class athletes, such as elite marathon runners and cross-country skiers, have $\dot{V}O_{2max}$ values as high as approximately 75 and 85 mL·kg⁻¹·min⁻¹, respectively. A few elite male endurance athletes achieve values as high as 94 to 96 mL·kg⁻¹·min⁻¹. Normative values for $\dot{V}O_{2max}$ for males and females ranging in age from 20 to 60 years are presented in Table 13-5. Maintaining a minimal $\dot{V}O_{2max}$ is important because a $\dot{V}O_{2max}$ below the 20th percentile is associated with a sedentary lifestyle and an increased risk of death from all causes.[9] $\dot{V}O_{2max}$, whether obtained from a laboratory test or a field test (field tests are discussed in subsequent sections), can be compared with the normative values presented in Table 13-5.

Table 13-5. Percentile Values for Maximal Aerobic Power

Percentile	$\dot{V}O_{2max}$ (mL·kg⁻¹·min⁻¹) by Age Range (Years)				
	20–29	30–39	40–49	50–59	60+
Men					
90	55.1	52.1	50.6	49.0	44.2
80	52.1	50.6	49.0	44.2	41.0
70	49.0	47.4	45.8	41.0	37.8
60	47.4	44.2	44.2	39.4	36.2
50	44.2	42.6	41.0	37.8	34.6
40	42.6	41.0	39.4	36.2	33.0
30	41.0	39.4	36.2	34.6	31.4
20	37.8	36.2	34.6	31.4	28.3
10	34.6	33.0	31.4	29.9	26.7
Women					
90	49.0	45.8	42.6	37.8	34.6
80	44.2	41.0	39.4	34.6	33.0
70	41.0	39.4	36.2	33.0	31.4
60	39.4	36.2	34.6	31.4	28.3
50	37.8	34.6	33.0	29.9	26.7
40	36.2	33.0	31.4	28.3	25.1
30	33.0	31.4	29.9	26.7	23.5
20	31.4	29.9	28.3	25.1	21.9
10	28.3	26.7	25.1	21.9	20.3

Reprinted with permission from American College of Sports Medicine. ACSM's Guidelines for Exercise Testing and Prescription, 7th ed. Philadelphia, PA: Lippincott Williams & Wilkins; 2005.

Heart Rate Measurement

Heart rate is used extensively as an indicator of aerobic exercise intensity and is useful in formulating aerobic exercise prescription (see Chapter 12). It is used extensively because it is noninvasive and convenient, especially due to the availability of accurate and reliable heart rate monitors. Heart rate is useful from a physiological perspective as an indicator of aerobic exercise intensity and aerobic or cardiovascular fitness because of several relationships:

- With increased aerobic fitness, resting heart rate and heart rate at an absolute submaximal workload decrease.
- Heart rate has a general linear relationship to $\dot{V}O_2$.

- Heart rate has a general linear relationship to mechanical power output, workload, and exercise intensity.

Long-term aerobic training and, to some extent, resistance training result in a decreased resting heart rate (see Chapter 12). A low resting heart rate or a decrease in resting heart rate due to training is generally accepted as an indicator of increased aerobic fitness. A decrease in resting heart rate with the maintenance of cardiac output is possible only if stroke volume increases (see Chapter 5) because cardiac output = heart rate × stroke volume. Thus, even though heart rate decreases, cardiac output is maintained because of an increase in stroke volume. This maintains blood supply, delivery of oxygen and nutrients, and removal of waste products from tissues despite a decrease in heart rate. Resting heart rate values of both men and women have a considerable range (Table 13-6), with the lowest values of approximately 35 bpm typically shown by international class aerobic athletes, such as marathon runners and road cyclists. The greater the aerobic or cardiovascular fitness of a person, the lower his or her heart rate at any given absolute (same power output) submaximal workload. Thus, a person in better aerobic fitness will have a lower heart rate than a less fit person at the same absolute submaximal workload, and aerobic training will result in a decrease in heart rate at a given absolute submaximal workload.

Heart rate's linear relationship to $\dot{V}O_2$, mechanical power output, workload, and exercise intensity dictates that heart rate will increase in response to elevations of those variables. There are, however, several factors to consider concerning these relationships. Although heart rate shows a general linear relationship to $\dot{V}O_2$ and exercise intensity, heart rate does not increase in a perfect linear fashion as exercise intensity increases. Heart rate plateaus at near maximal exercise intensities as it approaches its maximal value and generally

Table 13-6. Normal Values for Resting Heart Rate

Classification	Resting Heart Rate (bpm)	
	Men	Women
Low	35–56	39–58
Moderately low	57–61	59–63
Less than average	62–65	64–67
Average	66–71	68–72
Greater than average	72–75	73–77
Moderately high	76–81	78–83
High	82–103	84–104

bpm = beats per minute.
Data from Golding L. YMCA Fitness Testing and Assessment Manual. Champaign, IL: Human Kinetics Publishers; 2000.

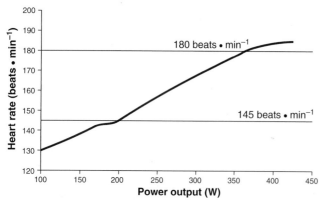

Figure 13-3. Heart rate has a linear relationship to power output only between approximately 145 and 180 bpm or approximately 40% and 80% of the maximal power output during cycle ergometry. Thus, heart rate best represents workload or intensity of aerobic exercise in this range.

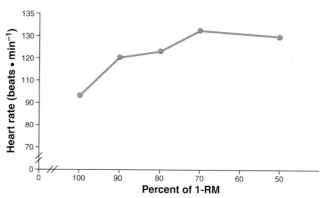

Figure 13-4. The relationship between maximal heart rate during sets of the knee extension exercise to concentric failure demonstrate that heart rate is not a good indicator of weight training intensity expressed as the percentage of one repetition maximum (1-RM). In fact, heart rate is lower when lifting 100% of 1-RM compared to lower percentages of 1-RM. (Data from Fleck SJ, Dean L. Previous resistance training experience and the pressor response during resistance exercise. J Appl Physiol. 1987;63:116–120.)

shows the most predictable and consistent relationship to exercise intensity and $\dot{V}O_2$ between 45% to 50% and 85% to 90% of maximal values.[6] For example, during an incremental exhaustive bicycle ergometry test, heart rate shows a plateau as the maximal workload is approached. The heart-rate-to-power-output relationship is linear only between approximately 145 and 180 bpm or 40% and 80% of the maximal power output (Fig. 13-3).

Some people, such as cardiac patients prescribed drugs such as beta blockers to treat hypertension and lower myocardial oxygen consumption, will demonstrate an abnormal heart-rate-to-aerobic workload or intensity relationship. Beta blockers result in a decreased heart rate at a given submaximal workload of 20% to 30%, depending on dosage, compared with normal and a decrease in maximal heart rate. This factor must be considered for these individuals when interpreting the exercise-intensity-to-heart-rate relationship and when prescribing aerobic exercise.

Heart rate, although a good indicator of aerobic exercise intensity, is not a good indicator of resistance training exercise intensity. Resistance training exercise intensity is many times indicated as a percentage of the maximal weight possible for one-repetition, or 1-RM (see Chapter 12). If the 1-RM for an exercise is lifted, a lower heart rate will result compared with lifting 50% to 90% of 1-RM to **concentric failure**, or performing an exercise until it is impossible to complete a repetition, which normally occurs in the concentric or lifting phase of the repetition. For example, in untrained people, peak heart rate at the end of a set to concentric failure at resistances less than 1-RM results in higher heart rates than 1-RM (Fig. 13-4).

In summary, resting heart rate and heart rate at an absolute submaximal workload can be used as indicators of aerobic fitness. Heart rate can be used as an indicator of aerobic fitness because of its linear relationship to $\dot{V}O_2$ and exercise intensity. However, heart rate is not a good indicator of resistance training exercise intensity.

Blood Pressure Measurement

Blood pressure is the force acting against the artery walls during (systole) and between (diastole) contraction of ventricles. Blood pressure at rest and during activity and the effect of training on blood pressure have already been discussed (see Chapter 5). Recall that higher-than-normal resting blood pressure is termed *hypertension* (see Box 13-3 for more information concerning hypertension), that physical training reduces resting blood pressure, and that during both endurance and strength training, blood pressure

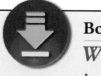

Box 13-3 DID YOU KNOW?
White-Coat Hypertension is Not Benign

White-coat hypertension refers to having high blood pressure when blood pressure is taken in a doctor's office or clinic. It is typically thought to be due to nervousness because of being in a doctor's office. Although nervousness may well explain part of a high-blood-pressure reading while in a doctor's office, white-coat hypertension is not a benign condition. People who demonstrate white-coat hypertension are at greater risk of becoming hypertensive. After 10 years, people who had white-coat hypertension were 2.5 times more likely to develop sustained hypertension (high blood pressure during 24-hour monitoring or taken at home) compared to people who did not demonstrate white-coat hypertension.

Mancia G, Bombelli M, Facchetti R, et al. Long-term risk of sustained hypertension in white-coat or masked hypertension. Hypertension. 2009;54:226–232.

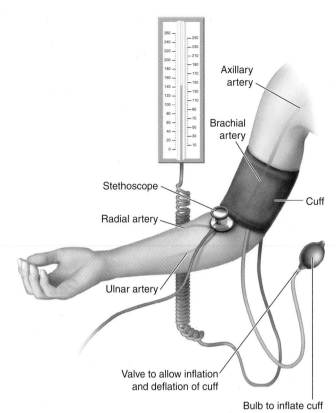

Figure 13-5. The typical arrangement to determine blood pressure by auscultation using an aneroid sphygmomanometer is shown. The cuff can be inflated and deflated using a rubber bulb and valve. The stethoscope is used to listen for the Korotkoff sounds.

increases, with the increase being greater during resistance training.

Blood pressure is normally measured in the brachial artery of the upper arm. Thus, normally, systemic blood pressure and not pulmonary blood pressure, which is substantially lower, is measured. Additionally, blood pressure varies throughout the systemic circulation, with the highest pressures within the aorta and the lowest within veins. Blood pressure is normally obtained using **auscultation**: listening for sounds from organs or tissue to aid in diagnosis of normal or abnormal function. Auscultation to measure blood pressure is accomplished using a **sphygmomanometer**, an instrument consisting of a pressure gauge and an inflatable rubber cuff, in conjunction with a stethoscope (Fig. 13-5). When the rubber cuff is inflated, it compresses the brachial artery and occludes all blood flow. The stethoscope is placed over the brachial artery distally to where flow is occluded. With blood flow occluded, no sound of blood flow can be heard. The pressure within the rubber cuff is then gradually released. As the pressure is released, blood flow through the occluded area will occur only during systole, when blood pressure is the highest. This intermittent blood flow is turbulent and creates a sound normally described as a sharp tapping. This sound is called the first **Korotkoff**

sound and is named after the man who developed this method of determining blood pressure in 1905. As pressure within the cuff is further reduced, turbulent flow decreases, resulting in a muffling of the sound, which is termed the fourth Korotkoff sound. As the pressure is reduced further, smooth or laminar flow occurs during both systole and diastole, resulting in no sound, which is termed the fifth Korotkoff sound. In someone who is normotensive, the first, fourth, and fifth Korotkoff sounds would occur at approximately 120, 90, and 80 mm Hg, with the first and fifth Korotkoff sounds representing systolic and diastolic blood pressure, respectively.

There are several types of sphygmomanometers. The American Heart Association regards a mercury sphygmomanometer as the most accurate and valid to measure blood pressure.[35] However, the aneroid sphygmomanometer, or pressure gauge sphygmomanometer, and automated sphygmomanometer are also commonly used. An automated sphygmomanometer automatically inflates and deflates the rubber cuff using a microphone and a computer program to determine the Korotkoff sounds.

In addition to measuring blood pressure at rest to determine whether someone is normotensive, hypotensive, or hypertensive, blood pressure is many times also measured during a stress test and during recovery from a stress test. As discussed above, during activity, blood pressure is most easily determined during a bicycle ergometer stress test as opposed to a treadmill stress test. The normal blood pressure response to a stress test is a gradual increase in systolic pressure with little or no change in diastolic blood pressure (Fig. 13-6). The systolic blood pressure

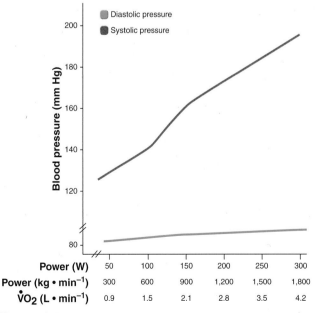

Power (W)	50	100	150	200	250	300
Power (kg • min⁻¹)	300	600	900	1,200	1,500	1,800
$\dot{V}O_2$ (L • min⁻¹)	0.9	1.5	2.1	2.8	3.5	4.2

Figure 13-6. The normal blood pressure response to cycle ergometry is depicted. Systolic blood pressure (*red line*) gradually increases as exercise workload increases while diastolic blood pressure (*blue line*) increases very little or not at all.

during cycle ergometry typically increases 6 to 9 mm Hg per 50 W of increased workload.[37] If the systolic blood pressure response is exaggerated or diastolic blood pressure increases substantially, an abnormal response to exercise is indicated. For example, normotensive adults typically reach a systolic pressure of 180 to 190 mm Hg during aerobic or endurance type exercise. If systolic pressure exceeds 240 mm Hg, it may indicate a susceptibility to hypertension. If systolic pressure decreases more than 10 mm Hg with an increase in workload or if it drops below the value obtained in the same position prior to testing, the test should be terminated as this may indicate a myocardial ischemic response.[37] Blood pressure often returns to preexercise levels within 5 to 8 minutes after cessation of exercise. However, it is not unusual for systolic blood pressure to drop temporarily to slightly below pre-exercise levels during recovery from exercise.

Exercise testing protocols and obtaining blood pressure measurements are used for diagnostic purposes and have been described extensively.[37] The major goal of obtaining blood pressure at rest, during exercise, and during recovery from exercise is for diagnostic purposes. Abnormal responses during exercise and during recovery from exercise indicate various types of cardiovascular problems, such as a myocardial ischemic response to exercise or a susceptibility to hypertension.

Electrocardiogram Measurement

A 12-lead ECG is typically obtained when stress testing individuals who show signs or symptoms of cardiovascular disease or who are thought to be at higher risk than normal for cardiovascular disease. The waveforms of an ECG represent contraction and relaxation of the cardiac chambers. The height, width, spacing, and shape of the waveforms indicate either normal or abnormal cardiac function (see Chapter 5). When stress testing individuals who are believed to be at increased risk for cardiovascular disease, the ECG is monitored throughout the test and examined for indications of abnormal cardiac function, such as ST-segment depression, which indicates myocardial ischemia (see Fig. 5-7).

Although the ECG is most often used to diagnose cardiovascular disease, it is also used in some situations when testing healthy athletes. For example, one adaptation to physical training is increased left ventricular mass, which is indicated on the ECG by increased height but normal shape of the waveform (QRS), representing ventricular contraction.

Heart rate is expressed as number of beats per minute, but there are variations in the exact time between heartbeats. This means that if the heart rate is 60 beats per minute, a heartbeat does not take place exactly every second. The variation in the time between heartbeats is termed **heart rate variability**. Heart rate variability can be determined by measuring the distance between QRS complexes and may be of value for diagnostic purposes.[5,28] Heart rate variability decreases with age, and low heart rate variability may be associated with increased mortality and may change with training (see Box 13-4). Additionally, changes in heart rate variability may be useful in diagnosing overtraining. Thus, heart rate variability is an aspect of the ECG that may be useful for diagnostic purposes among both sedentary individuals as well as athletes.

Box 13-4 APPLYING RESEARCH
Heart Rate Variability and Recovery Heart Rate

Heart rate variability is the measurement of variation in heart rate by accurately measuring the variation in time between the peak of QRS waveforms or R-R intervals on an ECG. Heart rate variability can be represented as a time component, graphing the R-R intervals (milliseconds) against time (seconds), or as a frequency component (the frequency at which the length of the R-R intervals change). Some data indicate heart rate variability increases with training; however, this has not been consistently shown. Heart rate variability may also change with overtraining. The lack of consistent results may relate to which measure of heart rate variability is being used and when heart rate variability is being determined. For example, either the time component or the frequency component could be determined at rest, during submaximal or maximal exercise and during recovery from exercise. Heart rate variability does show promise as a measure of training status and possibly to determine or predict if an athlete is overtrained. However, before any firm conclusions can be reached, further research is needed.

Recovery heart rate refers to how quickly heart rate returns toward resting values after an exercise bout. An increase in heart rate recovery, or returning to resting heart rate in a shorter period of time, is an adaptation to physical training, especially aerobic training. In contrast, a decrease in recovery heart rate is clearly associated with an increase in mortality. Thus, a decrease in resting heart rate and decreased heart rate during submaximal exercise are not the only physiological changes due to training or increased fitness.

Borresen J, Lambert MI. Autonomic control of heart rate during and after exercise measurements and implications for monitoring training status. Sports Med. 2008;38:1633–1646.

Perceived Exertion Measurement

The rating of perceived exertion (RPE) is a psychophysiological measure of exercise intensity. The RPE scale was developed by the Swedish psychologist Gunnar Borg and brought to the attention of exercise scientists in the United States by Bruce Noble, a professor and exercise physiologist at the University of Pittsburg. The classical RPE 6 to 20 scale provided a subjective, yet useful and easily obtainable, estimate of physical exertion during exercise.[11] The classical scale of 6 to 20 was intended to correspond to the person's heart rate (when multiplied by 10) and thus also corresponds to oxygen uptake during GXTs. Although RPE is a nonphysiological estimate of exercise intensity, research has found it to be a reliable tool and that the 6 to 20 scale corresponds with other more precise physiological indicators of cardiovascular and metabolic stress, as seen in Table 13-7. During graded exercise tests, RPE ratings should be obtained from the subject during the last 15 seconds of each stage, or workload. In addition, the key to optimal use of RPE scales is giving proper instructions to the patient or subject.

Test Termination Criteria

Exercise tests may be terminated for either clinical indications of an abnormal response or, if testing apparently healthy individuals or athletes, when physiological responses indicate that a maximal effort has been attained. When exercise testing is performed in a clinical setting, the test may be terminated due to a contraindication for continued exercise or due to volitional fatigue. Contraindications to exercise include any abnormal response to the exercise stress, such as the following:

- Angina or chest pain indicating myocardial ischemia
- Abnormal blood pressure response (as discussed above)
- Abnormal ECG response (as discussed above)
- Discomfort or pain in the extremities (normally the legs) indicating intermittent claudication (discussed further in Chapter 12 under "Peripheral Artery Disease")
- **Dyspnea**, or difficulty in breathing or labored breathing
- Dizziness or **syncope**

Table 13-7. RPE Scale and Associated Physiological Responses

RPE Scale	% Maximal Heart Rate	% $\dot{V}O_{2max}$	Blood Lactate (mmol·L^{-1})
6			
7 Very, very light			
8			
9 Very light			
10			
11 Fairly light	35–54	25–44	
12			
13 Somewhat hard	55–69	45–59	
14			
15 Hard	70–89	60–84	2.5
16			
17 Very hard	>90	≥85	
18			4.0
19 Very, very hard			
20	100	100	

Reprinted with permission from Tipton CM, ed. ACSM's Advanced Exercise Physiology. Baltimore: Lippincott Williams & Wilkins; 2006.

 Quick Review

- Cardiovascular endurance is normally quantified as the maximal amount of oxygen consumed in mitochondrial respiration during maximal exercise.
- Cardiovascular endurance can be tested in the laboratory setting with a graded exercise test.
- Many protocols exist to administer a graded exercise test. These protocols typically use a bicycle ergometer or a motorized treadmill.
- Heart rate is extensively used as an indicator of aerobic exercise intensity and is useful in formulating aerobic exercise prescription.
- Blood pressure is obtained during a stress test as an indicator of abnormal cardiovascular response.
- A 12-lead ECG is typically obtained when stress testing individuals showing signs or symptoms of cardiovascular disease or thought to be at higher risk than normal for cardiovascular disease.
- Perceived exertion (RPE) is used as an indicator of cardiovascular stress due to its relationship to other physiological variables (% maximal heart rate, % maximal oxygen consumption, blood lactate).
- In a clinical setting, graded exercise test termination criteria indicate an abnormal response to the exercise stress while test termination criteria for healthy individuals or athletes typically indicate attainment of maximal oxygen consumption.

Box 13-5 DID YOU KNOW?

What is the Error of Measuring Maximal Oxygen Consumption?

When measuring any variable, such as $\dot{V}O_{2max}$, we typically assume that the value determined is correct. If the correct equipment is used and calibrated, this is generally a good assumption. However, measurement of anything has some inherent error. Error in determination of $\dot{V}O_{2max}$ could be either due to technological or equipment error or biological variability due to day-to-day fluctuations in physiology. Determination of $\dot{V}O_{2max}$ several days apart has a variation of 2.2% to 5.6%. Of this variability it has been estimated that 90% is biological and 10% technological in nature. So, $\dot{V}O_{2max}$ determination does have some error. It could be hypothesized that such biological variation may in part explain a "good day" or a "bad day" for an athlete.

Katch VL, Sady SS, Freedson P. Biological variability in maximum aerobic power. Med Sci Sports Exerc. 1982;14:21–25.

Wisen AGM, Wohlfart B. Aerobic and functional capacity in a group of healthy women: Reference values and repeatability. Clin Physiol Funct Imaging. 2004;24:341–351.

The goal of many exercise tests for apparently healthy individuals or athletes is the determination of $\dot{V}O_{2max}$. For these types of tests, the primary indicator that peak oxygen consumption has been achieved is a plateau or slight decrease in oxygen consumption with an increase in workload.[6] For example, less than a 2.1 mL·kg^{-1}·min^{-1} increase in oxygen consumption occurs with an increase in running speed equal to 1 km·hr^{-1}. This indicates that $\dot{V}O_{2max}$ has been achieved, and to continue to perform the exercise, energy must be obtained from anaerobic sources. Even if this primary indicator is not met, $\dot{V}O_{2max}$ may still have been achieved if secondary criteria are met. Secondary criteria of achieving $\dot{V}O_{2max}$ are as follows:

- Blood lactate concentration of 8 to 12 mmol·L^{-1}
- Respiratory exchange ratio greater than 1:1
- Heart rate equal to at least 90% of predicted maximum (see Chapter 12 for equations to predict maximum heart rate)
- Volitional fatigue

One may terminate an exercise test when either clinical contraindications to continued exercise are present or physiological responses in apparently healthy people indicate attainment of peak oxygen consumption or a maximal effort. The criteria used to terminate an exercise test, therefore, depend on the goal of the test and the health status of the person being tested. Despite the fact that the best efforts of a healthy person to achieve $\dot{V}O_{2max}$ and meeting criteria indicating $\dot{V}O_{2max}$ have been reached, there is a small amount of variability in its determination (Box 13-5).

ESTIMATION OF CARDIOVASCULAR ENDURANCE CAPABILITIES

In some testing situations, such as when one needs to test many people quickly or when laboratory equipment to directly measure endurance capabilities is not available, an estimate of $\dot{V}O_{2max}$ may suffice as a measure of endurance capabilities. Estimates of $\dot{V}O_{2max}$ are normally based on the heart rate response to submaximal exercise. This approach works because of several assumptions:

- A general linear relationship exists between heart rate and workload and $\dot{V}O_2$.
- Attaining a maximal workload indicates attaining $\dot{V}O_{2max}$.
- A steady-state heart rate is obtained at each submaximal workload during a test, and this heart rate is consistent from day to day.
- Maximal heart rate for a given age is uniform among individuals.
- $\dot{V}O_2$ at a given workload (mechanical efficiency) is equivalent among individuals.
- Subjects performing a test are not on any medications that alter the heart rate response.

These assumptions could be used to predict $\dot{V}O_{2max}$ during many types of physical activity. The most commonly used activities to predict $\dot{V}O_{2max}$ are running, walking, stepping up and down onto a bench, and cycling. These tests have advantages and disadvantages that should be considered when choosing an exercise test to predict $\dot{V}O_{2max}$.

Run and Walk Tests

Run and walk tests are the most popular type of aerobic or cardiovascular field test. They are applicable to large numbers of people and require minimal equipment (Fig. 13-7). Here, the 12-minute run test, the 1.5-mile run test, the 20-meter shuttle run test, and the Rockport 1-mile fitness walking test are discussed.

12-Minute Run Test

This test involves running as far as possible in 12 minutes, although walking is allowed if necessary. This test can be used to predict $\dot{V}O_{2max}$ in all age groups if the individuals are apparently healthy. A shorter version of the test, the 9-minute run test,[2] can be used to predict $\dot{V}O_{2max}$ in

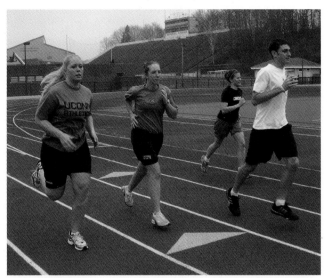

Figure 13-7. Run and walk tests to estimate maximal oxygen consumption can be performed on a 400-meter track. This allows easy determination of the distance run or the time to cover a specific distance, which is needed to estimate maximal oxygen consumption.

children 5 to 12 years old.[1] It is important that people performing the test pace themselves to run as far as possible in the allotted time. The test is normally performed on a standard 400-meter track. Accurately determining the distance run is important in estimating $\dot{V}O_{2max}$ and can be aided by placing cones or markers dividing the 400-meter track into eighths (50-meter lengths). The distance of 400 meters on a standard track applies only to the innermost lane, so those being tested should be encouraged to run in the innermost lane. The distance run significantly correlates with $\dot{V}O_{2max}$ ($r = 0.897$) and can be used in the following regression equation to predict $\dot{V}O_{2max}$[14]:

$$\dot{V}O_{2max} \text{ (mL·kg}^{-1}\text{·min}^{-1}) = (0.0268 \times \text{distance in meters run in 12 minutes}) - 11.3 \qquad (3)$$

For example, if a person completed 2400 meters (6 laps on a 400-meter track), their estimated $\dot{V}O_{2max}$ would be 53.02 mL·kg^{-1}·min^{-1}.

1.5-Mile Run Test

The 1.5-mile run test (2.4 kilometers) is very similar to the 12-minute run test except the goal for those taking the test is to run 1.5 miles in as short a period of time as possible. This test is appropriate for all ages if the participants are apparently healthy. However, a shorter version of the test, the 1.0-mile run test (1.6 km), can be used to predict $\dot{V}O_{2max}$ in children 5 to 12 years old.[1] The test is typically performed on a 400-meter track. To complete 1 mile on a 400-meter track requires covering 9.89 yards (9.0 meters) more than six complete laps. The time needed to complete 1.0 mile successfully correlates ($r = 0.90$) with $\dot{V}O_{2max}$ and can be used to estimate $\dot{V}O_{2max}$ using the following equations[14]:

Women:

$$\dot{V}O_{2max} \text{ (mL·kg}^{-1}\text{·min}^{-1}) = 88.020 - (0.1656 \times \text{body mass in kg}) - (2.767 \times 1.5\text{-mile time in minutes}) \qquad (4)$$

Men:

$$\dot{V}O_{2max} \text{ (mL·kg}^{-1}\text{·min}^{-1}) = 91.736 - (0.1656 \times \text{body mass in kg}) - (2.767 \times 1.5\text{-mile time in minutes}) \qquad (5)$$

For example, if a man and a woman completed 1.5 miles in 13 minutes and both had a body mass of 140 lb (63.6 kilograms), their predicted $\dot{V}O_{2max}$ measures would be 45.23 and 41.52 mL·kg^{-1}·min^{-1}, respectively.

20-Meter Shuttle Run Test

The 20-meter shuttle run test, also termed the multistage fitness test, involves running back and forth between two lines 20 meters apart at ever-increasing velocities until volitional fatigue. The test is performed using a CD (Australian Institute of Sport, http://www.ausport.gov.au/pubcat/) that indicates with verbal instructions and beeps the pace at which each 20-meter distance should be covered. The test has 21 levels, with each level being approximately 1 minute in length. Each level has multiple shuttles or 20-meter distances to be covered. For example, level 1 consists of seven shuttles, whereas level 21 consists of 16 shuttles.

To obtain the best result, the person taking the test must pace himself or herself to cover each 20-meter distance no faster than the prescribed pace. Only one foot must be placed on or over the 20-meter line for a shuttle to be successful. If a person fails to complete a shuttle in the prescribed time, he or she is warned to catch up to the prescribed pace. When the person can no longer maintain pace of the 20-meter shuttles, the test is terminated. The last successfully completed level and shuttle are the score for the test.

The level and shuttle number completed can be used as a marker of endurance capabilities or used to predict $\dot{V}O_{2max}$ ($r = 0.92$).[27,36] For example, successfully completing level 5, shuttle 2 predicts a $\dot{V}O_{2max}$ of 30.2 mL·kg^{-1}·min^{-1}, whereas completing level 14, shuttle 2 predicts a $\dot{V}O_{2max}$ of 61.1 mL·kg^{-1}·min^{-1}.

Rockport 1-Mile Fitness Walking Test

This test is similar to the 1.5-mile run test, except that 1 mile (1.6 kilometers) is walked on a 400-meter track as fast as possible. To complete 1 mile on a 400-meter track, requires covering 9.89 yards (9.0 meters) more than four complete laps. Morbidity and mortality are independently predicted (longer times equal higher morbidity and mortality) by the 1-mile walk test.[7] The 1-mile walk test may be more appropriate than run tests for people of low fitness levels, such as sedentary and older people or those suffering from a disease. The heart rate in the final minute of the test is used in conjunction with the time to complete the test to predict

$\dot{V}O_{2max}$. Depending on the age of the person, several equations ($r = 0.59$–0.88 to actual $\dot{V}O_{2max}$) can be used to predict $\dot{V}O_{2max}$:

Women (20–79 years of age)[20,25]:

$$\dot{V}O_{2max} \ (mL \cdot kg^{-1} \cdot min^{-1}) = 132.853 - (0.3877 \times age \ in \ years) - (0.3722 \times body \ mass \ in \ kg) - (3.2649 \times 1\text{-mile walk time in minutes}) - (0.1565 \times heart \ rate \ in \ bpm) \qquad (6)$$

Men (30–69 years in age)[25]:

$$\dot{V}O_{2max} \ (mL \cdot kg^{-1} \cdot min^{-1}) = 139.168 - (0.3877 \times age \ in \ years) - (0.3722 \times body \ mass \ in \ kg) - (3.2649 \times 1\text{-mile walk time in minutes}) - (0.1565 \times heart \ rate \ in \ bpm) \qquad (7)$$

For example, if a 30-year-old woman, 65 kilograms (143 lb) in body mass, completed the 1-mile walk in 15 minutes with a heart rate of 120 bpm in the last minute of the test, the predicted $\dot{V}O_{2max}$ would be 35.6 $mL \cdot kg^{-1} \cdot min^{-1}$.

Women (18–29 years in age)[18,21]:

$$\dot{V}O_{2max} \ (mL \cdot kg^{-1} \cdot min^{-1}) \ 88.768 - (0.2105 \times body \ mass \ in \ kg) - (1.4537 \times 1\text{-mile} \\ walk \ time \ in \ minutes) - (0.1194 \times \\ heart \ rate \ in \ bpm) \qquad (8)$$

Men (18–29 years in age)[18,21]:

$$\dot{V}O_{2max} \ (mL \cdot kg^{-1} \cdot min^{-1}) = 97.660 - (0.2105 \times body \ mass \ in \ kg) - (1.4537 \times 1\text{-mile} \\ walk \ time \ in \ minutes) - (0.1194 \\ \times heart \ rate \ in \ bpm) \qquad (9)$$

For example, if a 20-year-old male, 176 lb (80 kilograms), walked the mile in 13 minutes and had a heart rate of 120 bpm, the predicted $\dot{V}O_{2max}$ would be 47.59 $mL \cdot kg^{-1} \cdot min^{-1}$.

Step Tests

Step tests to predict $\dot{V}O_{2max}$ are convenient and inexpensive to perform and allow testing of relatively large groups at one time. Special precautions might be needed for people with balance problems. Additionally, performance of the test could be limited by leg strength in some populations, as one leg is used to step up onto and down from the bench (Fig. 13-8). The Queens College step test[30] involves stepping only for 3 minutes at a cadence of up-up-down-down at 22 complete step-ups per minute (88 foot placements per minute) for women and 24 step-ups per minute (96 foot placements per minute) for men. The bench height used for stepping is 41.28 centimeters (16.25 inches). The heart rate is taken immediately on completion of the 3 minutes of stepping and can be used with the following equations to predict ($r = -0.75$, inverse correlation, highest $\dot{V}O_{2max}$ associated with the lowest heart rate after the test) $\dot{V}O_{2max}$:

College-Age Women:
$$\dot{V}O_{2max} \ (mL \cdot kg^{-1} \cdot min^{-1}) = 65.81 - (0.1847 \times \\ heart \ rate \ immediately \ on \\ completion \ of \ the \ test) \qquad (10)$$

College-Age Men:
$$\dot{V}O_{2max} \ (mL \cdot kg^{-1} \cdot min^{-1}) = 111.33 - (0.42 \times heart \ rate \\ immediately \ on \ completion \ of \ the \ test) \qquad (11)$$

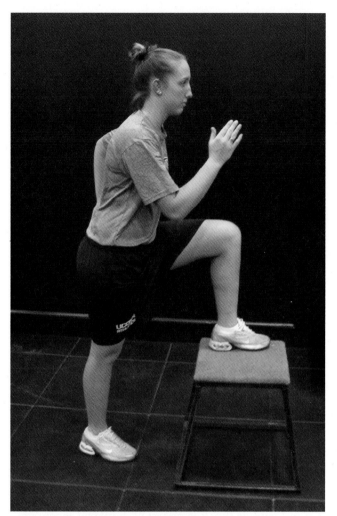

Figure 13-8. Step tests to predict maximal oxygen consumption are inexpensive and easy to perform. Care must be taken when performing step tests if a person has balance difficulties, and results of the test may be limited by leg strength in some populations.

Obtaining heart rate immediately on completion of the test (within 5–15 seconds) is important, because allowing the heart rate to recover after exercise will result in an overprediction of $\dot{V}O_{2max}$. If a college-age male and female had a heart rate of 160 bpm on completion of the test, the predicted $\dot{V}O_{2max}$ measures would be 36.26 and 44.13 $mL \cdot kg^{-1} \cdot min^{-1}$, respectively.

Bicycle Ergometry Tests

Bicycle ergometry tests to predict $\dot{V}O_{2max}$ require a laboratory-grade bicycle capable of maintaining a constant workload (Fig. 13-9). During bicycle ergometry, the workload depends on both the resistance to peddling and the cadence or rpm of peddling. On mechanically braked bicycle ergometers, in which the resistance to peddling is constant, this means maintaining a constant peddling rpm. On electromagnetically braked bicycle ergometers, the resistance to peddling is automatically adjusted to maintain a constant work rate, even if the rpm vary.

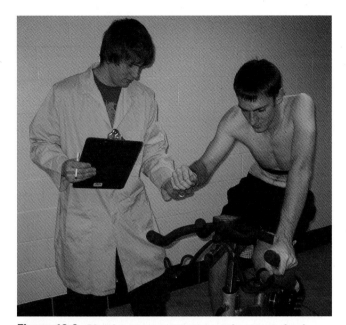

Figure 13-9. Bicycle ergometry tests to estimate maximal oxygen consumption require a laboratory grade ergometer. The ergometer must accurately control workload for an accurate prediction of maximal oxygen consumption.

The Astrand cycle test[3] is a popular cycle ergometry test that has been shown to give valid (10–15% error) predictions of $\dot{V}O_{2max}$.[3] The test consists of riding at 50 rpm against a constant resistance (10 kg·m·min^{-1}·kg body mass^{-1}) for 6 minutes. This workload is designed to result in a heart rate at the end of the test of approximately 150 bpm. Heart rate is obtained during each minute of the test. During the third minute of the test, if the heart rate is less than 139 bpm or greater than 150 bpm, the workload is adjusted so that heart rate will be approximately 150 bpm at the end of 6 minutes. The heart rate in the last 30 seconds of the test is used to predict $\dot{V}O_{2max}$ using two equations. Predicted oxygen consumption at the workload used during the test is calculated with the first equation, whereas the second equation (one version for males and one for females) predicts $\dot{V}O_{2max}$ in liters per minute. If the workload was adjusted at the end of the third minute of the test, the adjusted workload is used in the calculations.

Predicted oxygen consumption at the workload used during the test is calculated with the following equation:

$$\dot{V}O_{2max} \ (\text{L·min}^{-1}) = (\text{power in kg·m·min}^{-1} \times 0.002) + 0.3 \qquad (12)$$

Men:

$$\text{predicted } \dot{V}O_{2max} \ (\text{L·min}^{-1}) = \text{predicted oxygen consumption at the workload used (L·min}^{-1}) \times 220 - \text{age in years} - 61/\text{heart rate at the end of the test} - 61 \qquad (13)$$

Women:

$$\text{predicted } \dot{V}O_{2max} \ (\text{L·min}^{-1}) = \text{predicted oxygen consumption at the workload used (L·min}^{-1}) \times 220 - \text{age in years} - 72/\text{heart rate at the end of the test} - 72 \qquad (14)$$

Quick Review

- In some testing situations, such as when one needs to test many people quickly or when laboratory equipment to directly measure endurance capabilities is not available, an estimate of $\dot{V}O_{2max}$ may suffice as a measure of endurance capabilities.
- Estimates of $\dot{V}O_{2max}$ are normally based on the heart rate response to submaximal exercise.
- Although $\dot{V}O_{2max}$ can be estimated using cycling ergometry or step tests, running and walking tests are the most popular type of aerobic or cardiovascular field test.

For example, a 22-year-old woman with a body mass of 132 lb (60 kg) would use a workload of 600 kg·m·min^{-1} (100 W) to start the test. If the workload was not adjusted after the third minute of the test then the heart rate at the end of the test was 152 bpm. The predicted oxygen consumption at the workload used during the test would be 1.5 L·min^{-1}, and the predicted $\dot{V}O_{2max}$ would be 2.39 L·min^{-1} or 39.8 mL·kg^{-1}·min^{-1}.

LACTATE THRESHOLD

As exercise intensity increases, the rate at which ATP can be supplied solely through aerobic metabolism is exceeded, and further ATP demand must be met with anaerobic metabolism. The lactate threshold is the point at which blood lactate shows an inflection, that is, a nonlinear shift upward during exercise of gradually increasing intensity. In Figure 13-10, oxygen consumption in L·min^{-1} is depicted; however, exercise intensity could also be depicted as oxygen consumption in ml·kg^{-1}·min^{-1}, heart rate, velocity of running, or any other measure of exercise intensity. This is

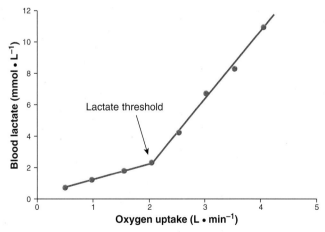

Figure 13-10. Lactate threshold occurs at the oxygen consumption or exercise intensity where blood lactate increases substantially relative to the intensity of work. To determine lactate threshold requires performing multiple workloads and obtaining a blood sample. (Modified from Faude O, Kindermann W, Meyer T. Lactate threshold concepts: How valid are they? Sports Med. 2009;39:469–490.)

different from the response of oxygen uptake during exercise of progressively greater intensity because oxygen uptake shows a straight or linear increase that parallels that of the increasing workload. Blood lactate, in contrast, remains stable during the earlier stages of the exercise session before demonstrating a sharp elevation that exceeds that of the increments of exercise intensity and oxygen uptake. In untrained people, lactate threshold occurs at about 50% to 60% of one's maximal oxygen uptake ($\dot{V}O_{2max}$). In well-trained athletes, however, lactate threshold can be as high as 80% to 90% of their $\dot{V}O_{2max}$.

Note that even under resting conditions, there is lactate present in the blood at a concentration of about 1 mmol·L^{-1}. During the early stages of gradually increasing exercise intensity, blood lactate levels remain stable. This occurs because, although the working muscles are producing more lactate, other organs such as the heart and liver (and even oxidative muscle fibers) take it up from the blood to either be oxidized as an energy substrate or converted to glucose. But at some point, as more lactate is produced by working muscles and released into the blood, its rate of uptake from the blood is exceeded, resulting in net increases in circulating lactate. The cause for this excessive rate of lactate release into the blood is complex and includes the following:

1. A greater reliance on carbohydrates, as opposed to lipids, as an energy substrate
2. The recruitment of fast-twitch muscle fibers that have high concentrations of glycolytic enzymes but poor oxidative function
3. Stimulation of the sympathetic nervous system, resulting in "fight-or-flight" responses that increase the activity of the glycolytic but not oxidative bioenergetic pathway, leading to an accumulation of pyruvate that must be converted to lactate to allow energy production to continue

To the athlete, the specific causes of blood lactate accumulation are not nearly as relevant as how it affects his or her performance. Simply stated, the pace, or work rate, that an endurance athlete can sustain is that which coincides with his or her lactate threshold. Thus, if the lactate threshold occurs at 75% of $\dot{V}O_{2max}$, that is the intensity (sometimes referred to as "performance $\dot{V}O_2$") that he or she can exercise at for an extended period of time.[24] This phenomenon is rooted in the fact that lactate, or more specifically the H$^+$ that was associated with it as lactic acid, will cause cellular pH disturbances, resulting in signs of muscular fatigue. Fortunately, for endurance athletes, the lactate threshold displays greater responsiveness to training than $\dot{V}O_{2max}$. Thus, it is possible to improve it and, accordingly, the pace that can be maintained during an endurance event.

Many treadmill protocols have been developed for specific groups of people, such as endurance athletes, and for specific purposes, such as determination of lactate threshold (Chapter 2) or ventilatory threshold (Chapter 6).

Protocols for those with good cardiovascular fitness may be preceded by a warm-up procedure, with the initial workload being greater than that in protocols for people who are less fit cardiovascularly. A protocol for determination of lactate threshold for an endurance athlete is depicted in Table 13-8. Blood lactate concentration, heart rate, and oxygen consumption are monitored throughout the test and used to establish pace and heart rate at, above, and below lactate threshold. This information can then be used to establish running paces above and below lactate threshold. The test was developed for an athlete with a 10-kilometer time of 33 minutes or an average pace during the race of 284 m·min^{-1} (5 minutes 40 seconds per mile), five speeds below average race pace are established at 10 m·min^{-1} intervals. This same change in speed is used to establish paces above race pace. Grade is 0% and workload is increased only by increasing speed. This is done to mimic as closely as possible the physiological stress encountered in a 10-kilometer race that is contested on a flat track. The initial stage is 4 minutes in length, with each successive stage being 3 minutes in length. This time frame is used so that, if possible, blood lactate concentrations are stabilized at the end of the stage. At the end of each stage, a small blood sample is obtained and immediately analyzed for blood lactate concentration. Once blood lactate concentration is greater than a value (5.0 mmol·L^{-1}), clearly indicating that the workload is above lactate threshold, the current workload is completed and the test terminated. If determination of $\dot{V}O_{2max}$ is desired, the athlete is allowed to rest 10 minutes. The treadmill is set at the second-to-last workload achieved in the lactate threshold determination protocol and the treadmill elevated 1% each minute until volitional fatigue.

A protocol to determine lactate threshold using a cycle ergometer is depicted in Table 13-9. For both males and females, workload is increased 150 kg·m·min^{-1} (50 Watts) at each stage of the test, with females starting at a lower workload compared with males (100 vs. 150 Watts). At

Table 13-8. Treadmill Protocol for Lactate Threshold for an Endurance Athlete

Stage	Speed (m·min^{-1})	Speed (miles·hr^{-1})	Duration (min)
1	234	8.7	4
2	244	9.1	3
3	254	9.5	3
4	264	9.8	3
5	274	10.2	3
6	284	10.6	3
7	294	11.0	3
8	304	11.3	3

Table 13-9.	Electronically Braked Bicycle Ergometry Protocol for Lactate Threshold for an Endurance Athlete		
Stage	**Male (W)**	**Female (W)**	**Duration (min)**
1	150	100	4
2	200	150	3
3	225	175	3
4	250	200	3
5	275	225	3
6	300	250	3
7	325	275	3
8	350	300	3

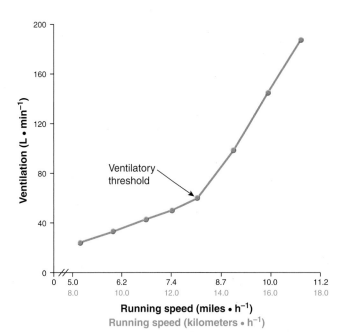

Figure 13-11. Ventilatory threshold can be estimated as the work intensity where $\dot{V}_E$ increases disproportionately relative to the intensity. Using ventilatory threshold to estimate lactate threshold does not require obtaining a blood sample.

the end of each workload, a blood sample is immediately analyzed for blood lactate. When blood lactate is clearly above a concentration (5.0 mmol·L^{-1}), indicating that lactate threshold has been surpassed, the workload being performed is completed and test terminated. Throughout the test, heart rate and $\dot{V}O_2$ are determined and used to design training paces. If it is desired to determine $\dot{V}O_{2max}$ after a 10-minute rest, the cycle ergometer is set to the second-to-last workload completed and workload is increased 75 m·min^{-1} (25 Watts) per minute until volitional fatigue.

An indirect method, termed *ventilatory threshold*, of estimating lactate threshold uses an analysis of ongoing ventilator measures with a metabolic cart. Determination of ventilatory threshold has been previously described using ventilatory equivalents of carbon dioxide and oxygen (see Chapter 6). Briefly, in the early stages of an increasingly difficult exercise session, minute ventilation ($\dot{V}_E$) and $\dot{V}O_2$ reveal parallel and linear inclines. But at some point, the gradually increasing exercise intensity elicits an uncoupling of the rise in $\dot{V}_E$ and $\dot{V}O_2$ in which minute ventilation displays a sharper, curvilinear elevation (Fig. 6-13). It is proposed that this disproportionate increment in $\dot{V}_E$ is due to a rather sudden increase in CO_2 production (it is arterial CO_2 blood concentration that has the greatest influence on ventilation), resulting from the buffering of lactate, or more specifically H$^+$, in the blood. Recall that lactic acid quickly dissociates to lactate and H$^+$ at a physiological pH. On entering the bloodstream, it binds with bicarbonate (HCO$_3^-$) that is present in the blood to form carbonic acid (H$_2$CO$_3$). Carbonic acid, in turn, is converted to H$_2$O and CO_2 by the enzyme carbonic anhydrase. It is this nonmetabolically produced CO_2 that drives the increase in $\dot{V}_E$, whereas $\dot{V}O_2$ remains unaffected. The exercise intensity at which the rise in $\dot{V}_E$ exceeds that of $\dot{V}O_2$ is referred to as the ventilatory threshold. Another estimate of ventilatory threshold can be obtained by graphing $\dot{V}_E$ versus workload. In Figure 13-11,

running velocity is depicted as the workload; however, workload could also be cycling velocity, swimming velocity, or any other measure of workload. With this method, when $\dot{V}_E$ increases disproportionately relative to velocity is the point at which ventilatory threshold is estimated to occur.

The ventilatory threshold method of estimating lactate threshold enjoys the benefits of being quantified continuously (when using a modern online metabolic system), rather than at specific intervals, and not requiring blood sampling. However, there have been some who have questioned its accuracy because it has been found that the ventilatory changes can occur before the inflection in blood lactate.[16] Moreover, other investigators have reported that, in addition to lactate and H$^+$, the presence of potassium in the blood acts to stimulate the brain's ventilatory control center, causing a sharp rise in $\dot{V}_E$ in the absence of exercise and anaerobic metabolism.[34,42]

Quick Review

- The lactate threshold is the point at which blood lactate shows an inflection, that is, a nonlinear shift upward during exercise of gradually increasing intensity.
- Estimates of lactate threshold can be obtained using ventilatory measures.
- During a test to determine lactate threshold, heart rate, oxygen consumption, and blood lactate are monitored throughout the test and used to establish pace and heart rate at lactate threshold. This information can then be used to establish running paces above and below lactate threshold.

ANAEROBIC CAPACITY

In contrast to the performance of endurance athletes, which will suffer with the accumulation of blood lactate as a result of excessive dependence on anaerobically produced ATP, the performance of some sporting events is directly linked to the capacity of the working muscles to function anaerobically. For example, long-distance sprint performances (e.g., 400 and 800 meters) are greatly influenced by the athlete's ability to synthesize ATP anaerobically and to withstand high levels of muscle and blood lactate. Indeed, any activity lasting between 30 seconds and 3 minutes that features all-out or near all-out muscular effort heavily depends on the athlete's ability to produce energy via the anaerobic, or glycolytic, bioenergetic pathway. The advantage of the glycolytic pathway is its capacity to rapidly generate ATP to meet the needs of the athlete's rapidly and powerfully contracting muscle fibers during short-duration, high-intensity events. But pyruvate is produced just as rapidly as is ATP during glycolysis. In fact, pyruvate can be generated at a pace that exceeds the rate at which it can be transported into the mitochondria and oxidized. Accordingly, there is a buildup of cytoplasmic pyruvate. To allow glycolysis to continue—along with ATP synthesis—the pyruvate must be converted to lactate. Thus, sprint-type events depend on intramuscular ATP and PC as well as the glycolytic pathway and, by extension, lactate production. The muscle fiber type of an athlete will affect their anaerobic capabilities. Specifically, those with more fast-twitch fibers (type II) will have a greater capacity for short-duration, high-intensity activity or anaerobic capacity than do those with a greater number of slow-twitch fibers (type I).

Testing of Anaerobic Capacity

Rather than measuring particular physiological parameters and/or markers, most tests of anaerobic capacity quantify performance in tasks that rely heavily on ATP synthesis, via the exercising muscles' phosphagen and glycolytic pathways. Perhaps the most popular test of anaerobic power is the **Wingate test**, developed by exercise scientists at the Wingate Institute in Israel. A cycle ergometer is used to perform this test. The person performing the test starts pedaling as fast as he or she can with minimal resistance. Once the maximal pedaling speed has been achieved, a specified resistance per kilogram of body mass is abruptly applied to begin the 30-second sprint test. The resistance for untrained males is kg = body mass (kg) × 0.090 and for females kg = body mass (kg) × 0.086.[19] These resistances are chosen because they give the untrained person the best possibility of achieving the highest peak power. For a trained athlete, the resistance can be increased while for other populations, such as seniors or children, the resistance is decreased. The person continues to pedal as fast as possible throughout the entire 30-second test. Both peak

and mean anaerobic power are derived using the resistance to peddling and the number of revolutions completed during the best 5-second interval (greatest number of revolutions completed) and the total 30 seconds, respectively. For untrained men, a peak power of about 9.5 $W\cdot kg^{-1}$ of body weight would be considered normal, whereas mean power might be approximately 7.5 $W\cdot kg^{-1}$ of body mass.[23] The average values for peak and mean power among untrained women are approximately 8.5 and 5.7 $W\cdot kg^{-1}$ of body mass, respectively.[23] Other measures can also be determined from the Wingate test. Such measures include total work performed during the entire 30-second test and fatigue index or the fatigue from the peak power to the lowest power during the test (peak power – lowest power/ peak power × 100).

One of the oldest and still more popular tests for assessing anaerobic power is the **Margaria step test**.[29] This test requires very little sophisticated equipment: a staircase (each step being 175 millimeters high) and two switch-mats that are connected to a time recorder that can measure up to hundredths of a second. The switch-mats are placed on the 8th and 12th steps of the staircase. The subject begins the test by running up the stairs as fast as possible using every other step. The time elapsed between contact with the 8th and 12th steps, vertical distance between the 8th and 12th steps, and body mass are used to calculate power. In untrained males, average power for the Margarita step test is about 15 $W\cdot kg^{-1}$ of body weight, whereas untrained females display values of approximately 12 $W\cdot kg^{-1}$ of body mass.[38]

Another method of quantifying anaerobic capacity that requires little sophisticated equipment is the **anaerobic treadmill test**.[15] This test assesses anaerobic power by running on a motorized treadmill set at a sharp (20%) grade at a speed of 8 miles·hr^{-1}. The subject begins the session by standing on the treadmill, which has already been set at the predetermined grade and speed, and straddling the moving belt. When ready, he or she quickly leaves the straddled position and begins running. The timed session begins with the first step and continues until exhaustion. When the subject is not able to keep pace any longer, he or she grabs the side rails of the treadmill and again straddles the moving belt until it can be brought to a stop. For safety, it is recommended that a spotter stand on each side of the treadmill to assist the subject in resuming the straddled position at the point of exhaustion. Anaerobic capacity is quantified by the number of seconds the participant is capable of running before exhaustion occurs. Data have shown that the average running time for untrained males is 52 seconds, whereas trained adult males can tolerate the severe grade and pace of the treadmill for 64 seconds.[15]

Perhaps the simplest and most popular way of measuring muscular power of the leg muscles is with the **vertical jump test**. This test can consist of measuring only vertical jump height or calculation of power produced. In its most sophisticated form, a force platform can be used to measure

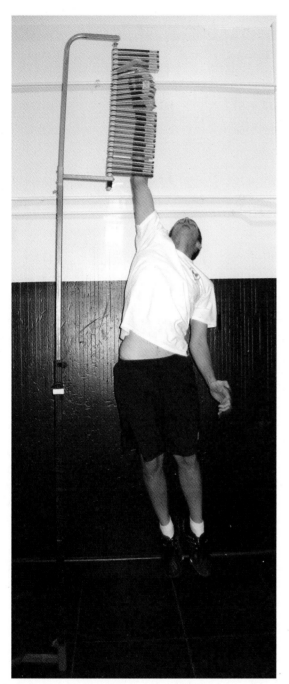

Figure 13-12. A piece of equipment (Vertec) with movable vanes can be used to determine jump height. The height of the vanes can be adjusted to accommodate people of various heights and of differing maximal vertical jump ability.

the highest vain possible, which is the reach height. The jump test described here is a noncountermovement jump during which the subject stands below the vanes, bends his or her knees to approximately 90° prior to jumping, and holds this position for 2 to 3 seconds prior to jumping. However, for some athletes, such as hitters in volleyball or basketball players, a jump using a several step approach can also be performed. When ready, the subject jumps from the 90° knee bend as high as possible using a normal jumping arm swing. At the top of the jump, the arms and fingers are fully extended and as many vanes as possible are touched and pushed to the side; this designates the maximal jump height. The distance in centimeters (cm) between the reach height and the maximum jump height is taken as the measure of the vertical jump. Three attempts are performed, with a 1-minute rest period between successive jumps. The single highest jump height achieved is typically used for analysis, rather than an average of the three attempts. Performance of this power test can be measured either by using the raw data, i.e., number of cm jumped, and comparing them to subject-appropriate norms, or by using a formula to convert cm jumped into watts. Several equations have been developed to estimate peak power from vertical jump height.[13,39] According to Sayers et al.,[39] results from a noncountermovement jump, as described here, can accurately gauge peak power with the use of the following equation:

$$\text{peak power (W)} = (60.7 \times \text{jump height in cm}) \\ + (45.3 \times \text{body mass in kg}) - 2055 \quad (15)$$

Thus, a 70-kg man who jumps 50 cm would display peak power of 4151 W, in that

$$4151 \text{ W} = (60.7 \times 50) + (45.3 \times 70) - 2055 \quad (16)$$

According to the norms found in Table 13-10, this would place a 20-year-old male in the "fair" category.

Peak power during a countermovement jump can be accurately calculated with the following equation[13]:

$$\text{peak power (W)} = 65.1 \times (\text{jump height cm}) \\ + 25.8 \times (\text{body mass kg}) - 1413.1$$

Thus, a 70-kg man who jumps 60 cm would display peak power in W, in that

$$4298.9 \text{ W} = 65.1 \times 60 \text{ cm} + 25.8 \times 70 \text{ kg} - 1413.1$$

The choice of which type of jump test to perform depends upon the purpose of testing. For general fitness, a noncountermovement or countermovement jump could be utilized. However, for athletes, the type of jump used in their sport typically is chosen for testing purposes.

Another commonly used method to assess speed and anaerobic muscle power is the running sprint test. This test simply records the amount of time it takes to cover a given distance while running with all-out effort. The 40-yard (36.7 meters) dash test is typically used because this distance is short enough to provide a valid measure of power and speed, as opposed to endurance. Any running

power, as well as other measures, such as rate of force development, while jumping. A simple piece of equipment (e.g., Vertec jump testing system, Vertec, Inc., Pensacola, FL) is frequently used to determine vertical jump height (Fig. 13-12). This equipment has movable vanes that can be set at a predetermined height. Standing below the vanes with feet approximately hip-width apart, the subject reaches up as high as possible with the dominant arm and touches

Table 13-10. Norms and Performance Classifications for the Noncountermovement Vertical Jump Test (W)

Age (sex)	Excellent	Very Good	Good	Fair	Poor
15–19					
Male	≥4644	4185–4643	3858–4184	3323–3857	≤3322
Female	≥3167	2795–3166	2399–3166	2156–2398	≤2155
20–29					
Male	≥5094	4640–5093	4297–4639	3775–4296	≤3774
Female	≥3250	2804–3249	2478–2803	2271–2477	≤2270
30–39					
Male	≥4860	4389–4859	3967–4388	3485–3966	≤3484
Female	≥3193	2550–3192	2335–2549	2147–2334	≤2146
40–49					
Male	≥4320	3700–4319	3242–3699	2708–3241	≤2707
Female	≥2675	2288–2674	2101–2287	1688–2100	≤1687

Source: The Canadian Physical Activity, Fitness & Lifestyle Appraisal: CSEP-Health & Fitness Programs Health-Related Appraisal and Counseling Strategy, 3rd ed., 2003. Reprinted with permission of the Canadian Society for Exercise Physiology.

sprint test can be performed in a field setting rather than in a laboratory, as it requires nothing more than a standard stopwatch or electronic timing system and a flat area with a surface that provides good traction when sprinting. As with all power tests in which muscles execute maximal, explosive contractions, it is important that the individual or athlete warms up properly before attempting the 40-yard dash test. Cones or markers are used to designate the start and finish lines of the test. Several types of starting positions can be utilized, depending upon what type of athlete is being tested. The typical "sprinter's start" position, with his or her hands on the starting line, one leg in a bent position with the knee beneath the chest, and the other leg in a near-full extension behind him or her, is commonly used. However, a standing start position, with the feet slightly staggered front to back, may be more appropriate for athletes who start sprinting from this position, such as American football wide receivers or soccer players. However, the typical American football three-point stance of offensive linemen is more appropriate for these athletes. Regardless of the starting position used, no body parts are to extend beyond the starting point. The tester, who is holding the stopwatch, stands at the finish line. The tester starts the 40-yard dash test by calling out the start command while simultaneously starting the stopwatch. The athlete runs as fast as possible through the finish line, whereupon the tester stops the stopwatch and records the time to the nearest 0.01 seconds. Generally, three sprints are completed, separated by 3- to 4-minute rest

intervals, and the best time is selected as representative of test performance. To provide a sense of average times for the 40-yard dash test, a man 16 to 18 years old would have to run 40 yards in 5.10 seconds, whereas a woman of the same age must have a time of 6.11 seconds to reach the 50th percentile.[22] There are also norms for various groups of athletes, for example, NCAA Division I women's volleyball players and Division III male soccer players have mean 40-yard sprint times of 5.62 and 4.73 seconds, respectively.[22]

Factors Affecting Anaerobic Power and Speed Tests

Although the tests described above are intended to quantify the capacity of skeletal muscles to generate power via anaerobic pathways, factors other than innate physical characteristics influence an individual's or athlete's performance. Some of these may even be psychological in origin, such as one's motivation to perform at his or her best. Moreover, skill at performing some of the movements may alter performance. This is particularly true of sprint tests, where proper body positioning at the starting line, as well as coming out of that position and transitioning into a full sprint speed quickly, are essential to optimal performance. Similarly, some degree of coordination is necessary during the vertical leap tests to ensure that the maximal height recorded occurs at the apex of the effort and is measured correctly. Another important variable that

- The performance of some sporting events is directly linked to the capacity of the working muscles to function anaerobically.
- Any activity that is of high-intensity, short-duration nature and that features all-out or near all-out muscular effort heavily depends on the athlete's ability to produce energy via the anaerobic pathways (intramuscular ATP and PC, glycolysis).
- Many tests can be used to measure an anaerobic performance, including vertical jump test, Wingate test, and running sprint tests.
- Other factors, such as individual motivation and skill, can impact performance in anaerobic speed and power tests.

contributes to power performance is muscle-fiber-type composition. Because power is an explosive or rapid expression of muscle force production, those with a high percentage of fast-twitch or type II fibers, particularly in the quadriceps muscles (which are usually emphasized during these tests), tend to display greater power.[23] And because many of these tests require the movement of the entire body while climbing, leaping, or sprinting, body composition is a factor, as it is a detriment to performance to have to move, or propel, a greater amount of noncontractile body mass. Thus, those with a better muscle-to-fat mass ratio have been found to perform better on most power tests.[26,33]

MUSCULAR STRENGTH

Simply defined, **strength** is the maximal amount of force exerted during a single maximal effort. Strength is perhaps the most regularly assessed parameter of fitness because it is a component of health-related fitness, as well as sports-related fitness. Unlike muscular power or speed, the expression of muscular strength does not require any movement or distance covered. Indeed, measurement of strength developed during an isometric contraction (no visible movement) is a commonly used method of quantifying strength. Simple pieces of equipment that feature force sensors can accurately gauge the strength exerted by contracting muscles. Hand grip dynamometers and tensiometers are good examples of devices used to ascertain strength during isometric contractions.

Other tests to measure strength, however, emphasize movement of specific body parts through a given range of motion. These may involve concentric (shortening) contractions or eccentric (lengthening) contractions

during these phases of a repetition of a resistance training exercise, or, more commonly, a combination of the two while completing a full repetition. Several types of equipment (with wide ranging costs) can be used to provide resistance and gauge the maximal force producing capacity of muscle(s). For example, free weights can be used effectively, as well as weight machines with stacked weights, machines that employ pneumatic resistance (e.g., Keiser), and even sophisticated, expensive isokinetic dynamometers (e.g., Biodex, Kin-Com).

One popular test of strength is the **grip dynamometer test** that measures force development by the finger flexors during an isometric action. This test has the advantages of ease of use; a simple, inexpensive testing device; and time efficiency. Moreover, although strength of the forearm and hand muscles is directly quantified, research has demonstrated that the results of the grip dynamometer test are significantly correlated with alternate measures of strength, although considerable variability may exist between grip strength and that of diverse muscle groups.[10] Nonetheless, results of the grip dynamometer test are commonly used as a practical and reliable measure of upper body strength.

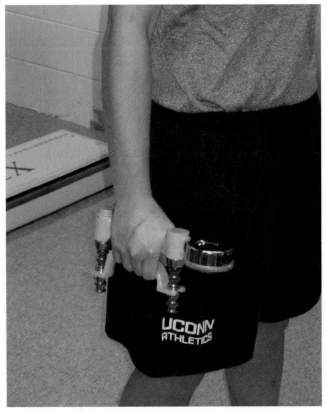

Figure 13-13. A grip dynamometer measures isometric force development of the finger flexors. The maximal scores for both hands can be added together to produce a final score and compared to normative values.

Table 13-11. Grip Strength (Kilograms) Norms by Age Groups and Sex for Combined Right and Left Hand

Age (years)	15–19		20–29		30–39		40–49		50–59		60–69	
Gender	M	F	M	F	M	F	M	F	M	F	M	F
Excellent	≥108	≥68	≥115	≥70	≥115	≥71	≥108	≥69	≥101	≥61	≥100	≥54
Very Good	98–107	60–67	104–114	63–69	104–114	63–70	97–107	61–68	92–100	54–60	91–99	48–53
Good	90–97	53–59	195–103	58–62	95–103	58–62	88–96	54–60	84–91	49–53	84–90	45–47
Fair	79–89	48–52	84–94	52–57	84–94	51–57	80–87	49–53	76–83	45–48	73–83	41–44
Needs Improvement	≤78	≤47	≤83	≤51	≤83	≤50	≤79	≤48	≤75	≤44	≤72	≤40

Source: The Canadian Physical Activity, Fitness & Lifestyle Appraisal: CSEP-Health & Fitness Programs Health-Related Appraisal and Counseling Strategy, 3rd ed., 2003. Reprinted with permission of the Canadian Society for Exercise Physiology.

To perform the test, the dynamometer must be properly adjusted to fit the size of the person's hand. The subject's hand and the dynamometer must be dry to prevent slipping when squeezing the dynamometer. The subject then clasps the grip dynamometer and, in a slightly bent-over position at the waist, extends the arm in front of him or her with a slight bend at the elbow, as shown in Figure 13-13. It is important that the arm does not contact any part of the body or anything else. When ready, the subject squeezes the dynamometer with maximal effort while keeping the body and arm stationary. Three attempts are made with each hand. The highest value (in kilograms) for the left hand can be added to the highest value for the right hand to produce a final score. Results can be assessed in absolute terms, i.e., total kilograms of force generated or, in relative terms, by taking that figure and dividing it by body mass in kilograms. Norms for grip strength test results in absolute terms are presented in Table 13-11.

Box 13-6 DID YOU KNOW?

Determination of 1-RM Requires a Specific Protocol

Although testing of one-repetition maximum (1-RM) appears to be relatively simple, it does require a specific protocol be followed if valid and reliable results are to be obtained. Typically, to determine test–retest reliability, or the accuracy of the test during repetitive testing, the test is performed on two or more separate occasions. For the test to have good test–retest reliability, little variation on successive tests should occur. The following testing protocol has been shown to have high test–retest reliability in both men and women.

No matter what exercise for which 1-RM is determined, there should be a familiarization period to the exercise and all testing procedures. During testing, successful completion of a repetition should be defined as the full range of motion of a normal repetition of the exercise and held constant whenever 1-RM is tested. All safety precautions for an exercise, such as spotters, should be followed during all testing. The following testing procedure can be used to determine 1-RM:

1. A warm-up set of 5 to 10 repetitions at 40% to 60% of the perceived 1-RM
2. A second warm-up-set of three to five repetitions at 60% to 80% of the perceived 1-RM

3. An attempt at the perceived 1-RM
4. If the 1-RM attempt is successful, increase the resistance and perform another attempt
5. If the 1-RM attempt is not successful, decrease the resistance and perform another attempt
6. Follow steps 4 and 5 for no more than four 1-RM attempts
7. If the 1-RM is not determined in four attempts, have the subject return another day for retesting
8. The warm-up sets and 1-RM attempts are separated by rest periods of 3 to 5 minutes

When someone performs 1-RM testing of an exercise for the first time, the perceived 1-RM can be estimated from previous training data or based on past experience of the tester. After the initial testing of the 1-RM, the perceived 1-RM is based on previous testing data.

Kraemer WJ, Ratamess NA, Fry AC, et al. Strength Training: Development and evaluation of methodology. In: Maud P, Foster C, eds. Physiological Assessment of Human Fitness, 2nd ed. Champaign, IL.: Human Kinetics, 2006:119–150.

Another test to quantify strength is the **1-RM**. As stated earlier, this is the maximal amount of weight or resistance that can be lifted through the entire range of motion for a single time in a given movement. This dynamic assessment of strength is often used with the bench press and leg press as measures of upper and lower body strength, respectively. Before performing these tests, the subject should become familiar with the exercise movements. Once comfortable with the equipment and the movement, the subject should complete some lighter resistance warm-up repetitions prior to successive heavier 1-RM attempts. Although the testing of 1-RM seems relatively simple, as with all tests, a protocol must be followed if valid and reliable results are to be obtained (Box 13-6).

In performing the 1-RM free weight bench press, the subject lies on his or her back on the bench. The barbell is supported on upright racks. The arms are extended upward to grasp the bar with an overhand grip, hands roughly shoulder-width apart. The bar is lifted off of the support racks and lowered in a controlled, deliberate manner until it comes in contact with the chest. The bar is then pressed back up until the arms are fully extended, completing the repetition. The greatest amount of weight that can be used while properly executing the full movement is considered the 1-RM. If the subject is using free weights, a spotter

---

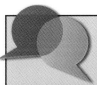

Box 13-7 EXPERT VIEW
Importance of Testing

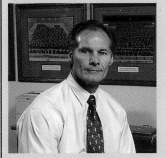

Boyd Epley, M.Ed, CSCS*D, MSCC, FNSCA
Director of Coaching Performance
National Strength and Conditioning Association
Colorado Springs, CO

Why Test?

Every conditioning program should begin with the testing and evaluation of each participant. By learning athletes' strengths and weaknesses, it is much easier to direct their training and achieve maximum results.

Testing also helps determine if the program is effectively achieving the goals desired and, most importantly, how the athlete is progressing.

Testing also serves as a great motivator. Many athletes, especially the younger ones, need positive proof that sports conditioning will benefit them before they are willing to put forth the effort needed to obtain maximum results. Once the athlete begins achieving goals, he or she will be eager to set higher goals. It is always better to pull back on an athlete who is motivated versus one who needs to be pushed.

Coaches who make the effort to test, evaluate, and set goals have results that can be documented. Some schools overlook the tremendous benefits of this four-step process and begin lifting or conditioning right away.

Validity

Each test must measure the component it is constructed to measure. Does the test used to measure performance potential correlate to the specific sport in which the athlete participates?

Reliability

Reliability is dependent upon the coach keeping testing conditions and results consistent each time. The testing results will be different if testing is done outside on the grass one time, then inside on the basketball court another time. The condition of the field, the time of day, wind, rain, temperature, etc., all have an effect on the testing results.

The order in which the tests are given will affect the results. The testing order needs to be the same each and every time, and the testing equipment needs to be the same each time. Have the same coaches administer the same test each time, if possible.

Annual Performance Test Cycle

The combination of testing periods forms an "Annual Test Cycle." Put a big emphasis on testing, but do it only three to four times a year. Hold testing sessions the week before the conditioning program starts and after each conditioning cycle.

Organize Equipment and Facility

The more you do in advance, the smoother the testing day will go. Determine the equipment and facilities that will be needed, and get them ready. Get permission to use the facility and secure all the equipment and make sure everything is in working order and calibrated. Draw a floor plan to help decide how the "stations" of the test will be organized. Use the floor plan to decide how the traffic will flow as the athletes move from one testing station to another, and share the plan with your coaches and athletes so that everyone knows the plan.

Develop Data Collection Cards

Have your athletes carry data collection cards with them to each station, on which the coach can record test results. The card should include all the tests being administered and personal information, such as name and date. The tests should be listed in the order in which they are to be performed so that there is no confusion.

CASE STUDY

Scenario

You are a sports scientist working with a group of elite distance runners. You have been asked to develop a test battery to help track training improvements and assist with establishing heart rate training zones for training. What types of tests and measurements will you use?

Options

The athletes would perform a treadmill running test to determine $\dot{V}O_{2max}$ and lactate threshold. A running test, as opposed to another type of test such as cycling, would be used because of the specificity of heart rate and other physiological responses to the mode of exercise. The lactate threshold test will be performed first, followed by the $\dot{V}O_{2max}$ test.

To individualize the lactate threshold test, the average pace during the athlete's primary running event would be determined. For example, for an athlete with a 10-kilometer time of 33 minutes, the average pace during the race is 284 m·min^{-1} (5 minutes 40 seconds per mile). To establish stages of a discontinuous treadmill test, five speeds below and several above average race pace would be established at 10 m·min^{-1} intervals. Grade would be 0% throughout the test to mimic the physiological stress of running on a flat track. So, workload would only be increased by increasing speed. The first stage of the treadmill test would be 4 minutes in length, with each successive stage 3 minutes in length. This length of stages would be used so that, if possible, blood lactate concentrations are stabilized at the end of the stage. Throughout the test, $\dot{V}O_2$ would be measured and, at the end of each stage, heart rate would be measured. Between stages, the athlete would straddle the treadmill so that a small blood sample could be obtained. The blood sample would be immediately analyzed for blood lactate concentration. Once blood lactate concentration was greater than 5.0 mmol·L^{-1}, which clearly indicates that the workload is above lactate threshold, the current workload would be completed and the test terminated. The blood lactates would be utilized to determine lactate threshold. The heart rate and treadmill speed would be used to establish paces above and below lactate threshold to assist in prescribing training paces. After a 10-minute rest, a test to determine

$\dot{V}O_{2max}$ would be performed. This test would start at the second-to-last workload achieved in the lactate threshold test and the treadmill would be elevated 1% each minute until volitional fatigue. With increased aerobic fitness, both lactate threshold and $\dot{V}O_{2max}$ would increase, and ideally $\dot{V}O_2$ at submaximal paces would decrease. So, these measures would be utilized to help determine improvements in aerobic fitness and whether the training program was bringing about the desired results.

Scenario

What type of graded exercise test would you utilize, and what would you monitor during the test, for a senior who has some difficulty with balance and some indicators of increased cardiovascular risk?

Options

This senior would perform a graded exercise test on a cycle ergometer with blood pressure, heart rate, ECG, perceived exertion (RPE), and $\dot{V}O_2$ monitored throughout the test. A cycle ergometer, as opposed to a treadmill, is chosen to help alleviate any potential problems with balance while performing the test. Cycle ergometry would also be chosen because this mode of exercise results in less artifact of the ECG and makes it easier to obtain blood pressure during the test. The workload would be elevated slowly during the test so that the blood pressure response and ECG could be monitored for indicators of a cardiovascular problem and the test terminated if needed. For example, it is expected that systolic blood pressure will increase as the test progresses, whereas a significant increase in diastolic blood pressure would indicate an abnormal cardiovascular response. However, ST-segment depression on the ECG would indicate a lack of blood flow to the heart. If either of these occurred, the test would be terminated. RPE during the test would be utilized to help establish aerobic training zones; it would also be used if a cardiovascular problem was used to establish aerobic training zones below a heart rate at which a problem was indicated. $\dot{V}O_2$ during the test would be used to help determine aerobic fitness and as a marker of a change in fitness over time.

should always be present to ensure the safety of the subject. Alternatively, a bench press machine with stacked weights can be used, which does not require the presence of a spotter.

A popular test to assess the strength of the lower body is the 1-RM leg press. This is performed using a leg press machine, rather than free weights. Again, the subject should first become accustomed to the machine and perform some warm-up repetitions prior to 1-RM

attempts. It should be noted that different devices (45° leg press, supine leg press) used to accomplish the leg press require the body's joints to be situated at different angles, resulting in a leg pressing motion at different angles in the vertical and horizontal planes. These differences affect the amount of resistance that can be used to complete one repetition. Regardless of the machine used, the subject should secure his or her position by grasping side handles attached to the seat of the machine. The range of motion should be from a 90° knee angle to a position where the knees are fully extended. Feet should be placed on the foot platform approximately hip-width apart. In both the 1-RM bench press and leg press, strength can be expressed in absolute terms (total amount lifted), or as a relative measure by dividing the amount lifted by the person's body mass. Due to the effect of the type of equipment used, norms for 1-RM determination are difficult to establish. However, for a machine bench press for men and women 20 to 29 years old, the 50th percentile for the 1-RM, in relative terms, is 1.06 and 0.40, respectively. In the 1-RM leg press, relative strength for 20- to 29-year-old men and women corresponding to the 50th percentile is 1.91 and 1.32, respectively.[41]

Although not practical in field settings, the 1-RM test of strength can also be carried out with an isokinetic dynamometer. This is a sophisticated, expensive piece of testing and rehabilitative equipment that is generally found in well-equipped human performance laboratories or in clinical settings such as physical therapy units. Isokinetic devices do not use external weights to provide resistance for the subject to attempt to overcome. Rather, the tester programs the device to permit the subject to complete a fixed range of motion at a constant velocity, regardless of how much force is applied. In short, the speed of movement at which the repetition is completed is determined ahead of time, not the amount of resistance to be lifted, as with free weights or machines with stacked weights. When force is exerted, it is quantified by a force transducer and recorded. Modern isokinetic dynamometers allow the testing of numerous different muscle groups, including the quadriceps, hamstrings, calf muscles, shoulders, and arms. However, these machines are designed to isolate single muscle groups during unilateral movements such as knee extensions/flexions, and elbow extensions/flexions, making it difficult, if not impossible, to test muscle strength during compound, or multi-joint, exercises such as leg presses or bench presses. Isokinetic dynamometers have the distinct advantage, though, of eliminating the trial-and-error approach of establishing the 1-RM that characterizes testing with free weights and machines with stacked weights. Instead, the tester determines which speed of movement will be used: even isometric contractions can be tested. After familiarization and warm-up, the subject exerts his or her maximal effort, which is measured with a very high level of precision and accuracy by the computerized isokinetic machine. Testing is important for the coach or practitioner to optimize programs and meet individual fitness goals (see Box 13-7).

CHAPTER SUMMARY

Testing the functional capacity of various physiological systems during maximal or submaximal intensity effort can play an important role in exercise physiology, fitness training, coaching, and conditioning. Determining how well different systems are capable of performing may help the athlete and the coach determine which sport, or even position, each athlete is best suited for. Coaches and conditioning specialists may want to test athletes and fitness clients at regular intervals to ascertain the efficacy of a training regimen. Moreover, athletes, coaches, and conditioning experts can use the results from these testing sessions as a motivational tool.

In clinical settings, testing is typically conducted not on highly trained athletes, but on people of all ages recovering from medical procedures and ailments, or simply to evaluate health status. The appraisal of physical fitness is often times incorporated into an overall testing battery used to determine which people are selected for certain jobs in public safety, and even for promotion to higher rank and pay grade in the military. Clearly, the testing of physiological function is ubiquitous and provides vital information for people of all levels of fitness, all ages, and many professions. Thus, the person responsible for selecting and conducting these tests must have an appropriate level of expertise in laboratory and field testing procedures.

Quick Review

- Strength is the maximal amount of force exerted during a single attempt of a movement.
- The grip dynamometer test is a popular test of strength.
- The 1-RM is another test to quantify strength. This is the amount of weight or resistance that can be lifted through the entire range of motion for a single time in a given movement.

REVIEW QUESTIONS

Fill-in-the-Blank

1. To measure blood pressure typically a _____ and a _____ are used.

2. _____ is force times vertical distance divided by time.

3. In untrained people, lactate threshold typically occurs at about _____% of that person's $\dot{V}O_{2max}$.

4. _____ is an enzyme responsible for converting carbonic acid (H_2CO_3) into water (H_2O) and carbon dioxide (CO_2).

5. Typically, the Wingate test of anaerobic power involves maximal effort cycling for _____ seconds.

Multiple Choice

1. Submaximal _____ can be used to estimate $\dot{V}O_{2max}$ because it has a linear relationship to oxygen consumption up to maximal workloads.
   a. heart rate
   b. lactate threshold
   c. strength
   d. blood pressure

2. The _____ and _____ Korotkoff sound represent systolic and diastolic blood pressure, respectively.
   a. fourth and fifth
   b. first and fourth
   c. first and fifth
   d. first and second

3. Female and male international class endurance athletes have $\dot{V}O_{2max}$ values of approximately _____, respectively.
   a. 30 and 45 mL·kg^{-1}·min^{-1}
   b. 60 and 70 mL·kg^{-1}·min^{-1}
   c. 75 and 85 mL·kg^{-1}·min^{-1}
   d. 90 and 95 mL·kg^{-1}·min^{-1}

4. Which of the following measurements would indicate attainment of maximal oxygen consumption during a GXT?
   a. Blood lactate concentration of 5 mmol·L^{-1} or greater
   b. Respiratory exchange ratio greater than 0.90
   c. Heart rate equal to at least 80% of age predicted maximum
   d. Plateauing or decrease in $\dot{V}O_2$ with an increase in workload

5. Which of the following tests accurately assesses anaerobic capacity of glycolysis?
   a. Vertical jump
   b. Wingate test
   c. Grip dynamometer
   d. 1-RM bench press

True/False

1. Work is defined as force exerted over distance.
2. Strength is the product of force multiplied by velocity.
3. An important disadvantage to using an isokinetic dynamometer to assess muscular strength is that it tends to test isolated muscles during unilateral movements.
4. The maximal amount of muscular force exerted during a single effort is referred to as work.

5. The primary advantage of the anaerobic metabolic pathway is that its use for energy production is not likely to result in muscle fatigue.

Short Answer

1. Explain the difference between work and power using a real-life example.
2. Explain when it may be appropriate to conduct a cardiovascular endurance test on an athlete using modes of exercise other than cycling or running.
3. Discuss typical maximal oxygen consumption values for different age groups, sexes, and athletes from different sports.
4. Discuss how auscultation using a stethoscope and sphygmomanometer can be used to determine blood pressure.
5. Describe the assumptions that allow estimation of cardiovascular endurance capabilities or $\dot{V}O_{2max}$ from field tests.

Critical Thinking

1. Discuss termination criteria of a cardiovascular endurance test for a healthy individual or athlete and for a person at increased risk of cardiovascular disease.
2. Discuss factors affecting anaerobic power and speed tests.

KEY TERMS

anaerobic treadmill test: determination of anaerobic capabilities as the time to exhaustion while running on a treadmill at a predetermined grade and speed
auscultation: listening for sounds from organs or tissue to aid in diagnosis of normal or abnormal function
concentric failure: performing an exercise until it is impossible to complete a repetition, which normally occurs in the concentric or lifting phase of the repetition
continuous protocol: exercise test during which exercise intensity is increased in stages with no rest or break between stages
discontinuous protocol: exercise test during which exercise intensity is increased in stages, but with a short rest period between stages
dyspnea: difficulty in breathing or labored breathing
graded exercise test (GXT): a test of cardiovascular endurance during which exercise intensity is progressively increased using a treadmill or cycle ergometer
grip dynamometer test: strength test that measures force development by the finger flexors during an isometric action
heart rate variability: the variation in time between heartbeats
Korotkoff sound: one of the sounds used to determine systolic and diastolic blood pressure when using auscultation to determine blood pressure
Margaria step test: a power test consisting of sprinting up a flight of stairs
power: force times distance divided by time, or work divided by time

sphygmomanometer: an instrument consisting of a pressure gauge and inflatable rubber cuff; used in conjunction with a stethoscope to determine blood pressure

strength: the amount of force generated during a single all-out effort

syncope: dizziness

$\dot{V}O_{2max}$: the maximal amount of oxygen that the body can consume; typically determined with an exercise test

vertical jump test: test of maximal vertical jump ability used to determine lower body power

Wingate test: 30-second maximal cycling ergometry test during which peak power, average power, anaerobic capacity, and fatigue index can be calculated

work: force times distance

REFERENCES

1. American Alliance for Health and Physical Education, Recreation, and Dance. Health Related Physical Fitness Test Manual. Washington, DC: AAHPERD; 1980.
2. American Heart Association. Heart disease and stroke statistics—2008 uptake: A report from the American Heart Association Statistics Committee and Stroke Statistics Subcommittee. Circulation. 2008;117:e25–e146.
3. Astrand PO. Work Tests With the Bicycle Ergometer. Varberg, Sweden: Monark Crescent AB, 1988.
4. Balke B, Ware RW. An experimental study of physical fitness of Air Force personnel. US Armed Forces Med J. 1959;10:675–688.
5. Berkoff D, Cairns CB, Sanchez LD, et al. Heart rate variability in a league American track-and-field athletes. J Strength Cond Res. 2007;21:227–231.
6. Billat V, Lopes P. Indirect methods for estimation of aerobic power. In: Maud PJ, Foster C. Physiological Assessment of Human Fitness, 2nd ed. Champaign, IL: Human Kinetics Publishers, 2006:19–37.
7. Bittner V, Weiner DH, Yusuf S, et al. Prediction of mortality morbidity with a 6-minute walk test in patients with less ventricular dysfunction. JAMA. 1993;270:1702–1707.
8. Blair S, Kampert JB, Kohl HW III, et al. Influences of cardiorespiratory fitness and other precursors on cardiovascular disease and all-cause mortality in men and women. JAMA. 1996;276:205–210.
9. Blair S, Kohl HW III, Barlow CE, et al. Changes in physical fitness and all-cause mortality. A prospective study of healthy and unhealthy men. JAMA. 1995;273:1093–1098.
10. Bohannon RW. Is it legitimate to characterize muscle strength using a limited number of measures? J Strength Cond Res. 2008;22:166–173.
11. Borg G. Perceived exertion as an indicator of somatic stress. Scand J Rehabil Med. 1970;2:92–98.
12. Buchfuhrer MJ, Hansen JE, Robinson TE, et al. Optimizing the exercise protocol for cardiopulmonary assessment. J Appl Physiol. 1983;55:558–564.
13. Canavan PK, Vescovi JD. Evaluation of power prediction equations: Peak vertical jumping power in women. Med Sci Sports Exerc. 2004;36:1589–1593.
14. Cooper KH. A means of assessing maximal oxygen intake. JAMA. 1968;203:201–204.
15. Cunningham DA, Faulkner JA. The effect of training on anaerobic and anaerobic metabolism during a short exhaustive run. Med Sci Sports Exerc. 1969;1:65–69.
16. Davis HA, Cass GC. The anaerobic threshold as determined before and during training: acidosis. Eur J Physiol Occup Physiol. 1981;47:141–149.
17. Davis JA, Kasch FW. Aerobic and anaerobic differences between maximal running and cycling in middle-aged males. Sports Med. 1975;7:81–84.
18. Dolgener FA, Hensley LD, Marsh JJ, et al. Validation out of the Rockport fitness walking test in college males and females. Res Q Exerc Sport. 1994;65:152–158.
19. Dotan R, Bar-Or O. Load optimization for the Wingate anaerobic test. Eur J Appl Physiol. 1983;51:409–417.
20. Fenstermaker KL, Plowman SA, Looney MA. Validation out of the Rockport fitness walking test in females 65 years and older. Res Q Exerc Sport. 1992;63:322–327.
21. George JD, Fellingham GW, Fisher AG. A modified version of the Rockport fitness walking test for college men and women. Res Q Exerc Sport. 1998;69:205–209.
22. Housh TJ, Cramer JT, Weir JP, et al. Physical Fitness Laboratories on a Budget. Scottsdale, AZ: Holcomb Hathaway, 2009.
23. Inbar O, Bar-Or O, Skinner JS. The Wingate Anaerobic Test. Champaign, IL: Human Kinetics, 1996.
24. Joyner MJ, Coyle EF. Endurance exercise performance: The physiology of champions. J Physiol. 2008;586:35–44.
25. Kline GM, Porcari JP, Hintermeister R, et al. Estimation of $\dot{V}O_{2max}$ from a one-mile track walk, gender, age and body weight. Med Sci Sports Exerc. 1987;19:253–259.
26. Lafortuna CL, Agosti F, Marinone PG, et al. The relationship between body composition and muscle power output in men and women with obesity. J Endocrinol Invest. 2004;27:854–861.
27. Leger LA, Lambert J. A maximal multistage 20 m shuttle run test to protect VO_2 max. Eur J Appl Physiol. 1982;49:1–5.
28. Lopes PL, White J. Heart rate variability: Measurement methods and practical applications. In: Maud PJ, Foster C . Physiological Assessment and Human Fitness, 2nd ed. Champaign, IL: Human Kinetics Publishers, 2006:39–62.
29. Margaria R, Aghemo P, Rovelli E. Measurement of muscular power (anaerobic) in man. J Appl Physiol. 1966;21:1662–1664.
30. McArdle WD, Katch FI, Pecher GS, et al. Reliability and interrelationships between maximal oxygen intake, physical work capacity, and step-test scores in college women. Med Sci Sports Exerc. 1972;4:182–186.
31. Meyers J, Prakash M, Froelichier V, et al. Exercise capacity and mortality among man referred for exercise testing. N Engl J Med. 2002;4:793–801.
32. Midgley AW, Bentley DJ, Luttikholt H, et al. Challenging a dogma of exercise physiology does an incremental exercise test for valid $\dot{V}O_{2max}$ determination really need to last between 8 and 12 minutes? Sports Med. 2008;38:441–447.
33. Nedeljkovic A, Mirkov DM, Pazin N, et al. Evaluation of Margaria staircase test: The effect of body size. Eur J Appl Physiol. 2007;100:115–120.
34. Paterson DJ, Friedland JS, Bascom DA, et al. Changes in arterial K+ and ventilation during exercise in normal subjects and subjects with McArdle's syndrome. J Physiol. 1990;429:339–348.
35. Pickering TG, Hall JE, Appel LJ, et al. Recommendations for blood pressure measurement in humans from the subcommittee of professional and public education of the American Heart Association Council on high blood pressure research. Circulation. 2005;111:697–716.
36. Ramsbottom R, Brewer J, Willimas C. A progressive shuttle run test to estimate maximal oxygen uptake. Sports Med. 1988;22:141–145.
37. Robinson TE, Sue DY, Huszczuk A, et al. Intra-arterial and cuff blood pressure responses during incremental cycle ergometry. Med Sci Sports Exerc. 1988;20:142–149.
38. Sawka MN, Tahamont MV, Fitzgerald PI, et al. Alactic capacity and power: Reliability and interpretation. Eur J Appl Physiol Occup Physiol. 1980;45:109–116.
39. Sayers SP, Harackiewicz DV, Harman EA, et al. Cross-validation of three jump power equations. Med Sci Sports Exerc. 1999;31:572–577.
40. Spirduso WW, Francis KL, MacRae PG. Physical of Dimensions of Aging. Champaign, IL: Human Kinetics, 1997:95–121.
41. Whaley MH, Brubaker PH, Otto RM. ACSM's Guidelines for Exercise Testing and Prescription, 7th ed. Philadelphia, PA: Lippincott Williams & Wilkins, 2007.
42. Yoshida T, Chida M, Ichioka M, et al. Relationship between ventilation and arterial potassium concentration during incremental exercise and recovery. Eur J Appl Physiol Occup Physiol. 1990;61:193–196.

Suggested Readings

Housh TJ, Cramer JT, Weir JP, et al. Physical Fitness Laboratories on a Budget. Scottsdale, AZ: Holcomb Hathaway, 2009.

Maud PJ, Foster C. Physiological Assessment of Human Fitness, 2nd ed. Champaign, IL: Human Kinetics, 2006.

Midgley AW, Bentley DJ, Luttikholt H, et al. Challenging a dogma of exercise physiology: does an incremental exercise test for valid $\dot{V}O_{2max}$ determination really need to last between 8 and 12 minutes? Sports Med. 2008;38:441–447.

Whaley MH. ACSM's Guidelines for Exercise Testing and Prescription, 7th ed. Baltimore, MD: Lippincott Williams & Wilkins, 2006 .

Classic References

Astrand PO. Work Tests With the Bicycle Ergometer. Varberg, Sweden: Monark Crescent AB, 1988.

Borg G. Perceived exertion as an indicator of somatic stress. Scand J Rehabil Med. 1970;2:92–98.

Knuttgen HG, Kraemer WJ. Terminology and measurement in exercise performance. J Appl Sport Sci Res. 1987;1:1–10.

14

Ergogenics in Exercise and Sport

After reading this chapter, you should be able to:

1. Describe and critique ergogenic aid research
2. Explain the physiological basis of oxygen delivery aids
3. Discuss and compare different types of oxygen delivery aids
4. Explain the proposed mechanisms of supplements that are used to delay fatigue
5. Describe the possible effects on physical performance of hormone supplements commonly used by athletes

6. Discuss the use of oral contraceptives by female athletes and potential impacts on performance
7. Explain the underlying physiological mechanisms of prohormones and why athletes might choose to use them
8. Critique the impact of the effectiveness of drugs on performance
9. Discuss different types of drugs used by athletes
10. Discuss nutritional supplements use by athletes, including type and rationale

A general definition of an **ergogenic aid** is a substance, training practice, or phenomenon that may increase physical performance. In the Olympic Games or world championships for specific sports, the difference in performance between winning gold, silver, or bronze medals or finishing in the top 5 to 10 athletes can be as small as 1% to 2%. Due to the fame and potential monetary rewards associated with winning for elite athletes, it is easy to understand the allure of ergogenic aids for elite athletes. However, some ergogenic aids have also become popular among fitness enthusiasts. Some ergogenic aids are banned for use by professional athletes and those competing in international competitions. Not all ergogenic aids are illegal, but many of the chemical substances that artificially elevate performance and have negative side effects have been banned. To find out the status of a drug or supplement for use by athletes in the Olympic Games, Pan American Games, or Paralympic Games, see the Web site of the U.S. Anti-Doping Agency (http://www.usada.org/dro/).

The list of potential ergogenic aids is quite long and includes nutrients, drugs, training practices such as a warm-up or altitude training, and even biomechanical aids, such as swimsuits that reduce drag. The effects of some ergogenic aids have already been discussed: carbohydrate and protein supplementation (Chapter 8), sufficient fluid ingestion (Chapter 9), altitude training (Chapter 10), and a warm-up (Chapter 2). In this chapter, additional ergogenic aids will be discussed that are popular and have been sufficiently researched to allow conclusions concerning their effectiveness. Ergogenic aids typically increase performance by affecting endurance capabilities, strength or power, or body composition.

ERGOGENIC AID RESEARCH

Many ergogenic aids become popular because an elite or professional athlete uses an ergogenic aid and then becomes successful. This results in the athlete directly or indirectly giving a testimonial that the ergogenic aid did increase his or her performance. Thus, the ergogenic aid becomes popular in the sport in which the athlete competes and possibly other sports. Although the ergogenic aid may have contributed to the athlete's success, many other factors could also have contributed to the athlete's success. Such testimonials do not constitute scientific research substantiating the effectiveness of an ergogenic aid.

Factors Related to the Application of Research

Drawing conclusions from ergogenic aid research concerning the effectiveness of an ergogenic aid can be difficult. The ability to apply conclusions from research to actual competitions depends in part on the similarities between the controlled laboratory setting and the athletic competition, where environmental factors may be different from the controlled laboratory setting. Several factors and considerations can enter into the applicability of research conclusions to athletic competition, including the following:

- **Testing specificity:** The laboratory test used to evaluate the effectiveness of an ergogenic aid may not accurately represent its effect in athletic competition. For example, sometimes a maximal 30-second sprint cycling test (Wingate test) is used to examine whether an ergogenic aid increases sprint ability. However, whether the results from a cycling test represent the ability in a running sprint on a track or in a game, such as American football, could be questioned.

- **Task specificity:** The ergogenic aid may increase performance in very short-term, high-power anaerobic events, such as Olympic weightlifting, but not in longer term high-power events, such as 200-meter sprinting and endurance events or vice versa. This makes it necessary to limit conclusions concerning the effectiveness of an ergogenic aid to specific types of tests and tasks.

- **Subjects:** Most research projects use untrained or moderately trained subjects, so it is questionable whether the results apply to athletes and, particularly, elite athletes. An ergogenic aid may increase performance in untrained subjects because they have not made training adaptations that athletes have, due to their training regimes.

- **Dosage:** Too little or too much of the ergogenic aid may show no effect on performance, with too much also potentially resulting in unwanted side effects that could negatively affect performance or health. Some athletes and coaches prescribe to the axiom, "if some is good, more is better." This results in the dosage of some ergogenic aids used by athletes being excessive and not reproducible in a controlled laboratory setting due to health and safety concerns.

- **Acute versus chronic use:** The acute effect of an ergogenic aid in subjects not accustomed to the ergogenic aid may be positive on performance. However, long-term use may result in an accommodation or lack of a positive response to the aid because it is no longer a novel stimulus, resulting in no effect on performance.

- **Statistical significance:** Scientists evaluate the results of projects on the basis of whether a statistically significant difference or change occurs. A 0.5% increase in performance may not be statistically significant, but a change of this magnitude could make the difference to athletes between winning or losing in many events.

All of these factors make it necessary to limit comments regarding the effectiveness of an ergogenic aid to specific types of tests and tasks, to specific populations, such as trained or untrained subjects, to specific dosages of the ergogenic aid, and to whether the effects, if any, are acute or chronic. Thus, it is necessary for exercise and sport scientists to carefully design projects investigating the effect of ergogenic aids and carefully interpret research results.

Placebo Effect

If an athlete or the subject in a research project believes that the ergogenic aid will increase his or her performance, it is likely that performance will, in fact, increase. In such cases, the increase in performance can be due to the psychological effects of believing that the ergogenic aid will be effective and not due to a physiological effect of the ergogenic aid, a phenomenon known as the "placebo effect." Thus, a **placebo**, or a "look-alike" substance or treatment that has no physiological effect, needs to be included in research projects to account for psychological effects.

It is also possible that a researcher believes that the ergogenic aid will have a positive effect on performance. This could result in unconscious behaviors by the researcher that could affect the outcome of the study, such as offering slightly more encouragement to subjects during testing. This problem is controlled by a **double-blind research design**, in which neither the researchers nor the subjects know who is receiving the ergogenic aid versus the placebo. With this type of research design, subjects are randomly assigned to either receiving substance or treatment A or B, representing the placebo or ergogenic aid, with neither the researchers nor the subjects knowing whether the subject is receiving the ergogenic aid or placebo. Only after completion of the research project and statistical analysis of the data to determine whether the ergogenic aid was effective are the researchers informed whether A or B was the ergogenic aid. Although these types of research designs are complex and difficult to perform, they are necessary to decrease the chance of the placebo effect for

Quick Review

- Ergogenic aid research is difficult to apply to athletes and field settings because of test specificity, task specificity, use of untrained or moderately trained subjects, dose-specific effects, chronic versus acute use, and differences between statistical and practical significance.
- The placebo effect can affect ergogenic aid research.
- To account for the placebo effect, researchers need to use appropriate research designs, such as double-blind research projects.

both the subjects and researchers. (See Chapter 1 as to how science creates knowledge in exercise and sport science.)

OXYGEN DELIVERY AIDS

Oxygen is necessary for aerobic metabolism and for recovery after an anaerobic event (EPOC; see Chapter 2). Oxygen delivery aids increase oxygen availability for metabolism during activity or during recovery from activity. If oxygen availability during activity is increased, performance may be increased, especially for aerobic or endurance activities. Also, if oxygen availability is increased during the recovery period after activity, the recovery may be enhanced and the ability to perform successive bouts of activity may be increased. Below, we will explore several forms of increasing oxygen availability during and after activity, including blood doping, erythropoietin (EPO), and oxygen supplementation. Other aids are currently being developed and may never be used by athletes because they would be easily detectable, but may be used to treat various disease states. These will not be discussed in depth here but include the following[18]:

- **Hematide:** a synthetic protein that stimulates red blood cell production (by binding to EPO receptors)
- **Gene doping:** modulation of genes to increase red blood cell production (stimulate EPO production) or other factors related to aerobic capabilities (aerobic enzymes)
- **Blood oxygen enhancers:** artificial substances that transport oxygen within the blood (hemoglobin-based oxygen carriers, perfluorocarbon emulsions)
- **Modulators of hemoglobin:** substances that decrease the affinity of hemoglobin for oxygen, thus increasing oxygen release to tissues (clofibrate, bezafibrate)

Blood Doping

Blood doping refers to any means by which total blood volume or red blood cell mass is increased above normal. All forms of blood doping were banned for use in the Olympic Games in 1984. The original method of blood doping involved infusion of red blood cells with the goal of increasing red blood cell number. This was accomplished either by an **autologous transfusion,** in which red blood cells previously withdrawn from the same person were infused, or **homologous transfusion,** in which red blood cells obtained from someone else were infused. Both methods resulted in an increase in blood volume and red blood cell number. The goal of blood doping, when used by athletes, is to increase red blood cell mass so that the ability to transport and deliver oxygen to muscle tissue increases. Blood doping primarily affects endurance performance, not anaerobic performance such as weightlifting or short sprints.

As early as 1972, a study showed that withdrawal of 800 to 1200 milliliters of red blood cells, refrigeration of the cells for 4 weeks, and then reinfusion resulted in considerable improvement in endurance performance markers.[32] The reinfusion of red blood cells resulted in a 9% increase in treadmill $\dot{V}O_{2peak}$ and a 23% increase in treadmill performance time. Other studies after 1972 showed inconsistent results, with some showing no effect and others significant improvement in endurance performance markers with blood doping. In 1980, a study using autologous transfusions started to reveal why blood doping showed inconsistent results concerning endurance performance.[20] In this study, highly trained distance runners were tested at the following times:

1. Before blood withdrawal
2. Shortly after blood withdrawal (before the withdrawn red blood cells could be replaced by the body by normal physiological means)
3. After a placebo infusion of saline after blood withdrawal
4. After reinfusion of 900 milliliters of blood that had been stored by freezing
5. After the amount of red blood cells had returned to normal after the reinfusion of blood

The results on $\dot{V}O_{2peak}$ and running time to exhaustion are shown in Figure 14-1. The results clearly show that the placebo reinfusion of saline had little effect. However, $\dot{V}O_{2peak}$ remained elevated for up to 16 weeks after the blood transfusion, and running time to exhaustion, although still elevated 16 weeks after the transfusion, gradually declined from 1 day after the transfusion.

Why did the study cited above start to explain why inconsistent results concerning endurance performance and blood doping were shown during the 1970s? Some studies in the 1970s did not infuse a sufficient amount of blood and infused the blood too early after blood withdrawal.[37] It appears that at least 900 milliliters of blood must be reinfused and at least 5 to 6 weeks and possibly up to 10 weeks must be allowed after blood withdrawal for the body to reestablish normal blood volume so that the infusion of blood results in above-normal red blood cell number. If these two factors are not met, little or no increase in $\dot{V}O_{2peak}$ or endurance performance will occur.

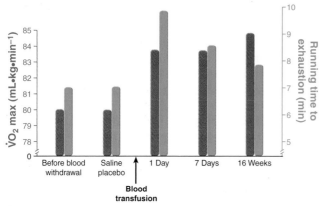

Figure 14-1. Effects of blood doping using blood reinfusion. Reinfusion of blood results in increased V̇O2max and running time to exhaustion. *Orange* bars, V̇O2max; *Blue* bars, running time to exhaustion. *Significantly different than the control value. (Adapted from Buick FJ, Gledhill N, Froese AB, et al. Effect of induced erythrocythemia on aerobic were capacity. J Appl Physiol. 1980;48:636–642.)

Another important factor is how the blood was stored prior to reinfusion. Both the 1972 study, which showed no change in performance, and the 1980 study, which showed improved performance, used autologous transfusions to increase blood volume. However, the 1972 study stored the blood using refrigeration, and the 1980 study stored the blood by freezing after withdrawal. Refrigeration of blood results in approximately 40% of red blood cells being destroyed, and blood can only be stored for approximately 5 weeks using refrigeration. Freezing of blood results in only approximately 15% of the red blood cells being destroyed and can be used to store blood for much longer periods of time. Thus, studies that refrigerated blood for long periods of time did not show increased endurance performance, whereas studies freezing blood did show increases in endurance performance. If blood doping is performed correctly, increases in V̇O2peak and endurance performance do take place.

How much of an increase in performance can be expected with blood doping? Autologous transfusions of 920 milliliters of blood in experienced distance runners decreased the time of 5-mile (8 kilometers) simulated runs on a treadmill by 51 seconds or 2.7% compared with an infusion of 920 milliliters of a saline placebo.[96] Most of this decrease in time occurred in the last 2.5 miles (4 kilometers), where blood doping resulted in a 33-second (3.7%) decrease in time compared with the saline placebo. Additionally, the results indicate that improvement with blood doping is in large part due to the increase in red blood cell number and not due to an expansion of total blood volume (saline placebo), which could increase cardiac output.

Blood doping, especially when performed using a homologous transfusion, does have some inherent risks. Increasing red blood cell count could result in the blood becoming too viscous or clotting, possibly causing heart

failure or stroke. Homologous transfusions do carry several additional risks compared with autologous transfusions. Mismatching the blood type of the donor and recipient could result in an allergic reaction, and there are risks of infection, such as hepatitis, human immunodeficiency virus (HIV), or any other bloodborne pathogen. Blood doping does increase endurance performance but is banned in athletic events. A newer form of blood doping using the hormone EPO is explored in the next section.

Erythropoietin

Eryhtropoietin (EPO) is a naturally occurring hormone that stimulates red blood cell production by bone marrow (see Chapter 10). When hypoxia, or lack of sufficient oxygen in the blood, is sensed by receptors in the kidneys, EPO is produced and released into the bloodstream. Small amounts of EPO are also produced by the liver (less than 10% of the total amount) and very small amounts by the brain.[18,76] The EPO circulates to the bone marrow, where it binds to specific receptors that stimulate erythropoiesis, or formation of red blood cells, and to the surface of erythroblasts or immature red blood cells, which increases the ability of erythroblasts to survive and mature into red blood cells. The mature red blood cells, or erythrocytes, are released into the blood, increasing the total amount of red blood cells. This improves oxygen delivery to the tissues producing EPO as well as other tissues. Without the stimulus of hypoxia, production of EPO by the kidneys, liver, and brain ceases.

Recombinant human EPO (rHuEPO) became available in 1985 and was banned from use by the International Olympic Committee (IOC) Medical Commission in 1990. Endurance athletes, however, have continued to attempt to use EPO to increase endurance capabilities. rHuEPO was originally developed to treat various disease states, such as anemia and cancer. However, the possible effects of rHuEPO injection on healthy humans were shown as early as 1991.[31] rHuEPO administration clearly increases V̇O2peak and endurance exercise performance in both untrained[83] and endurance-trained subjects.[14] In one study, 6 weeks after low-dose subcutaneous injection of rHuEPO in moderately trained to well-trained subjects, the following occurred:

- V̇O2peak increased 6% to 8%
- Time to exhaustion on a treadmill increased 13% to 17%
- Both hemoglobin concentration and hematocrit increased approximately 10%

Injection of rHuEPO in well-trained male endurance athletes three times per week for 30 days or until hematocrit reached 50% resulted in the following:

- Hematocrit increased 18.9% (42.7–50.8%)
- Cycling time to exhaustion increased 9.4% (12.8–14.0 min)
- Cycling V̇O2peak increased 7% (63.8–68.1 mL·kg⁻¹·min⁻¹)

rHuEPO administration was terminated in this study once a 50% hematocrit was reached. However, hematocrit levels can drastically exceed this level with rHuEPO administration. Extreme increases in hematocrit as well as other side effects can occur with rHuEPO administration.

Up to 18 deaths in competitive cyclists in the late 1980s were reportedly linked to rHuEPO use.[1] Like all hormones, once an artificial hormone is released into the bloodstream, the consequences are difficult to control or predict. Adverse side effects associated with rHuEPO injections include the following:

- Increased blood viscosity
- Increased platelet adhesion
- Increased platelet count
- Arterial hypertension
- Headache
- Muscle cramps
- Upper respiratory tract infections
- Posttreatment anemia
- Convulsion
- Incomplete development of red blood cells

These side effects place an athlete who chooses to use rHuEPO at considerable risk for a heart attack or stroke and other circulatory problems.

Although the primary mechanism by which rHuEPO increases endurance performance is by affecting red blood cell count, other actions of EPO may also increase endurance capabilities. For example, in rats, EPO administration alone or in conjunction with treadmill running results not only in increased hematocrit, but also in the following:

- Increased metabolic enzyme concentrations (cytochrome c oxidase, citrate synthase, phosphofructokinase)
- Muscle contractile changes (increased slow myosin heavy chains associated with type I muscle fibers)[22]

The effects of EPO administration and endurance training on these factors in rats is additive. This means that rats that received EPO and did not exercise showed positive changes in all the above factors, whereas those that received EPO and did exercise showed even greater responses in all of the above factors.

Oxygen Supplementation

Oxygen supplementation refers to increasing the oxygen content or barometric pressure of inspired air, both of which increase the partial pressure of oxygen. Increasing the partial pressure of oxygen potentially increases the oxygen carried by the blood and so the amount of oxygen available for aerobic metabolism. Oxygen supplementation could be used immediately before, during, or immediately after a work bout. Some professional athletes, such as American football players, use oxygen supplementation during games, believing it will increase performance or aid recovery.

Oxygen supplementation immediately prior to a work bout might aid performance by increasing the amount of oxygen in the bloodstream, which could reduce dependence on anaerobic energy sources. The oxyhemoglobin disassociation curve (Chapter 6) ensures that, at altitudes close to sea level, red blood cells are close to 100% saturated with oxygen. Thus, supplemental oxygen at altitudes close to sea level would be of little value to increase oxygen saturation of hemoglobin. Supplemental oxygen may slightly increase the amount of oxygen dissolved in plasma. However, only a small amount of oxygen is dissolved in plasma, so an increase would be of minimal value in increasing oxygen availability.

Supplemental oxygen immediately after a work bout potentially aids recovery (Chapter 2) by increasing the oxygen available for aerobic metabolism during recovery (EPOC). But research suggests that similar to oxygen supplementation initially prior to a work bout at altitudes close to sea level, supplementation immediately after a work bout would minimally affect oxygen availability for aerobic metabolism. Breathing 100% oxygen or normal air for 4 minutes after a treadmill run to exhaustion lasting approximately 6 minutes did not result in lower blood lactate concentrations after 4 minutes of recovery.[98] There was also no difference in the time (approximately 2 minutes) of a second run to exhaustion after the recovery period of breathing either normal air or 100% oxygen. Although the information available is minimal, it does indicate that breathing 100% oxygen in a recovery period does not aid recovery or performance in the next work bout.

It has long been known that oxygen supplementation during exercise increases performance. In 1954, the same year that Roger Bannister became the first person to run a mile in less than 4 minutes, this physician researcher demonstrated that increasing the percent of oxygen in inspired air to greater than the normal 21% increased running time to exhaustion.[8] In well-trained road cyclists, off-road cyclists, and triathletes, increasing the percent of oxygen in inspired air while at moderate altitude (1860 meters) also increases performance.[93,94] The athletes performed six cycling intervals while completing a fixed amount of work (100 kilojoules), with the goal of completing the intervals as fast as possible. The total mean time needed to complete the six intervals when inspiring 21% oxygen was 6 minutes and 17 seconds. When breathing 26% oxygen and 60% oxygen, total mean time needed decreased by 5% and 8%, respectively. It is interesting to note that the 26% oxygen results in the same partial pressure of oxygen as at sea level at the altitude (barometric pressure) at which the intervals were performed.

Some athletes living and training at moderate altitude and higher for long periods of time lose the ability to maintain sea-level race pace due to loss of peripheral and neuromuscular adaptations. Supplemental oxygen can be used (as shown by the Wilber et al. studies cited above) during training sessions while at moderate altitude to offset the loss of ability to maintain sea-level race pace, and thus help to increase sea-level performance after training

- Oxygen delivery aids potentially increase available oxygen for aerobic metabolism during activity and for recovery processes.
- Use of transfusions when the blood is properly stored and when a sufficient amount of red blood cells are infused results in increased red blood cell number and blood volume that does significantly increase aerobic capabilities and performance.
- EPO use not only can increase red blood cell number, aerobic capabilities, and endurance performance, but can also have severe side effects.
- Oxygen supplementation between work bouts appears to be of little value to aid recovery and performance in subsequent work bouts. However, it is of value to maintain training intensity when training at altitude, which aids endurance performance on returning to sea level.

at altitude. Supplemental oxygen during training bouts at altitude has been shown to benefit sea-level performance in elite rowers,[64] endurance athletes,[70] and track sprinters.[66] Thus, although supplemental oxygen before and after an exercise bout may not significantly change performance, using supplemental oxygen while training at altitude does appear to be of value for increasing performance on returning to sea level.

SUPPLEMENTS THAT DELAY FATIGUE

Many different types of supplements have been used to limit fatigue and enhance performance, with success depending on the specific conditions of the exercise stress. These types of supplements typically buffer acidity resulting from metabolism, which may delay fatigue. These supplements may work in some situations and not in others, based on the exact effects of the supplement on the mechanisms resulting in fatigue in the complex fatigue process.[80]

Blood Buffering

The body tightly regulates blood pH, but under conditions of fatigue or extreme exercise blood pH drops from the normal pH range of 7.35 to 7.45. Exercise will cause a decrease in blood pH, with severe exercise causing a blood pH of approximately 7.1 (muscle can go to 6.8 pH). In some cases, blood pH can decrease even lower in highly anaerobically conditioned athletes. The decrease in pH is due to the metabolic production of hydrogen ions and other acids, such as lactic acid, pyruvic acid, and acetic acid. However, an increase in acidity depends not just on the production of acids, but also on buffering systems, or **blood buffers**.[75] The bicarbonate buffering system is the most important buffering system in the blood and helps to maintain a constant

pH. In the blood and body fluids, the chemical involved in the bicarbonate buffering system is sodium bicarbonate.

A number of reactions can take place involving the bicarbonate ion that affect blood pH.

1. The bicarbonate ion is really the conjugate base of carbonic acid:
$$H^+ + HCO_3^- \leftrightarrow [H_2CO_3]; pKa = 6.14 \qquad (1)$$
[Nonenzymatic acid–base reaction]

2. Carbonic acid, however, is very rapidly converted to CO_2 and water by carbonic anhydrase, making it a benign species:
$$[H_2CO_3] \leftrightarrow CO_2 + H_2O; pKa = 6.14 \qquad (2)$$
[Enzymatic reaction]

3. The products of carbonic anhydrase action, which are water and CO_2, are benign. Water can be absorbed into the body systems, and CO_2 can be expired.

4. HCO_3^- and H^+ can be regulated by physiological mechanisms operating in the kidney.

In a comprehensive review, McNaughton and colleagues examined the basis for using sodium bicarbonate as an ergogenic aid to help buffer the dramatic effects of exercise on blood pH and how this might translate to increased performance.[59] Typically, 0.3 g·kg body mass^{-1} mass is the dose used. Higher doses have many adverse symptoms, such as diarrhea, which limits the practicality of the use of higher doses.[80] As pointed out in this review, the effects on performance are due to the dose, timing of ingestion, and toleration. Approximately 10% of subjects do not tolerate bicarbonate supplementation. In addition, dehydration and the associated susceptibility to heat stress are factors that must be monitored. However, sodium bicarbonate supplementation can be effective in enhancing various types of performances in which decreased blood pH might be associated with the fatigue process.[59] The effects of bicarbonate on performance can be small but are significant. Table 14-1 shows the typical responses in different types of activities.

Phosphate Loading

Although a minor pH buffer in skeletal muscle, inorganic phosphate does contribute to buffering mechanisms. Other buffers in skeletal muscle include the amino acid histidine and carnosine. If extracellular and intracellular inorganic phosphate levels are increased, more phosphate is available for aerobic metabolism and for use as a buffer (like bicarbonate). (Remember that aerobic production of adenosine triphosphate (ATP) requires hydrogen and thus lowers acidity.) This has led to the concept of using a supplement containing P_i to augment these processes. Few data exist on this type of supplement, and the efficacy of such a dietary supplement is limited by the highly controlled regulation of inorganic phosphate by the kidney. In a study by Kraemer et al., highly trained road cyclists performed four

Table 14-1. Effects of Sodium Bicarbonate on Performance

Author	Exercise Mode or Sport-Specific Exercise	Dose (g·kg body mass^{-1})	Loading Time Before Exercise	Reported Ergogenic Effect
Single-Bout Exercise (Listed by Publish Date)				
Lindh et al., 2007	200-m freestyle swim	0.3	60–90 min	↓mean performance times in NaHCO$_3$ trial (~1 s)
Siegler et al., 2007	Cycle to exhaustion at 120% of PPO	0.3	60 min	No difference in TTE
Robergs et al., 2005	Cycle to exhaustion at 110% of PPO	0.2 NaHCO$_3$ + 0.2 NaCitrate	60 min	No difference in TTE
Van Montfoort et al., 2004	Run to exhaustion (range 19–23 km·hr^{-1})	0.3 NaHCO$_3$ or 0.525 NaCitrate or 0.4 NaLactate	90 min	↑NaHCO$_3$ trial (~2.7%) ↑NaCitrate trial (~2.2%) ↑NaLactate trial (~1.0%)
Raymer et al., 2004	Forearm exercise to fatigue	0.3	90 min	↑TTE and PPO in NaHCO$_3$ trial (~12%)
Gordon et al., 1994	90 s Wingate test at 0.05 kg·kg body mass^{-1}	0.3 g or	45 min	No difference
	Multiple-Bout Exercise			
Matsuura et al., 2007	Ten 10-s RS interspersed with passive recovery (range 30–360 s)	0.3 divided into six ingestion periods every 10 min	60 min	No difference in peak or mean power output
Artioli et al., 2007	Simulated judo performance (assessed in number of throws)	0.3	120 min	5.1% more throws in NaHCO$_3$ trial as well as ↑average power in Wingate test for upper limps
Mero et al., 2004	Interval swim (2 × 100 m with 10 min passive rest between intervals)	0.3	60 min	↓second swim time (~0.9 s) in NaHCO$_3$ trial[a]
Bishop et al., 2004	Series of five 6-s RS (4:1 work to rest ratio)	0.3	90 min	↑in total work and ↑ in work and PO in sprints 3 to −5
Aschenbach et al., 2000	Eight 15-s intervals of maximal forearm exercise (20-s active recovery between sets)	0.3	Split into equal doses at 90 and 60 min	No difference
	Endurance Performance			
Bishop and Claudius, 2005	Two 36-min "halves" of intermittent field hockey specific activity	0.2 twice	Split at 90 and 20 min	No difference in total work over 72 min; ↑work performed in 7 of 18 second half sprints
Price et al., 2003	Two 30-min intermittent cycling trials	0.3	60 min	↑average related PO during maximal spring efforts
Stephens et al., 2002	30-min continuous cycling at ~ 70% $\dot{V}O_{2max}$ followed by a performance ride (time to complete 469 ± 21 kJ work)	0.3 (60 min ingestion time)	90 min	No difference in performance
	Chronic Loading			
Douroudos et al., 2006	30-s Wingate (0.075 kg·kg body mass^{-1})	0.5 for 5 d 0.3 for 5 d	None on day of trial	↑average power in 0.5 g NaHCO$_3$ only
Edge et al., 2006	6–12 2-min cycle intervals at 140–170% of LT (in addition to regimented training)	0.2 twice	90 and 30 min	↑ performance at LT after 8 wk of training on NaHCO$_3$

[a]Additional use of creatine (Cr) supplementation but did not have a Cr only trial included in the methodology.

PPO: peak power output; PO: power output; TTE: time to exhaustion; RS: repeated sprint; LT: lactate threshold.

Adapted with permission and modified from: McNaughton LR, Siegler J, Midgley A. Ergogenic effects of sodium bicarbonate. Curr Sports Med Rep. 2008;7(4):230–236.

30-second cycling sprint tests (Wingate test) separated by 2 minutes, with and without a multibuffer supplement containing predominantly inorganic phosphate, bicarbonate, and carnosine.[50] The major findings were that this dietary supplement did not impact acid–base balance and did not improve Wingate test performances. It did appear to help some markers of recovery between sprints (increased postexercise levels of 2,3-DPG and the 2,3-DPG/Hb ratio). Thus, phosphate loading does not appear to be a very effective way to enhance high-intensity performance.

HORMONES

Hormones occur naturally within the body. Some hormones affect muscle protein synthesis and metabolic substrate use, possibly resulting in increased muscle mass. The increased muscle mass potentially results in increased maximal strength. This makes some hormones attractive as possible ergogenic aids to athletes. Hormone ingestion is also used to control the menstrual cycle, which could also affect physical performance. How hormones exert their influence on bodily function has been previously discussed (Chapter 7) and will not be extensively discussed here. The possible effects on physical performance of the most commonly used hormones by athletes are discussed in the following section.

Steroids

A recent comprehensive review of the use of anabolic steroids and growth hormone (GH) was published as a position stand by the *National Strength and Conditioning Association*.[44] Testosterone has both androgenic (secondary sex characteristics) and anabolic (to build or promote growth) properties. The many synthetic forms abused by athletes are all forms of the male hormone testosterone (Fig. 14-2). Due to the many alterations in testosterone now available, the term now used is androgen use or abuse. As discussed in detail in Chapter 7, testosterone is the primary hormone in males that stimulates the secondary sex characteristics during puberty and signals anabolic effects with exercise training. Testosterone stimulates anabolic effects via the androgen receptor on a regulatory element of the cell's DNA. Testosterone concentrations are 20 to 30 times lower in women. Although it is still very effective and uses the same mechanisms, the lower concentration makes its role in women less pronounced. The low concentration in women is one reason women who train naturally do not have to worry about getting extremely large muscles. However, with such low concentrations in the body, the use of synthetic androgens is extremely effective in women, producing changes in many body tissues that may be irreversible (e.g., secondary sex characteristics). Thus, the use of androgens in women has serious consequences.

Clearly, the use of synthetic androgens with a resistance training program dramatically enhances strength, power, and muscle size. In addition, it helps to enhance recovery from exercise and competition stress. The combination of benefits is well known to coaches and athletes and has made use of these anabolic drugs tempting for many years.[44] The side effects and risks of androgen use are likewise well known and include being banned from competition, ending careers, and losing hero status in their sports (e.g., loss of hall-of-fame nominations, medals and titles being removed, loss of income from endorsements, etc.). However, new designer androgens, such as tetrahydrogestrinone (TGH), are still appearing on the scene that do not test positively in commonly used drug tests and are not discovered by the agencies that perform advanced drug testing until after some athletes have already used them. In addition, searching for new ways to avoid detection of anabolic drugs in drug testing also continues. So, combating such illegal drug use in sports continues to be a challenge for governing bodies in sports. Many of the side effects for different types of androgens have been noted and are related to the type of synthetic androgen abused.[44] The National Institute of Drug Abuse has documented some of the major negative effects of synthetic androgen use, and they are as follows:

- Steroid abuse can lead to serious, even irreversible health problems. Some of the most dangerous include liver damage, jaundice (yellowish pigmentation of skin, tissues, and body fluids), fluid retention, high blood pressure, increases in LDL-C (bad cholesterol), and decreases in HDL-C (good cholesterol). Other reported effects include renal failure, severe acne, and trembling. In addition, there are some gender- and age-specific adverse effects:
  - For men—shrinking of the testicles, reduced sperm count, infertility, baldness, development of breasts, increased risk for prostate cancer
  - For women—growth of facial hair, male-pattern baldness, changes in or cessation of the menstrual cycle, enlargement of the clitoris, deepened voice
  - For adolescents—stunted growth due to premature skeletal maturation and accelerated puberty changes; adolescents risk not reaching their expected height if they take anabolic steroids before the typical adolescent growth spurt
- In addition, people who inject anabolic steroids run the added risk of contracting or transmitting HIV/acquired immunodeficiency syndrome (AIDS) or hepatitis, which causes serious damage to the liver.

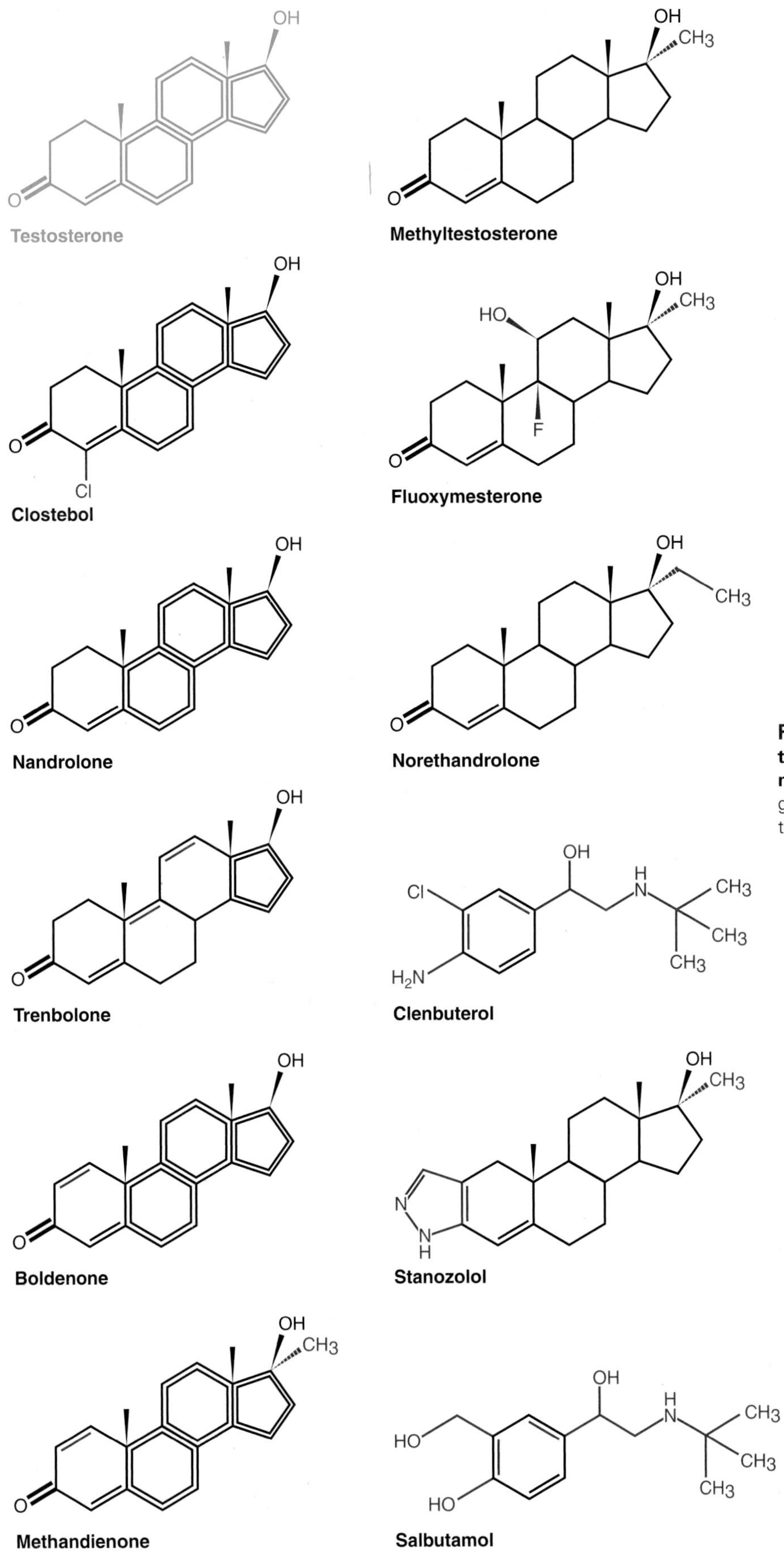

Testosterone

Methyltestosterone

Clostebol

Fluoxymesterone

Nandrolone

Norethandrolone

Figure 14-2. The male sex hormone testosterone (upper left corner) has been modified in many ways. The modifications generally maintain the basic ring structure of testosterone and mimic its physiological actions.

Trenbolone

Clenbuterol

Boldenone

Stanozolol

Methandienone

Salbutamol

Human Growth Hormone

Growth hormone (GH), often called human growth hormone (HGH) when talking about it as a drug supplement has received a lot of attention in athletics over the past 5 years.[49] With the increased sophistication of tests for synthetic androgen use, HGH had become a drug of choice among some athletes in the attempt to avoid drug testing and gain some benefits of an anabolic drug. However, now a test for GH use has been developed and has been used (see Chapter 7). Many coaches and athletes are not aware that HGH can be taken only via an injection and that it must be kept cold or it will degrade, making it ineffective. Its physiological role is linear bone growth in children, by actions at the epiphysis (growth plates) and the differentiation of the osteoblasts, and to promote anabolic (tissue building) metabolism, resulting in an altered body. GH actions include the hepatic and local synthesis and release of its main mediator, insulin-like growth factor-I (IGF-I). It shares some of these roles with IGF-I, meaning that the direct effect of GH and/or local production of IGF-I are both required for optimal growth. As discussed in Chapter 7, GH is a family of polypeptides and not a single hormone. However, the 22-kD, 191-amino acid form is what is made by the DNA and is what the pharmaceutical companies make and modify for its use clinically. Many of the actions of GH may be attributed to a variant of GH or an aggregate of GH with binding proteins thus making a test for GH use challenging from an analytical and legal perspective. However, as noted in Chapter 7, a new test for GH doping has been implemented by the World Anti-Doping Agency and has been used by to detect GH use in athletes.[49]

With conventional doses, it has been shown that HGH does not appear to be an effective anabolic substance for younger people, or anti-aging agent in the elderly, making its use even more suspect.[55,56] One study by Graham et al., however, did show short-term improvements in muscle force production and protein metabolism with acute 6-day use in untrained people.[41] A study by Meinhardt et al.[61] examined HGH (2 mg·day^{-1} injected subcutaneously) supplementation for 6 weeks in men and women. They also in men alone examined GH and testosterone (250 mg·wk^{-1} injected intramuscularly), or combined treatments. The authors stated "First, body cell mass at baseline was correlated with all measures of physical performance. Second, growth hormone significantly reduced fat mass, increased lean body mass through an increase in extracellular water, and increased body cell mass when given with testosterone. Third, growth hormone led to statistically significant improvements in sprint capacity that were not maintained after a 6-week washout period in a pooled group of men and women, and the improvements were greater when growth hormone was co-administered with testosterone to men. Finally, changes in body cell mass did not correlate with improvement in sprint capacity, except when growth hormone was co-administered with testosterone." The extent of use and doses of HGH used by athletes are difficult to ascertain.[49] The benefits are still equivocal and may not be worth the risks associated with the side effects that accompany its use, especially since its real impact comes with the concomitant use of testosterone. Side effects, especially of high doses of HGH, include the following:

- **Acromegaly** a disease of abnormal bone growth and gigantism. Interestingly, many bodybuilders require plastic surgery to correct some of the anatomical changes, especially women (e.g., ear, nose procedures). Side effects related to this disease include the following:
  - Coarse, oily, thickened skin
  - Extreme sweating and body odor
  - Small outgrowths of skin tissue (skin tags)
  - Exhaustion and muscle weakness
  - A deepened, husky voice due to enlarged vocal cords and sinuses
  - Severe snoring due to obstruction of the upper airway
  - Impaired vision; headaches
  - A puffy tongue
  - Pain and limited joint mobility
  - Menstrual cycle irregularities in women
  - Puffed-up liver, heart, kidneys, spleen, and other organs
  - Increased chest size (barrel chest)
- **Hypoglycemia:** low concentration of blood glucose. Some people with hypoglycemia have too much insulin, which causes the uptake of glucose into the cells. GH stimulates insulin release from the pancreas, and insulin mediates the lower concentrations of blood glucose by stimulating its entry into cells.
- **Belly distension due to internal organ growth**
- **Carpal tunnel syndrome:** a nerve impingement in the wrist, which leads to pain, created by induced bone growth
- **Joint pain:** this can occur due to the growth promoting actions in the connective tissue of joints

Insulin

As discussed in Chapter 7, insulin is important for hormone replacement in patients whose pancreas cannot produce insulin (type I diabetes). Athletes use this drug in an attempt to improve body composition or performance based on its growth-promoting properties as a natural hormone secreted in response to meals and exercise. The hormone's primary role is the tight regulation of blood glucose. It is assisted in this function by its antagonistic hormone glucagon. However, it has also been viewed as an anabolic drug, with little data to support its use for this purpose. Its mediating effects for protein synthesis in cells is due to receptor-mediated signaling systems for stimulating protein synthesis as well as glucose uptake. The effectiveness of this hormone as a drug remains unclear due to its dramatic effect on glucose metabolism and its redundancy with other anabolic hormones, which are not so tightly regulated. Side effects can be severe, including long-term hypoglycemic states, death due to insulin shock, and brain damage.

Insulin-Like Growth Factors

Similar to GH, IGF-I has been thought to be an ergogenic aid based on its known role in muscle tissue anabolism.[9] As noted in Chapter 7, its multiple roles in various target tissues make the side effects potentially dramatic (e.g., cancers). Owing to its relationship to GH, its negative impact on normal GH release and function is compromised.[35] At present, there is little or no experimental data to understand the efficacy of IGF-I supplementation in athletes.

Oral Contraceptives

The use of oral contraceptives (OCPs) has become increasingly popular among female athletes, and it is now estimated that their use is as common among athletes as among the general population.[13] In large part, this popularity is attributed to refinements in the dosages and types of exogenous estrogens and progesterones (progestogen) used. In general, dosages used today are much less than they were when OCPs first became available, so secondary effects are similarly less pronounced. Depending on the dosages of sex steroids contained in them, as well as the timing of when peak dosages occur, OCPs can be broadly assigned to three categories: monophasic, biphasic, and triphasic. Of the three, monophasic and triphasic OCPs are by far the most commonly prescribed today. **Monophasic oral contraceptive pills** are formulated to hold estrogen and progestogen levels constant throughout the 28-day menstrual cycle. In contrast, **triphasic oral contraceptive pills** dispense three different doses of estrogen, and usually progestogen, throughout the 28-day cycle. As a result, circulating levels of these steroid hormones vary accordingly during a 4-week interval. Because women may respond quite differently to specific types of OCPs, and so many variations of both monophasic and triphasic OCPs exist, it is difficult to reach broad, encompassing conclusions regarding the impact of OCPs on athletic performance.

A primary concern of women taking OCPs is that they may cause water retention and thus weight gain. Indeed, reports of feeling bloated are common among athletes as well as nonathletes, regardless of whether they are taking monophasic or triphasic OCPs. Despite the consistency of claims of feeling bloated, research indicates that the training status may determine whether weight gain actually occurs. Specifically, the limited research available suggests that trained women may experience a significant weight gain of as much as 2 kilograms over the course of 6 months, whereas untrained women show no alteration in body weight.[65] Furthermore, changes in body composition may accompany the use of OCPs. In particular, triphasic OCPs have been associated with an increased percentage of body fat if they are taken for

at least 4 months.[21,53] This increased fat mass, typically 3% to 10%, may be problematic in sports that usually encourage minimal body mass and fat, such as distance running and gymnastics.

Because even endogenous progesterone is known to influence core temperature regulation, it is not surprising that its synthetic analog, progestogen, which is used in OCPs, also impacts the internal temperature of females taking OCPs. Indeed, when progestogen concentrations are highest during the 28-day cycle of the OCP prescription, core temperature also peaks. This is most obvious when using triphasic OCPs, in which progestogen dosages vary over a 28-day interval. In monophasic OCPs, in which the dose of progestogen remains steady, so does temperature, but at higher values than those of controls who were not prescribed OCPs. In sports in which proper thermoregulation is essential for optimal performance, such as distance running or soccer, the OCP-induced increase in core temperature may have detrimental effects. Recent research, however, seems to contradict this assumption. Armstrong et al. found that women taking OCPs adapted to the stress of endurance training and heat acclimation as well as women not taking them.[4]

In addition to temperature regulation, another area in which the OCPs appear to exert a substantial influence is substrate utilization. Both at rest and during exercise, trained and untrained women taking OCPs demonstrate an increased reliance on lipids for ATP production and, as a result, a glycogen-sparing effect.[17,60] Of course, this glycogen-sparing effect would be of benefit in long-duration events such as the marathon. As of yet, however, this benefit has not been confirmed scientifically.

In women taking monophasic OCPs, in which sex steroid endocrine status is held constant throughout the 28-day cycle, research has yielded conflicting results concerning the effect of OCPs on $\dot{V}O_{2max}$. Although one study examining peak aerobic capacity over 6 months documented a significant decline in $\dot{V}O_{2max}$ of ~8%,[65] another study examining short-term (3 weeks) effects of monophasic OCPs failed to identify any variability in aerobic capacity.[57] In addition to differences in the duration of OCP use, it is also important to note that the women who experienced decrements in aerobic fitness were physically active, whereas those who did not were untrained.

Unlike the lack of evidence with monophasic OCPs, the impact of triphasic OCPs on maximal aerobic capacity is quite clear. Research consistently shows that women taking triphasic OCPs exhibit significant decreases in $\dot{V}O_{2max}$.[21] Over the course of two full OCP cycles, the decrement in peak aerobic capacity was ~5%, but after six cycles it was found to be ~15%. At this point, the data suggest that monophasic OCPs would better suit female endurance athletes.

Although monophasic OCPs do not appear to influence anaerobic performance, there is some evidence that, when using the triphasic formulations, short-term, all-out exercise is most impressive during the 28-day cycle when estrogen and progestogen levels are at their lowest.[74] It has been suggested that these improvements in anaerobic performance are linked to an improved buffering capacity of lactate and thus pH regulation in contracting muscles.

Unlike that of anaerobic performance, the literature regarding the interaction of muscle strength and OCPs is consistent. Neither monophasic nor triphasic OCPs alter the maximal force production of muscles.[63] This is true both in female athletes and untrained women.

Because of the many variations of OCPs, it is difficult to arrive at firm conclusions concerning their influence on athletic performance. The most consistent findings seem to be the following:

- Strength is not sensitive to the fluctuations in hormonal status brought about by OCPs.
- Anaerobic performance may vary throughout the 28-day cycle of triphasic—but not monophasic—OCPs, such that performance peaks when sex steroids are at their lowest.
- Aerobic fitness declines with the use of triphasic OCPs.

PROHORMONES

In the body's own natural biosynthetic pathways that lead to the production of testosterone—which has potent muscle building effects—there are intermediate products. Each intermediate product or substance is referred to as a **prohormone**. Because these naturally occurring steroid precursors are eventually converted by various enzymes to testosterone, many athletes take synthetically produced prohormones under the assumption that, once introduced into the body, they will properly enter the steroid pathways, leading to increased endogenous testosterone secretion. Until recently, these agents could be purchased without a prescription at nutrition centers as legal dietary supplements. But in 2005, the U.S. Food and Drug Administration (FDA) included the most commonly used prohormones in their list of controlled substances, and they can now be sold only with a medical prescription.

DHEA

The testosterone precursor **dihydroepiandrosterone (DHEA)** is naturally produced in the body, mainly by the adrenal glands, and is an important intermediate in the pathway leading to testosterone. Accordingly, DHEA has been marketed as an effective ergogenic aid leading to increased muscle mass and strength. Although, theoretically, it would seem that introducing artificially synthesized DHEA would, indeed, act to enhance endogenous testosterone levels and thus promote anabolic (muscle building) effects, research has not been able to support this conjecture. In fact, a number of studies have demonstrated that no changes in circulating testosterone can be detected, although oral consumption of even large doses (i.e., 1600 grams per day) of DHEA may cause dramatic increases of its own concentration in the bloodstream. Not surprisingly then, it has been determined that large daily doses of DHEA for as long as 4 weeks failed to alter body weight, lean body mass, or body composition.[92] And when prolonged DHEA supplementation was combined with a robust resistance training program, it did nothing to amplify the strength and muscle mass gains demonstrated by the group of subjects who completed the same training regimen without taking DHEA.[19] In general, scientific investigation into the efficacy of DHEA supplementation to increase muscle mass and strength has failed to identify a notable ergogenic effect. DHEA is an intermediary not only for testosterone production, but also for estrogen production. In fact, some studies show an increase in estrogen in males taking DHEA.

Androstenedione

Perhaps the most popular prohormone supplement among strength training athletes is **androstenedione**. Like DHEA, it is naturally produced by the body along the biosynthetic pathway, ultimately leading to the production of testosterone. Commonly known as "Andro," this steroid intermediate gained notoriety in 1998 when, still available commercially, major league baseball player Mark McGwire admitted to using it during his chase to break what was then the single-season home run record of 61 (he finished with 70). Controlled trials testing its efficacy, however, have contradicted anecdotal reports of its ability to increase muscle mass and thus strength. When taken in dosages suggested by the manufacturer, it appears that circulating values of testosterone remain unaffected by androstenedione supplements. Moreover, a resistance training program augmented with androstenedione ingestion was found to be no more effective in promoting muscle

Quick Review

- Prohormones potentially increase muscle mass and performance by increasing testosterone levels.
- The prohormones androstenedione and DHEA do not appear to have any notable ergogenic effects.

and strength gains than the same training protocol when a placebo was taken.[48] These results have been replicated by other more recent studies, leading to the conclusion that androstenedione is not effective either in amplifying circulating levels of testosterone or in promoting gains in muscle mass and strength.

Overall, the evidence clearly indicates that neither DHEA nor androstenedione exhibits ergogenic effects. Importantly, these prohormones are now considered illegal without a medical prescription and are banned by

most sports organizations, including the IOC, resulting in disqualification if detected in athletes.

DRUGS

Many drugs offer potential performance-enhancing ability. Most drugs, however, are banned by the IOC and other governing bodies for use by professional and collegiate athletes. Some drugs are not banned for use by athletes when prescribed at specified dosages by a physician for a specific medical condition (Box 14-1).

Drawing conclusions concerning whether a drug enhances performance can be difficult due to several factors. The dosage of the drug and the timing of when performance is measured after drug ingestion can affect whether performance enhancement occurs. Many drugs show a great deal of individual variability concerning their effects, so performance may be enhanced in one

Box 14-1 PRACTICAL QUESTIONS FROM STUDENTS

What Ergogenic Substances Are Banned for Use by Collegiate Athletes?

The NCAA has a Web site (www.NSCA.org/health-safety) where the list of banned substances for college athletes can be found. The NCAA also warns athletes that some nutritional and dietary supplements also contain banned substances. The following is a list of drug classes that are banned for use by athletes by the NCAA, with some examples.

Anabolic Agents

- Androstenedione
- Boldenone
- DHEA
- Nandrolone
- Testosterone
- THG
- 19-Norandrostenedione

Stimulants

- Cocaine
- Ephedrine (Ma Huang)
- Methamphetamine
- Synephrine

Street Drugs

- Heroin
- Marijuana
- Tetrahydrocannabinol (THC)

Diuretics and Urine Manipulators

- Bumetanide
- Probenecid
- Finasteride

Peptide Hormones and Analogues

- EPO
- Human growth hormone (HGH)

Anti-Estrogens

- Clomiphene (Clomid)
- Tamoxifen

Products Containing Banned Substances (Medical Exception may be Granted for Required Use with a Prescription)

- Adderall
- Anadrol
- Androgel
- Cylert
- Dexedrine
- Epogen
- Lasix
- Oxandrin
- Ritalin
- Testoderm

Nonprescription Medications

- Bronkaid (ephedrine)
- Primatene tablets (ephedrine)

person and unchanged in another person, even at the same dosage. Even with double-blind placebo-controlled studies, controlling for the placebo effect may be difficult if the drug has effects that are easily noticeable, such as increased heart rate. Such effects would allow subjects to discern whether they received the drug or placebo. Here we will discuss several drugs that are used by athletes and have potential performance-enhancing characteristics.

Amphetamines

Amphetamines stimulate the central nervous system by increasing dopamine release and are also a **sympathomimetic amine** drug, meaning that they mimic the effects of catecholamines. Amphetamines are also known as "speed" and "pep pills." They are readily absorbed in the small intestine. Their effects start to appear within 30 minutes and peak 2 to 3 hours after ingestion but can last as long as 24 hours. Once in the bloodstream, amphetamines bind to receptors for epinephrine and norepinephrine (alpha and beta adrenergic receptors), mimicking the effects of these hormones by causing increased blood pressure, heart rate, metabolic rate, and plasma free fatty acid concentration. They also supposedly increase alertness, self-confidence, and muscle force, and increase the capacity to perform work by masking fatigue. Due to these effects, they are thought to increase performance in a wide variety of sports and activities.

Amphetamines could increase performance by the catecholamine effect of mobilizing free fatty acids, thus sparing muscle glycogen, or by masking fatigue. This drug does appear to mask pain or fatigue and improve performance in some people.[25] However, timing of when performance takes place after drug ingestion may be important. Some studies not showing a change in performance measured performance 30 to 60 minutes after ingestion. Other studies, measuring performance 2 to 3 hours after ingestion, however, showed an increase in performance.[25] As with all drugs, dosage may also be important. Some studies using lower doses did not show performance effects, whereas studies using higher doses did show performance effects.[25] Additionally, there is some indication that the effects of amphetamines may be more apparent in trained athletes compared with untrained people.[25]

In a double-blind placebo study in which an amphetamine was ingested 2 to 3 hours prior to performance, 73% of runners, 85% of weight throwers, and 67% to 93% of swimmers performed better after amphetamine ingestion compared with placebo.[78] The improvements in performance ranged from 0.6% to 4%. Another double-blind placebo study, in which testing took place 2 hours after amphetamine or placebo ingestion by former high school athletes who were currently not training, also showed positive results in a wide variety of tests.[23] The former athletes were tested three times after placebo ingestion and

three times after amphetamine ingestion. They showed, on average, the following significant increases:

- 22.6% in isometric knee extension
- 3.8% in acceleration during a 30-yard (27.3-meter) sprint
- 4.4% in treadmill running time to exhaustion
- 8.3% in peak plasma lactate
- 2.1% in maximal heart rate after amphetamine ingestion compared with placebo

However, other performance measures, although increased after amphetamine ingestion, did not show significant changes compared with placebo, including cycling peak leg power (3.0%), isometric elbow flexion force (6.3%), and maximal oxygen consumption ($L \cdot min^{-1}$, 0.3%).

Increased performance due to amphetamine use does have potential dangerous side effects, including the following:

- Masking of pain or fatigue, resulting in injury
- Masking of pain, contributing to heat-related injury, especially in hot, humid environments
- Long-term use resulting in emotional or physiological drug dependency
- Need for larger doses with prolonged use, which could increase the possibility of any other side effect
- General side effects of agitation, confusion, headache, and dizziness

It does appear that amphetamine use at the proper dosage and with the correct timing of performance after ingestion can increase performance in a wide variety of physical performance measures in many people.[25] However, there is a great deal of individual variability in the effects of amphetamine. Also, side effects can be dangerous, and the psychological effects of agitation and confusion could possibly reduce performance in sports requiring quick decisions during competition.

Ephedrine

Ephedrine is a sympathomimetic amine drug and a central nervous stimulant. It is found in various antiasthmatic and cold or cough medications in pill, tablet, and inhaler forms. Ephedrine is also found within dietary supplements and herbal teas containing Ma Huang, also termed Chinese ephedra or herbal ephedrine. Ephedrine has a chemical structure similar to that of amphetamine and stimulates receptors for epinephrine and norepinephrine (alpha and beta receptors). Thus, it has similar effects on the cardiovascular and metabolic systems as amphetamine. It is also used for weight loss because it supposedly curbs the appetite and increases metabolic rate. Ephedrine, especially when combined with aspirin or caffeine, appears to increase body weight loss in obese people. However, it does not act as a fat burner in people who are lean and, therefore, is of little value to promote body fat loss in athletes.[25]

Literature reviews in the late 1990s concluded that ephedrine has no effect on physical performance.[25,95] However, recent double-blind placebo studies indicate that ephedrine can increase some types of physical performance. In one study, ephedrine was ingested 2 hours prior to performing three sets to exhaustion of the leg press (80% of one-repetition maximum [1-RM]) and bench press (70% of 1-RM). It resulted in a significantly greater number of repetitions per set in the first set of the bench press (13.3 vs. 12.3) and leg press (16.3 vs. 12.5), but not in the second and third sets compared with a placebo.[46] In another study, power output in the first 10 seconds of a 30-second maximal cycling test (Wingate test) was improved significantly by approximately 1% when ephedrine was ingested 1.5 hours prior to the test compared with a placebo.[10] Both of these studies indicate increases in power capabilities and/or local muscular endurance capabilities due to ephedrine ingestion.

In a double-blind study, ephedrine ingestion 1.5 hours prior to a cycling test to exhaustion did not significantly increase time to exhaustion compared with a placebo.[11] However, ephedrine ingestion 1.5 hours prior to a simulated 10-kilometer run (6.25 miles) in a double-blind placebo comparison showed a significant decrease (45.5 vs. 46.8 min) in time after ephedrine ingestion, indicating that ephedrine may possibly increase performance in endurance-oriented events.[12] Several of these more recent studies do show increases in resting heart rate and resting blood pressure. These studies conclude that increases in performance, when present, are related to central nervous system stimulation as well as the cardiovascular and metabolic effects of ephedrine.

Ephedrine has similar side effects, such as headache, agitation, and gastrointestinal distress, as amphetamine.[95] Also, similar to amphetamine, there is a large individual variability in the response to ephedrine use for both performance and side effects. Ephedrine is banned by the IOC and other sport-controlling bodies.

Pseudoephedrine

Pseudoephedrine is a sympathomimetic amine found in over-the-counter decongestants used to treat sinus and nasal congestion associated with the common cold, sinusitis, and allergic rhinitis. As with other sympathomimetic amines, its actions are due to binding to norepinephrine and epinephrine receptors (primarily alpha-adrenergic receptors). Side effects of pseudoephedrine include insomnia, nervousness, irritability, light-headedness, increased heart rate, and increased blood pressure.

Ingestion by athletes of pseudoephedrine 1 to 2 hours prior to testing at the normal dosage or two times the normal dosage does not significantly affect cycling time to exhaustion, 40-kilometer time trial performance, $\dot{V}O_{2peak}$, maximal isometric strength or power, or work measures during a maximal 30-second (Wingate test) cycling test.[36,82]

Ingestion of the normal dose six times during a 36-hour period also did not significantly change $\dot{V}O_{2peak}$ or 5,000-meter (3.12 miles) run time in trained runners.[24] However, ingestion by trained athletes at three times the normal dosage 70 minutes prior to testing resulted in a 2.1% improvement in 1,500 meters (0.93 miles).[42] Thus, there is some evidence that pseudoephedrine at greater-than-normal therapeutic dosages can improve performance. Similar to ephedrine, timing of ingestion prior to physical performance may be important, as pseudoephedrine exerts its effects starting at approximately 1 hour after ingestion, with peak plasma concentrations occurring 2 hours after ingestion.

Diuretics

Diuretics are drugs that induce body weight loss by increasing urine production. Diuretics were developed to treat certain pathological conditions, including hypertension. They are used by athletes in weight-class sports, such as boxing, wrestling, and weightlifting, and in sports in which a lower body mass may offer an advantage, such as gymnastics. Diuretics are banned for use in the Olympics, Pan American Games, and Paralympics. All diuretics increase urine output and loss of some electrolytes. There are three major types of diuretics:

- Thiazide diuretics: They block sodium reabsorption in the distal tubules of the kidney's nephron and increase sodium, chloride, and potassium excretion.
- Loop diuretics: They slow sodium chloride transport in the kidney's ascending loop of Henle and increase sodium, chloride, and potassium loss.
- Potassium-sparing diuretics: They increase sodium and chloride loss in the kidney's distal tubules without an accompanying potassium loss.

There is no question that diuretics decrease body mass due to water weight loss as urine. Up to 3% to 4% of total body mass can be lost during 24 hours using diuretics.[25] One goal of using diuretics to decrease total body mass is to increase strength or power relative to body mass, which could be an advantage in some sports. For example, having less body mass to accelerate during a short sprint or a vertical jump could increase performance. This idea is supported by an increase in vertical jump height after body mass loss due to a diuretic.[84] Loss of too much water weight, however, results in decreased aerobic performance and anaerobic performance due to decreases in plasma volume, hyperthermia, decreased glycolytic ability, and decreased ability to buffer hydrogen ions produced during metabolism (see Chapter 9). However, whether body weight loss due to diuretic use is detrimental to performance is controversial and may depend on the sport in question.

Track and field athletes who lost approximately 2% of total body mass due to diuretic use showed increases in 1,500-, 5,000-, and 10,000-meter race times of approximately 3%,

7%, and 7%, respectively, thus decreasing performance.[3] The decrease in performance in the 1,500-meter distance was not statistically significant, and performance decreased to a greater extent in the longer distances compared with the 1,500-meter distance. However, an approximately 2% loss of body mass due to using a diuretic did not significantly change 50-, 200-, or 400-meter sprint time or vertical jump height in former sprinters.[91]

Aerobic activities may show a greater decrease in performance due to the use of diuretics than anaerobic activities or activities dependent on maximal strength and power. This disparity occurs because body mass loss due to dehydration of as little as 2% to 3% affects aerobic capabilities, but body mass loss of 5% due to dehydration may be needed to affect anaerobic capabilities (see Chapter 9). Another factor affecting whether the use of diuretics will affect performance is how much time an athlete has between having to make weight (be at a certain body mass) and when competition begins. In some sports, such as wrestling, an athlete may have from 5 to 20 hours between weigh in and competition, allowing time for intake of fluids and rehydration.

Diuretics do have potential side effects, including dizziness, decreased potassium within the body resulting in neurological problems, muscle weakness, cramps, and dehydration resulting in thermoregulatory problems, especially in hot, humid environments. Bodybuilders who use diuretics have shown hypotension, hyperkalemia (above-normal levels of potassium in the blood), muscle weakness, and cramps.[25] Thus, diuretics may increase performance for some athletes in some sports, but they are banned for use in the Olympics, Pan American Games, and Paralympics.

Caffeine

Caffeine is one of the most consumed substances worldwide and has both pharmacological and psychoactive effects. Caffeine is considered a "xanthine alkaloid" and is found in varying concentrations in foods such as coffee beans, tea leaves, chocolate, and cocoa. Thus, we take in caffeine from everything from soft drinks (37–71 milligrams) to painkillers (e.g., two tablets of Extra Strength Excedrin, 130 milligrams). In this high-energy society, we seem to be obsessed with attaining "energy bursts," and these typically involve the use of caffeine.

The levels of caffeine in foods vary greatly depending on preparation. Coffee, tea, and cola (i.e., soft drinks), respectively, contain approximately 60 to 150, 40 to 60, and 40 to 50 milligrams of caffeine per cup.[79] The FDA has limited the amount of caffeine for cola and other soft drinks to 71 milligrams per 12 oz.

Caffeine, though having no nutritional value, has attracted the attention of many competitive athletes and recreational fitness enthusiasts as a legal ergogenic. Endurance athletes became interested in caffeine in the late 1970s due to early pioneering studies showing improvements in endurance

capacity.[27,45] Caffeine is included in many multicomponent supplements to optimize both energy and mood states before a workout.[51]

The underlying mechanisms of action are diverse and depend on the demands of the exercise (Fig. 14-3). Caffeine has many effects on the central nervous system as well as cognitive effects. It also impacts hormonal, metabolic, muscular, cardiovascular, pulmonary, and renal functions during rest and exercise. For example, it stimulates bronchodilation of alveoli, vasodilatation of blood vessels, neural activation of muscle contraction, blood filtration in the kidneys, catecholamine secretion, and lipolysis. These metabolic, physiologic, and hormonal effects of caffeine lower the respiratory exchange ratio, peripheral fatigue, rating of perceived exertion (RPE), and the threshold for exercise-induced cortisol and β-endorphin release. They also increase oxygen uptake, cardiac output, ventilation, circulating levels of epinephrine, metabolic rate, and fat oxidation during endurance exercise in trained and untrained people.[79] Interestingly, one long-term myth is that caffeine can cause dehydration, but this is not the case.[5]

As discussed in a review, caffeine can significantly increase performance up to several percent in a wide variety of tasks.[79] Caffeine studies involving endurance exercise have shown increased work output and time to exhaustion. Caffeine also enhances performance during intense, short-term cycling and running events of approximately 5 minutes.

However, positive ergogenic effects were equivocal during sprint and power exercise lasting less than 3 minutes, possibly because of the limited number of investigations and different protocols used. In sprint and power events that rely mainly on the phosphagen system (≤10 seconds), caffeine improved peak power output, speed, and isokinetic strength. However, in events that heavily rely on the glycolytic system (15 seconds to 3 minutes), no improvements were found with caffeine use. In fact, it may have been detrimental to performance during repeated bouts of exercise.

In addition, ingestion of varying levels of caffeine doses exerted no ergogenic effect on maximal strength and endurance during isokinetic strength testing of 15 repetitions. In tennis, an individual sport requiring concentration and skill, caffeine increased hitting accuracy, running speed, agility, and overall playing success, possibly because it improved reaction time and mental alertness. Tennis players also reported higher energetic drive during the last hours of play.[79] The following practical applications for caffeine can be put forth[79]:

1. Nonusing athletes who are considering caffeine as an ergogenic aid will be unaccustomed to its cognitive and physiologic effects. Nonusers therefore should test its effects before implementing a caffeine strategy for training or competition.

2. Because caffeine cessation decreases exercise performance, habituated athletes may consider ingesting lower doses

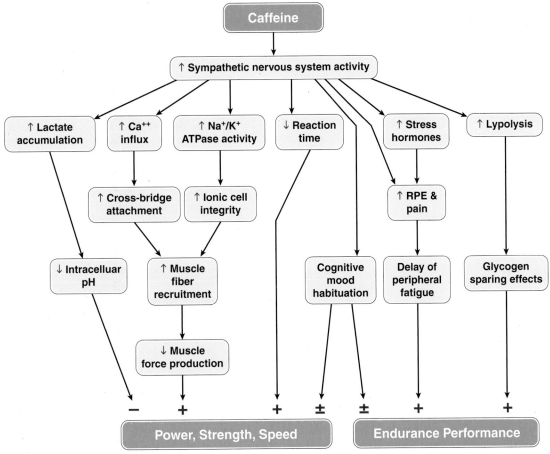

Figure 14-3. Caffeine has many mechanisms by which it can affect performance. Its many effects result in the ability to increase performance in a wide variety of activities. (From Sökman B, Armstrong LE, Kraemer WJ, et al. Caffeine use in sports: Considerations for the athlete. J Strength Cond Res. 2008;22:978–986.)

($\leq$3 mg·kg^{-1}) of caffeine to avoid the undesirable withdrawal symptoms associated with complete cessation. In fact, lower doses may be as effective.

3. If an athlete decides to stop consuming caffeine before competition to increase its ergogenic effects during competition, he or she should reduce caffeine consumption at least 1 week before competition to be completely free from withdrawal effects. To avoid potential negative symptoms, the dose should be gradually reduced over 3 to 4 days, instead of quitting abruptly. Resuming caffeine on the day of competition will provide the desired ergogenic effects, as it would for a nonuser.

4. Caffeine ingestion can benefit high-volume or intense endurance training. Three or four days of consecutive low levels of caffeine intake, during a period of heavy training days, can serve as an ergogenic aid in preparing for competition.

5. The half-life of caffeine is approximately 4 to 6 hours, and plasma concentration has been shown to peak in 30 to 60 minutes. Therefore, caffeine should be ingested, at the latest, 3 hours before power, sprint, and short endurance events or 1 hour before prolonged endurance events.

6. Acute redosing with caffeine does not necessarily improve performance; however, if the events are more than 6 hours apart, it may be beneficial.

7. Because caffeine increases plasma lactate levels and decreases intracellular pH, it may be contraindicated for athletes in sprint events that last 30 seconds to 3 minutes. Further research is warranted.

β-Blockers

The sympathetic branch of the autonomic nervous system is responsible for eliciting the well-known "fight-or-flight" response. This response is characterized by increases in heart rate, blood pressure, and cardiac output, as well as more peripheral responses such as amplified sweat rates, blood flow to skeletal muscle, and substrate availability to skeletal muscles. In large part, the sympathetic nervous system achieves this overall excitatory effect by releasing its neurotransmitter, norepinephrine, and by stimulating the adrenal glands to secrete the hormone epinephrine. Both of these ligands then interact with β-adrenergic receptors located on target cells in the heart, lungs, blood vessels, and skeletal muscle.[28] Pharmacological agents known as β-**blockers** are routinely used in legitimate clinical treatments to control racing heart rates and inappropriately elevated cardiac outputs in those with adrenergic dysfunction. However, some athletes have used the same antagonists to induce a calming effect, in general, and, in particular, to improve control of fine muscle contractions and thus steadiness of hand motions, which can be useful in sports such as archery or pistol and rifle shooting. Indeed, research has established that shooting accuracy in those sports can be enhanced following the consumption of β-blockers. Accordingly, these substances have been banned by athletic organizations such as the IOC and the National Collegiate Athletic Association (NCAA).

Alcohol

Another substance that acts as a physiological depressant, thereby eliciting an overall calming effect on the body, is alcohol, or more specifically ethanol. This is the form of alcohol that is found in beverages or spirits. The presumed neutralizing effect of alcohol on muscular tremors has been cited by some athletes of shooting sports as providing a potential ergogenic effect. There is, however, no empirical evidence to support that claim.

For many years, athletes in some sports have contended that consumption of small amounts of alcohol not long before a sports event may improve performance by "calming the nerves." But rather than improving performance, data from controlled studies indicate that alcohol actually imparts an "ergolytic" or performance-limiting effect. This is most obvious during sports relying on aerobic capacity, because alcohol impairs the function of the Krebs cycle and increases lactate production. Furthermore, alcohol has a well-known diuretic effect, and during prolonged endurance exercise, it may induce dehydration. Dehydration, in turn, may lead to thermoregulatory disturbances, again hampering performance. In a position stand put forth by the American College of Sports Medicine, experts concluded that low-to-moderate levels of

> ### Quick Review
>
> - Determining whether a drug has ergogenic effects can be difficult because of dosage, timing of when the drug is ingested and performance measured, and individual differences in response to the drug.
> - Amphetamine can increase performance in a wide variety of activities; however, there are potential dangerous side effects.
> - Older research indicates that ephedrine does not increase performance. Newer research, however, indicates small but significant increases in both strength and endurance measures.
> - Pseudoephedrine at normal dosages does not increase performance, but ingestion at greater-than-normal dosages may increase some types of physical performance.
> - Diuretics do result in weight loss due to increased urine production and may increase performance in both endurance and anaerobic activities.
> - Caffeine has both physiological and psychological effects and can increase performance in wide variety of tasks, ranging from endurance to short-term, high-power activities. It may have little effect on activities relying heavily on glycolysis, however.
> - β-Blockers, used by some athletes to slow heart rate and produce a calming effect, may enhance performance in sports requiring fine motor control.
> - Alcohol in low dosages may produce a calming effect, but does not have any ergogenic effects and is detrimental to many physical tasks.

alcohol intake offered no performance-enhancing benefits but may, in fact, have detrimental effects by slowing reaction time, disturbing eye–hand coordination, impairing balance, and even limiting muscle strength. The major points made in that position stand are presented in Box 14-2.

Box 14-2 APPLYING RESEARCH

Major Points Made in the American College of Sports Medicine's Position Stand "The Use of Alcohol in Sports"

1. The acute ingestion of alcohol can exert a harmful effect on many psychomotor skills, such as reaction time, hand–eye coordination, accuracy, balance, and complex coordination.
2. Acute ingestion of alcohol will not substantially influence metabolic or physiological functions essential to physical performance, such as energy metabolism, maximal oxygen consumption ($\dot{V}o_{2max}$), heart rate, stroke volume, cardiac output, muscle blood flow, arteriovenous difference, or respiratory dynamics. Alcohol consumption may impair body temperature regulation during prolonged exercise in a cold environment.
3. Acute alcohol ingestion will not improve and may decrease strength, power, local muscular endurance, speed, and cardiovascular endurance.

4. Alcohol is the most abused drug in the United States and is a major contributing factor to accidents and their consequences. Also, it has been documented widely that prolonged excessive alcohol consumption can elicit pathological changes in liver, heart, brain, and muscle, which can lead to disability and death.
5. Serious and continuing efforts should be made to educate athletes, coaches, health and physical educators, physicians, trainers, the sports media, and the general public regarding the effects of acute alcohol ingestion on human physical performance and on the potential acute and chronic problems of excessive alcohol consumption.

NUTRITIONAL SUPPLEMENTS

A **nutritional supplement** is a substance found in a normal diet that has been proposed to have ergogenic effects. Several nutritional supplements have received considerable publicity and undergone sufficient research to warrant their inclusion as possible ergogenic aids. The ergogenic effects of protein and carbohydrate have already been discussed (Chapter 8). Here, other nutritional supplements that have possible ergogenic effects and have been sufficiently researched to determine their efficacy will be discussed.

Creatine

Creatine is one of the most successful, because it enhances strength and power, yet misunderstood (e.g., it is not a steroid or amino acid) nutritional supplements on the market today. Creatine was discovered in 1835 by a French scientist and philosopher, Michel-Eugène Chevreu; so it has been known for almost two centuries. **Creatine** (methylguanidino acetic acid) is a nonessential, naturally occurring, organic, nitrogen-containing compound synthesized in the liver from three amino acids: arginine, glycine, and methionine. Ninety-five percent or more of the body's creatine is stored in skeletal muscle. Therefore, skeletal muscle is a primary target for supplementation, especially when enhanced physical performance is the goal (see Box 14-3). Figure 14-4 shows creatine metabolism under normal dietary conditions (panel A) and when one uses supplementation (panel B).

Typically, about 1 gram a day is obtained though normal dietary intakes (e.g., red meat and fish), and although one may increase dietary intake of those sources, it is difficult to ingest creatine at the levels needed to increase muscle concentrations. Creatine concentration in muscle can be increased with either a rapid-loading regime (5 days ingesting 4×5 grams a day) or slow-loading regime (30 days ingesting 2×5 grams a day). Typically, after a loading regime, a maintenance (3 to 5 grams per day) dose is ingested to maintain elevated muscle creatine concentrations.

Although the exact mechanism(s) that mediate the positive effects of creatine on physical performance remain

Box 14-3 AN EXPERT VIEW
Creatine Supplementation

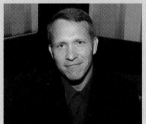

Jeffrey R. Stout, PhD, FACSM, FNSCA
Associate Professor
Department of Health and
Exercise Science
University of Oklahoma
Norman, OK

Creatine is one of the most researched ergogenic aids with over 350 human studies conducted. Unfortunately there has been a great deal of misinformation regarding the safety and efficacy of creatine supplementation. Contrary to the published science, the media have suggested that "supplementing with creatine is harmful to the liver and kidneys and may cause dehydration and cramping." In truth, creatine is intimately involved in energy metabolism, performance, and training adaptations.

Creatine is an energy compound that is made by the body from the amino acids arginine, methionine, and glycine. Creatine can also be obtained through the diet from foods, such as fish and beef. Elevating skeletal muscle creatine levels through supplementation has been shown in several studies to increase the hydration status of cells, protein synthesis, sports performance, training intensity, slow- and fast-twitch muscle hypertrophy, and muscle mass.[1]

When evaluating the peer-reviewed published studies on creatine supplementation, there are several factual assertions that can be made. Below are the statements about creatine supplementation based on the available science.[2]

- Creatine monohydrate is the most effective erogenic nutritional supplement currently available to athletes in terms of increasing high-intensity exercise capacity and lean body mass during training.
- Creatine monohydrate supplementation is not only safe, but possibly beneficial in regard to preventing injury and/or management of a number of select medical conditions when taken within recommended guidelines.
- There is no evidence that short- or long-term use of creatine monohydrate has any detrimental effects on otherwise healthy individuals.
- At present, creatine monohydrate is the most extensively studied and clinically effective form of creatine for use in nutritional supplements in terms of muscle uptake and ability to increase high-intensity exercise capacity.
- The quickest method of increasing muscle creatine stores appears to be through the consumption of ~0.3 g·kg body mass^{-1}·day^{-1} of creatine monohydrate for at least 3 days, followed by 3–5 g·day^{-1} thereafter to maintain elevated stores. Ingesting smaller amounts of creatine monohydrate (e.g., 2–3 g·day^{-1}) will increase muscle creatine stores over a 3- to 4-week period; however, the performance effects of this method are less supported.

References

1. Buford TW, Kreider RB, Stout JR, et al. International Society of Sports Nutrition position stand: Creatine supplementation and exercise [published online ahead of print August 30, 2007]. J Int Soc Sports Nutr. 2007;4:6.
2. Stout JR, Antonio J, Kalman D. (Eds.). Essentials of Creatine in Sports and Health. Totowa, NJ: Humana Press, 2007.

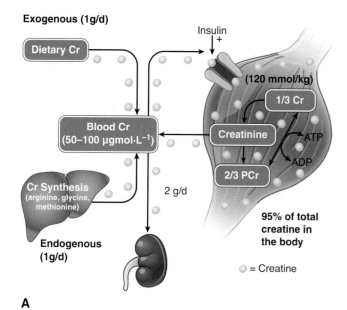

Exogenous (1g/d)

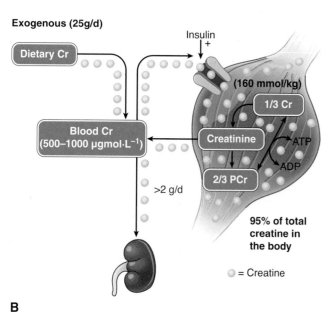

Exogenous (25g/d)

Figure 14-4. As illustrated in **A**, about 1 gram of creatine per day is obtained through normal exogenous dietary intake (e.g., red meat and fish) while natural production by the liver (i.e., endogenous) is also about 1 g·day⁻¹. But, as depicted in **B**, a greater daily intake of exogenous creatine (about 25 grams) is needed to increase creatine storage in skeletal muscle (Figure courtesy of Dr. Jeff Volek, University of Connecticut).

a topic of study, the primary mechanism appears to be related to its support of phosphagen metabolism helping in the production of ATP (see Chapter 2). The creatine pool impacts the amount of phosphocreatine (PCr) that is available and can be broken down to its basic components of creatine and phosphate. In this process, energy is produced that can be used to bond a phosphate molecule to an adenosine diphosphate (ADP) molecule, making ATP, the energy compound needed for muscular contraction. Thus, the influence of creatine supplementation on energy production appears to be one of the primary mechanisms

by which increased concentrations of creatine in skeletal muscle affects performance. Figure 14-5 depicts the effect of mechanisms by which supplementation increases performance.

Reviews conclude that creatine is a safe and effective supplement for improving strength and power.[87,90] Early in its study, creatine had been blamed for muscle cramping, but if one is properly hydrated, cramps and heat toleration have been shown not to differ from placebo conditions.[89] After loading, a person typically gains 2 to 3 pounds (0.9–1.4 kilograms) of body mass, which is thought to be due to increases in the amount of body water retained in muscle to maintain normal osmotic gradients. Along with this weight gain, improvements in strength, power, and local muscular endurance also occur. This has led investigators, coaches, and athletes to conclude that the quality of a workout can be improved with supplementation.[86,87,88] An improvement in physical performance has even been observed in older men and women.[39,40]

The improvement in the quality of a resistance training workout or the amount of weight that can be lifted after supplementation may lead to a more rapid improvement in strength and power with resistance training.[86] Although supplementation generally results in increased strength and power, there is a variable response due to the fact that some people have naturally higher levels of resting creatine in their muscles. Those with high resting muscle creatine concentrations show little change in muscle creatine concentration and little weight gain with supplementation and are nonresponders to supplementation. The average increase in muscle strength (1-, 3-, or 10-RM) following creatine supplementation while resistance training is 8% greater than the average increase in muscle strength following placebo ingestion while resistance training (20% vs. 12%).[72] However, the increase in strength does have a wide range. For example, bench press 1-RM increases from 3% to 45% with supplementation. Thus, it is clear that creatine supplementation can increase strength in healthy people. Interestingly, it has recently been reported that creatine supplementation may influence cerebral function.[69]

It should, however, be noted that the performance benefits associated with creatine supplementation are relegated to specific types of muscular activity. That is, due to its role in the rephosphorylation of ADP to ATP upon the hydrolysis of PCr, the benefits of creatine consumption are most apparent with high intensity, sprint-type activities, especially when repeated efforts are involved. Likewise, the effect of creatine supplementation during resistance training is manifested during repeated sets consisting of multiple repetitions. In contrast, performance of a single repetition of a resistance exercise, or a single, brief, all-out effort, like a shot put attempt, is not likely to directly improve with creatine supplementation as the muscle contains enough ATP to satisfy the demands of such brief efforts. But improvement may occur over time as a result of the enhanced training volumes enabled by creatine

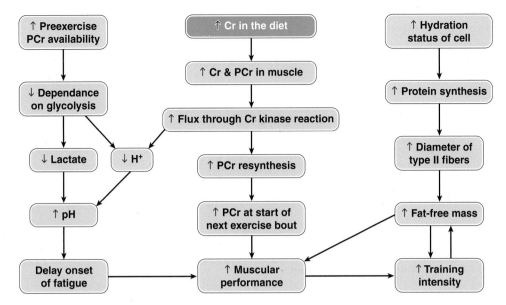

Figure 14-5. Mechanisms by which creatine supplementation improves physical performance. The increased muscle concentrations of creatine improve maximal strength and the quality of weight training sessions, resulting in increased fat-free mass over time, which further increases maximal strength.

supplementation. For those athletes who rely on aerobic metabolism, creatine consumption confers no advantages, even over time.

Beta-Hydroxy Beta-Methylbutyrate

Beta-hydroxy beta-methylbutyrate (HMB) is synthesized in the human body and is a metabolite of the amino acid leucine and its keto acid, alpha-ketoisocaproate. HMB as a nutritional supplement became known over 15 years ago at an experimental biology meeting in Washington, DC. Its proposed ergogenic effect was to increase muscle mass and decease muscle catabolism.[47] Foods (e.g., grapefruit, catfish) contain very limited amounts of HMB, and, therefore, supplementation appears to be the most efficient way in which significant amounts can be obtained. It appears that HMB is safe in the typical doses studied, which range from 1.5 to 6 grams per day. In a comprehensive and critical review, Wilson et al.[97] suggested that the primary mechanisms of action for enhancing muscle mass and decreasing muscle loss appear to be related to the following:

1. Increased sarcolemmal integrity (due to conversion to HMG-CoA reductase)
2. Enhanced muscle protein synthesis (by stimulating the mTOR—mammalian target of rapamycin—pathway)
3. Decreased muscle protein degradation (by inhibition of the ubiquitin pathway)

Each of these mechanisms would contribute to a reduction in muscle protein wasting and positively influence protein synthesis, increasing muscle mass over time.

Studies examining the efficacy of HMB as an ergogenic aid have shown conflicting results. The conflicting results have been partly attributed to differences in experimental designs and doses used.[97] To date, studies have been of a short duration, ranging from 3 to 9 weeks until a study by Kraemer et al. (see ref in Box 14-4) examined 12 weeks

of supplementation (Box 14-4). During most of this 3 to 9 week time frame, neural adaptation is a major factor in bringing about strength gains, making the role of increased protein synthesis in response to resistance training difficult to interpret. Nevertheless, studies have shown 15% to 20% improvements in strength measures compared with placebo and increases in fat-free mass of 2.6 to 6.6 pounds (1.2–3 kilograms) (see Box 14-4). These results support HMB's intended purposes of increasing muscle mass and decreasing muscle degradation. It does appear that HMB may be more effective in untrained people, who have a greater potential for muscle mass and strength gains, than in highly trained athletes, because the window of gain may be much greater.[43,67,68,97] Thus, untrained people and older people may well find greater benefits from HMB supplementation.[34] Furthermore, various wasting pathologies (e.g., cancer, AIDS, injury trauma) may respond in a positive manner to HMB supplementation, due to the need for optimizing protein synthesis or minimizing protein loss in these diseases.[52]

Antioxidants

In chemical terms, a free radical is a molecule that contains at least one unpaired electron, thus resulting in an electrical charge to that molecule. As a result, free radicals are highly unstable and reactive with other substances, because unpaired electrons are attracted to, and react with, other particles that express charges. In living systems, including humans, these free radicals are formed during the reduction of oxygen to water and are called reactive oxygen species (ROS).[26] In particular, ROS are produced during aerobic respiration, or oxidative phosphorylation, within mitochondria. Thus, as aerobic respiration increases, so does the appearance of ROS. This is of concern because, due to their high reactivity with other substances, they have been found to cause structural and, thus, functional damage to proteins, membranes, and DNA, all essential components of biological cells.

Box 14-4 DID YOU KNOW?
Weight Training and HMB Supplementation

HMB may very well influence muscle hypertrophy in men eating a normal diet of protein, carbohydrates, and fat when performing a periodized heavy resistance training program. In a study by Kraemer and colleagues[1], it was shown that HMB may in fact augment weight training adaptations. In a randomized, double-blind, placebo-controlled design, one group ingested Muscle Armor™ (MA) (Abbott Laboratories) and the other group ingested an isonitrogenous control twice daily during a 12-week resistance training protocol. Both groups with the training program demonstrated significant improvements in lean body mass, muscle strength, and muscle power. However, MA supplementation augmented these responses to a significantly greater extent when compared with the control group. The supplementation promoted increases in resting and exercise-induced testosterone and resting GH concentrations. In addition, MA reduced preexercise cortisol concentrations. Throughout the training protocol, MA attenuated circulating creatine kinase and malondealdehyde compared with the control group, suggesting that MA might have influenced a reduction in muscle damage. No negative side effects were observed during the study. It was concluded that the supplement beneficially affected training-induced changes in lean body mass, muscle strength, and power, as well as hormonal responses and markers of muscle damage in response to 12 weeks of resistance exercise training in young men when compared with an isonitrogenous (equal protein basis with the only difference being the HMB content) control.

Reference

1. Kraemer WJ, Hatfield DL, Volek JS, et al. Effects of amino acids supplement on physiological adaptations to resistance training. Med Sci Sports Exerc. 2009;41(5):1111–1121.

Research has shown that during exercise—primarily, but not exclusively, aerobic—contracting muscles exhibit elevated levels of ROS. And due to their enriched mitochondrial content, type I muscle fibers display more pronounced ROS concentrations than do type II fibers. As a result of exercise-induced elevations of ROS, muscle fibers undergo damage of the contractile proteins (myosin and actin), disturbances in membrane integrity at the mitochondrial and cellular levels, and even DNA mutations. Muscle fatigue and soreness accompany these cellular and molecular disruptions. In short, then, the production of ROS can directly contribute to impaired exercise performance.[33]

To protect against the damaging effects of ROS, the body is capable of employing a potent antioxidative system of defense. This system comprises both endogenous and exogenous **antioxidants**, or substances that can neutralize free radicals. The endogenous ones are enzymes synthesized in muscle, the liver, and other organs in the body. The exogenous antioxidants are typically consumed in the diet as micronutrients and vitamins. For example, tocopherol (vitamin E), ascorbic acid (vitamin C), and retinol (vitamin A) are well-known antioxidants, as are minerals such as zinc, copper, selenium, and iron. In both humans and animals, these important dietary constituents have been shown to exert antioxidant effects and can effectively decrease—at least when consumed in proper amounts—damage caused by ROS.

In well-trained athletes, the enzymes functioning as naturally produced antioxidants are expressed in high amounts compared with untrained controls. Moreover, it has been demonstrated that sedentary people who start participating in an endurance (i.e., aerobic) training program display a greater content of antioxidative enzymes by the end of that program. As a result, although the increased aerobic metabolism of regular exercise training amplifies ROS production, the trained muscles are more adept at preventing ROS-induced damage because the endogenous antioxidant defense system is bolstered. However, it seems that periods of unusually demanding training may result in a disproportionate production of ROS and thus overwhelm the body's antioxidant defense mechanisms, resulting in muscle damage, soreness, and decreased performance. Indeed, it has been suggested that this imbalance between the body's ROS production and its antioxidative capacity is central to the condition of overtraining.[33]

To guard against the negative effects of ROS, many athletes regularly take mineral and vitamin supplements. Although these supplements do effectively increase the amounts of important antioxidants in the body and decrease markers of oxidative stress, the preponderance of evidence indicates that they do not significantly improve exercise performance. Yet, by ensuring adequate amounts of these micronutrients and vitamins in the diet, it has been suggested that athletes stay healthy and accordingly can withstand the rigorous training necessary to optimize athletic performance. In contrast, consumption of excessive amounts of antioxidant supplements can impair peak performance.[33]

Quick Review

- Creatine supplementation does increase muscle concentrations of creatine and maximal strength in many people.
- HMB may be effective for increasing maximal strength and muscle mass; however, it may be more effective in untrained compared with trained people.
- Antioxidants do neutralize ROS or free radicals. However, in a properly nourished person, supplementation does not appear to enhance physical performance.

CASE STUDY

Scenario

You are an athletic trainer for a successful high school football program. The football coach approaches you and notes that while watching a college game, he observed several players donning oxygen masks on the sideline following long runs. He asks if the trainer can arrange to have oxygen tanks and masks available on the sideline for this Saturday's game. The coach believes that by providing oxygen supplementation following long runs when the players appear winded, they will be able to recover faster and return to action more quickly.

Questions

- Is the coach correct in believing that oxygen tanks on the sidelines will help players' performance?
- Is there any reason to make oxygen available on the sideline during the game?

Options

You tell the coach that although it may have a placebo effect for some players, oxygen supplementation during recovery provides no real physiological benefit. In young athletes with normal, healthy respiratory systems, arterial blood is already virtually fully saturated with oxygen. That is, the red blood cells are already carrying as much oxygen as they can. As a result, providing supplemental oxygen while athletes recover between plays is useless since no more oxygen can be delivered to the muscles than is already occurring while simply breathing ambient air. You suggest that there is no need to add oxygen tanks to the side line, but if he believes that it will give the players a psychological boost, you will consider it since there is no danger involved.

Scenario

A freshman javelin thrower on the university's track and field team believes that he could improve his performance if he could put on a few more pounds of muscle mass, so he is considering taking creatine supplements. Since you are the strength and conditioning coach of the team, he asks you what you think of his idea.

Questions

- Is there any reason to believe that taking creatine supplements will help this young athlete?
- Is there anything else you should tell the athlete about the use of creatine supplements as an ergogenic aid?

Options

Although there is evidence that creatine supplements may be beneficial to strength/power athletes, there are some limitations of its use. You first point out that early weight gains that may be evident when taking creatine supplements are more likely to be from water retention than from muscle hypertrophy (creatine is osmotically active and draws water to it). Further, the athlete must understand that by itself, creatine intake will not lead to increases in muscle size and strength; it must be coupled with a properly designed resistance training program. And although creatine itself will not stimulate gains in muscle size (it is not an anabolic agent), its bioenergetic properties will make it possible to do, perhaps, a couple of extra repetitions per set while lifting weights. This results in a more potent training stimulus, and in turn, will enhance (moderately) gains in muscle mass and strength.

CHAPTER SUMMARY

In summary, many of the ergogenic aids discussed in this chapter are effective for increasing physical performance. However, many ergogenic aids are banned for use by athletes by the IOC and the NCAA. This leaves a relatively short list of ergogenic aids discussed in this chapter that may be effective to increase physical performance and that are not banned for use by athletes. Included in this list are OCPs, caffeine, creatine, HMB, and antioxidants. Athletes also need to be aware that some over-the-counter sport supplements may also contain banned substances.

REVIEW QUESTIONS

Fill-in-the-Blank

1. Steroid use _____ the risk for prostate cancer in men.

2. Hypoglycemia can be a side effect of taking _____.

3. DHEA is a precursor for _____.

4. Two of the side effects of pseudoephedrine are _____ and _____.

5. EPO stimulates the formation of red blood cells in the _____.

Multiple Choice

1. This ergogenic technique involves increasing total blood volume, or red blood cell count to levels above that which are considered normal.
   a. Oxygen supplementation
   b. Blood buffering
   c. Blood doping
   d. Insulin supplementation

2. β-Blockers cause what effect in the body?
   a. Increase muscle protein synthesis
   b. Make you really excited

c. Dampen one's "fight-or-flight" response

d. a and b

3. Reactive oxygen species (ROS) would increase the most with which sport?

a. Football

b. 1500-meter run

c. Marathon

d. Shot put

4. $\dot{V}_{O_{2max}}$ decreases with which type of oral contraceptive?

a. Monophasic

b. Biphasic

c. Triphasic

d. None of these; $\dot{V}_{O_{2max}}$ is not affected by contraceptives

5. Endurance training, in proper intensities and volumes, will

a. Have no effect on the body's natural protection of antioxidants

b. Decrease the body's natural protection of antioxidants

c. Increase the body's natural protection of antioxidants

d. Have a variable effect, depending on the exact volume and intensity

True/False

1. Erythropoietin (EPO) is a synthetic substance that can only be artificially produced in a laboratory.
2. An ergogenic aid is a supplement that may increase physical performance.
3. Double-blind design helps prevent bias in ergogenic aid research.
4. One of the most dangerous side effects of steroid use is liver damage.
5. Caffeine is not a drug and has no adverse effects.

Short Answer

1. Name and describe two methods of blood doping.
2. What is the normal role and effect of growth hormone?
3. What are the three types of oral contraceptives? How are they different from each other?
4. Why is growth hormone so popular with athletes as a drug when it seems that it really has little or no effect on performance?
5. How does creatine work to enhance strength and power performances?

KEY TERMS

amphetamine: a drug that stimulates the central nervous system and mimics the effects of catecholamines

androstenedione: a prohormone, or intermediate, in the biosynthetic pathway leading to the synthesis of the male sex steroid testosterone

antioxidant: a substance that neutralizes free radicals, or reactive oxygen species (ROS), which can have damaging effects on proteins, DNA, and membranes

autologous transfusion: a transfusion in which red blood cells previously withdrawn from the same person are reinfused

β-blocker: a pharmaceutical agent that inhibits the excitatory effects elicited by the body's sympathetic nervous system

beta-hydroxy beta-methylbutyrate (HMB): a metabolite of the amino acid leucine and its keto acid, alpha-ketoisocaproate

blood buffers: a substance that increases the ability to decrease acidity

blood doping: any means by which total blood volume or red blood cell number is increased above normal

creatine: a nonessential, naturally occurring, organic, nitrogen-containing compound synthesized in the liver from three amino acids: arginine, glycine, and methionine

dehydroepiandrosterone (DHEA): a prohormone, or intermediate, in the biosynthetic pathway leading to the synthesis of the male sex steroid testosterone

diuretics: drugs that induce body weight loss by increasing urine production

double-blind research design: research performed where neither the researchers nor the subjects know when they are receiving the ergogenic aid or the placebo

ephedrine: a sympathomimetic amine drug and a central nervous stimulant that has a chemical structure similar to amphetamine

ergogenic aid: a substance, training practice, or phenomenon that may increase physical performance

erythropoietin (EPO): a naturally occurring hormone that stimulates red blood cell production by bone marrow

homologous transfusion: a transfusion in which red blood cells obtained from someone else are infused

monophasic oral contraceptive pill: an oral contraceptive pill that releases the female sex steroids (estrogens, progestogens) in a steady or unchanging pattern throughout the 28-day menstrual cycle

nutritional supplement: a substance found in a normal diet that has been proposed to have ergogenic effects

oxygen supplementation: any method of increasing the oxygen content of inspired air or increasing the barometric pressure, both of which increase the partial pressure of oxygen, which potentially increases the oxygen carried by the blood

placebo: a substance or treatment that has no physiological effect but may have a psychological effect of causing a subject to believe that it will have a positive impact on performance

prohormone: a substance that is an intermediate product in the synthesis of testosterone

pseudoephedrine: a sympathomimetic amine found in over-the-counter decongestants

sympathomimetic amine: a drug that mimics the effects of catecholamines

triphasic oral contraceptive pill: an oral contraceptive pill that releases the female sex steroids (estrogens, progestogens) in three different dosages throughout the 28-day menstrual cycle

REFERENCES

1. American College of Sports Medicine Position Stand. The use of blood doping as an ergogenic aid. Med Sci Sports Exerc. 1996;28:i–xii.
2. American College of Sports Medicine Position Stand. The use of alcohol in sports. Med Sci Sports Exerc. 1982;14:ix–xi.
3. Armstrong LE, Costill DL, Fink WJ. Influenced out of diuretic-induced dehydration on competitive running performance. Med Sci Sports Exerc. 1985;17:456–461.
4. Armstrong LE, Maresh CM, Keith NR, et al. Heat acclimation and physical training adaptations of young women using different contraceptive hormones. Am J Physiol Endocrinol Metab. 2005;288:E868–E875.
5. Armstrong LE, Pumerantz AC, Roti MW, et al. Fluid, electrolyte and renal indices of hydration during eleven days of controlled caffeine consumption. Int J Sport Nutr Exerc Metab. 2005;15:252–265.
6. Artioli GG, Gualano B, Coelho DF, et al. Does sodium bicarbonate ingestion improve simulated judo performance. Int J Sport Nutr Exerc Metab. 2007;17:206–217.
7. Aschenbach W, Ocel J, Craft L, et al. Effect of oral sodium loading on high-intensity arm ergometry in college wrestlers. Med Sci Sports Exerc. 2000;32:669–675.
8. Bannister RG, Cunnimgham JC. The effects of the respiration and performance during exercise of adding oxygen to the inspired air. J Physiol. 1954;125:118–137.
9. Barroso O, Mazzoni I, Rabin O. Hormone abuse in sports: The anti-doping perspective. Asian J Androl. 2008;10:391–402.
10. Bell DG, Jacobs I, Ellerington K. Effect of caffeine and ephedrine ingestion on an aerobic exercise performance. Med Sci Sports Exerc. 2001;33:1399–1403.
11. Bell DG, Jacobs I, Zamecnik J. Effects of caffeine, ephedrine and their combination on time to exhaustion during high-intensity exercise. Eur J Appl Physiol. 1998;77:427–433.
12. Bell DG, McLellan TM, Sabiston CM. Effect of ingesting caffeine and ephedrine on 10-km from performance. Med Sci Sports Exerc. 2002;34:344–349.
13. Bennell K, White S, Crossley K. The oral contraceptive pill: A revolution for sportswomen? Br J Sports Med. 1999;33:231–238.
14. Birkeland KI, Stray-Gundersen J, Hemmersbach P, et al. Effect of rhEPO administration on serum levels of sTfR and cycling performance. Med Sci Sports Exerc. 2000;32:1238–1243.
15. Bishop D, Edge J, Davis C, et al. Induced metabolic alkalosis affects muscle metabolism and repeated-sprint ability. 2004;36:807–813.
16. Bishop D, Claudius B. Effects of induced metabolic alkalosis on prolonged intermittent-sprint performance. Med Sci Sports Exerc. 2005;37:759–767.
17. Bonen A, Haynes FW, Graham TE. Substrate and hormonal responses to exercise in women using oral contraceptives. J Appl Physiol. 1991;70:1917–1927.
18. Borrione P, Mastrone A, Salvo RA, et al. Oxygen delivery enhancers: Past, present, and future. J Endocrinol Invest. 2008;31:185–192.
19. Brown GA, Vukovich MD, Sharp RL, et al. Effect of oral DHEA on serum testosterone and adaptations to resistance training in young men. J Appl Physiol. 1999;87:2274–2283.
20. Buick FJ, Gledhill N, Froese AB, et al. Effect of induced erythrocythemia on aerobic work capacity. J Appl Physiol. 1980;48:636–642.
21. Casazza GA, Suh SH, Miller BF, et al. Effects of oral contraceptives on peak exercise capacity. J Appl Physiol. 2002;93:1698–1702.
22. Cayla JL, Maire P, Duvallet A, et al. Erythropoietin induces a shift of muscle phenotype from fast glycolytic to slow oxidative. Int J Sports Med. 2008;29:460–465.
23. Chandler JV, Blair SN. The effect of academy on selected physiological component related to athletic success. Med Sci Sports Exerc. 1980;12:65–69.
24. Chester N, Reilly T, Mottram DR. Physiological, subjective and performance effects of pseudoephedrine and phenylpropanolamine during endurance running exercise. Int J Sports Med. 2003;24:3–8.
25. Clarkson PM, Thompson HS. Drugs and sport research findings and limitations. Sports Med. 1997;24:366–384.
26. Clarkson PM, Thompson HS. Antioxidants: What role do they play in physical activity and health? Am J Clin Nutr. 2000;72:637S–646S.
27. Costill DL, Dalsky GP, Fink WJ. Effects of caffeine ingestion on metabolism and exercise performance. Med Sci Sports. 1978;10:155–158.
28. Davis E, Loiacono R, Summers RJ. The rush to adrenaline: Drugs in sport acting on the beta-adrenergic system. Br J Pharmacol. 2008;154:584–597.
29. Douroudos II, Fatouros IG, Gourgoulis V, et al. Dose-related effects of prolonged $NaHCO_3$ ingestion during high-intensity exercise. Med Sci Sports Exerc. 2006;38:1746–1753.
30. Edge J, Bishop D, Goodman C. Effects of chronic $NaHCO_3$ ingestion during interval training on changes to muscle buffer capacity, metabolism, and short-term endurance performance. J Appl Physiol. 2006;101:918–925.
31. Ekblom B, Berglund B. Effect of erythropoietin administration on maximal aerobic power. Scand J Med Sci Sports. 1991;1:88–93.
32. Ekblom B, Goldbarg AN, Gullbring B. Response to exercise after blood loss and reinfusion. J Appl Physiol. 1972;33:175–180.
33. Finaud J, Lac G, Filaire E. Oxidative stress: Relationship with exercise and training. Sports Med. 2006;36:327–358.
34. Flakoll P, Sharp R, Baier S, et al. Effect of beta-hydroxy-beta-methylbutyrate, arginine, and lysine supplementation on strength, functionality, body composition, and protein metabolism in elderly women. Nutrition. 2004;20:445–451.
35. Gibney J, Healy ML, Sönksen PH. The growth hormone/insulin-like growth factor-I axis in exercise and sport. Endocr Rev. 2007;28:603–624.
36. Gilles H, Derman WE, Noakes TD, et al. Pseudoephedrine is without ergogenic effect during prolonged exercise. J Appl Physiol. 1996;81:2611–2617.
37. Gledhill N. The influence of older blood volume and oxygen transport capacity on aerobic performance. Exerc Sports Sci Rev. 1985;13:75–93.
38. Gordon SE, Kraemer WJ, Vos NH, et al. Effect of acid-base balance on the growth hormone response to acute high-intensity cycle exercise. J Appl Physiol. 1994;76:821–829.
39. Gotshalk LA, Kraemer WJ, Mendonca MA, et al. Creatine supplementation improves muscular performance in older women. Eur J Appl Physiol. 2008;102:223–231.
40. Gotshalk LA, Volek JS, Staron RS, et al. Creatine supplementation improves muscular performance in older men. Med Sci Sports Exerc. 2002;34:537–543.
41. Graham MR, Baker JS, Evans P, et al. Physical effects of short-term recombinant human growth hormone administration in abstinent steroid dependency. Horm Res. 2008;69:343–354.
42. Hodges K, Hancock S, Currell K, et al. Pseudoephedrine enhances performance in 1500-m runners. Med Sci Sports Exerc. 2006;38:329–333.
43. Hoffman JR, Cooper J, Wendell M, et al. Effects of beta-hydroxy beta-methylbutyrate on power performance and indices of muscle damage and stress during high-intensity training. J Strength Cond Res. 2004;18:747–752.
44. Hoffman JR, Kraemer WJ, Ratamess NA, et al. Position stand on androgen and growth hormone use. J Strength Cond Res. 2009;23 (5 Suppl):S1–S59.
45. Ivy JL, Costill DL, Fink WJ, et al. Influence of caffeine and carbohydrate feedings on endurance performance. Med Sci Sports 1979;11:6–11.
46. Jacobs I, Pasternak H, Bell DG. Effects of ephedrine, caffeine and their combination on muscular endurance. Med Sci Sports Exerc. 2003;35:987–994.
47. Jówko E, Ostaszewski P, Jank M, et al. Creatine and beta-hydroxy-beta-methylbutyrate (HMB) additively increase lean body mass

and muscle strength during a weight-training program. Nutrition. 2001;17:558–566.

48. King DS, Sharp RL, Vukovich MD, et al. Effect of oral androstenedione on serum testosterone and adaptations to resistance training in young men: A randomized controlled trial. JAMA. 1999;281:2020–2028.

49. Kraemer WJ, Dunn-Lewis C, Comstock BA, et al. Growth hormone, exercise, and athletic performance: a continued evolution of complexity. Curr Sports Med Rep. 2010, 9(4):242–252.

50. Kraemer WJ, Gordon SE, Lynch JM, et al. Effects of multibuffer supplementation on acid–base balance and 2,3-diphosphoglycerate following repetitive anaerobic exercise. Int J Sport Nutr. 1995;5:300–314.

51. Kraemer WJ, Hatfield DL, Spiering BA, et al. Effects of a multinutrient supplement on exercise performance and hormonal responses to resistance exercise. Eur J Appl Physiol. 2007;101:637–646.

52. Kuhls DA, Rathmacher JA, Musngi MD, et al. Beta-hydroxy-beta-methylbutyrate supplementation in critically ill trauma patients. J Trauma. 2007;62:125–131.

53. Lebrun CM, Petit MA, McKenzie DC, et al. Decreased maximal aerobic capacity with use of triphasic oral contraceptive in highly active women: A randomised controlled trial. Br J Sports Med. 2003;37:315–320.

54. Lindh AM, Peyrebrune MC, Ingham SA, et al. Sodium bicarbonate improves swimming performance. Int J Sports Med. 2008;29:519–523.

55. Liu H, Bravata DM, Olkin I, et al. Systematic review: The effects of growth hormone on athletic performance. Ann Int Med. 2008;148:747–758.

56. Liu H, Bravata DM, Olkin I, et al. Systematic review: The safety and efficacy of growth hormone in the healthy elderly. Ann Int Med. 2007;146:104–115.

57. Lynch NJ, De Vito G, Nimmo MA. Low dosage monophasic oral contraceptive use and intermittent exercise performance and metabolism in humans. Eur J Appl Physiol. 2001;84:296–301.

58. Matsuura R, Arimitsu T, Kimura T, et al. Effect of oral administration of sodium bicarbonate on surface EMG activity during repeated cycling sprints. Eur J Appl Physiol. 2007;101:409–417.

59. McNaughton LR, Siegler J, Midgley A. Ergogenic effects of sodium bicarbonate. Curr Sports Med Rep. 2008;7:230–236.

60. McNeill AW, Mozingo E. Changes in the metabolic cost of standardized work associated with the use of an oral contraceptive. J Sports Med Phys Fitness. 1981;21:238–244.

61. Meinhardt U, Nelson AE, Hansen JL, et al. The effects of growth hormone on body composition and physical performance in recreational athletes: a randomized trial. Ann. Intern. Med. 2010;152(9):568–577.

62. Mero AA, Keskinen KL, Malvela MT, et al. Combined creatine and sodium bicarbonate supplementation enhances interval swimming. 2004;18:306–310.

63. Nichols AW, Hetzler RK, Villanueva RJ, et al. Effects of combination oral contraceptives on strength development in women athletes. J Strength Cond Res. 2008;22:1625–1632.

64. Nielson HB, Boushel R, Madsen P, et al. Cerebral desaturation during exercise reversed by O_2 supplementation. Am J Physiol. 1999;277:H1045–H1052.

65. Notelovitz M, Zauner C, McKenzie L, et al. The effect of low-dose oral contraceptives on cardiorespiratory function, coagulation, and lipids in exercising young women: A preliminary report. Am J Obstet Gynecol. 1987;56:591–598.

66. Nummela AT, Hamalainen IT, Rusko HK. Effect of hyperoxia on metabolic responses and recovery in intermittent exercise. Scand J Med Sci Sports. 2002;12:309–315.

67. O'Connor DM, Crowe MJ. Effects of six weeks of beta-hydroxy-beta-methylbutyrate (HMB) and HMB/creatine supplementation on strength, power, and anthropometry of highly trained athletes. J Strength Cond Res. 2007;21:419–423.

68. Palisin T, Stacy JJ. Beta-hydroxy-beta-methylbutyrate and its use in athletics. Curr Sports Med Reports. 2005;4:220–223.

69. Pan JW, Takkahashi K. Cerebral energetic effects of creatine supplementation in humans. Am J Regul Integr Comp Physiol. 2007;292:R1745–R1750.

70. Peltonen JE, Tikkanen HO, Rusko HK. Cardiorespiratory responses to exercise an acute hypoxia, hyperoxia and normoxia. Eur J Appl Physiol. 2001;85:82–88.

71. Price M, Moss P, Rance S. Effects of sodium bicarbonate ingestion on prolonged intermittent exercise. Med Sci Sports Exerc. 2003;35:1303–1308.

72. Rawson ES, Volek JS. Effects of creatine supplementation and resistance training on muscle strength and weightlifting performance. J Strength Cond Res. 2003;17:822–831.

73. Raymer GH, Marsh GD, Kowalchuk JM, et al. Metabolic effects of induced alkalosis during progressive forearm exercise to fatigue. J Appl Physiol. 2004;96:2050–2056.

74. Redman LM, Scroop GC, Westlander G, et al. Effect of synthetic progestin on the exercise status of sedentary young women. J Clin Endocr Metab. 2005;90:3830–3837.

75. Roberts RA, Ghiasvand F, Parker D. Biochemistry of exercise-induced metabolic acidosis. Am J Physiol Regul Integr Comp Physiol. 2004;287:R502–R516.

76. Robinson N, Giraud S, Saudan C, et al. Erythropoietin and blood doping. Br J Sports Med. 2006;40(Suppl 1):i30–i34.

77. Siegler JC, Keatley S, Midgley AW, et al. Pre-exercise alkalosis and acid-base recovery. Int J Sports Med. 2008;29:545–551.

78. Smith GM, Beecher HK. Amphetamine sulfate and athletic performance. JAMA. 1959;170:542–557.

79. Sökmen B, Armstrong LE, Kraemer WJ, et al. Caffeine use in sports: Considerations for the athlete. J Strength Cond Res. 2008;22:978–986.

80. Spriet LL, Perry CG, Talanian JL. Legal pre-event nutritional supplements to assist energy metabolism. Essays Biochem. 2008;44:27–43.

81. Stephens TJ, McKenna MJ, Canny BJ, et al. Effect of sodium bicarbonate on muscle metabolism during intense endurance cycling. Med Sci Sports Exerc. 2002;43:614–621.

82. Swain RA, Harsha DM, Baenziger J, et al. Do pseudoephedrine or phenylpropanolamine improve maximum oxygen uptake and time to exhaustion? Tech J Sport Med. 1997;7:168–173.

83. Thomsen JJ, Rentsch RL, Robach P, et al. Prolonged administration of recombinant erythropoietin increases the submaximal performance more than maximal aerobic capacity. Eur J Appl Physiol. 2007;101:481–486.

84. Viitasalo JT, Kryolainen H, Bosco C, et al. Effects of rapid weight reduction on force production and vertical jumping height. Int J Sports Med. 1987;8:281–285.

85. Van Montfoort MC, Van Dieren L, Hopkins WG, et al. Effects of ingestion of bicarbonate, citrate, lactate, and chloride on sprint running. Med Sci Sports Exerc. 2004;36:1239–1243.

86. Volek JS, Duncan ND, Mazzetti SA, et al. Performance and muscle fiber adaptations to creatine supplementation and heavy resistance training. Med Sci Sports Exerc. 1999;31:1147–1156.

87. Volek J, Kraemer WJ. Creatine supplementation: Its effect on human muscular performance and body composition. J Strength Cond Res. 1996;10:200–210.

88. Volek JS, Kraemer WJ, Bush JA, et al. Creatine supplementation enhances muscular performance during high-intensity resistance exercise. J Am Diet Assoc. 1997;97:765–770.

89. Volek JS, Mazzetti SA, Farquhar WB, et al. Physiological responses to short-term exercise in the heat after creatine loading. Med Sci Sports Exerc. 2001;33:1101–1108.

90. Volek JS, Rawson ES. Scientific basis and practical aspects of creatine supplementation for athletes. Nutrition. 2004;20:609–614.

91. Watson G, Judelson DA, Armstrong LE, et al. Influence of diuretic-induced dehydration on competitive sprint and power performance. Med Sci Sports Exerc. 2005;37:1168–1174.

92. Welle S, Jozefowicz R, Statt M. Failure of dehydroepiandrosterone to influence energy and protein metabolism in humans. J Clin Endocrinol Metab. 1990;71:1259–1264.

93. Wilber RL, Holm PL, Morris DM, et al. Effect of FIO2 on physiological responses and cycling performance at moderate altitude. Med Sci Sports Exerc. 2003;35:1153–1159.

94. Wilber RL, Holm PL, Morris DM, et al. Effect of FIO2 on oxidative stressed during interval training at moderate altitude. Med Sci Sports Exerc. 2004;36:188–1894.

95. Williams MH. The Ergogenic Edge. Champaign, IL: Human Kinetic Publishers, 1997.

96. Williams MH, Wesseldine S, Somma T, et al. The effect of induced erythrocythemia upon 5-mile treadmill run time. Med Sci Sports Exerc. 1981;13:169–175.

97. Wilson GJ, Wilson JM, Manninen AH. Effects of beta-hydroxy-beta-methylbutyrate (HMB) on exercise performance and body composition across varying levels of age, sex, and training experience: A review. Nutr Metab (Lond). 2008;3:5–11.

98. Winter FD, Snell PG, Stray-Gundersen J. Effects are 100% oxygen on performance of a professional soccer players. JAMA. 1989;262:227–229.

Suggested Readings

Barroso O, Mazzoni I, Rabin O. Hormone abuse in sports: The antidoping perspective. Asian J Androl. 2008;10:391–402.

Clarkson PM, Thompson HS. Drugs and sport research findings and limitations. Sports Med. 1997;24:366–384.

Cooper CE. The biochemistry of drugs and the methods used to enhance aerobic sport performance. Essays Biochem. 2008;44:63–83.

Finaud J, Lac G, Filaire E. Oxidative stress: Relationship with exercise and training. Sports Med. 2006;36:327–358.

Hoffman JR, Kraemer WJ, Bhasin S, et al. Position stand on androgen and growth hormone use. J Strength Cond Res. 2009;23(Suppl): S1–S59.

Gledhill N. The influence of older blood volume and oxygen transport capacity on aerobic performance. Exerc Sports Sci Rev. 1985;13: 75–93.

Sökmen B, Armstrong LE, Kraemer WJ, et al. Caffeine use in sports: Considerations for the athlete. J Strength Cond Res. 2008;22:978–986.

Spriet LL, Perry CG, Talanian JL. Legal pre-event nutritional supplements to assist energy metabolism. Essays Biochem. 2008;44:27–43.

Williams MH. The Ergogenic Edge. Champaign, IL: Human Kinetic Publishers, 1997.

Williams MH. Facts and fallacies of purported ergogenic amino acid supplements. Clin Sports Med. 1999;18:633–649.

Wilson GJ, Wilson JM, Manninen AH. Effects of beta-hydroxy-beta-methylbutyrate (HMB) on exercise performance and body composition across varying levels of age, sex, and training experience: A review. Nutr Metab (Lond). 2008;3:5–11.

15

Training Considerations for Special Populations

After reading this chapter, you should be able to:

1. Appreciate that not everyone one should be presented with the same exercise stimulus, i.e., intensity, frequency, duration, mode.

2. Understand that due to certain physiological conditions or health concerns, exercise regimens may need to be customized for some groups of people.

3. Appreciate that the capacity of special populations of people to respond (short-term) and/or adapt (long-term) to exercise may be altered.

4. Conclude how exercise training may be of even greater benefit for some groups of people than for the normal population.

5. Be cognizant of the limitations that pregnancy may place on a woman's capacity to safely exercise.

6. Understand what factors must be considered when designing exercise programs for children and the aged.

7. Recognize how exercise may be used to manage certain diseases such as asthma and diabetes.

Although health experts recommend a program of regular exercise training for virtually everyone, there are segments of the population that merit special considerations in their need for exercise, how they may respond to it, and the design of their training regimens. Of special concern are women, children, the aged, and people with clinical pathologies such as diabetes, arthritis, chronic obstructive pulmonary disease, and special genetic conditions. We will begin this chapter by discussing female athletes.

WOMEN AND EXERCISE

Over the past 20 to 30 years, women have become increasingly involved with athletic participation and exercise training. The passage of Title IX in 1972 has had far-reaching effects, not only by providing more varsity sport opportunities for women but also by attracting more women to engage in personal fitness programs. Although women display positive physiological adaptations to exercise training similar to that of men—both endurance training and resistance training—there are some gender-specific anatomical and physiological factors that must be taken into account when examining the effects of exercise on women.

Inherent Differences in Female and Male Anatomy and Physiology

Despite many similarities in physiological adaptations between men and women, there are also inherent differences in anatomy and physiology. These differences are related to body composition, strength, power, endurance, and aerobic capacity.

With respect to body composition, women typically have lower whole-body and muscle mass, but a higher percentage of body fat than men, as seen in Figure 15-1. The lower muscle mass noted among women is mainly accounted for by the decreased size of muscle fibers in women compared with men. This is evident in each of the three major muscle fiber types (I, IIA, and IIX) that are found in adult human skeletal muscle. Although men and women demonstrate comparable muscle fiber type composition, it appears that at least in the thigh muscles, type I fibers occupy the greatest proportion of muscle mass in women, whereas in men, type IIA fibers account for the largest amount of muscle mass.[110]

As a result of less total muscle mass, women are not capable of generating as much absolute force as men, particularly in the upper body, where they may be about 50% weaker than men. However, when strength is expressed relative to muscle size or mass, these sex-related differences are minimized or even eliminated. Indeed, in a recent study examining the contractile characteristics of isolated muscle fibers obtained from human muscle biopsy samples, specific tension—force produced per cross-sectional area of the fiber—was not different between young men and women.[126]

In the other two indices of muscle function, power and endurance, research on the impact of gender has yielded contrasting results. That is, women have consistently demonstrated more impressive muscle endurance than men,[18,31,44] whereas it is typically reported that men exhibit greater muscle power than women.

Aerobic performance is also influenced by gender. Even after controlling for differences in lean body mass, the maximal oxygen uptake ($\dot{V}O_{2max}$) of women is 5% to 15% less than that of men.[15] Because the skeletal muscles of women have the same degree of capillarity as those of men, as well as similar mitochondrial content and aerobic enzyme activity,[88,96,115] the decrement in $\dot{V}O_{2max}$ observed in women is most likely related to a reduced capacity to deliver oxygen to the working muscles.

Indeed, compared with men of equivalent size, women have a reduced maximal stroke volume—amount of blood ejected per heart beat—and thus cardiac output, or the amount of blood pumped per minute.[89,124] A lower blood volume in women contributes to those diminutions in cardiac function during high-intensity endurance exercise. In addition, hematocrit, or the percentage of whole blood made up of red blood cells, is lower in women than men (42% vs. 45%). Thus, women have less hemoglobin and oxygen-carrying capacity.[15] This, in turn, is accounted for by the lower concentrations of the hormone **testosterone** noted among women. Testosterone, often referred to as the male sex steroid, has anabolic effects and stimulates the development of the male secondary sexual (androgenic) characteristics (see Chapter 7). However, it also stimulates the production of the hormone erythropoietin, which triggers the formation of red blood cells in bone marrow.

The innate gender-related differences described earlier directly translate to disparities in endurance performance between men and women. In time to exhaustion while exercising at a submaximal intensity,[101] as well as in times to complete a marathon, women suffer from a disadvantage of as little as 6% to as great as 15%.[16,85] Even among highly trained, elite athletes, the performance times of women are not as impressive as those of their male counterparts, as displayed in Figure 15-2.

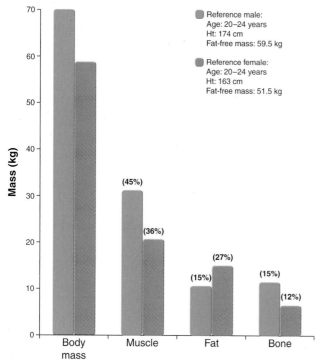

Figure 15-1. Anthropometric differences between men and women. (Modified from Behnke AR, Wilmore JH. Evaluation and Regulation of Body Building and Composition. Englewood Cliffs, NJ: Prentice-Hall, 1974.)

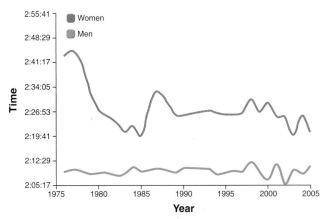

Figure 15-2. Comparison of best times of marathon races completed by male and female American athletes each year from 1976 to 2005. (Modified from Pate RR, O'Neill JR. American women in the marathon. Sports Med. 2007;37:294–298.)

Adaptations to Exercise Training

Despite the presence of inherent anatomical and physiological differences between men and women, adaptability to exercise training does not appear to be notably influenced by sex. That is, when presented with the same exercise stimulus with respect to intensity, frequency, and duration, men and women undergo similar improvements in functional capacity. This is true of both resistance training (e.g., weight lifting, strength training) and endurance training.

Adaptations to Resistance Training in Women

Although it has only been for the past 20 to 30 years that females have been encouraged to perform resistance training, it has been scientifically determined that women are capable of experiencing strength gains that are equal to those observed among similarly trained men. Despite the fact that initial strength levels are lower among women, relative improvements in muscle force production do not differ from those detected in men, i.e., more than doubling in some muscles.[61,111] Accompanying these strength gains are hypertrophic responses at the whole muscle and muscle fiber levels that, too, are not sex-specific. Because women show the same relative increases in strength and muscle size men do, the prescription of resistance training programs does not differentiate between men and women, and the same recommendations in the design of weight training regimens can be applied to both sexes.

Adaptations to Aerobic Training in Women

As with resistance training, there do not appear to be gender-specific adaptations to endurance training. When properly and similarly trained, both men and women can expect about a 20% improvement in cardiovascular capacity (i.e., $\dot{V}O_{2max}$). In both sexes, those improvements are due to increases in stroke volume, cardiac output, and oxygen extraction (i.e., arteriovenous oxygen [a-vO$_2$] difference) by the working muscle of the blood delivered to it. Of interest, however, is the fact that at any prolonged, submaximal effort, women rely to a greater extent on lipids as an energy substrate than do men, who show greater utilization of carbohydrate energy sources.[115] This occurs in both trained and sedentary males and females. Finally, because both men and women experience similar relative adaptations to endurance training, exercise prescription guidelines for cardiovascular fitness are applicable to both genders.

The Effect of the Menstrual Cycle on Exercise Performance

Because of the physiological variations that occur throughout the normal 28-day menstrual cycle, it was assumed for some time that athletic performance would also vary in accordance with those changes. Indeed, a considerable amount of research has been devoted to determine whether phases of the menstrual cycle (the follicular portion of the menstrual cycle after ovulation, or early luteal portion of the cycle) affect athletic performance in females. In general, the most tightly controlled research indicates that physical performance is independent of the menstrual cycle and that there is no need to adjust either training schedules or competitive events to accommodate the stage of the menstrual cycle. For example, neither muscular strength nor muscular endurance has been found to vary during the menstrual cycle, and no correlation was established between muscle function and circulating concentrations of **progesterone**, the female sex hormone produced by the ovaries that stimulates the luteal phase of the menstrual cycle, and **estrogen**, the female ovarian hormones.[48] It is these two female sex steroid hormones that demonstrate sharp fluctuations within the phases of the menstrual cycle.

Research has also confirmed that $\dot{V}O_{2max}$ also remains constant throughout the menstrual cycle.[48] Although maximum oxygen uptake obtained during a relatively short (8–12 minutes), high-intensity testing session is resistant to fluctuations of female sex steroids, there is some concern that prolonged, moderate-intensity endurance exercise may be subject to variation within the menstrual cycle. Resting body temperature is elevated by about 0.5°C (0.9°F) during the luteal phase. Also, during the luteal phase, endurance exercise results in a commensurately increased temperature and thus a higher temperature than at other times of the cycle.[54] As a result, the process of thermoregulation, which includes sweating, the loss of blood plasma volume, and a greater amount of blood flow to the skin, presents a greater cardiovascular challenge during the luteal phase. As a result of an exaggerated loss of plasma volume, the cardiovascular system is more strained

Box 15-1 APPLYING RESEARCH
Menstrual Cycle and Exercise

Many female athletes and their coaches are concerned about the impact that the menstrual cycle may have on exercise performance. In particular, they wonder whether hormonal fluctuations that occur during different phases of the cycle cause similar variance in the athletic performance of women. This seems to be a reasonable concern since the female sex steroids estrogen and progesterone influence a number of physiological variables including substrate utilization and body temperature. However, although there have been anecdotal reports from female athletes that their performance is altered by different phases

of the menstrual cycle, scientific evidence does not support these claims. The consensus among exercise scientists is that aerobic performance, anaerobic performance, and muscular strength do not consistently or significantly vary at different stages of the menstrual cycle. Accordingly, coaches and athletes should not be concerned that because an athletic event is to be held during a specific phase of an athlete's menstrual cycle, her performance will either suffer or be enhanced. Of course, if menses, or the menstrual phase of blood loss, is accompanied by pain and cramping, performance might be impacted.

in meeting the working muscles' demand for blood flow.[87] This is particularly evident when prolonged endurance exercise is performed under unfavorable (i.e., hot, humid) conditions. However, it has yet to be confirmed that endurance performance is, in fact, compromised during the luteal phase (see Box 15-1).

The Female Athlete Triad

Although most investigations have concluded that the menstrual cycle does not alter exercise performance, large volumes of endurance training can, indeed, impact the menstrual cycle. As shown in Figure 15-3, there appears to be a relationship between the number of miles run and the incidence of **amenorrhea**, or the cessation of menstrual periods, in female endurance athletes.

In fact, what is most critical to the onset of amenorrhea is an insufficient availability of energy—calories—brought

about by excessive energy expenditure, inadequate consumption via food intake, or a combination of these two factors. This disturbed menstrual function is one of the symptoms of a condition termed the **female athlete triad**, which presents a serious clinical condition in far too many young women. The amenorrhea associated with excessive weight-bearing exercise, such as running and ballet, and/or inadequate energy intake results in declines in the production of leuteinizing hormone and follicle-stimulating hormone. These hormones are essential for the maintenance of normal menstrual function and thus the production of estrogen by the ovaries. During amenorrhea, estrogen is deficient, which leads to decreased bone mineral density and, if severe enough, to **osteoporosis**, a condition typically associated with postmenopausal women. A consequence of the decreased bone mineral density, which occurs at a rate of 2% to 6% a year, is an increased incidence of bone stress fractures, as has been detected among serious female athletes. In female athletes, particularly those in sports that emphasize thinness, this interrelationship between insufficient energy availability, amenorrhea, and decreased bone density have been described as in Figure 15-4.

According to the position stand on the female athlete triad recently published by the American College of Sports Medicine, the primary treatment for the condition involves increasing energy intake and/or reducing training volume so that energy availability becomes sufficient to permit normal menstrual function and female sex steroid synthesis.[80]

Pregnancy and Exercise

Not too many years ago, women were discouraged from exercising out of concern that it may reduce the chance of becoming pregnant when desired, impair normal growth of the fetus during pregnancy, or increase the risk of having a difficult delivery during childbirth. But in the last 20 to 25 years, attitudes have dramatically changed and for good reason. Research has shown that trained women have no

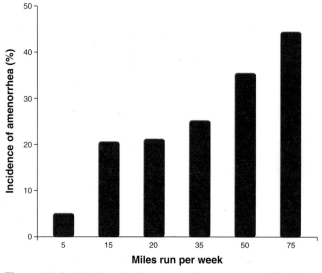

Figure 15-3. Relationship between miles run per week and incidence of amenorrhea in women. (Modified from Brooks GA, Fahey TD, Baldwin KM. Exercise Physiology: Human Bioenergetics and Its Applications, 4th ed. Boston, MA: McGraw Hill, 2005.)

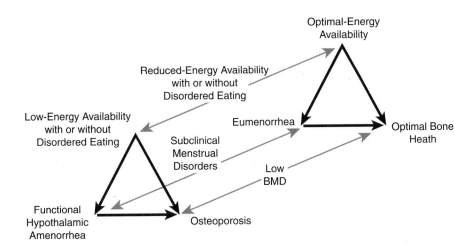

Figure 15-4. Relationship between energy availability, menstrual status, and bone health. Bone mineral density (BMD) is defined as the amount of mineral in any given volume of bone. (Reprinted with permission from Nattiv A, Loucks AB, Manore MM, et al. American College of Sports Medicine position stand. The female athlete triad. Med Sci Sports Exerc. 2007;39:1867–1882.)

more trouble becoming pregnant than sedentary women. Moreover, exercise training during pregnancy can provide beneficial effects to the mother and even reduce the incidence of fetal morbidities.[5] Indeed, so compelling is this favorable evidence that the American College of Obstetricians and Gynecologists recommends that, barring medical contraindications, pregnant women perform 30 minutes or more of moderate-intensity exercise on most, if not all, days of the week. In essence, the same exercise recommendations put forth in a joint statement by the American College of Sports Medicine and the Centers for Disease Control and Prevention for all healthy adults, both male and female, are applicable to pregnant women.

The main benefit of exercising during pregnancy is reduced risk of **gestational diabetes mellitus (GDM)**—insulin resistance during pregnancy—and **preeclampsia**—high blood pressure manifested in some women during pregnancy. During pregnancy, most women experience insulin resistance, making it more difficult to properly manage blood glucose levels. In some women, this increased resistance to the effect of insulin becomes severe enough to lead to the onset of GDM. Up to 7% of pregnant women in the United States suffer from GDM, which can lead to health concerns for the mother (infection, excess weight gain, and postpartum hemorrhaging) and the child (jaundice, birth trauma, and low blood sugar). Several studies have shown that moderate exercise before and/or during pregnancy significantly reduces the risk of GDM.[20,21,22] One study involving almost 1,000 pregnant women revealed that those who were minimally active before becoming pregnant enjoyed a 56% decreased risk of GDM, whereas those who exercised at a moderate intensity for at least 4 hr·wk[-1] before pregnancy demonstrated a 76% decrease in the incidence of GDM.[22]

Preeclampsia is another common condition that afflicts pregnant women, again identified in about 7% of that population. It is a hypertensive disorder that has been associated with liver failure, kidney failure, blood clots, and cerebral hemorrhaging in mothers. As a result, preeclampsia accounts for 15% of all maternal deaths in the United States. Research has shown that exercise is an effective tool in managing this potentially lethal condition. Depending on the amount of energy expended during daily physical activity during the first 20 weeks of pregnancy, women can expect a 40% to 70% decrease in the risk of developing preeclampsia.[69,100] Women who are regularly physically active the year before becoming pregnant enjoy similar protective benefits.[108]

In addition to the effect of exercise before or during pregnancy on the health of the mother, there is the issue of the effect of maternal exercise on fetal outcomes. Commonly, those outcomes are described in terms of birth weight, time of delivery, and mode of delivery. Regarding birth weight of the baby, it has been established that women performing vigorous endurance exercise during the first two trimesters of pregnancy deliver children that weigh no more or less than children born to sedentary mothers.[107] However, there is evidence that women who continue to perform vigorous exercise into their third trimester of pregnancy deliver infants with birth weights that are 200 to 400 g less than those delivered by sedentary mothers. The caloric intake of those mothers that exercised vigorously throughout their pregnancy was not assessed. It has been suggested that increasing dietary intake, i.e., calories, may correct for the lower birth weights of mothers who exercised vigorously.[59]

Another important fetal outcome relates to how far into pregnancy exercising women are when their children are born. Research studies have reported either no difference in the risk of preterm labor, or the gestational age at which babies are born, or even a reduction in the incidence of early births among women who continue to exercise through their second trimester of pregnancy.[29,47,60]

Finally, mode of delivery, vaginal or cesarean, in mothers who are inactive compared with those who participate in vigorous activity while pregnant is another fetal outcome of interest. The best information available at this time indicates that there is a decrease in the number of cesarean deliveries among mothers who participate in vigorous activity while pregnant (see Box 15-2).[41]

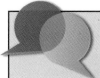

Box 15-2 AN EXPERT VIEW
Gestational Diabetes and Exercise

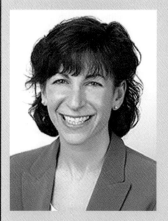

Lisa Chasan-Taber, ScD, FACSM

Associate Professor
Division of Biostatistics and
Epidemiology
Department of Public Health
University of Massachusetts
Amherst, MA

Gestational diabetes mellitus (GDM) is the onset or first recognition of diabetes during pregnancy.[3] Women diagnosed with GDM are at substantially increased risk of developing type 2 diabetes and obesity, currently at epidemic rates in the United States. Their children are at increased risk of adverse perinatal outcomes, including stillbirth, macrosomia, and, in the long term, obesity and glucose intolerance.

Exercise and Prevention of GDM

The American College of Obstetricians and Gynecologists recommends that pregnant women without medical or obstetrical complications engage in 30 minutes of moderate-intensity physical activity (e.g., brisk walking) during most days of the week.[1] According to observational epidemiologic studies, women who report exercising before pregnancy have a reduced risk of GDM. Studies examining women who exercise during pregnancy are less consistent with some observing significant protective effects and others supporting this trend, but not significantly so.

Although sparse, ongoing intervention studies have been designed to investigate the impact of exercise on GDM among women at high risk of this disorder. For example, the Behaviors Affecting Baby and You (B.A.B.Y.) Study is an intervention study in Western Massachusetts designed to investigate the effects of a motivationally targeted, individually tailored exercise intervention on risk of GDM.[5] The FitFor2 Study is an intervention study in Amsterdam, The Netherlands, designed to assess whether a prenatal exercise program will improve insulin sensitivity and fasting plasma glucose levels.[9]

In summary, evidence-based exercise prevention programs for GDM with guidelines for frequency, intensity, duration, and type of activity remain to be established. Ongoing and future well-controlled intervention studies in this area will inform programs designed to prevent the incidence of GDM in women at risk of this disorder.

Exercise and Control of GDM

In 2006, the Cochrane Review reviewed randomized controlled treatment trials among pregnant women diagnosed with GDM comparing any exercise program to no specific exercise program.[4] A total of four trials met the eligibility criteria. In these studies, women were recruited during the third trimester and the exercise intervention was performed for approximately 6 weeks. Programs ranged from regular exercise on a cycle ergometer, arm ergometer, or circuit-type resistance exercise.[2] The review found no significant differences between the exercise and control groups for all the outcomes evaluated and concluded that there was insufficient evidence to recommend, or advise against, enrollment in exercise programs for pregnant women with GDM.[6,7]

However, more recent trials have found a beneficial impact of, for example, structured walking programs, on mean glucose concentrations, suggesting an effective role for exercise among women with GDM. In combination with other small treatment studies, which did not qualify for the review, exercise intervention studies to date suggest that moderate exercise may be effective in lowering maternal glucose concentrations in women with GDM.[8] In summary, additional controlled clinical trials are necessary to determine the effectiveness of structured exercise programs and to identify the appropriate type, duration, and intensity of such exercise.

Conclusion

As long-term follow-up studies reveal that a significant proportion of women with GDM go on to develop diabetes outside of pregnancy, especially during the first decade after the pregnancy, GDM offers an important opportunity for the development, testing, and implementation of clinical strategies for diabetes prevention. Pregnant women more readily seek medical care and are highly motivated to make healthy lifestyle changes, making pregnancy a critical opportunity for both short- and long-term behavior modification.

References

1. ACOG Committee Obstetric Practice. ACOG Committee opinion. Number 267, January 2002: exercise during pregnancy and the postpartum period. Obstet Gynecol. 2002;99:171–173.
2. Brankston GN, Mitchell BF, Ryan EA, et al. Resistance exercise decreases the need for insulin in overweight women with gestational diabetes mellitus. Am J Obstet Gynecol. 2004;190:188–193.
3. Buchanan TA, Xiang A, Kjos SL, et al. What is gestational diabetes? Diabetes Care. 2007;30 Suppl 2:S105–S111.
4. Ceysens G, Rouiller D, Boulvain M. Exercise for diabetic pregnant women. Cochrane Database Syst Rev. 2006;3:CD004225. Online.
5. Chasan-Taber L, Marcus BH, Stanek E, et al. A Randomized controlled trial of prenatal physical activity to prevent gestational diabetes: design and methods. J Womens Health. 2009;18:851–859.
6. Dempsey JC, Butler CL, Williams MA. No need for a pregnant pause: physical activity may reduce the occurrence of gestational diabetes mellitus and preeclampsia. Exerc Sport Sci Rev. 2005;33:141–149.
7. Kim C, Newton KM, Knopp RH. Gestational diabetes and the incidence of type 2 diabetes: a systematic review. Diabetes Care. 2002;25:1862–1868.
8. Mottola MF. The role of exercise in the prevention and treatment of gestational diabetes mellitus. Curr Sports Med Rep. 2007;6:381–386.
9. Oostdam N, van Poppel MNM, Eekhoff EMW, et al. Design of FitFor2 study: the effects of an exercise program on insulin sensitivity and plasma glucose levels in pregnant women at high risk for gestational diabetes. BMC Pregnancy Childbirth. 2009;9:1–9.

- Women show anthropometric differences from men, such as decreased muscle mass, decreased muscle fiber size, and increased body fat.
- When expressed relative to unit of muscle mass (i.e., specific tension), there is no difference in strength between men and women
- The aerobic capacity, or $\dot{V}O_{2max}$, of women is 5% to 15% less than that of men when expressed in relative terms (i.e., $mL \cdot kg^{-1} \cdot min^{-1}$).
- Women have a lower hematocrit level than men, contributing to decreased oxygen-carrying capacity of their blood.
- Endurance exercise performance (e.g., marathon) of women is less than that of men.
- When performing resistance training of the same intensity and duration, there is no difference in relative strength gains or muscle hypertrophy in men and women.
- Women and men experience similar improvements in aerobic fitness (i.e., $\dot{V}O_{2max}$) when they participate in endurance training of the same relative intensity and duration.
- Neither muscle strength nor muscle endurance varies during the course of the 28-day menstrual cycle in women.
- Healthy women who exercise during pregnancy lower their risk of experiencing gestational diabetes and preeclampsia.
- Exercise during pregnancy has little effect on fetal outcomes.

CHILDREN AND EXERCISE

For generations, children were viewed simply as miniature versions of adults. We know now that the physiology of a child and his or her responses to an acute bout of exercise, as well as adaptations to an extended training regimen, are, in many ways, different from those of adults. These differences must be taken into account when prescribing exercise for children. Also, the manner in which exercise might impact the natural growth and development of children must be considered.

Effect of Exercise Training on Growth

Infancy comprises the time from birth through the first year of life. During this period, significant growth of the neonate's trunk and legs occur, resulting in body-to-head proportions that more closely mimic those of an adult. The end of infancy marks the beginning of **childhood**— first birthday to onset of adolescence, which then lasts until the onset of **adolescence**—beginning of puberty to the onset of physical maturity. During childhood, significant physical growth takes place, the rate of which is similar in boys and girls. In fact, with the obvious

exception of primary sexual characteristics (i.e., gonads), there are virtually no physical differences between boys and girls during this stage, and on average, they are equal in height, weight, muscle mass, and body fat. Accordingly, during childhood, boys and girls are encouraged to play together and even compete with one another in sporting events.

Childhood ends with the onset of puberty and thus the beginning of adolescence. Generally, puberty begins in girls at about the age of 8–13 years and in boys at approximately 9–14 years of age. A sharp increase in the rate of skeletal growth, or height, occurs during puberty, reaching its peak at 12 and 14 years old in girls and boys, respectively. By the end of adolescence—the beginning of adulthood—the average boy in the United States stands 69.5 inches (111.2 cm) tall, and the average girl is 64 inches (102.4 cm) tall. And due to the dramatic change in the circulating hormones of adolescence, we see a greater increase in the development of muscle mass in men than women so that, by the end of this period, skeletal muscle comprises 40% of total body weight in men, but only 32% of total body weight in women. In contrast, body fat is added to a greater extent in women than in men. By the point of reaching adulthood, body fat accounts for approximately 25% of the woman's total body weight, whereas young men are composed of about 15% fat. Because of these differences in growth rate and muscle mass accumulation, and resultant disparities in strength, adolescent males and females can no longer compete fairly in sports and we see a separation of boys' and girls' athletic teams. The period of adolescence is typically completed at 19 years old in females and 22 years old in males, at which time adulthood is achieved.

Based mainly on anecdotal reports, some have expressed concern that exercise training may slow the natural rate of growth in children and perhaps even delay the onset of puberty. There are data showing that young female gymnasts participating in regular and rigorous training achieve a smaller stature at adulthood and that **menarche** (i.e., first menstrual period), which generally occurs about 2 years after the onset of puberty, takes place later than it typically does in girls. However, a thorough review of the literature determined that genetics, not intense training, was probably the main factor for the gymnasts' smaller stature and delayed menarche. The mothers of those athletes also tended to be of smaller size and had themselves experienced delayed onsets of menarche.[67] Athletes, both boys and girls, participating in other sports were found to display the same rates of growth in height and weight as nonathletes.[68] However, natural growth rates can be attenuated in some sports in which athletes—particularly females—are encouraged to restrict caloric intake to maintain an abnormally low body weight and body fat content. Experts have concluded that adequate caloric intake must be sustained in prepubertal and pubertal athletes to ensure proper growth and sexual development.[95]

Box 15-3 APPLYING RESEARCH

Guidelines of the American Academy of Pediatrics for Resistance Training by Children and Adolescents

1. Strength training programs for preadolescents and adolescents can be safe and effective if proper resistance training techniques and safety precautions are followed.
2. Preadolescents and adolescents should avoid competitive weight lifting, power lifting, body building, and maximal lifts until they reach physical and skeletal maturity.
3. When pediatricians are asked to recommend or evaluate strength training programs for children and adolescents, the following issues should be considered:
   a. Before beginning a formal strength training program, a medical evaluation should be performed by a pediatrician. If indicated, a referral may be made to a sports medicine physician who is familiar with various strength training methods as well as risks and benefits in preadolescents and adolescents.
   b. Aerobic conditioning should be coupled with resistance training if general health benefits are the goal.
   c. Strength training programs should include a warm-up and cool-down component.
   d. Specific training exercises should be learned initially with no load (resistance). Once the exercise skill has been mastered, incremental loads can be added.
   e. Progressive resistance exercise requires successful completion of 8 to 15 repetitions in good form before increasing weight or resistance.
   f. A general strengthening program should address all major muscle groups and exercise through the complete range of motion.
   g. Any sign of injury or illness from strength training should be evaluated before continuing the exercise in question.

Reprinted with permission from Committee on Sports Medicine and Fitness, American Academy of Pediatrics. Strength training by children and adolescents. Pediatrics. 2001;**107**:1470–1472.

With the growing popularity of resistance training, or weight lifting, as a conditioning technique among athletes, some have voiced concerns regarding the efficacy or safety of that mode of training among children and adolescents. Research has shown that children can effectively gain strength as a result of resistance training, although muscle hypertrophy is less than in older individuals, with greater improvements in hypertrophy as the child approaches puberty. Similar to adults, improvements in the capacity of the nervous system to recruit, or activate, muscle tissue account for a large portion of training-induced strength gains among children.

In addition to strength improvements, resistance training among children has been documented to enhance bone density and health among children and adolescents. Regarding concerns that resistance training will cause injuries in children, a review of the literature reveals that, when properly instructed and supervised, the incidence of injury was minimal—far less than one per 100 participant hours—and none were catastrophic in nature. Indeed, the American Academy of Pediatrics and the National Strength and Conditioning Association have concluded that resistance training, when using proper technique, is safe in healthy children and adolescents.[41,74] Recommendations for safe and effective resistance training among children and adolescents are presented in Box 15–3.

Cardiovascular Capacity and Exercise Responses

Because of their smaller body size, children have smaller hearts and lower blood volumes than adults. As a result, the child's maximal cardiac output, stroke volume, and oxygen uptake is less impressive than that of an adult.[81,119] However, when scaled to the child's smaller body surface area, maximal stroke volume and cardiac output no longer differ between children and adults.[121] Similarly, when maximal oxygen uptake is expressed relative to body mass (i.e., $mL \cdot kg^{-1} \cdot min^{-1}$), there is no appreciable difference between adults, adolescents, and children.

Heart rates at rest as well as during aerobic exercise of all intensities are higher in children than in adults.[119] The higher heart rate compensates for the lower absolute stroke volumes mentioned earlier. Also, children more thoroughly perfuse their working muscles with blood flow, resulting in more effective oxygen extraction from the blood by the active muscle mass. At rest and for any given exercise intensity, blood pressure has been found to be lower in children than in adults.[52,120] But as children grow and their physical dimensions increase, a gradual reduction in heart rate and increase in blood pressure are evident at rest and during aerobic exercise.

When participating in similarly robust endurance training regimens, the increment in $\dot{V}O_{2max}$, expressed as $mL \cdot kg^{-1} \cdot min^{-1}$ observed in children is only about 10%. Adults, however, generally experience improvements in maximal aerobic power on the order of 20% to 25%. This training-induced difference is mainly attributed to the smaller heart size and blood volume that is inherent in children. Regarding endurance performance, it has been noted that, when running, the amount of oxygen consumed (i.e., $mL \cdot kg^{-1} \cdot min^{-1}$) by a child at any given pace is significantly higher than that by adults. This diminished "running economy" detected among juveniles is best explained by the fact that their legs, and thus stride lengths, are shorter than those of adults. Accordingly, to maintain the same running pace of an adult, children must take more steps (i.e., increase stride frequency), resulting in more frequent muscle contractions and thus increased oxygen consumption.

Anaerobic Capacity and Exercise Responses

Research has demonstrated that, compared with adults, the potential of children to perform anaerobic muscular activity is limited. This is true even when anaerobic power is expressed relative to body mass. In both maximal effort 30-second resisted sprint cycling (i.e., the Wingate test) and the Margaria step test, anaerobic power is lower in children than in adults.[6,43] Moreover, during submaximal- and maximal-intensity endurance exercise, blood and muscle lactate concentrations are lower in children than in adults, again suggesting decreased anaerobic metabolic activity in children. These differences are related to the attenuated glycogen content detected in the muscle of children along with diminished glycolytic enzyme activity in their muscle tissue.

Thermoregulation

The sweating mechanism in children is not as efficient as in adults because their sweat glands are less responsive to elevations in temperature and secrete less sweat. As a result, many have expressed concern that children are more susceptible to hyperthermia and heat illness during exercise and physical activity. However, because of their smaller size, the ratio of skin surface area to body mass is greater in children than in adults. This is advantageous in that it enhances the capacity of the available sweat to evaporate and heat to dissipate into the surrounding environment, promoting cooling. It has also been reported that, during exercise, children have greater blood flow to the skin than do adults, also enabling greater heat loss from the exercising tissue to the environment.[104]

The amount of heat lost to the surrounding environment is directly linked to the temperature gradient between the body and its surrounding environment. So, when exercising under unfavorable environmental conditions of high humidity and heat—particularly if ambient temperature exceeds that of the body—the larger skin surface–to–body mass ratio of the child may actually increase the risk of hyperthermia. This increased risk occurs because heat may be gained from, rather than lost to, the surrounding environment. In children, as with people of all ages, the danger posed by exercising in a hot environment must be recognized and appropriate precautions, such as ensuring ample hydration and reducing exercise intensity and duration, must be taken.

Obesity

The epidemic of **obesity** observed in most Western societies, including the United States, is apparent not only

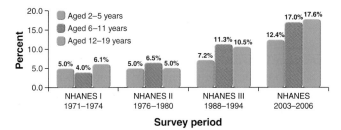

Figure 15-5. Prevalence of being overweight among American children and adolescents from 1971 to 2006. The National Health and Nutrition Examination Survey is a survey research program that is conducted by the National Center for Health Statistics to assess the health and nutritional status of adults and children in the United States and to track changes over time. (From Centers for Disease Control and Protection. Trends in Childhood Obesity. Atlanta, GA: Centers for Disease Control and Protection. Available at http://www.cdc.gov/nchs/nhanes.htm.)

among adults but also among children. Indeed, data collected by the Centers of Disease Control and Prevention (CDC) indicate that, in 2006, the percentage of American children and adolescents considered to be obese had risen to 16%. This trend continues to grow (Fig. 15-5).

The increase in childhood obesity is a major health concern, especially as it corresponds with a similar elevation in the incidence of type II, or "adult-onset," diabetes in children. Other diseases or conditions associated with obesity include high blood pressure, respiratory problems, heart disease, and even depression. According to the CDC, factors that contribute to this disturbing trend in obesity

Quick Review

- Participation in sports and exercise training does not affect the rate of physical growth and maturation in either boys or girls, as long as proper caloric intake is maintained.
- A properly designed resistance training program emphasizing correct technique results in strength gains—with little muscle hypertrophy—in boys and girls without undue risk of injury.
- When expressed in relative terms (i.e., $mL \cdot kg^{-1} \cdot min^{-1}$), there is no significant difference in the maximal aerobic capacity, or $\dot{V}O_{2max}$, of children compared with adults.
- During endurance exercise of the same intensity, the heart rate of children is higher than that of adults, but the working muscles of children are more effective in extracting oxygen from the blood delivered to them.
- Even when participating in endurance training programs of the same intensity and duration, improvements in $\dot{V}O_{2max}$ are lower in children compared with adults, mainly due to differences in heart size and blood volume.
- The anaerobic exercise performance of children is less than that of adults. This is explained by the lower glycogen content and glycolytic enzyme capacity in the muscles of children.

among children include an increase in sedentary leisure-time activities and a decrease in structured and unstructured physical activity. A recent policy statement released by the American Association of Pediatrics strongly urges that more opportunities be provided for children to regularly participate in physical activity in school, after-school programs, and various community settings and that children and their parents make healthier dietary decisions.[56]

THE AGED AND EXERCISE

Demographic data clearly indicate that the populations of nations throughout the world, including the United Sates, are growing older (Fig. 15-6). According to the U.S. Census Bureau, it is estimated that by the year 2050, approximately 90 million Americans will be considered aged (i.e., at least 65 years old). By comparison, in the year 2000, fewer than 40 million U.S. citizens fell within that age category. To improve the health of and decrease medical costs among this growing segment of our population, all major health organizations, including the American College of Sports Medicine, the Centers for Disease Control and Prevention, and the U.S. Surgeon General's Office, recommend that older people regularly engage in physical activity and exercise.

Physiological Effects of Aging

The aging process has physiological effects on the whole body. Here, we will consider effects on the cardiovascular system, skeletal muscle, and skeletal system.

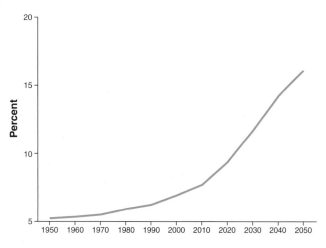

Figure 15-6. There is a growing number of aged (≥65 years) among the global population. (From the Centers for Disease Control and Protection. Young Children and Older People as Percentage of Global Population. Atlanta, GA: Centers for Disease Control and Protection. Available at http://www.nia.nih.gov/NR/rdonlyres/9E91407E-CFE8-4903-9875-D5AA75BD1D50/0/WPAM_finalpdftorose3_9.pdf.)

Cardiovascular System

Although it can be difficult to isolate the effects of aging from those of physical inactivity, some changes among the aged are consistently observed. For example, cardiovascular fitness, typically assessed as $\dot{V}O_{2max}$ (mL·kg^{-1}·min^{-1}), declines with aging at a rate of 8% to 10% per decade from its peak value, reached at approximately 25 years of age. Although the loss of muscle tissue and gain of fat mass that accompany aging explain some of the decrement in $\dot{V}O_{2max}$, it has been found that, even when maximal aerobic power is expressed relative to lean body mass, it is still lower among the aged than the young.[90] The primary factor for this decline in $\dot{V}O_{2max}$ is a similar decrement in maximal cardiac output.[50,83] The inevitable and gradual decrease in maximal heart rate beginning at about 20 years of age contributes to this decline, but evidence demonstrates that the reduction in maximal stroke volume is the principal factor.[83] The decreased maximal stroke volume detected among the aged is related to reductions in left ventricular contractility—and thus a lower ejection fraction when the heart beats—along with a smaller blood volume. Arterial wall stiffness is greater among the aged, contributing to the higher mean arterial pressure observed among older people during both maximal- and submaximal-intensity exercise. This results in elevations in systolic, as well as diastolic, blood pressure.[70] Along with increased blood pressure during exercise, due to a decrease in the ability to redistribute blood flow to active muscle, the amount of blood delivered to the contracting muscles is reduced in the aged.[91]

In addition to the age-related disadvantages of cardiovascular function, other mechanisms related to the body's ability to maximally consume oxygen are hindered with aging. That is, the capacity of working muscle tissue to extract oxygen from the blood delivered to it is decreased, resulting in a decreased a-vO$_2$ difference in older people. The lower capillarity and mitochondrial density detected in aged skeletal muscle can account for its diminished a-vO$_2$ difference.

Skeletal Muscle

Similar to the reduction in cardiovascular capacity displayed by the aged, skeletal muscle strength also declines at a rate of roughly 10% per decade. However, this begins at a later age—50 years old—than the decline in $\dot{V}O_{2max}$. The loss of strength noted with aging, though, accelerates after the sixth decade of life, reaching a rate of approximately 15% per decade. In fact, recent longitudinal data studying the same people over time suggest that, after the age of 60 years, strength may decrease as rapidly as 3% to 5% annually.[4,30] The age-related loss of muscle power, or "explosive strength," begins at about 40 years of age and generally declines more quickly than strength. This is of particular concern because, more so than strength, the loss of muscle power is linked with the greater incidence of accidental falls and the resultant injuries among older people.[106]

Age-related declines in muscle strength and power are mainly accounted for by the loss of muscle mass and a greater proportion of the remaining muscle being occupied by slow-twitch fibers (type I). The term **sarcopenia** refers to the loss of skeletal muscle tissue that accompanies aging (Box 15-4). This loss of tissue is evident in the whole muscle and its constituent fibers. The rate of the decline of muscle mass mirrors the loss of muscle strength that occurs during aging. Like strength, muscle mass is well maintained from its peak in the midtwenties through the fifth decade of life.

During these years, muscle atrophies a total of only 10%. However, beyond 50 years of age, muscle atrophy occurs at a rate of 10% per decade.[62] This loss in muscle mass results from atrophy of individual fibers, with type II or fast-twitch fibers being most affected, as well as a decrease in the number of fibers comprising the muscle. Indeed, it is the decline in muscle fiber count that principally accounts for sarcopenia.[62]

There is strong evidence that this **apoptosis**, or cell death, of fibers is triggered by an age-related denervation

Box 15-4 AN EXPERT VIEW

Resistance Exercise: The Secret to Maintaining Strength, Function, and Independence Into Old Age

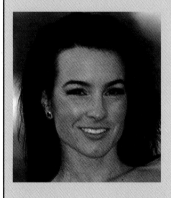

Maren S. Fragala, PhD, CSCS*D
Research Fellow
Center on Aging
University of Connecticut Health Center
Farmington, CT

After the age of 30, muscle strength declines by about 10% to 15% per decade,[10,20] with the rate accelerating after age 50–60.[10,17,20] Losses in muscle mass and muscle quality accompany this decline.[18,19] This age-related loss in muscle mass and function is termed *sarcopenia*.[9,16,22,25] Sarcopenia is common in about a quarter of adults older than age 65, and the prevalence increases with age.[13] Not only is sarcopenia associated with the inability to perform activities of daily living,[3,12] such as getting out of a chair, climbing stairs, bathing, or dressing independently, but is also associated with another state of vulnerability, termed *frailty*. Frailty is characterized by unintentional weight loss, physical exhaustion, muscle weakness, slow walking speed, and low physical activity.[6] Frailty represents a concerning state of decreased resilience in older adults and predisposition to catastrophic events, such as a fall or influenza.[2,7,8,21,23,29]

Luckily, the development of sarcopenia and frailty can be postponed, and the onset of disability can be delayed with the proper interventions. Successful intervention strategies involve resistance exercise training. Several studies have demonstrated the benefits of resistance training programs for older adults to not only increase muscle strength and muscle mass[11,24,26] but also improve functional performance and quality of life measures, and reduce the risk of frailty.[1,4,14,27] Resistance exercise has also been shown beneficial to management of other chronic conditions in older adults such as obesity, osteoporosis, osteoarthritis, and diabetes by decreasing both total and intra-abdominal fat, maintaining bone mineral density,

increasing muscle quality, and reducing pain and insulin resistance.[5,15,28]

Although special considerations exist in resistance training for older adults, including health ailments such as dementia, cardiovascular disease, osteoporosis, balance issues, or medication side effects, training an older adult in resistance exercise is like training a world-class athlete. Both have goals of maximizing performance, which vary drastically in level (i.e., the ability to climb a flight of stairs vs. cutting a fraction of a second off of a 40-yd sprint). Similar principles and considerations apply: all focused on the *individual*. Like training athletes, exercise programs for older adults should be closely tailored based on the initial needs analysis, considering fitness level and experience, injuries, health concerns, goals, access to facilities, motivation, and barriers.

- Prescribed exercises should be *specific* to the goals of the individual; if stair climbing and rising out of a chair are a challenge, exercises that mimic these muscle actions and involve the same muscle groups and joints are important, such as step-ups (varying levels of height and balance support) or modified squats (chair rises).
- Exercises should work all major muscle groups (upper body, lower body, and trunk) and should include all major muscle actions (push, pull, lift, lower, bend, reach, rotate).
- Modifications to any exercise can be made to better accommodate varying levels of ability. For example, some older adults may be comfortable getting on the floor to perform a full push-up, while others may prefer remaining standing and could try a push-up with the hands against the wall.
- The range of motion should remain within a range of motion that is pain free.
- The load or resistance used should be selected cautiously to ensure proper form and technique and reduce unnecessary pain or soreness.
- *Progression* should be gradual, based on individual advancement, while considering that some challenge is needed to generate a stimulus to elicit adaptation.

(Continued)

Unlike younger adults, older adults most frequently report health concerns as the predominant barrier to exercise. Moreover, when an individual possesses any "risk factor" (of which age alone is considered a risk factor), physician clearance is required before beginning a resistance training program. Thus, physician support is necessary to ensure safety, set restrictions, and alleviate the common notion of older adults that, "My health is just too poor for me to exercise," so that more older adults can reap the benefits of resistance exercise.

Older adults should carefully communicate with their physicians and health care providers to discuss the muscle and functional benefits of resistance exercise against the restrictions and limitations of any underlying health ailment to maximize quality of life, well-being, and independence. Thus, resistance exercise training may be the secret to keeping aging muscles young and aging adults functional and independent. With the proper encouragement, older adults should participate in safe, comfortable, individualized, and enjoyable resistance exercise training programs as an important therapy to achieve enhanced quality of life during advanced years.

References

1. Binder EF, Yarasheski KE, Steger-May K, et al. Effects of progressive resistance training on body composition in frail older adults: results of a randomized, controlled trial. J Gerontol A Biol Sci Med Sci. 2005;60:1425–1431.
2. Campbell AJ, Borrie MJ, Spears GF. Risk factors for falls in a community-based prospective study of people 70 years and older. J Gerontol. 1989;44:M112–M117.
3. Estrada M, Kleppinger A, Judge JO, et al. Functional impact of relative versus absolute sarcopenia in healthy older women. J Am Geriatr Soc. 2007;55:1712–1719.
4. Evans WJ. Exercise training guidelines for the elderly. Med Sci Sports Exerc. 1999;31:12–17.
5. Fatouros IG, Chatzinikolaou A, Tournis S, et al. Intensity of resistance exercise determines adipokine and resting energy expenditure responses in overweight elderly individuals. Diabetes Care. 2009;32:2161–2167.
6. Fried LP, Tangen CM, Walston J, et al. Frailty in older adults: evidence for a phenotype. J Gerontol A Biol Sci Med Sci. 2001;56:M146–M156.
7. Fried LP, Walston JD, Ferrucci L. Frailty. In: Halter J, ed. Hazzard's Geriatric Medicine and Gerontology. New York, NY: McGraw-Hill, 2009.
8. Frontera WR, Hughes VA, Lutz KJ, et al. A cross-sectional study of muscle strength and mass in 45- to 78-yr-old men and women. J Appl Physiol. 1991;71:644–650.
9. Greenlund LJ, Nair KS. Sarcopenia—consequences, mechanisms, and potential therapies. Mech Ageing Dev. 2003;124:287–299.
10. Hakkinen K, Hakkinen A. Muscle cross-sectional area, force production and relaxation characteristics in women at different ages. Eur J Appl Physiol Occup Physiol. 1991;62:410–414.
11. Hakkinen K, Kraemer WJ, Pakarinen A, et al. Effects of heavy resistance/power training on maximal strength, muscle morphology, and hormonal response patterns in 60–75-year-old men and women. Can J Appl Physiol. 2002;27:213–231.
12. Hyatt RH, Whitelaw MN, Bhat A, et al. Association of muscle strength with functional status of elderly people. Age Ageing. 1990;19:330–336.
13. Iannuzzi-Sucich M, Prestwood KM, Kenny AM. Prevalence of sarcopenia and predictors of skeletal muscle mass in healthy, older men and women. J Gerontol A Biol Sci Med Sci. 2002;57:M772–M777.
14. Judge JO, Kenny AM, Kraemer WJ. Exercise in older adults. Conn Med. 2003;67:461–464.
15. Judge JO, Kleppinger A, Kenny A, et al. Home-based resistance training improves femoral bone mineral density in women on hormone therapy. Osteoporos Int. 2005;16:1096–1108.
16. Lamberts SW, van den Beld AW, van der Lely AJ. The endocrinology of aging. Science. 1997;278:419–424.
17. Larsson L, Grimby G, Karlsson J. Muscle strength and speed of movement in relation to age and muscle morphology. J Appl Physiol. 1979;46:451–456.
18. Larsson L, Li X, Yu F, et al. Age-related changes in contractile properties and expression of myosin isoforms in single skeletal muscle cells. Muscle Nerve. 1997;5:S74–S78.
19. Lexell J. Human aging, muscle mass, and fiber type composition. J Gerontol A Biol Sci Med Sci. 1995;50:11–16.
20. Lindle RS, Metter EJ, Lynch NA, et al. Age and gender comparisons of muscle strength in 654 women and men aged 20–93 yr. J Appl Physiol. 1997;83:1581–1587.
21. Muhlberg W, Sieber C. Sarcopenia and frailty in geriatric patients: implications for training and prevention. Z Gerontol Geriatr. 2004;37:2–8.
22. Proctor DN, Balagopal P, Nair KS. Age-related sarcopenia in humans is associated with reduced synthetic rates of specific muscle proteins. J Nutr. 1998;128:351S–355S.
23. Rantanen T, Guralnik JM, Ferrucci L, et al. Coimpairments: strength and balance as predictors of severe walking disability. J Gerontol A Biol Sci Med Sci. 1999;54:M172–M176.
24. Sallinen J, Pakarinen A, Fogelholm M, et al. Serum basal hormone concentrations and muscle mass in aging women: effects of strength training and diet. Int J Sport Nutr Exerc Metab. 2006;16:316–331.
25. Sehl M, Sawhney R, Naeim A. Physiologic aspects of aging: impact on cancer management and decision making, part II. Cancer J. 2005;11:461–473.
26. Sillanpaa E, Hakkinen A, Punnonen K, et al. Effects of strength and endurance training on metabolic risk factors in healthy 40–65-year-old men. Scand J Med Sci Sports. 2008;19:885–895.
27. Spirduso WW, Cronin DL. Exercise dose-response effects on quality of life and independent living in older adults. Med Sci Sports Exerc. 2001;33(6 Suppl):S598–S608.
28. Valkeinen H, Häkkinen A, Hannonen P, et al. Acute heavy-resistance exercise-induced pain and neuromuscular fatigue in elderly women with fibromyalgia and in healthy controls: effects of strength training. Arthritis Rheum. 2006;54:1334–1339.
29. Walston J, Hadley EC, Ferucci L, et al. Research agenda for frailty in older adults: toward a better understanding of physiology and etiology: summary from the American Geriatrics Society/National Institute on Aging Research Conference on Frailty in Older Adults. J Am Geriatr Soc. 2006;54:991–1001.

process that begins within the central nervous system. As motor neurons demonstrate necrotic damage and withdraw from the muscle fibers that they innervate, the newly abandoned fibers must be reinnervated by nearby, healthy motor neurons or they will first atrophy, then die. This process results in a smaller number of motor units per muscle, but those that remain in the aged muscle are larger (i.e., more fibers per motor neuron).[58] This denervation process equally affects type I (slow-twitch) and type II (fast-twitch) fibers so that fiber-type composition

(% of each fiber type) is unchanged with aging. However, the selective atrophy of type II fibers observed among aged muscles results in a greater proportion of the entire muscle mass being occupied by type I fibers.

Skeletal System

Another major health concern associated with aging is the well-documented loss of bone mineral density and, accordingly, bone strength. This age-related decline in bone mineral density is most pronounced among women, although it also is apparent to a lesser extent among men. In fact, osteoporosis, a degenerative disease characterized by bone mass loss and architectural deterioration consequently resulting in bone fragility, afflicts 10% of U.S. citizens aged 50 years or more. U.S. medical costs associated with osteoporotic bone fractures are estimated to be as high as $20 billion annually.[32] The age-related decline of bone mineral density has been shown to track the loss of muscle mass and strength detected among the aged. This relationship has led to the saying among gerontologists and exercise physiologists that, "strong muscles equal strong bones." Thus, they recommend weight-bearing exercise, as well as resistance training, for the effective strengthening of not only muscles but also the bones to which they are attached.

Adaptations to Exercise Training

Fortunately, the aged can significantly counteract the age-related declines discussed earlier through aerobic and resistance training. In this section, we consider cardiovascular, muscular, and skeletal adaptations to exercise among the aged.

Cardiovascular System

When subjected to endurance training programs of the same intensity, frequency, and duration as young adults, the aged experience relative improvements (i.e., percent increase from pretrained baseline) in $\dot{V}O_{2max}$ that do not differ from the 20% to 25% increases shown among the young.[53,102] Although those improvements occur in both sexes, they appear to be derived from different adaptations among aged men and women. In aged men, training-induced increases in $\dot{V}O_{2max}$ are mainly attributed to the central adaptations of greater cardiac output and stroke volume. Among aged women, however, peripheral adaptations, specifically improved oxygen extraction by the working skeletal muscle, account for increases in maximal oxygen uptake.[109] In both aged men and women, endurance training results in a lower heart rate and mean arterial pressure at rest, as well as during submaximal-intensity exercise.[19,36] And, as in younger people, an endurance training program lasting several months can reduce body fat by up to 3 kg, or around 4% of body mass.

Skeletal Muscle

Early investigations suggested that aged people had less potential to respond to resistance training and only minimally improved their strength and muscle size. However, these studies had many methodological shortcomings, such as using inadequately robust training regimens. In more recent studies, older people have completed training programs featuring the same intensity, frequency, and duration that are prescribed for young adults. The results of these studies clearly demonstrate that the aged are capable of significantly improving their strength and undergoing muscle hypertrophy. Despite some exceptions, most of the available data indicate that, when presented with the same resistance training stimulus, the aged experience strength gains that are equally impressive as those detected among the young.[38,39,77,123] Depending on the testing methods used, the type of muscle contraction performed (i.e., isotonic, isometric, isokinetic), the specific muscle(s) trained, and the duration of the resistance training program, these improvements can be on the order of 25% to more than doubling pretraining strength values.

Like studies of strength, those investigating the effect of resistance training on hypertrophy in the aged yield somewhat conflicting results. When assessing muscle hypertrophy as an expansion of whole-muscle volume, it appears that similarly trained young and aged adults display about the same degree of hypertrophy.[47,14] In contrast, when changes in size or cross-sectional areas of either the whole muscle or its constituent fibers are examined as a measure of hypertrophy, the data suggest that although the aged demonstrate significant hypertrophy, it is less pronounced than that exhibited by young adults.[38,123,55] Similar to endurance training, resistance exercise also significantly improves body composition among the aged, albeit with different mechanisms. Endurance training elicits reductions in fat mass with minimal effects on lean body mass, whereas resistance training both increases lean body mass and decreases fat mass.

Skeletal System

Because osteoporosis is more likely to afflict women than men, most investigations determining the potential of exercise training to improve bone mineral density and health have been conducted on postmenopausal women. In general, those studies indicate that endurance training significantly enhances bone mineral density, but those improvements are only observed on the weight-bearing bones and joints of the lower body. Although the increases in bone mineral density resulting from resistance training are no more impressive than those from endurance training (i.e., 1%–3%), those improvements are found at more numerous sites throughout the body, including the spine (see Box 15-5).[26,71,72,114]

Box 15-5 PRACTICAL QUESTIONS FROM STUDENTS

Is It Safe to Recommend Exercise Among the Aged, and If So, Will It Be Effective?

Not only is exercise training safe for the aged (assuming the absence of preexisting contraindications such as orthopedic and cardiovascular issues), it is also effective. In fact, virtually every major health and geriatric organization recommends that older people engage in a properly designed physical conditioning program. A multitude of investigations have demonstrated that in relative terms (i.e., percent increase from initial values), aged people improve their cardiovascular fitness to the same extent as younger people when participating in endurance training programs featuring the same intensity, frequency, and duration of training. It

also is now recognized that the aged can, and should, participate in resistance training on a regular basis. Similar to cardiovascular fitness, when the aged perform resistance training of appropriate intensity, frequency, and duration, they will show gains in strength and muscle fitness that are not unlike those detected among young adults. A proper exercise training program for the aged should include both cardiovascular training, so that risk of a cardiovascular event or stroke is reduced, and resistance training, to decrease the risk of type 2 diabetes and accidental falls and to enhance bone health and body composition.

Exercise Prescription

Most evidence suggests that, despite having lower initial levels of fitness, older people should follow the same exercise prescription guidelines as recommended for young adults.[49] This is true of endurance training intended to improve cardiovascular fitness, as well as resistance training designed to enhance musculoskeletal fitness. Of course, there are exceptions for those who may have pre-existing medical conditions that limit or even preclude exercise training. Also, exercise prescription guidelines for those aged people considered to be physically frail are modified so that intensity and total volume of training are decreased. The rate of progression of the long-term training program also may be more moderate for those people. In addition to endurance training and resistance training increasing the functional capacities of the cardiovascular and musculoskeletal systems, activities of daily living (e.g., rising out of chairs, climbing stairs, carrying bags of groceries) also become less stressful to the aged as a result of exercise training.

A unique aspect of exercise prescription for the aged is its inclusion of exercises that are designed specifically to improve balance and coordination. This is done in response

to the high frequency of accidental falls suffered among the aged and due to weakened bones and increased likelihood of bone fractures and other morbidities that result from those falls. Hip fractures are of particular concern among the aged because data reveal that, in over 20% of those cases, mortality will occur within 1 year of the injury.[40] Although balance training is typically included in overall fitness programs for the aged, there is little scientific evidence to either support or refute the effectiveness of balancing exercises, by themselves, in preventing falls (see Box 15-6).

Box 15-6 DID YOU KNOW?

Senior Olympics

The first Senior Olympics were held in 1970 and consisted of only three sports (swimming, track and field, and diving), with only 200 people competing. Today, the U.S. Senior Olympics features more than 30 events with several thousand athletes participating in both summer and winter Olympics. To compete in these contests, the only criterion you must meet is to be at least 50 years of age.

Quick Review

- People who are considered aged, that is, ≥65 years old, comprise the fastest growing segment of the U.S. population.
- Aerobic fitness, or $\dot{V}O_{2max}$, peaks at about 25 years of age before steadily declining at a rate of 8% to 10% per decade. This decrease is mainly accounted for by reductions in maximal stroke volume.
- Declines in muscle strength begin at about 50 years of age and proceed at a rate of roughly 10% per decade.
- Similar to strength, the loss of muscle mass beyond 50 years of age occurs at a rate of 10% per decade.
- Age-related muscle atrophy affects fast-twitch fibers more than slow-twitch ones.
- When participating in an endurance training program of similar intensity and duration, the aged experience improvements in cardiovascular fitness that match those of the young (i.e., 20%–25%).
- The aged display increases in muscle strength and size that are similar to those of the young when performing the same resistance training regimen.

ASTHMA AND EXERCISE

Asthma is a condition characterized by labored breathing, wheezing, and tightness of the chest. These symptoms are brought on by contraction of the smooth musculature surrounding the air pathways of the bronchiole network. This bronchoconstriction typically is triggered by exposure to environmental allergens, which cause an inflammatory response when mast cells located on the airway surface release histamine, prostaglandins, and leukotrienes. Asthma can affect people of all ages, but it most commonly is identified among children and adolescents because they are more regularly exposed to environments where allergens can be found. These include not only outdoor playing and sports fields but also swimming pools and ice-skating rinks, where, respectively, chlorine and ice-resurfacing chemicals and gaseous emissions provoke allergic responses among some.

Nonallergy Causes

Because the rise in the number of people afflicted with asthma coincides with the sharp increase in childhood obesity over the last three to four decades, it has recently been postulated that obesity may contribute to the onset of asthma.[13,112] It appears that the greater burden of breathing among the obese limits the deep breathing necessary to maintain the optimal size of airway passages. Over time, those passages reduce their diameter, thus increasing resistance to the flow of air through the ventilatory pathways. It has also been suggested, however, that irrespective of obesity, the steady decline in physical activity observed among children since the mid-twentieth century may be a powerful cause of the rise in asthma during those years.[46,94] As with obesity, the lack of regular deep breathing that accompanies a sedentary life style eventually leads to reduced dimensions of airway passages, which brings about the symptoms of asthma.

Effects of Exercise

Because the stimulus of exercise, which can increase minute ventilation many fold, may bring about wheezing, dyspnea, and coughing among those with asthma, historically it has been recommended that asthmatics avoid physical exertion. More recently, however, it has been proved that exercise training can benefit asthmatics. Results are mixed regarding the capacity of aerobic exercise to control the incidence and severity of asthma attacks. However, it has been consistently demonstrated that aerobic fitness and measures of quality of life (e.g., hospital visits, absenteeism from work or school) are improved along with psychological well-being (e.g., improved self-confidence) following exercise training. Also important is the fact that, with increased physical fitness, the ventilatory load required to carry out any physical task is lowered and, accordingly, less likely to stimulate an asthmatic episode. This in itself is a vital benefit.

Rather than discouraging exercise among asthma patients, experts in the field now advocate the inclusion of aerobic exercise training as part of an overall treatment program. Indeed, both the American College of Sports Medicine and the American Thoracic Society recommend that those with asthma participate in regular and vigorous activity, assuming, of course, that they are controlling their condition with medications, such as inhaled corticosteroids. The American Academy of Pediatrics guidelines for exercise among children with asthma are summarized in Box 15-7.

Exercise-Induced Asthma

In large part, the reason for recommending that asthmatics avoid exercise, the stance espoused by experts years ago, is that physical activity requiring a marked increase in ventilatory load serves as a robust trigger to the onset of asthma's symptoms. Indeed, up to 90% of those diagnosed with asthma experience what is termed "exercise-induced asthma," or EIA.[93] However, even those who are not asthma patients may experience EIA. As many as 13% of those who otherwise show no symptoms of asthma suffer from bronchospasm along with coughing, wheezing, and labored breathing associated with EIA.[99] In particular, endurance exercise, such as running, cycling, and swimming, has been shown to elicit EIA. However, any mode of exercise performed at an intensity of 80% or more of a person's maximum oxygen uptake is capable of evoking EIA in those who are susceptible. At particular risk are swimmers, who may be allergic to the chlorine used to treat water, and athletes from ice sports, who may be sensitive to emissions released by ice-resurfacing machines.

Etiology

Typically, bronchospasm (airway tightening) occurs 10 to 15 minutes following the start of exercise. The reason for this delay is that the inflammatory response leading to the constriction of airway smooth muscle takes some time to become fully activated. As exercise begins and ventilation increases, water that moistens internal air evaporates at a greater rate, acting to dehydrate and cool the surface of the airway network. The greater the increase in ventilation, the more severe the dehydration and cooling of the airway surface. When the mast cells located in the walls of the airways dry out and become hypertonic, they release leukotrienes and histamine, triggering an inflammatory response and bronchoconstriction, which impedes the flow of air in and out of the lungs.[3] Because cold air also tends to be dry, outdoor winter sport athletes are especially vulnerable to EIA. This risk can be significantly reduced when those athletes wear face masks to trap the moisture in expired air so that it can humidify and warm the cold, dry, inspired air before it reaches the bronchiole network.

Box 15-7 APPLYING RESEARCH
Guidelines for Exercise Prescription for Children With Asthma

The American Academy of Pediatrics' guidelines for sports participation in children states the following: "with proper medication and education, only athletes with the most severe asthma will need to modify their participation."

Preexercise

Warm-up: keep at low-to-moderate intensity, heart rate <75% predicted maximum for a few minutes; do not use intermittent sprinting.

Premedication: take 200 μg salbutamol (albuterol) or equivalent via large-volume spacer at least 10 min before starting warm-up; long-acting bronchodilator medication may be useful for children where exercise is unplanned.

Preferred Activities

- Swimming (but note possible chlorine sensitivity), cycling, and walking
- Other aerobic activities (e.g., running and playing games)

- Competitive sports (e.g., soccer and basketball)

Monitoring

- Children should be encouraged to "listen to their bodies" and learn how to take their heart rate and monitor signs of both exertional breathlessness and asthma.
- Further "rescue" medication should be available.
- Children should be encouraged to take appropriate rests during high-intensity competitive sports (e.g., basketball).

Contraindications

Same as for normal recommendations: fever and headache, but especially respiratory infections.

Reprinted with permission from Welsh L, Kemp JG, Roberts RGD. Effects of physical conditioning on children and adolescents with asthma. Sports Med. 2005;35:127–141.

Preventative Measures

Both pharmacological and nonpharmacological measures can be taken to help prevent EIA. These are discussed below.

Pharmacological Measures

Those athletes who have been diagnosed with asthma should consider inhaled corticosteroids, which suppress inflammatory responses of the airway passages, to be a first line of defense against EIA. As the anti-inflammatory effects of glucocorticosteroids are fairly long lasting, they can be taken several hours before exercise (or according to their typical daily administration) and remain effective during exercise in patients with mild asthma. Surprisingly, little is known about the efficacy of daily dosages of glucocorticosteroids in athletes prone to EIA attacks, but who are not considered to be asthma patients.

Particularly effective in virtually all (~95%) athletes suffering from EIA, asthmatics and nonasthmatics alike, is a class of agents termed short-acting β-agonists. These drugs can also be inhaled and serve as effective bronchodilators for up to 3 hours, with maximum effects seen 15 to 60 minutes following administration.[8] Accordingly, these agents should be taken about 15 minutes before the onset of exercise to prevent EIA symptoms. More recently, long-lasting β-agonists have been developed that can provide bronchodilatory effects for 9 to 12 hours following inhalation.[10]

Finally, leukotriene inhibitors have been shown to be effective in preventing the onset of EIA, even though they have limited capacity to manage long-term, or chronic, asthma. A caveat is in order here. Some of the variants of the drugs mentioned earlier have been outlawed by sports oversight committees because of their potential ergogenic effects. Competitive athletes should find out which ones are illegal and consult with their coaches and physicians to find asthma medications that will not disqualify them from participating in sports events.

Nonpharmacological Measures

Because exercise itself acts as a bronchodilator, it is important that those affected by EIA warm-up properly before working out or competing. This warm-up should include short bursts of high-intensity exercise to stimulate the release of catecholamines, which elicit bronchodilation. At the cessation of exercise, when the symptoms of EIA are often manifested, it is advisable to gradually cool down. Managing the environment in which the athlete practices and competes may also contribute to the effective prevention of EIA. For those who have reactions to pollen or other naturally occurring allergens in the air, simply avoiding freshly cut grass or fields may be helpful. And although the warm, humid air found in indoor swimming pool areas can actually reduce the chance of an EIA attack, those who are sensitive to the chlorine used to treat the water should consider how much is used and at what times it is dispensed.

- Asthma is caused by contraction of the smooth muscle tissue found in the bronchiole tubes leading into the lungs.
- Specific allergens dispersed in inspired air trigger asthmatic episodes.
- The rise in childhood obesity is paralleled by an increased incidence of asthma, as the increased pressure of excess body mass reduces the diameter of respiratory passageways.
- Medical associations recommend that those with asthma participate in a program of aerobic-type exercise on a regular basis.
- EIA may afflict even those who have not been diagnosed with asthma. In particular, endurance exercise may bring about symptoms such as wheezing, coughing, and labored breathing.
- EIA is more likely to occur in settings where allergens are prevalent, such as outdoor playing fields, indoor skating rinks, and indoor swimming pools.

For cold-weather athletes, a face mask can help warm and humidify inhaled air before it enters the air passages, in the manner described earlier. Those who perform on indoor ice-skating rinks must consider the power source of ice-resurfacing devices. Those that are electrically powered do not spew out potentially allergy-triggering fumes.

Finally, exercise training itself can assist in the treatment of EIA. Although improving aerobic fitness ($\dot{V}O_{2max}$) will not cure EIA, it decreases the ventilatory load posed by any particular physical task, thus reducing the chance of triggering an attack of EIA. With appropriate treatment strategies, including pharmacological and nonpharmacological interventions, medical experts estimate that 90% of those who have displayed EIA symptoms can participate in even vigorous physical activity and sports.[76]

DIABETES MELLITUS AND EXERCISE

Diabetes mellitus, more simply called **diabetes**, is rapidly increasing in incidence along with the "graying" or aging of most Western societies. Diabetes is a disease characterized by one's inability to maintain blood glucose levels within its normal limits as a result of the failure of the pancreas to produce and secrete the hormone insulin into the bloodstream (type 1) or decreased sensitivity of the hormone's target tissues (i.e., liver and skeletal muscle) (type 2). Indeed, in the United States, the incidence of diabetes increases according to age (Fig. 15-7). Perhaps more alarming is the more than doubling in the prevalence of diabetes since 1980, even when changes in aging demographics are accounted for. As of 2007, the Centers for Disease Control and Prevention estimates that nearly 8% of the American population, or 23.6 million people, can be considered diabetics. Accordingly, this affliction poses a significant financial burden on the country's healthcare system. In addition to the $116 billion annual price tag of the direct medical costs attributed to the treatment of diabetes, the Centers for Disease Control and Prevention estimates that another $58 billion is lost through indirect costs, such as missed work, disability, and premature mortality.

The distinguishing feature of diabetes is the patient's inability to maintain blood glucose levels within its normal

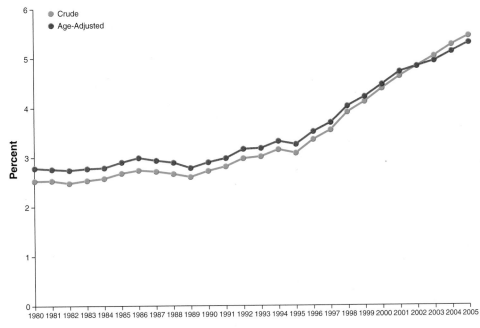

Figure 15-7. Crude and age-adjusted prevalence of Americans diagnosed with diabetes per 100 population (%) from 1980 to 2005. (From the Centers for Disease Control and Protection. Available at http://www.cdc.gov/diabetes/statistics/prev/national/figage.htm.)

limits. This can be the result of the failure of the pancreas to produce and secrete insulin into the bloodstream, which is known as **type 1 diabetes,** or insulin-dependent diabetes. This condition can also be caused by decreased sensitivity of the hormone's target tissues (i.e., liver and skeletal muscle), which is known as **type 2 diabetes,** or non–insulin-dependent diabetes. In both cases, the outcome is that the body lacks the capacity to store dietary carbohydrates in the target tissue to either be used as an energy source when increased metabolic activity may require it (skeletal muscle) or be released as glucose into the bloodstream when those levels are inadequate (liver). If left unchecked, diabetes can result in severe health complications, including heart disease and stroke, hypertension, blindness, kidney disease, nervous system disease, and dental disease. The vascular disease that often accompanies diabetes can be blamed for over 60% of the nontraumatic lower-limb amputations performed in the United States each year.

Type 1 Diabetes

Currently, insulin-dependent diabetes accounts for 10% to 15% of all cases of diabetes in the United States. This form of diabetes is sometimes called "child-onset" diabetes because it typically manifests itself in younger people, although people of all ages can display the first symptoms of the disease. Despite the growing trend of children displaying the symptoms of type 2 diabetes, it is the type 1 form that accounts for as much as 85% of the diagnosed cases of diabetes among children and adolescents each year.[63] These symptoms include excess urine production (polyuria), sugar in the urine, constant thirst, and elevated blood sugar (hyperglycemia) after eating a meal. Generally, the inability of the β-cells of the pancreas to synthesize insulin is the outcome of autoimmunity, in which the body's own immune system mistakenly identifies those cells as foreign and destroys them.[1] Consequently, exogenous insulin must be administered on a regular basis, most commonly via injections, but in some cases by a steadily releasing pump. In addition to insulin therapy, those with type 1 diabetes must learn to carefully control their diet so that carbohydrates are regularly consumed throughout the day. With the advent of affordable automated blood glucose monitors, patients can now periodically self-monitor their glucose levels to adjust insulin therapy and dietary intake as needed.

Increased use of glucose by working muscles during exercise may lead to hypoglycemia and its effects on the central nervous system, such as confusion, loss of coordination, and even loss of consciousness. Because of this, many with type 1 diabetes avoid sports and working out. Yet, despite reservations that exercise may unduly lower blood glucose, exercise has traditionally been, and continues to be, a vital component of the therapeutic strategy prescribed for those with diabetes. In its most recent position stand on this issue, the American Diabetes Association states that, "All levels of physical activity, including leisure activities, recreational sports, and competitive professional performance, can be performed by people with type 1 diabetes who do not have complications and are in good blood glucose control."[34]

Although all types of activities are encouraged, the different energy demands of various sporting events require that the measures taken to regulate blood glucose be adapted to those different demands. For example, to maintain normoglycemic conditions during moderate-intensity endurance-type activities, such as running, cycling, and swimming, preexercise insulin dosages should be reduced and carbohydrates should be eaten before workouts. This is to compensate for the decline in blood glucose that occurs during exercise as the working muscle takes up blood sugar at a rate that exceeds the rate of glucose release into the blood by the liver. It is also important to monitor blood glucose following exercise and, if necessary, consume additional carbohydrates, as hypoglycemia can persist with type 1 diabetes for up to 3 hours after exercise.[65] On the other hand, when high-intensity ($>80\%$ $\dot{V}O_{2max}$) and shorter-duration exercise is performed, athletes with insulin-dependent diabetes experience increased blood sugar levels. This hyperglycemia is also of concern and is a consequence of increased hepatic glucose production and release stimulated by augmented catecholamine and cortisol concentrations, which accompany higher-intensity exercise.[92] This hyperglycemia is most evident after exercise, when muscles are no longer using glucose at greater rates, but the effects of catecholamines and cortisol are still causing a greater-than-normal release of glucose into the bloodstream. Under these conditions, it is appropriate to administer a small dose of insulin after exercise and to avoid eating carbohydrates at that time.[34]

Like the spontaneous play of children, most sports played by adolescents and young adults feature short bursts of maximal effort interspersed by longer periods of mild- to moderate-intensity activity. This intermittent, high-intensity exercise is exemplified by some of our most popular sports, including soccer, basketball, racquetball, etc. Relatively little is known regarding how this type of exercise modifies blood glucose levels. However, the few available data suggest that, because of the influence of glucose-producing hormones (i.e., catecholamines, glucagon, cortisol), which are released during the bursts of high-intensity activity, hypoglycemia does not seem to be a concern during or after exercise.[35] Consequently, it is advised that, compared with moderate-intensity exercise, there is no need to alter preexercise insulin dosage or carbohydrate consumption to maintain proper glucose values during and after intermittent, high-intensity exercise.[34] However, each athlete must consult with his or her physician and coach and learn from experience what steps should be taken to maintain desired blood glucose levels during and following exercise.

Box 15-8 APPLYING RESEARCH

Guidelines to Help Regulate Glycemic Response to Physical Activity Among Those With Type 1 Diabetes

1. Metabolic control before physical activity
   a. Avoid physical activity if fasting glucose levels are >250 mg·dL^{-1} and ketosis is present, and use caution if glucose levels are >300 mg·dL^{-1} and no ketosis is present.
   b. Ingest added carbohydrate if glucose levels are <100 mg·dL^{-1}.
2. Blood glucose monitoring before and after physical activity
   a. Identify when changes in insulin or food intake are necessary.

   b. Learn the glycemic response to different physical activity conditions.
3. Food intake
   a. Consume added carbohydrate as needed to avoid hypoglycemia.
   b. Carbohydrate-based foods should be readily available during and after physical activity.

Reprinted with permission from Physical Activity/Exercise and Diabetes, a position statement by the American Diabetes Association. Diabetes Care. 2004;27(Suppl 1):S58–S62.

People with type 1 diabetes enjoy many health benefits as a result of exercise training, including improved blood lipid profiles, lower blood pressure, enhanced cardiovascular fitness, and even psychological well-being. However, exercise training does not directly improve the body's glucoregulatory capacity. That is, regardless of training status, those with type 1 diabetes will always have to take exogenous insulin, carefully watch what they eat, and monitor their blood glucose levels. The American Diabetes Association's guidelines for regulating glucose for those who are physically active are presented in Box 15-8.

Type 2 Diabetes

This form of diabetes is primarily identified by decreased insulin sensitivity of skeletal muscle and hepatic tissue, as well as an impaired capacity of the pancreas to secrete insulin. Type 2 diabetes accounts for 85% to 90% of all diabetes cases diagnosed in the United States each year. Traditionally, this non–insulin-dependent diabetes has also been referred to as "adult-onset" diabetes because most patients diagnosed with it are at least 18 years of age. Although the past 20 to 30 years have witnessed a sharp increase in the incidence of type 2 diabetes among children and adolescents, type 1 diabetes still comprises as much as 85% of the cases of clinically diagnosed diabetes in those populations.[63]

The marked increase in type 2 diabetes in the United States and throughout the world over the last two to three decades has been called an "epidemic" by some and is viewed with alarm by medical and healthcare experts. By the year 2025, it is expected that over 300 million people worldwide will have type 2 diabetes. This is of great concern because this condition is associated with elevated rates of mortality and serious morbidities, such as blindness, kidney failure, neuropathy, and vascular complications that can result in cardiovascular disease (see Box 15-9).[42]

Obesity as a Risk Factor

The growth in the prevalence of type 2 diabetes parallels that of obesity in modern, industrialized nations. In fact, obesity is considered the outstanding risk factor for the development of the disease, particularly the diminished ability of the pancreas to produce and release insulin. This is related to the fact that adipose tissue, especially visceral fat, secretes proinflammatory cytokines (i.e., TNF-α, IL-6, IL-8), which destroy the pancreatic β-cells that synthesize insulin. It has been estimated that more than half of the body's β-cells have been eradicated by the time a patient is actually diagnosed with type 2 diabetes.[11]

In addition to reduced insulin production, those with type 2 diabetes show a decreased sensitivity of the target tissue to

Box 15-9 DID YOU KNOW?

Consequences of Uncontrolled Type 2 Diabetes

The health consequences of having uncontrolled type 2 diabetes can be extremely diverse and sometimes fatal. For example, blindness, lack of sensation (particularly in the extremities), gangrene and the resultant amputation of limbs, heart attacks, and strokes all can result from unmanaged type 2 diabetes. How can so many seemingly different ailments be due to the same root cause condition? The problem is that if blood sugar remains consistently elevated for prolonged periods of time it can build up and damage the vascular system and nerves. Any tissues or organs that are dependent on proper blood supply and neural input by those blocked blood vessels and nerves suffer damage and can become nonfunctional.

the insulin circulating in the bloodstream. This is particularly true of the liver and skeletal muscle, the two principal sites for carbohydrate storage (i.e., glycogen). Obesity, especially among those with an "android" deposition of fat, resulting in an "apple" rather than a "pear" appearance, is also a major factor in this insulin resistance. It appears that, due to the high levels of free fatty acids released by visceral fat into the circulation, some of them are deposited into the cells of the liver (hepatocytes) and skeletal muscle (myocytes). This provokes a blunted response to insulin in those organs by disturbing intracellular signaling pathways.[66,103] Research has demonstrated that reductions in body fat can weaken this insulin resistance. In one investigation, it was reported that in obese people with type 2 diabetes, a mere 7% loss in body weight yielded a greater than 50% improvement in insulin sensitivity,[117] although other studies have showed less pronounced responses. Thus, it appears that obesity is a factor in the development of both the decreased insulin sensitivity of target tissue and the limited pancreatic insulin production that characterizes type 2 diabetes. It is also clear that reducing fat content, particularly visceral adipose, is an effective nonpharmacological intervention in the treatment and prevention of this increasingly common disease.

Lack of Physical Activity as a Risk Factor

Lack of physical activity is the second major risk factor for the onset of type 2 diabetes, which, unlike type 1 diabetes, develops gradually over time. Along with obesity, the rising trend in the prevalence of non–insulin-dependent diabetes is coupled with a gradual and significant decline in the amount of daily physical activity. The relationship is based on the fact that, like insulin, muscle contractile activity recruits GLUT 4 transporters to the muscle fiber's membrane, facilitating the uptake of glucose from the blood into the working muscle. Indeed, the effect of muscle contractions on glucose uptake persists for up to 48 hours following the cessation of exercise.[75] Furthermore, long-term exercise training augments the total number of transporters residing within the muscle fiber that can be recruited to the sarcolemma (membrane) during an acute bout of exercise, thereby promoting greater total glucose uptake during and following exercise.[33] More recently, it has been demonstrated that, like endurance exercise, resistance training (weight lifting) also effectively increases glucose uptake by contracting muscles.[28] Because of the improved sensitivity of skeletal muscle to insulin induced by contractile activity, exercise also eases the burden on pancreatic β-cells to produce insulin in attempts to maintain proper blood sugar levels.

Additional Risk Factors

In addition to obesity and physical inactivity, other important risk factors may predispose people to the onset of type 2 diabetes. For example, family history has been identified as a nonmodifiable risk factor in that up to 80% of those afflicted by the disease share it with at least one immediate relative.[73] Although lifestyle habits common to family members may be partly responsible for this, a strong genetic component appears to be in effect that is independent of behavior and lifestyle.

Ethnicity also contributes to the incidence of non–insulin-dependent diabetes. Those who are particularly vulnerable are Native Americans, followed by African-Americans, and then Hispanic Americans.[73] However, the disease has been identified in every ethnic group, including Caucasians and Asian-Americans.

Data suggest that in adults, sex plays no role in the occurrence of diabetes; this is true of all age groups between 18 and 79 years. In minors, however, it appears that girls are more prone to type 2 diabetes than boys are. And in adults and minors, the incidence of the disease increases with age.

Exercise and Type 2 Diabetes

Unlike type 1 diabetes, in which exercise can only play a role in managing the condition, type 2 diabetes can not only be treated but also prevented with exercise.[118] As mentioned previously, exercise augments the sensitivity of target tissue to insulin, thereby improving the uptake of blood glucose. Accordingly, exercise reduces the stress on the pancreas to produce inordinate amounts of insulin in efforts to compensate for insulin resistance. Other benefits accrued from exercise training are related to the cardiovascular risk factors commonly associated with type 2 diabetes. Regular sessions of aerobic exercise help reduce the hypertension, poor blood lipid profiles (i.e., high cholesterol and triglycerides), and poor body composition typically identified among those with type 2 diabetes. Indeed, the risk of death from cardiovascular disease and its complications is up to four times higher in those with diabetes than in the general population.[10] It has been estimated that including regular physical activity as part of a healthier lifestyle might decrease this risk by more than 50%.[84]

What should an exercise program for those with type 2 diabetes include? Aerobic exercise, which can effectively control blood pressure and blood lipids, as well as manage body weight and body composition, is an essential component. Because repetitive contractile activity recruits GLUT 4 transporters to the sarcolemma for only about 48 hours after exercise, endurance exercise must be performed on a regular basis, not separated by more than 2 days. Because the neuropathy that oftentimes accompanies type 2 diabetes can impair sensation in the feet, which may result in damage to them, it is wise to include non–weight-bearing exercises, such as swimming and cycling. Because people with non–insulin-dependent diabetes tend to have poor fitness levels, a beginning program should feature intensities as low as 40% of $\dot{V}_{O_{2max}}$ in its initial stages. But as cardiovascular fitness progresses, the intensity of workouts can be gradually increased to 50% to 70% of $\dot{V}_{O_{2max}}$. As with intensity, the duration of individual workouts should accommodate the low initial fitness observed in those with diabetes and begin in the range of 10 to 15 minutes. Over time, and as fitness improves, workouts should be at least 30 minutes in duration, and if weight loss is a primary objective, then 60-minute workouts of low-to-moderate intensity are appropriate.

Resistance training should also be included in the fitness program, as it has been shown to effectively recruit GLUT 4 transporters and enhance glucose uptake. Moreover, it increases muscle mass and carbohydrate-storing capacity, thus improving blood glucose regulation. The American College of Sports Medicine recommends that those with type 2 diabetes perform resistance training at least twice a week. It is also suggested that each weight-lifting workout feature 8 to 10 exercises involving large muscle groups, with at least one set per exercise consisting of 10 to 15 repetitions completed to the point of near fatigue.[2] The American Diabetes Association, while also recommending resistance training exercises that stimulate all major muscle groups, prefers that three workouts per week be conducted, with the number of sets increasing to three sets per exercise, and that each set consists of 8 to 10 repetitions.[105] Both organizations emphasize that, before engaging in an exercise training regimen, patients with type 2 diabetes should undergo a thorough medical screening and consultation with a physician.

Quick Review

- Diabetes affects nearly 8% of the American population.
- The principal distinguishing characteristic of diabetes is an inability to maintain proper concentrations of blood glucose.
- Type 1 diabetes occurs because the pancreas is incapable of producing insulin.
- Type 2 diabetes occurs because the tissues that normally take up blood glucose and store it as glycogen show decreased sensitivity to insulin.
- Medical experts recommend that those with either type 1 or type 2 diabetes participate in a program of exercise training for the various health benefits that can be derived.
- The incidence of type 2 diabetes has risen dramatically over the past 20 to 30 years, closely tracking a similar increase in the incidence of obesity.
- Like obesity, lack of physical activity has been identified as a major risk factor for the development of type 2 diabetes.
- For those with type 1 diabetes, exercise serves to manage the disease, but in type 2 diabetes, exercise can actually prevent the disease.

METABOLIC SYNDROME

Closely related to type 2 diabetes is a condition referred to as **metabolic syndrome,** or syndrome x. This is distinguished by the presence of a number of interrelated conditions, but principal among them are obesity, hypertension, a poor blood lipid profile, and insulin resistance. The accumulation of these disturbances increases the risk of eventually developing cardiovascular disease and/or type 2 diabetes. Indeed, statistics indicate that men and women with metabolic syndrome have more than twice the chance of dying from cardiovascular disease than those without it.[45] And metabolic syndrome increases the likelihood of developing type 2 diabetes more than ninefold.[57] The incidence of metabolic syndrome has rapidly expanded over the last two to three decades, and it is estimated that currently 23% of people residing in the United States are affected by the condition.[29]

Etiology

The rise in the number of cases of metabolic syndrome tracks the increase in obesity over the same time period. In fact, obesity is considered the primary risk factor for metabolic syndrome. In particular, central obesity with a high prevalence of visceral versus subcutaneous fat contributes mightily to the development of metabolic syndrome.[64] This visceral adipose tissue has a greater disposition to release free fatty acids into the blood, which affects the liver, reducing its responsiveness to insulin. Furthermore, this insulin resistance, both at the liver and skeletal muscle, is most commonly proposed to be the underlying cause of metabolic syndrome.

Additional risk factors for the onset of metabolic syndrome include age and physical inactivity. In addition, high carbohydrate diets may also contribute to the syndrome.[122] Data clearly confirm that the incidence of metabolic syndrome increases with age. Although this condition has been identified in less than 5% of adolescents, it is evident in 7% of those between 20 and 29 years old and in more than 40% of those at least 60 years of age. Regarding the effects of physical inactivity, a recent longitudinal study determined that the presence of metabolic syndrome was more than twice as high among the inactive as it was among those who were categorized as physically active.[125]

Management of Metabolic Syndrome

Because obesity and inactivity are the two strongest predictors of metabolic syndrome, experts consider lifestyle modifications to be the most effective treatment options. Weight reduction should be safely and effectively achieved by reducing daily caloric intake by 500 to 1,000 calories per day while aiming to lose 7% to 10% of body weight over a 6- to 12-month period.[25] In addition to reducing total caloric intake, the composition of the diet should be modified. An appropriate diet would focus on greater

Box 15-10 AN EXPERT VIEW
Micronutrients and Chronic Diseases

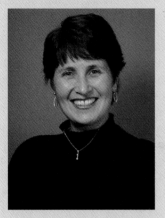

Stella Lucia Volpe, PhD, RD, LDN, FACSM

Division of Biobehavioral and Health Sciences
University of Pennsylvania
Philadelphia, PA

Total energy intake is important for health and especially important for athletes. Much of my research has focused on mineral supplementation and its potential effect on weight loss and/or type 2 diabetes mellitus, as well as mineral metabolism during exercise. In this "Expert View," I will share some of my research on minerals, exercise, and weight loss with you.

Chromium Supplementation and Weight Loss

Obesity and type 2 diabetes mellitus have increased dramatically over the past 30 years. All age groups have been affected, and the obesity epidemic is certainly a result of many different influences: decreased planned exercise, decreased leisure-time exercise, increased food consumption (mostly increased portion sizes), increased television watching and computer use, to name a few. Thus, one "magic bullet" will not solve this epidemic. However, in an attempt to research specific areas that may impact obesity and weight loss, I have evaluated mineral supplementation on weight loss.

My research team and I conducted a study on the effect of chromium picolinate on weight loss. Chromium is an active component of the protein chromodulin, which potentiates the effects of insulin to do its job in promoting glucose uptake. In the early 1990s, research had been conducted on chromium supplementation, mostly in male athletes, and without use of more accurate measures of body composition assessment (e.g., skinfold measurements). Thus, my research team and I conducted a randomized, placebo-controlled, double-blind trial on the effects of 400 mg·day^{-1} of chromium picolinate compared to an identical-looking

placebo in 44 overweight and obese women, who were placed on a supervised weight training and walking program for 12 weeks. Resting metabolic rate was measured, as was body composition via underwater weighing. Blood and urine were collected to evaluate chromium status, zinc and iron status, blood lipid levels, and serum insulin, glucagon and glucose concentrations. There was no effect of chromium supplementation on any of the measures—that is, we found no differences between the chromium-supplemented group and the placebo group.[3]

Magnesium and the Metabolic Syndrome

One of the studies that my research team and I are now conducting is an NIH-funded randomized controlled, double-blind, placebo-controlled trial on the effects of magnesium on metabolic syndrome. The metabolic syndrome is defined as a person having at least three of the following five characteristics: elevated waist circumference, elevated triglyceride levels, reduced high-density lipoprotein levels, elevated blood pressure, and elevated blood glucose levels (for more details, please see Grundy et al.[2] Circulation, 112(17), 2005). There are data that suggest that magnesium may prevent the metabolic syndrome and/or ameliorate type 2 diabetes mellitus.[1,2] The goal of the Magnesium and Metabolic Syndrome Trial is to evaluate if magnesium supplementation will improve insulin resistance in individuals with the metabolic syndrome. Though there are no results to present at the moment, we hope that this trial may shed some light on the effects of magnesium on the metabolic syndrome. Our next step would then be to evaluate the mechanism of how magnesium affects the metabolic syndrome.

References

1. Harris Rosenzweig P, Volpe SL. Effect of iron supplementation on thyroid hormone levels and resting metabolic rate in two college female athletes: a case study. Int J Sport Nutr Exerc Metab. 2000;10:434–443.
2. Maxwell C, Volpe SL. Effect of zinc supplementation on thyroid hormone function: a case study of two college females. Ann Nutr Metab. 2007;51:188–194.
3. Volpe SL, Huang HW, Larpadisorn K, et al. Effect of chromium supplementation on body composition, resting metabolic rate, and selected biochemical parameters in moderately obese women following an exercise program. J Am Coll Nutr. 2001;20:293–306.

consumption of fruits, vegetables, and whole grains while decreasing the intake of simple sugars and fats. More specifically, the consumption of saturated fats, trans fats, and cholesterol must be limited if higher levels of carbohydrate are ingested. It has been recently shown that carbohydrate restriction may be a very effective method of managing metabolic syndrome.[122]

Regular exercise training, especially of an aerobic nature, has been shown to be effective in managing

each constituent of metabolic syndrome. That is, an exercise regimen can have favorable effects on obesity, hypertension, insulin resistance, and blood lipids. Exercise prescription guidelines should be similar to those recommended to treat and prevent cardiovascular disease and should focus on moderate-intensity, sustained (≥30 min) sessions of endurance exercise, such as walking, jogging, cycling, and swimming (see Box 15-10).[25,116]

HIV/AIDS AND EXERCISE

The condition of HIV/AIDS is defined by the Centers of Disease Control and Prevention as when HIV infection has been identified, irrespective of whether the condition has progressed to the stage of AIDS. According to the Centers of Disease Control and Prevention, approximately 56,000 people a year in the United States become infected with HIV.[34] Through the year 2006, the cumulative estimated number of cases of AIDS in the United States was over one million. Because of the recent development of highly active antiretroviral therapy (HAART), the average lifespan of those afflicted with HIV/AIDS has significantly increased so that the condition is now considered more of a long-term chronic disease, rather than an acutely life-threatening one. But, as a downside of these new treatment options, patients now undergo a slower disease progression that is accompanied by numerous disabilities, such as neuropathy, cardiovascular disease, increased body fat, and myopathy. Also apparent is an increase in fatigability, making the performance of typical activities of daily living more challenging, along with muscle wasting and weakness. Moreover, research has revealed that cardiovascular fitness, quantified as $\dot{V}O_{2max}$, may be as much as 40% lower than what is observed in those without the disease.[12,51] In large part, it appears that the lower $\dot{V}O_{2max}$ exhibited by those with HIV/AIDS can be explained by mitochondrial damage in skeletal muscle. The result is an impaired ability of the exercising muscles to extract oxygen from the blood supply and to produce ATP via oxidative pathways. The reduced aerobic fitness of HIV/AIDS patients limits their aptitude to perform activities of daily living and the recreational activities that contribute to their overall quality of life. Therefore, scientists have wondered whether these patients can improve their fitness with exercise training. Several studies have shown that people diagnosed with HIV/AIDS are, in fact, capable of responding to properly designed endurance training programs and experience improvements in $\dot{V}O_{2max}$ that are similar (20%–30%) to those detected in people without the disease.[82,113] It is equally important to note that the performance of aerobic training posed no health risks to those with HIV/AIDS; neither viral load nor CD4 (immune cells) count was altered by training. Furthermore, psychological well-being was improved (i.e., increased satisfaction and decreased depression) following endurance training.[17]

In addition to decreased cardiovascular fitness, HIV/AIDS is often associated with a condition referred to as "wasting," even among those being treated with HAART. This wasting is characterized by a decline in body weight of at least 10% over a 12-month period. Not only does this loss of mass—most of it being skeletal muscle—decrease the person's functional capacity by reducing strength, research has shown that there is a strong association between wasting and disease progression leading to mortality. Several approaches have been experimented with to counter this muscle wasting. These include nutritional counseling and intervention, hormone therapy, and pharmacological agents. All, however, have serious drawbacks, such as nausea and high cost, which render them impractical for use on a large scale.[24] One intervention that has proved successful and presents few, if any, disadvantages is resistance training. A number of investigations have confirmed that people diagnosed with HIV/AIDS are capable of accruing improvements in muscle function and increased muscle mass that are similar to those observed in nondiseased, sedentary controls. For example, Roubenoff et al.[97] reported 31% to 50% increases in strength of all muscle groups tested following an 8-week training regimen using loads of 50% to 80% of one-repetition maximum for three sets of eight repetitions, along with a significant increase in lean body mass. In a later study, HIV/AIDS patients with wasting demonstrated 60% increases in muscle strength and a 5% increase in lean body mass as a result of progressive resistance exercise. These patients also reported that their physical functioning capacity during normal daily life was significantly enhanced as a result of resistance training.[98] As with aerobic training, participation in resistance training did nothing to compromise the health of HIV/AIDS patients or accelerate disease progression, thus proving it to be safe, as well as effective.[7]

EPILEPSY AND EXERCISE

Epilepsy is a condition that affects more than two million people in the United States, or about 1% of its population. The defining characteristic of epilepsy is the presence of recurring episodes of seizures. It is important to note that suffering a single seizure does not constitute a diagnosis of epilepsy.

Etiology

There is no single cause that can account for all cases of epilepsy, and in fact, almost half of all seizures have no known cause. Simply put, anything that results in the hyperactivity of clusters of neurons in the brain can be viewed as a cause of epilepsy. But in studying this perplexing disease, scientists have identified a number of factors that contribute to the onset of epilepsy. For example, genetic factors resulting in the expression of defective ion channels of the brain's neurons, leaving them with an abnormally high level of excitability and low threshold of stimulation, can cause epilepsy.

Brain damage stemming from tumors, alcoholism, drug abuse, and traumatic head injury also has been associated with the development of epilepsy. Moreover, any event or condition depriving the brain of an adequate oxygen supply may be viewed as a cause for the onset of epilepsy. Indeed, almost one-third of all newly diagnosed cases of epilepsy among adults occur as a result of cerebrovascular disease, which impairs blood flow to the brain. Other causative factors such as exposure to high levels of lead or carbon monoxide have been identified, especially among children. Finally, infectious conditions such as AIDS, meningitis, and encephalitis may lead to neuronal hyperactivity and epilepsy.

Despite the efficacy of modern drugs in controlling the symptoms of epilepsy, it is still possible for seizures to occur in those afflicted with this condition. So what is it that might act to trigger an epileptic seizure? Although patients with epilepsy may have different degrees of sensitivity to various stimuli, some of the more common triggers include fatigue, alcohol consumption, rhythmically flickering lights, cigarette smoke, and sleep deprivation. But perhaps the most commonly reported stimulus for the onset of an epileptic seizure is stress.[78] Because of this, it has been suggested that exercise training, which has been shown to be effective in stress management, may reduce the number of seizures experienced by those diagnosed with epilepsy (see Box 15-11).

Exercise and Epilepsy

Many people with epilepsy are unfit and unhealthy in large part because they believe that the stress of physical exertion will induce a seizure. This might be a legitimate concern as about 10% of the patient population will experience a seizure as a result of participating in exercise or sports.[79] However, up to 40% of that same population will experience fewer episodes because of exercising on a regular basis. There are numerous factors that may account for the disparate effects of exercise on epileptic seizures. It does appear that high-intensity, exhaustive exercise may increase the likelihood of seizures, especially among those who are not familiar with intense exercise, or are unfit. Another reason that may explain why exercise induces seizures in some relates to the psychological stress accompanying physical activity. This type of stress, alone, results in increased electrical activity within the brain. This activity combined with the baseline hyperactivity and low stimulation threshold of neurons within specific brain regions of epilepsy patients leads to uncontrolled firing of those neurons and seizure. Thus, it appears that the amount of psychological stress experienced by the patient before and during exercise is critical in determining whether exercise increases or decreases the chance of suffering a seizure. Because they are accustomed to exercise and it evokes less psychological stress, people who exercise on a regular basis are less likely to have an episode while exercising or playing sports. Physiologically, those who exercise regularly show an attenuated response of the sympathetic nervous system and decreased release of the stress hormone cortisol.[23] A lowered amount of cortisol delivered to the brain also reduces the incidence of exercise-induced epileptic seizures. It has also been postulated that the exercise-induced release of β-endorphins, which have an opioid-like relaxing effect, also decreases the activity of the neurons responsible for seizures.[2] It has also been suggested that the high degree of mental concentration required during exercise and sports may have a calming influence on those regions of the brain responsible for the onset of seizures.

It is the current thinking of medical experts that moderate-intensity exercise performed on a regular basis will have a stress-reducing effect on patients with epilepsy and accordingly will decrease the incidence of seizures in them. Moreover, people afflicted with epilepsy will enjoy the many other health benefits to be gained from exercise training and thus improve their quality of life. But for those who do

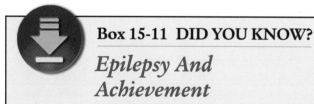

Box 15-11 DID YOU KNOW?

Epilepsy And Achievement

Although some people with mental disabilities also have epilepsy, the two conditions do not necessarily go hand in hand. In fact, a number of well-known, highly intelligent, accomplished people have been afflicted with epilepsy. Among others, this list includes Julius Caesar, Socrates, Napoleon Bonaparte, the actor Danny Glover, the singer Neil Young, and Olympic track star Florence Griffith Joyner.

engage in exercise and sports activities, it is important to get enough sleep, stay well hydrated, maintain proper electrolyte levels, avoid sports where head injuries may occur, and be aware that medications used to treat epilepsy can cause fatigue and vision problems and reduce bone mass.

HYPERTENSION AND EXERCISE

The presence of high blood pressure, or hypertension, is a very common health concern, especially among western cultures where it is most prevalent. Indeed, in the United States alone, over 58 million adults are hypertensive, meaning that they have a resting systolic blood pressure of 140 mm Hg or higher and/or a resting diastolic pressure of at least 90 mm Hg.[37] This is worrisome because hypertension has been significantly linked with an increased likelihood of stroke, heart disease, peripheral arterial disease, renal complications, and all-cause and cardiovascular mortality.[86] There are methods of effectively managing hypertension, however, including the use of antihypertensive medications and lifestyle modifications. One of those lifestyle changes is exercise training, although by itself, exercise is effective only among those with mild-to-moderate degrees of hypertension.

Exercise and Resting Blood Pressure

For many years, it has been known that exercise training can impart a positive effect on the resting blood pressure of hypertensive people. This is true for both men and women, who, research has shown, show similar incidences of hypertension. The most effective mode of exercise in treating hypertension is aerobic-type endurance exercise such as walking, jogging, cycling, and swimming. Most research demonstrates that when such activity is performed at a moderate intensity (i.e., <70% of $\dot{V}o_{2max}$) for 30–60 minutes per session over a period of several weeks, resting systolic and diastolic blood pressure decreases by 7.4 and 5.8 mm Hg, respectively, among hypertensive patients.[27] These changes were noted to be significantly greater than those experienced by people with normal resting blood pressure performing the same exercise routine.

With the increasing popularity of resistance exercise training, it has also been examined whether a program of weight lifting can also modify resting blood pressure among hypertensive people. To date, the evidence suggests that although a program of resistance training does reduce resting blood pressure, it does so to a lesser degree than a program of endurance training. Indeed, although they were found to be statistically significant, resistance training–induced declines in both systolic and diastolic pressures under resting conditions were only about 3 mm Hg. Still, even those minor reductions in blood pressure may reduce the incidence of stroke and heart disease by as much as 14% among patients with hypertension.

Exercise and Acute and Postexercise Responses

Although fewer studies have investigated how exercise training impacts blood pressure responses during exercise, some important results have been collected. In general, it appears that when people with hypertension complete a multiweek endurance training program, their acute blood pressure responses to moderate-intensity, aerobic-type exercise was decreased by about 7 mm Hg, while their heart rate during exercise declined by 6 beats per minute.[9] This implies not only improved fitness but also a lowered risk of cardiovascular injury during exercise among hypertensive patients.

There is even more compelling evidence, however, that similar to normotensives, there is a significant postexercise decrease in blood pressure among hypertensive patients, in fact, an even greater one. Both groups show what has been termed "postexercise hypotension," or a drop in both systolic and diastolic blood pressure, for up to 22 hours following the cessation of moderate-intensity endurance exercise. Importantly, it is thought by some experts that these repeated episodes of postexercise hypotension may have a cumulative effect and explain the training-induced declines in resting blood pressure among hypertensive and normotensive people.

CASE STUDY

Scenario

You are a 25-year-old woman and you have just learned that you are pregnant. You are delighted with this news, but after being inactive since high school, you only recently started a fitness program and you are concerned that you will now have to stop working out. What should you do?

Options

You express your concerns to your physician at your next appointment. She tells you that while taking into account that you are now pregnant, there is no need to stop exercising since you have no contraindications such as vaginal bleeding or history of preterm labor. In fact, your doctor tells you that not only is it safe to exercise when you are pregnant, there are actually health benefits to be gained by both the mother and baby. You learn that the chances of suffering gestational diabetes or preeclampsia—two common pregnancy-related health conditions—actually are reduced in women who regularly exercise while they are pregnant. Also, evidence shows that the risk of an early birth of the child or delivery by cesarean section is decreased among women who exercise while they are pregnant. Your doctor recommends that you participate in 30 minutes of moderate-intensity endurance exercise such as walking, swimming, or cycling on most, or even all, days of the week. She tells you that you can continue this exercise regimen into your third trimester of pregnancy, but that you should avoid high-impact exercises, or those that involve bouncing activities.

Scenario

You are the father of a 12-year-old boy who will be trying out for his middle school's football team in the fall. He comes to you and asks if he can start lifting weights to build strength and muscle size in preparation for the upcoming season. What should you do?

Options

You do a little research on your own and find out that it is safe for kids to engage in resistance training. You also learn that because of your son's age and stage of physical maturity, he may not gain much muscle mass with resistance training. However, with a properly designed resistance training program using correct exercise techniques during his training sessions it is possible for him to significantly improve his strength. To be sure that your son receives appropriate coaching and advice on resistance training, you bring him to a local fitness facility (e.g., YMCA, community recreation center) and enroll him for training sessions supervised by a certified strength and conditioning specialist.

Overall, it appears that by itself, exercise training, particularly that of an aerobic nature including rhythmic contractions of large muscle groups performed at moderate intensity for a period of weeks, can lead to significantly lower blood pressure at rest and during exercise in patients diagnosed with mild-to-moderate hypertension. This is true for men and women of all ages, irrespective of race.

An appropriate exercise prescription for these patients would be much like the same one recommended for the general adult population, emphasizing endurance exercise of a moderate intensity, for a duration of 30 to 60 minutes, performed most, if not all, days of the week, which is to be supplemented with resistance exercise two to three times per week.

CHAPTER SUMMARY

The benefits of exercise training can be enjoyed by virtually everyone. However, some groups of people may have certain considerations and/or priorities to bear in mind as they design and engage in their exercise regimens. Women obviously can exercise at the same intensity and frequency as men and enjoy positive adaptations of the same scale. Research shows that the capacity to exercise or perform athletic events is not modified by the menstrual cycle. Similarly, exercise can, and should, be performed during pregnancy, assuming that the woman is healthy and that no contradictory medical conditions exist. Daily physical activity is also recommended for children, and more structured exercise training regimens are entirely appropriate for adolescents. Among the aged, exercise training can bring about a host of important health benefits, and resistance training can be of particular benefit. With proper medical supervision, even those with conditions such as asthma and diabetes are urged to regularly participate in exercise. Patients diagnosed with HIV/AIDS enjoy significant benefits from exercise, especially resistance training to control the muscle wasting that typically occurs with that condition. Most people with epilepsy can exercise safely, allowing them to enjoy exercise-related health benefits, and they may even see a decline in the number of seizures due to reduced stress. Finally, research has clearly shown that people with mild-to-moderate hypertension can, and should, participate in an exercise training program mainly focusing on aerobic-type activities to effectively manage their condition.

REVIEW QUESTIONS

Fill-in-the-Blank

1. The absence of menstrual periods is termed
   _____.

2. The persistent condition of hypertension experienced by some women during pregnancy is termed
   _____.

3. _____ is the period of time extending from the birth of a child until his or her first birthday.

4. Running economy is _____ in children compared with adults.

5. The increasing number of children considered obese is of concern, in part, because it has been linked to the increased incidence of _____.

6. The term _____ refers to the loss of muscle mass that occurs with aging.

7. _____ diabetes results when the cells that produce insulin have been destroyed, usually by the immune system.

8. Those with type 2 diabetes who are beginning a resistance training program should perform _____ repetitions per set.

9. _____ is an increasingly common condition that is characterized by a cluster of disturbances including obesity, hypertension, insulin resistance, and poor blood lipids.

10. To a large extent, the loss of cardiovascular (aerobic) fitness that occurs in those with HIV/AIDS is due to _____ within skeletal muscle fibers.

Multiple Choice

1. Which muscle fiber type occupies the largest amount of total muscle size in women?
   a. Type I
   b. Type IIA
   c. Type IIX
   d. There is no difference between fiber types

2. Which muscle fiber type occupies the largest amount of total muscle size in men?
   a. Type I
   b. Type IIA
   c. Type IIX
   d. There is no difference between fiber types

3. Specific tension, or the force produced normalized to muscle size, is
   a. greater in men than women
   b. greater in women than men
   c. the same for men and women

4. Muscle endurance, or the ability to resist muscle fatigue, is
   a. greater in men than women
   b. greater in women than men
   c. the same for men and women

5. Research typically finds that muscle power, or "explosive strength," is
   a. greater in men than women
   b. greater in women than men
   c. the same for men and women

6. During endurance, or aerobic, exercise, women
   a. rely more on fats as an energy substrate than men do
   b. rely more on carbohydrates as an energy substrate than men do
   c. rely more on proteins as an energy substrate than men do
   d. show the same use of specific energy substrates as men do

7. On average, the peak rate of physical growth (increased height) during the woman's adolescent phase occurs at
   a. 10 years old
   b. 12 years old
   c. 14 years old
   d. 16 years old

8. When expressed in relative terms (i.e., ml·kg^{-1}·min^{-1}), maximal oxygen uptake is
   a. higher in adults
   b. higher in adolescents
   c. higher in children
   d. similar among adults, adolescents, and children

9. The sweat glands of children
   a. are more responsive to increased temperature than those of adults
   b. have a greater capacity to produce sweat than those of adults
   c. have a lower capacity to produce sweat than those of adults
   d. produce a more dilute sweat than those of adults

10. The increasing number of children considered obese is of concern, at least in part, because it has been closely linked with the growing incidence of which disease?

    a. Osteoporosis

    b. Anemia

    c. Type 1 diabetes

    d. Type 2 diabetes

11. Which of the following factors is the primary reason that maximal oxygen uptake is reduced among the aged?

    a. Decreased stroke volume

    b. Decreased myoglobin content in muscle

    c. Decreased capillarity of muscle

    d. Increased maximal heart rate

12. The age-related decline in muscular strength begins at what age?

    a. 40 years

    b. 50 years

    c. 60 years

    d. 70 years

13. The age-related decline in muscular power begins at what age?

    a. 40 years

    b. 50 years

    c. 60 years

    d. 70 years

14. Which of the following types of exercise would be most effective in preventing osteoporosis, or loss of bone mass?

    a. Swimming

    b. Cycling

    c. Arm cranking

    d. Walking or jogging

15. Just as with young adults, when older adults participate in a properly designed endurance (aerobic) training program, they experience how much improvement in their maximal oxygen uptake?

    a. 0% to 5%

    b. 10% to 15%

    c. 20% to 25%

    d. 30% to 40%

16. Which disease is characterized by wheezing, difficult breathing, and tightness of the chest?

    a. Hypertension

    b. Asthma

    c. Type 2 diabetes

    d. Osteoporosis

17. The most effective type of exercise to help those with asthma is

    a. resistance training

    b. balance training

    c. agility training

    d. prolonged aerobic training resulting in deep breathing

18. Which disease is best characterized by an inability to maintain blood glucose concentrations within normal limits?

    a. Diabetes

    b. Osteoporosis

    c. Asthma

    d. HIV/AIDS

19. Along with increased obesity, which of the following has been associated with the increased incidence of type 2 diabetes?

    a. Decreased consumption of dietary carbohydrates

    b. Increased consumption of dairy products

    c. Increased amount of daily physical activity and exercise

    d. Decreased amount of daily physical activity and exercise

20. The defining characteristic of epilepsy is

    a. recurring seizures

    b. high blood pressure

    c. decreased sensitivity to insulin

    d. a body mass index (BMI) equal to or greater than 30

True/False

1. The maximal oxygen uptake of women is 5% to 15% less than that of men.

2. When presented with the same resistance training stimulus, women experience the same relative improvements (% increase from baseline) in strength as men.

3. Research has conclusively demonstrated that strength varies according to the phase of the menstrual cycle.

4. If left uncontrolled, preeclampsia can result in death to pregnant women.

5. Skeletal muscle comprises a greater percentage of total body weight in women than in men.

6. With proper training and technique, resistance training can be safely performed by children.

7. In general, anaerobic power is less in children than in adults.

8. During the loss of muscle size that occurs with aging, it is type I muscle fibers that demonstrate the greatest amount of atrophy.

9. It is a decrease in the number of muscle fibers, rather than a decrease in their size, that principally accounts for the loss of muscle mass that occurs with aging.

10. In general, when presented with the same resistance training stimulus (intensity, duration, frequency, mode), the relative training-induced strength gains (% increases from baseline) detected among the aged are similar to those of young adults.

11. Health and medical organizations, such as the American Thoracic Society and the American College of Sports Medicine, recommend that those with asthma should not participate in a program of regularly performed exercise.

12. Even those who do not have asthma may experience the symptoms of EIA.

13. According to the American Diabetes Association, people with properly managed type 1 diabetes are capable of performing even highly intense physical activity and sports.

14. Exercise training can help prevent and treat both type 1 and type 2 diabetes.

15. It is typically recommended that those diagnosed with HIV/AIDS perform resistance training on a regular basis.

Short Answer

1. Is it safe for pregnant women to exercise?
2. Is it true that it is dangerous for kids to participate in resistance training?
3. Is it too dangerous for people with hypertension to exercise?
4. What is the difference between type 1 and type 2 diabetes?
5. Given the frail physical state of those afflicted with HIV, is it wise for them to exercise?

Critical Thinking

1. What are the differences and similarities in the skeletal muscle tissue of men and women, and how might athletic performance be affected by them?
2. Why is osteoporosis such a health concern among the aged, and what can be done to prevent, or even treat, it?

KEY TERMS

adolescence: the period between the beginning of puberty and the onset of physical maturity

amenorrhea: the absence of a menstrual period

apoptosis: biologically programmed cell death

asthma: a condition of labored breathing, often accompanied by wheezing and coughing, that is caused by a spasm and constriction of the bronchial tubes

childhood: interim between the first birthday and the onset of adolescence

diabetes: a disease characterized by one's inability to maintain blood glucose levels within its normal limits as a result of the failure of the pancreas to produce and secrete the hormone insulin into the bloodstream (type 1) or decreased sensitivity of the hormone's target tissue (i.e., liver and skeletal muscle) (type 2)

estrogen: a female sex steroid hormone primarily produced by the ovaries. In addition to its role in promoting conception, it is responsible for the development of female secondary sexual characteristics

female athlete triad: a combination of three medical problems found in women – caloric deficit (through increased exercise and dieting), amenorrhea, and decreased bone mineral density

gestational diabetes mellitus (GDM): a form of diabetes, or insulin resistance, that occurs during pregnancy in some women

infancy: the period of time from birth until the child's first birthday

menarche: a woman's first menstrual period, occurring during puberty

menopause: a woman's final menstrual period, marking the end of her reproductive years

metabolic syndrome: a cluster of a number of health conditions, principal among them being hypertension, obesity, dyslipidemia, and insulin resistance

obesity: the condition of excess body fat; it is sometimes identified as having a body mass index of 30 or greater

osteoporosis: a condition of decreased bone mineral density leading to an increased risk of fracture; most common among postmenopausal women

preeclampsia: high blood pressure manifested in some women during pregnancy

progesterone: a female sex steroid hormone mainly produced by the ovaries. Its concentration fluctuates throughout the menstrual cycle, affecting core temperature.

sarcopenia: the loss of skeletal muscle that occurs among the aged

testosterone: the primary male sex steroid hormone. It is produced mainly in the testes in men and the ovaries in women. It not only stimulates development of the male secondary sexual (androgenic) characteristics, but also has anabolic (muscle-building) effects

type 1 diabetes: sometimes called "child-onset" diabetes, a condition in which a person is unable to produce insulin

type 2 diabetes: sometimes referred to as "adult-onset" diabetes, a condition characterized by insulin resistance and often by decreased insulin production

REFERENCES

1. Abdi R, Fiorina P, Adra CN, et al. Immunomodulation by mesenchymal stem cells: a potential therapeutic strategy for type 1 diabetes. Diabetes. 2008;57:1759–1767.
2. Albrecht H. Endorphins, sport and epilepsy: getting fit or having one? N Z Med J. 1986;99:915.
3. Anderson SD, Daviskas E. The mechanism of exercise-induced asthma is …. J Allergy Clin Immunol. 2000;106:453–459.
4. Aniansson A, Hedberg M, Henning GB, et al. Muscle morphology, enzymatic activity, and muscle strength in elderly men: a follow-up study. Muscle Nerve. 1986;9:585–591.
5. Artal R, Catanzaro RB, Gavard JA, et al. A lifestyle intervention of weight-gain restriction: diet and exercise in obese women with gestational diabetes mellitus. Appl Physiol Nutr Metab. 2007;32:596–601.

6. Beneke R, Hutler M, Jung M, et al. Modeling the blood lactate kinetics at maximal short-term exercise conditions in children, adolescents, and adults. J Appl Physiol. 2005;99:499–504.

7. Bhasin S, Storer TW. Exercise regimens for men with HIV. JAMA 2000;284:175–176.

8. Bierman CW, Spiro SG, Petheram I. Characterization of the late response in exercise-induced asthma. J Allergy Clin Immunol. 1984;74:701–706.

9. Blumenthal JA, Sherwood A, Gullette EC, et al. Exercise and weight loss reduce blood pressure in men and women with mild hypertension: effects on cardiovascular, metabolic, and hemodynamic functioning. Arch Intern Med. 2000;160:1947–1958.

10. Bronsky EA, Yegen U, Yeh CM, et al. Formoterol provides long-lasting protection against exercise-induced bronchospasm. Ann Allergy Asthma Immunol. 2002;89:407–412.

11. Butler AE, Janson J, Bonner-Weir S, et al. Beta-cell deficit and increased beta-cell apoptosis in humans with type 2 diabetes. Diabetes. 2003;52:102–110.

12. Cade WT, Peralta L, Keyser RE. Aerobic capacity in late adolescents infected with HIV and controls. Pediatr Rehabil. 2002;5:161–169.

13. Camargo CA Jr, Weiss ST, Zhang S, et al. Prospective study of body mass index, weight change, and risk of adult-onset asthma in women. Arch Intern Med. 1999;159:2582–2588.

14. Cannon J, Kay D, Tarpenning KM, et al. Comparative effects of resistance training on peak isometric torque, muscle hypertrophy, voluntary activation and surface EMG between young and elderly women. Clin Physiol Funct Imaging. 2007;27:91–100.

15. Charkoudian N, Joyner MJ. Physiologic considerations for exercise performance in women. Clin Chest Med. 2004;25:247–255.

16. Cheuvront SN, Carter R, Deruisseau KC, et al. Running performance differences between men and women: an update. Sports Med. 2005;35:1017–1024.

17. Ciccolo JT, Jowers EM, Bartholomew JB. The benefits of exercise training for quality of life in HIV/AIDS in the post-HAART era. Sports Med. 2004;34:487–499.

18. Clark BC, Manini TM, The DJ, et al. Gender differences in skeletal muscle fatigability are related to contraction type and EMG spectral compression. J Appl Physiol. 2003;94:2263–2272.

19. Cononie CC, Graves JE, Pollock ML, et al. Effect of exercise training on blood pressure in 70- to 79-yr-old men and women. Med Sci Sports Exerc. 1991;23:505–511.

20. Damm P, Breitowicz B, Hegaard H. Exercise, pregnancy, and insulin sensitivity—what is new? Appl Physiol Nutr Metab. 2007;32:537–540.

21. Dempsey JC, Butler CL, Sorensen TK, et al. A case–control study of maternal recreational physical activity and risk of gestational diabetes mellitus. Diabetes Res Clin Pract. 2004;66:203–215.

22. Dempsey JC, Sorensen TK, Williams MA, et al. Prospective study of gestational diabetes mellitus risk in relation to maternal recreational physical activity before and during pregnancy. Am J Epidemiol. 2004;159:663–670.

23. Duclos M, Corcuff JB, Rashedi M, et al. Trained versus untrained men: different immediate post-exercise responses of pituitary adrenal axis. A preliminary study. Eur J Appl Physiol Occup Physiol. 1997;75:343–350.

24. Dudgeon WD, Phillips KD, Carson JA, et al. Counteracting muscle wasting in HIV-infected individuals. HIV Med. 2006;7:299–310.

25. Eckel RH, Grundy SM, Zimmet PZ. The metabolic syndrome. Lancet. 2005;365:1415–1428.

26. Engelke K, Kemmler W, Lauber D, et al. Exercise maintains bone density at spine and hip EFOPS: a 3-year longitudinal study in early postmenopausal women. Osteoporos Int. 2006;17:133–142.

27. Fagard RH. Exercise characteristics and the blood pressure response to dynamic physical training. Med Sci Sports Exerc. 2001;33:S484–S492; discussion S93–S94.

28. Fenicchia LM, Kanaley JA, Azevedo JL Jr, et al. Influence of resistance exercise training on glucose control in women with type 2 diabetes. Metabolism. 2004;53:284–289.

29. Ford ES, Giles WH, Dietz WH. Prevalence of the metabolic syndrome among US adults: findings from the third National Health and Nutrition Examination Survey. JAMA. 2002;287:356–359.

30. Frontera WR, Hughes VA, Fielding RA, et al. Aging of skeletal muscle: a 12-yr longitudinal study. J Appl Physiol. 2000;88:1321–1326.

31. Fulco CS, Rock PB, Muza SR, et al. Slower fatigue and faster recovery of the adductor pollicis muscle in women matched for strength with men. Acta Physiol Scand. 1999;167:233–239.

32. Geusens P, Dinant G. Integrating a gender dimension into osteoporosis and fracture risk research. Gend Med. 2007;4 Suppl B:S147–S161.

33. Goodyear LJ, Hirshman MF, Valyou PM, et al. Glucose transporter number, function, and subcellular distribution in rat skeletal muscle after exercise training. Diabetes. 1992;41:1091–1099.

34. Guelfi KJ, Jones TW, Fournier PA. New insights into managing the risk of hypoglycaemia associated with intermittent high-intensity exercise in individuals with type 1 diabetes mellitus: implications for existing guidelines. Sports Med. 2007;37:937–946.

35. Guelfi KJ, Jones TW, Fournier PA. The decline in blood glucose levels is less with intermittent high-intensity compared with moderate exercise in individuals with type 1 diabetes. Diabetes Care. 2005;28:1289–1294.

36. Hagberg JM, Graves JE, Limacher M, et al. Cardiovascular responses of 70- to 79-yr-old men and women to exercise training. J Appl Physiol. 1989;66:2589–2594.

37. Hajjar I, Kotchen TA. Trends in prevalence, awareness, treatment, and control of hypertension in the United States, 1988–2000. JAMA. 2003;290:199–206.

38. Hakkinen K, Kallinen M, Izquierdo M, et al. Changes in agonist–antagonist EMG, muscle CSA, and force during strength training in middle-aged and older people. J Appl Physiol. 1998;84:1341–1349.

39. Hakkinen K, Newton RU, Gordon SE, et al. Changes in muscle morphology, electromyographic activity, and force production characteristics during progressive strength training in young and older men. J Gerontol A Biol Sci Med Sci. 1998;53:B415–B423.

40. Haleem S, Lutchman L, Mayahi R, et al. Mortality following hip fracture: trends and geographical variations over the last 40 years. Injury. 2008;39:1157–1163.

41. Hall DC, Kaufmann DA. Effects of aerobic and strength conditioning on pregnancy outcomes. Am J Obstet Gynecol. 1987;157:1199–1203.

42. Hays NP, Galassetti PR, Coker RH. Prevention and treatment of type 2 diabetes: current role of lifestyle, natural product, and pharmacological interventions. Pharmacol Ther. 2008;118:181–191.

43. Hebestreit H, Mimura K, Bar-Or O. Recovery of muscle power after high-intensity short-term exercise: comparing boys and men. J Appl Physiol. 1993;74:2875–2880.

44. Hicks AL, Kent-Braun J, Ditor DS. Sex differences in human skeletal muscle fatigue. Exerc Sport Sci Rev. 2001;29:109–112.

45. Hu G, Qiao Q, Tuomilehto J, et al. Prevalence of the metabolic syndrome and its relation to all-cause and cardiovascular mortality in nondiabetic European men and women. Arch Intern Med. 2004;164:1066–1076.

46. Huovinen E, Kaprio J, Laitinen LA, et al. Social predictors of adult asthma: a co-twin case–control study. Thorax. 2001;56:234–236.

47. Ivey FM, Roth SM, Ferrell RE, et al. Effects of age, gender, and myostatin genotype on the hypertrophic response to heavy resistance strength training. J Gerontol A Biol Sci Med Sci. 2000;55:M641–M648.

48. Janse de Jonge XA. Effects of the menstrual cycle on exercise performance. Sports Med. 2003;33:833–851.

49. Judge JO, Kenny AM, Kraemer WJ. Exercise in older adults. Conn Med. 2003;67:461–464.

50. Julius S, Amery A, Whitlock LS, et al. Influence of age on the hemodynamic response to exercise. Circulation. 1967;36:222–230.

51. Keyser RE, Peralta L, Cade WT, et al. Functional aerobic impairment in adolescents seropositive for HIV: a quasiexperimental analysis. Arch Phys Med Rehabil. 2000;81:1479–1484.

52. Knecht SK, Mays WA, Gerdes YM, et al. Exercise evaluation of upper- versus lower-extremity blood pressure gradients in pediatric and young-adult participants. Pediatr Exerc Sci. 2007;19: 344–348.

53. Kohrt WM, Malley MT, Coggan AR, et al. Effects of gender, age, and fitness level on response of $\dot{V}O_{2max}$ to training in 60–71 yr olds. J Appl Physiol. 1991;71:2004–2011.

54. Kolka MA, Stephenson LA. Control of sweating during the human menstrual cycle. Eur J Appl Physiol Occup Physiol. 1989;**58**:890–895.

55. Kosek DJ, Kim JS, Petrella JK, et al. Efficacy of 3 days/wk resistance training on myofiber hypertrophy and myogenic mechanisms in young vs. older adults. J Appl Physiol. 2006;101:531–544.

56. Krebs NF, Jacobson MS. Prevention of pediatric overweight and obesity. Pediatrics. 2003;112:424–430.

57. Laaksonen DE, Lakka HM, Niskanen LK, et al. Metabolic syndrome and development of diabetes mellitus: application and validation of recently suggested definitions of the metabolic syndrome in a prospective cohort study. Am J Epidemiol. 2002;156:1070–1077.

58. Larsson L. Motor units: remodeling in aged animals. J Gerontol A Biol Sci Med Sci. 1995;50 Spec No:91–95.

59. Leet T, Flick L. Effect of exercise on birthweight. Clin Obstet Gynecol. 2003;46:423–431.

60. Leiferman JA, Evenson KR. The effect of regular leisure physical activity on birth outcomes. Matern Child Health J. 2003;7:59–64.

61. Lemmer JT, Hurlbut DE, Martel GF, et al. Age and gender responses to strength training and detraining. Med Sci Sports Exerc. 2000;32:1505–1512.

62. Lexell J, Taylor CC, Sjostrom M. What is the cause of the ageing atrophy? Total number, size and proportion of different fiber types studied in whole vastus lateralis muscle from 15- to 83-year-old men. J Neurol Sci. 1988;84:275–294.

63. Liese AD, D'Agostino RB Jr, Hamman RF, et al. The burden of diabetes mellitus among US youth: prevalence estimates from the SEARCH for Diabetes in Youth Study. Pediatrics. 2006;118: 1510–1518.

64. Lorenzo C, Serrano-Rios M, Martinez-Larrad MT, et al. Central adiposity determines prevalence differences of the metabolic syndrome. Obes Res. 2003;11:1480–1487.

65. MacDonald MJ. Postexercise late-onset hypoglycemia in insulin-dependent diabetic patients. Diabetes Care. 1987;10:584–588.

66. Machann J, Haring H, Schick F, et al. Intramyocellular lipids and insulin resistance. Diabetes Obes Metab. 2004;6:239–248.

67. Malina RM, Ryan RC, Bonci CM. Age at menarche in athletes and their mothers and sisters. Ann Hum Biol. 1994;21:417–422.

68. Malina RM. Weight training in youth-growth, maturation, and safety: an evidence-based review. Clin J Sport Med. 2006;16:478–487.

69. Marcoux S, Brisson J, Fabia J. The effect of leisure time physical activity on the risk of pre-eclampsia and gestational hypertension. J Epidemiol Community Health. 1989;43:147–152.

70. Martin WH III, Ogawa T, Kohrt WM, et al. Effects of aging, gender, and physical training on peripheral vascular function. Circulation. 1991;84:654–664.

71. Martyn-St James M, Carroll S. High-intensity resistance training and postmenopausal bone loss: a meta-analysis. Osteoporos Int. 2006;17:1225–1240.

72. Martyn-St James M, Carroll S. Meta-analysis of walking for preservation of bone mineral density in postmenopausal women. Bone. 2008;43:521–531.

73. Mayer-Davis EJ. Type 2 diabetes in youth: epidemiology and current research toward prevention and treatment. J Am Diet Assoc. 2008;108:S45–S51.

74. McCambridge TM, Stricker PR. Strength training by children and adolescents. Pediatrics. 2008;121:835–840.

75. Mikines KJ, Sonne B, Farrell PA, et al. Effect of physical exercise on sensitivity and responsiveness to insulin in humans. Am J Physiol. 1988;254:E248–E259.

76. Milgrom H, Taussig LM. Keeping children with exercise-induced asthma active. Pediatrics. 1999;104:e38.

77. Moritani T, deVries HA. Potential for gross muscle hypertrophy in older men. J Gerontol. 1980;35:672–682.

78. Nakken KO, Solaas MH, Kjeldsen MJ, et al. Which seizure-precipitating factors do patients with epilepsy most frequently report? Epilepsy Behav. 2005;6:85–89.

79. Nakken KO. [Should people with epilepsy exercise?]. Tidsskr Nor Laegeforen. 2000;120:3051–3053. In Norwegian.

80. Nattiv A, Loucks AB, Manore MM, et al. American college of sports medicine position stand. The female athlete triad. Med Sci Sports Exerc. 2007;39:1867–1882.

81. Nottin S, Vinet A, Stecken F, et al. Central and peripheral cardiovascular adaptations during a maximal cycle exercise in boys and men. Med Sci Sports Exerc. 2002;34:456–463.

82. O'Brien K, Nixon S, Tynan AM, et al. Effectiveness of aerobic exercise in adults living with HIV/AIDS: systematic review. Med Sci Sports Exerc. 2004;36:1659–1666.

83. Ogawa T, Spina RJ, Martin WH III, et al. Effects of aging, sex, and physical training on cardiovascular responses to exercise. Circulation. 1992;86:494–503.

84. Orchard TJ, Temprosa M, Goldberg R, et al. The effect of metformin and intensive lifestyle intervention on the metabolic syndrome: the Diabetes Prevention Program randomized trial. Ann Intern Med. 2005;142:611–619.

85. Pate RR, O'Neill JR. American women in the marathon. Sports Med. 2007;37:294–298.

86. Pescatello LS, Franklin BA, Fagard R, et al. American College of Sports Medicine position stand. Exercise and hypertension. Med Sci Sports Exerc. 2004;36:533–553.

87. Pivarnik JM, Marichal CJ, Spillman T, et al. Menstrual cycle phase affects temperature regulation during endurance exercise. J Appl Physiol. 1992;**72**:543–548.

88. Porter MM, Stuart S, Boij M, et al. Capillary supply of the tibialis anterior muscle in young, healthy, and moderately active men and women. J Appl Physiol. 2002;92:1451–1457.

89. Proctor DN, Beck KC, Shen PH, et al. Influence of age and gender on cardiac output–VO_2 relationships during submaximal cycle ergometry. J Appl Physiol. 1998;84:599–605.

90. Proctor DN, Joyner MJ. Skeletal muscle mass and the reduction of $\dot{V}O_{2max}$ in trained older subjects. J Appl Physiol. 1997;82:1411–1415.

91. Proctor DN, Koch DW, Newcomer SC, et al. Leg blood flow and VO_2 during peak cycle exercise in younger and older women. Med Sci Sports Exerc. 2004;36:623–631.

92. Purdon C, Brousson M, Nyveen SL, et al. The roles of insulin and catecholamines in the glucoregulatory response during intense exercise and early recovery in insulin-dependent diabetic and control subjects. J Clin Endocrinol Metab. 1993;76:566–573.

93. Randolph C. Exercise-induced asthma: update on pathophysiology, clinical diagnosis, and treatment. Curr Probl Pediatr. 1997;27:53–77.

94. Rasmussen F, Lambrechtsen J, Siersted HC, et al. Low physical fitness in childhood is associated with the development of asthma in young adulthood: the Odense schoolchild study. Eur Respir J. 2000;16:866–870.

95. Roemmich JN, Richmond RJ, Rogol AD. Consequences of sport training during puberty. J Endocrinol Invest. 2001;24:708–715.

96. Roepstorff C, Schjerling P, Vistisen B, et al. Regulation of oxidative enzyme activity and eukaryotic elongation factor 2 in human skeletal muscle: influence of gender and exercise. Acta Physiol Scand. 2005;184:215–224.

97. Roubenoff R, McDermott A, Weiss L, et al. Short-term progressive resistance training increases strength and lean body mass in adults infected with human immunodeficiency virus. AIDS. 1999;13: 231–239.

98. Roubenoff R, Wilson IB. Effect of resistance training on self-reported physical functioning in HIV infection. Med Sci Sports Exerc. 2001;**33**:1811–1817.

99. Rupp NT, Brudno DS, Guill MF. The value of screening for risk of exercise-induced asthma in high school athletes. Ann Allergy. 1993;70:339–342.

100. Saftlas AF, Logsden-Sackett N, Wang W, et al. Work, leisure-time physical activity, and risk of preeclampsia and gestational hypertension. Am J Epidemiol. 2004;160:758–765.

101. Sargent C, Scroop GC. Plasma lactate accumulation is reduced during incremental exercise in untrained women compared with untrained men. Eur J Appl Physiol. 2007;101:91–96.

102. Seals DR, Hagberg JM, Hurley BF, et al. Endurance training in older men and women. I. Cardiovascular responses to exercise. J Appl Physiol. 1984;57:1024–1029.

103. Seppala-Lindroos A, Vehkavaara S, Hakkinen AM, et al. Fat accumulation in the liver is associated with defects in insulin suppression of glucose production and serum free fatty acids independent of obesity in normal men. J Clin Endocrinol Metab. 2002;87:3023–3028.

104. Shibasaki M, Inoue Y, Kondo N, et al. Thermoregulatory responses of prepubertal boys and young men during moderate exercise. Eur J Appl Physiol Occup Physiol. 1997;75:212–218.

105. Sigal RJ, Kenny GP, Wasserman DH, et al. Physical activity/exercise and type 2 diabetes: a consensus statement from the American Diabetes Association. Diabetes Care. 2006;29:1433–1438.

106. Skelton DA, Kennedy J, Rutherford OM. Explosive power and asymmetry in leg muscle function in frequent fallers and non-fallers aged over 65. Age Ageing. 2002;31:119–125.

107. Snyder S, Pendergraph B. Exercise during pregnancy: what do we really know? Am Fam Physician. 2004;69:1053, 1056.

108. Sorensen TK, Williams MA, Lee IM, et al. Recreational physical activity during pregnancy and risk of preeclampsia. Hypertension. 2003;41:1273–1280.

109. Spina RJ, Ogawa T, Kohrt WM, et al. Differences in cardiovascular adaptations to endurance exercise training between older men and women. J Appl Physiol. 1993;75:849–855.

110. Staron RS, Hagerman FC, Hikida RS, et al. Fiber type composition of the vastus lateralis muscle of young men and women. J Histochem Cytochem. 2000;48:623–629.

111. Staron RS, Karapondo DL, Kraemer WJ, et al. Skeletal muscle adaptations during early phase of heavy-resistance training in men and women. J Appl Physiol. 1994;76:1247–1255.

112. Stenius-Aarniala B, Poussa T, Kvarnstrom J, et al. Immediate and long term effects of weight reduction in obese people with asthma: randomised controlled study. BMJ. 2000;320:827–832.

113. Stringer WW, Berezovskaya M, O'Brien WA, et al. The effect of exercise training on aerobic fitness, immune indices, and quality of life in HIV+ patients. Med Sci Sports Exerc. 1998;30:11–16.

114. Suominen H. Muscle training for bone strength. Aging Clin Exp Res. 2006;18:85–93.

115. Tarnopolsky MA. Gender differences in substrate metabolism during endurance exercise. Can J Appl Physiol. 2000;25:312–327.

116. Thompson PD, Buchner D, Pina IL, et al. Exercise and physical activity in the prevention and treatment of atherosclerotic cardiovascular disease: a statement from the Council on Clinical Cardiology (Subcommittee on Exercise, Rehabilitation, and Prevention) and the Council on Nutrition, Physical Activity, and Metabolism (Subcommittee on Physical Activity). Circulation. 2003;107:3109–3116.

117. Toledo FG, Menshikova EV, Ritov VB, et al. Effects of physical activity and weight loss on skeletal muscle mitochondria and relationship with glucose control in type 2 diabetes. Diabetes. 2007;56:2142–2147.

118. Tuomilehto J, Lindstrom J, Eriksson JG, et al. Prevention of type 2 diabetes mellitus by changes in lifestyle among subjects with impaired glucose tolerance. N Engl J Med. 2001;344:1343–1350.

119. Turley KR, Wilmore JH. Cardiovascular responses to treadmill and cycle ergometer exercise in children and adults. J Appl Physiol. 1997;83:948–957.

120. Turley KR. The chemoreflex: adult versus child comparison. Med Sci Sports Exerc. 2005;37:418–425.

121. Vinet A, Nottin S, Lecoq AM, et al. Cardiovascular responses to progressive cycle exercise in healthy children and adults. Int J Sports Med. 2002;23:242–246.

122. Volek JS, Phinney SD, Forsythe CE, et al. Carbohydrate restriction has a more favorable impact on the metabolic syndrome than a low fat diet. Lipids. 2009;44:297–309.

123. Welle S, Totterman S, Thornton C. Effect of age on muscle hypertrophy induced by resistance training. J Gerontol A Biol Sci Med Sci. 1996;51:M270–M275.

124. Wiebe CG, Gledhill N, Warburton DE, et al. Exercise cardiac function in endurance-trained males versus females. Clin J Sport Med. 1998;8:272–279.

125. Yang X, Telama R, Hirvensalo M, et al. The longitudinal effects of physical activity history on metabolic syndrome. Med Sci Sports Exerc. 2008;40:1424–1431.

126. Yu F, Hedstrom M, Cristea A, et al. Effects of ageing and gender on contractile properties in human skeletal muscle and single fibres. Acta Physiol (Oxf). 2007;190:229–241.

Suggested Readings

Anderson SD. How does exercise cause asthma attacks? Curr Opin Allergy Clin Immunol. 2006;6:37–42.

Faigenbaum AD, Kraemer WJ, Blimkie CJ, et al. Youth resistance training: updated position statement paper from the national strength and conditioning association. J Strength Cond Res. 2009;23:S60–S79.

Goodman LR, Warren MP. The female athlete and menstrual function. Curr Opin Obstet Gynecol. 2005;17:466–467.

Hawley JA, Lessard SJ. Exercise training-induced improvements in insulin action. Acta Physiol. 2008;192:127–135.

Hollman W, Struder HK, Tagarakis CVM, et al. Physical activity and the elderly. Eur J Cardiovasc Prev Rehabil. 2007;14:730–739.

Lamberrt CP, Evans WJ. Adaptations to aerobic and resistance exercise in the elderly. Rev Endocr Metab Disord. 2005;6:137–143.

Lucas SR, Platts-Mills TAE. Physical activity and exercise in asthma: relevance to etiology and treatment. J Allergy Clin Immunol. 2005;115:928–934.

Praet SFE, van Loon LJC. Optimizing the therapeutic benefits of exercise in Type 2 diabetes. J Appl Physiol. 2007;103:1113–1120.

Tanaka H, Seals DR. Endurance exercise performance in Masters athletes: age-associated changes and underlying physiological mechanisms. J Physiol. 2008;586:55–63.

Vereeke West R. The female athlete: the triad of disordered eating, amenorrhea and osteoporosis. Sports Med. 1998;26:63–71.

Index

Note: Page numbers followed by *b*, *f* and *t* indicate boxes, figures and tables respectively